2

Springer Series in Biomaterials Science and Engineering

For further volumes:
http://www.springer.com/series/10955

Series Editor

Prof. Min Wang
Department of Mechanical Engineering
The University of Hong Kong
Pokfulam Road, Hong Kong
e-mail: memwang@hku.hk

Aims and Scope

The Springer Series in Biomaterials Science and Engineering addresses the manufacture, structure and properties, and applications of materials that are in contact with biological systems, temporarily or permanently. It deals with many aspects of modern biomaterials, from basic science to clinical applications, as well as host responses. It covers the whole spectrum of biomaterials – polymers, metals, glasses and ceramics, and composites/hybrids – and includes both biological materials (collagen, polysaccharides, biological apatites, etc.) and synthetic materials. The materials can be in different forms: single crystals, polycrystalline materials, particles, fibers/wires, coatings, non-porous materials, porous scaffolds, etc. New and developing areas of biomaterials, such as nano-biomaterials and diagnostic and therapeutic nanodevices, are also focuses in this series. Advanced analytical techniques that are applicable in R & D and theoretical methods and analyses for biomaterials are also important topics. Frontiers in nanomedicine, regenerative medicine and other rapidly advancing areas calling for great explorations are highly relevant.

The Springer Series in Biomaterials Science and Engineering aims to provide critical reviews of important subjects in the field, publish new discoveries and significant progresses that have been made in both biomaterials development and the advancement of principles, theories and designs, and report cutting-edge research and relevant technologies. The individual volumes in the series are thematic. The goal of each volume is to give readers a comprehensive overview of an area where new knowledge has been gained and insights made. Significant topics in the area are dealt with in good depth and future directions are predicted on the basis of current developments. As a collection, the series provides authoritative works to a wide audience in academia, the research community, and industry.

Besim Ben-Nissan
Editor

Advances in Calcium Phosphate Biomaterials

Springer

Editor
Besim Ben-Nissan
Chemistry and Forensic Science
University of Technology
Sydney, NSW, Australia

ISSN 2195-0644 ISSN 2195-0652 (electronic)
ISBN 978-3-642-53979-4 ISBN 978-3-642-53980-0 (eBook)
DOI 10.1007/978-3-642-53980-0
Springer Heidelberg New York Dordrecht London

Library of Congress Control Number: 2014936420

Printed on acid-free paper

Springer is part of Springer Science+Business Media (www.springer.com)

This book is dedicated to Professor Racquel Z. LeGeros, who has taught us and contributed so much in both research and education for the advancement of calcium phosphates and biomaterials. She will be greatly missed.

Tribute to Racquel

I ran across a simple note when cleaning out our offices from someone I really don't remember. It goes like this:

> Dear Dr Racquel. I really wish to thank you for everything you have done for me to advance my career. You really did not know me, and I had difficulty understanding why you would help me until I got to know you and observed that it was your nature to be kind and helpful to everyone in your path.

John P. LeGeros, Ph.D.

Preface

"Cogito Ergo Sum"
René Descartes 1644

I would like to tell a story that all these years I seldom talked about.

It was on one of those dark sunsets of October 1973 that I found myself wounded in one of those conflicts that unfortunately never ended.

A number of doctors were busy trying to help me and other wounded soldiers under the harsh dangers of the front line. These doctors and following surgeries in hospital helped me to realise how "life was at the edge of a fine line" that separated our existence from death. In reality this happens in many instances throughout human history; on one side, humanity tries to exterminate each other and on the other it tries to save or repair life.

This was my first intimate and personal encounter with the medical field, and I admire those individuals that sacrificed themselves to help. It opened a new thinking in my mind to use my knowledge to help to preserve and improve life. It became a search for solutions to problems within medical science, which opened up new avenues for future endeavours.

After a few months, I found a number of people–at that time–that were the backbones of the "biomedical materials field pioneering research" with their new inventions and ground-breaking research. Dr. Charnley in the UK was one of those orthopaedic surgeons that understood well both biomechanics and materials in addition to his surgical skills. He was an excellent inventive thinker and was experimenting on the total hip joint designs that set the benchmark that we still use today. Professor Weis was working on the first blade-type titanium dental implants in the USA.

On the scientific side of the biomaterials field, Drs. Racquel and John LeGeros were active and initiated the basic chemistry and substitutions of calcium phosphates for bone regeneration and repair. Dr. Larry Hench was a young inventor with unique scientific approach to chemistry and ceramic synthesis to introduce the bioglass and other inventions that motivated generations that followed, and still do. Dr. Samuel Hulbert and his PhD student Dr. Klawitter postulated that porous ceramics can be used as scaffolds, and produced a list of materials that till today is the golden standard of biocompatible materials. Dr. Aoki pioneered and set the synthesis methods for calcium phosphates that motivated me and others to follow his footsteps and all these giants mentioned in the field. During the late 1970s and the early 1980s, in Asia and specifically in Japan, Drs. Kawahara, Yamamuro, Oonishi and Kokubo and in Europe Klaas de Groot, Ducheyne, Rey and Dacusi and others were experimenting on a range of calcium phosphate bioceramics that further opened new avenues into which many of us built our research.

My motivation and involvement in bioceramics goes back to these researchers and their pioneering research efforts mentioned above. I have admired and have respect for all of the new small steps that many scientists contributed during the years and having motivated us with their work. I was thrilled when Prof. Min Wang proposed that I should edit a book on the "Advances in Calcium Phosphate Biomaterials" for Springer. Immediately, I contacted Prof. Racquel LeGeros to ask her to share with me the pleasure of partially writing and editing this book. Although very busy, she graciously agreed. At the Bioceramics 24 meeting last year in Kyushu, Japan, we prepared the basic structure and the list of authors we aimed to invite to contribute.

We were interested in calcium phosphate-based biomaterials and specifically "apatites" that since the early days have taken a role of passive scaffold for bone regeneration and repair. We were observing that during the last two decades, the concept has changed from passive participation to active involvement to stimulate the body to regenerate and repair the tissue. New-generation calcium phosphate scaffolds are designed to stimulate specific cellular responses in the nanoscale level utilising biogenic additives such as bone morphogenic proteins and stem cells to help release the ionic dissolution products and activate the cells in contact with the biomaterials. With the appropriate microbiological, biochemical and biomechanical stimulation, the cells produce additional growth factors that in turn stimulate generation of growing cells to self-assemble to the required tissues. Taking to account all these factors, we aimed in this book to bring these new concepts, mechanisms and methods by experienced and well-known and young academics, clinicians and researchers to forward their knowledge and expertise on calcium phosphate and related materials and their clinical applications. The general aim was directed not only to cover the fundamentals but also to open new avenues to meet the challenges of the future in research and clinical applications. Both Racquel and I were going to share the responsibility of inviting and co-authoring a few chapters, but it was not meant to be. A few months after sending invitation letters to authors, I received the sad, unexpected and hurting news from Prof. Dacusi that Racquel passed away in France, during her visit, where she usually helped students in their research efforts on calcium phosphates and related materials.

It was a very difficult decision to continue with the book without her guidance and support. However, we felt that this was probably what Racquel would have wanted us to do.

We received 17 chapters, and many others apologised that due to their heavy academic load they could not meet the timeline. This book is therefore their story that covers the advances in calcium phosphate materials from its modern characterisation methods to tissue-biomaterial interactions, from bioglass to biocomposites, from marine structures to drug delivery and from its history to new orthopaedic and maxillofacial applications.

To meet various needs of research, education and clinical applications, each chapter provides clear and fully detailed descriptions, theoretical and experimental issues, discussions and future considerations. This in-depth, practical coverage should also assist the recent graduates and the medical professionals in the calcium phosphate and in general in the biomedical materials field.

Throughout history, science never ceased "advancing", and I trust that this reference book conveys the intensity of this fast "advancing calcium phosphate" field in an enthusiastic way to generate further research and their medical applications to further help the well-being of humans.

Sydney, NSW, Australia Besim Ben-Nissan, Ph.D.

Acknowledgements

First of all, I would like to acknowledge the contributions of Prof. Racquel Z. LeGeros to this book during its inception and for setting the tone. During the last five decades, she has inspired many of us to work and publish in the calcium phosphate field, and she set directions in which future generations will take the field further.

It was her unfortunate departure that left me alone to complete what we started together. To achieve this goal, two individual colleagues have contributed on every step of preparing this book, Dr. Andy H. Choi and Mr. Innocent Jacob Macha; without their hard work, persistence and contribution and visions, this book could not have been completed.

Contents

Contributors

Alexandre A. Barros 3B's Research Group – Biomaterials, Biodegradables and Biomimetics, University of Minho, Taipas, Guimarães, Portugal

ICVS/3B's – PT Government Associate Laboratory, Braga, Guimarães, Portugal

Besim Ben-Nissan School of Chemistry and Forensic Science, University of Technology, Sydney, NSW, Australia

Faculty of Science, University of Technology, Sydney, NSW, Australia

Chris C. Berndt Industrial Research Institute Swinburne (IRIS), Swinburne University of Technology, Hawthorn, VIC, Australia

Department of Materials Science and Engineering, Stony Brook University, Stony Brook, NY, USA

Luiz E. Bertassoni Biomaterials Science Research Unit, Department of Dental Biomaterials, Faculty of Dentistry, University of Sydney, Surry Hills, NSW, Australia

Andy H. Choi School of Chemistry and Forensic Science, Faculty of Science, University of Technology, Sydney, NSW, Australia

Joshua Chou Faculty of Pharmacy, Research Institute of Pharmaceutical Science, Musashino University, Nishi-Tokyo, Tokyo, Japan

Faculty of Science, University of Technology, Sydney, NSW, Australia

Christèle Combes CIRIMAT-Carnot Institute, University of Toulouse, UMR CNRS-UPS-INPT 5085, ENSIACET, Toulouse, France

Richard C. Conway School of Chemistry and Forensic Science, Faculty of Science, University of Technology, Sydney, NSW, Australia

Guy Daculsi Inserm U791, University of Nantes and Inserm CIC-IT 802, Hospital of Bordeaux LIOAD Inserm Université de Nantes UMR U791, Faculté de Chirurgie Dentaire Pl A. Ricordeau, Nantes cedex, France

Sergey Dorozhkin Kudrinskaja sq. 1-155, Moscow 123242, Russia

Christophe Drouet CIRIMAT-Carnot Institute, University of Toulouse, UMR CNRS-UPS-INPT 5085, ENSIACET, Toulouse, France

Hunida M. Elfallah Biomaterials Science Research Unit, Department of Dental Biomaterials, Faculty of Dentistry, University of Sydney, Surry Hills, NSW, Australia

Borhane Hakim Fellah Oniris, National Veterinary School, Nantes, France

David W. Green School of Chemistry and Forensic Science, University of Technology, Sydney, NSW, Australia

Faculty of Dentistry, The University of Hong Kong, Hong Kong, China

David Grossin CIRIMAT-Carnot Institute, University of Toulouse, UMR CNRS-UPS-INPT 5085, ENSIACET, Toulouse, France

Yoshifumi Hanaoka, M.D. H. Oonishi Memorial Joint Replacement Institute, Tominaga Hospital, Osaka, Japan

Jia Hao Oral Implantology and Regenerative Dental Medicine, Tokyo Medical and Dental University, Tokyo, Japan

Md. Fahad Hasan Industrial Research Institute Swinburne (IRIS), Swinburne University of Technology, Hawthorn, VIC, Australia

Larry L. Hench, Ph.D. Department of Biomedical Engineering, Florida Institute of Technology, Melbourne, FL, USA

Kunio Ishikawa Department of Biomaterials, Faculty of Dental Science, Kyushu University, Fukuoka, Kyushu, Japan

Atsuo Ito Human Technology Research Institute, National Institute of Advanced Industrial Science and Technology (AIST), Tsukuba, Ibaraki, Japan

Ryoko Iwata, Ph.D. Olympus Terumo Biomaterials Corporation, Tokyo, Japan

Ikuo Kawahara, M.D. H. Oonishi Memorial Joint Replacement Institute, Tominaga Hospital, Osaka, Japan

Feza Korkusuz, M.D. Department of Sports Medicine, Hacettepe University Faculty of Medicine, Ankara, Turkey

Petek Korkusuz, M.D., Ph.D. Department of Histology and Embryology, Hacettepe University Faculty of Medicine, Ankara, Turkey

Racquel Z. LeGeros Department of Biomaterials and Biomimetics, New York University College of Dentistry, New York, NY, USA

Álvaro J. Leite 3B's Research Group – Biomaterials, Biodegradables and Biomimetics, University of Minho, Taipas, Guimarães, Portugal

ICVS/3B's – PT Government Associate Laboratory, Stony Brook University, Braga, Guimarães, Portugal

Innocent J. Macha School of Chemistry and Forensic Science, Faculty of Science, University of Technology, Sydney, NSW, Australia

João F. Mano 3B's Research Group – Biomaterials, Biodegradables and Biomimetics, University of Minho, Taipas, Guimarães, Portugal

ICVS/3B's – PT Government Associate Laboratory, Braga, Guimarães, Portugal

Olivier Marsan CIRIMAT-Carnot Institute, University of Toulouse, UMR CNRS-UPS-INPT 5085, ENSIACET, Toulouse, France

Bruce Milthorpe Faculty of Science, University of Technology, Sydney, NSW, Australia

Thomas Miramond LIOAD Inserm Université de Nantes UMR U791, Faculté de Chirurgie Dentaire Pl A. Ricordeau, Nantes cedex, France

Hirotsugu Ohashi, M.D., Ph.D. Department of Orthopaedic Surgery, Saiseikai Nakatsu Hospital, Osaka, Japan

Hironobu Oonishi, M.D., Ph.D. H. Oonishi Memorial Joint Replacement Institute, Tominaga Hospital, Osaka, Japan

Hiroyuki Oonishi Jr., M.D. H. Oonishi Memorial Joint Replacement Institute, Tominaga Hospital, Osaka, Japan

Akiyoshi Osaka Faculty of Engineering, Okayama University, Tsushima, Okayama-shi, Japan

Makoto Otsuka Faculty of Pharmacy, Research Institute of Pharmaceutical Science, Musashino University, Nishi-Tokyo, Tokyo, Japan

Ayako Oyane Nanosystem Research Institute, National Institute of Advanced Industrial Science and Technology (AIST), Tsukuba, Ibaraki, Japan

Ricardo A. Pires 3B's Research Group – Biomaterials, Biodegradables and Biomimetics, University of Minho, Taipas, Guimarães, Portugal

ICVS/3B's – PT Government Associate Laboratory, Braga, Guimarães, Portugal

Rui L. Reis 3B's Research Group – Biomaterials, Biodegradables and Biomimetics, University of Minho, Taipas, Guimarães, Portugal

ICVS/3B's – PT Government Associate Laboratory, Braga, Guimarães, Portugal

Christian Rey CIRIMAT-Carnot Institute, University of Toulouse, UMR CNRS-UPS-INPT 5085, ENSIACET, Toulouse, France

Stéphanie Sarda CIRIMAT-Carnot Institute, University of Toulouse, UMR CNRS-UPS-INPT 5085, ENSIACET, Toulouse, France

K.-P. Schmitz Institute for Biomedical Engineering, University of Medicine, University of Rostock, Rostock, Germany

Mahdi Shahmoradi Biomaterials Science Research Unit, Department of Dental Biomaterials, Faculty of Dentistry, University of Sydney, Surry Hills, NSW, Australia

Michael Swain Biomaterials Science Research Unit, Department of Dental Biomaterials, Faculty of Dentistry, University of Sydney, Surry Hills, NSW, Australia

U. Tietz Industrial Research Institute Swinburne (IRIS), Swinburne University of Technology, Hawthorn, VIC, Australia

Muharrem Timuçin, Ph.D. Department of Metallurgical and Materials Engineering, Middle East Technical University, Ankara, Turkey

Xiupeng Wang Human Technology Research Institute, National Institute of Advanced Industrial Science and Technology (AIST), Tsukuba, Ibaraki, Japan

Abbreviations

ACP	Amorphous calcium phosphate
ALP	Alkaline phosphatase
ASC	Embryonic stem cells
BCP	Biphasic calcium phosphate
BMP	Bone morphogenetic protein
CDA	Calcium-deficient apatite
CFA	Carbonate- and fluoride-containing apatite
CHA	Carbonate hydroxyapatite
CPPD	Calcium pyrophosphate dehydrate
DCPD	Dicalcium phosphate dehydrate
ECM	Extracellular matrix
HAp	Hydroxyapatite
HCA	Hydroxyl-carbonate apatite
hMSCs	Human mesenchymal stem cells
IBBC	Interface bioactive bone cement
LPD	Liquid phase deposition
MCPM	Monocalcium phosphate monohydrate
OCP	Octacalcium phosphate
SBF	Simulated body fluid
TCP	Tricalcium phosphate

Chapter 1
Introduction to Synthetic and Biologic Apatites

Racquel Z. LeGeros and Besim Ben-Nissan

Abstract In the early 1970s, bioceramics were employed to perform singular, biologically inert roles, such as to provide parts for bone replacement. The realization that cells and tissues perform many other vital regulatory and metabolic roles has highlighted the limitations of synthetic materials as tissue substitutes. Demands of bioceramics have changed from maintaining an essentially physical function without eliciting a host response to providing a more integrated interaction with the host. This has been accompanied by increasing demands from medical devices to improve the quality of life, as well as extend its duration. Bioceramics especially hydroxyapatite incorporating biologic additives can be used as body interactive materials, helping the body to heal or promoting regeneration of tissues, thus restoring physiological functions. The crystallography and characterization of biologic and synthetic apatites are very complex. This chapter attempts to cover over four decades of research on one of the most intriguing and fascinating fields of research.

Keywords Bioceramic • Biologic apatite • Coralline HAp • Biomimetic • Nanocrystals

---

R.Z. LeGeros
Department of Biomaterials and Biomimetics, New York University College of Dentistry, New York, NY, USA

B. Ben-Nissan (✉)
School of Chemistry and Forensic Science, Faculty of Science, University of Technology, Broadway, Ultimo, PO BOX 123, Sydney, NSW 2007, Australia
e-mail: Besim.Ben-Nissan@uts.edu.au; b.ben-nissan@uts.edu.au

B. Ben-Nissan (ed.), *Advances in Calcium Phosphate Biomaterials*, Springer Series in Biomaterials Science and Engineering 2, DOI 10.1007/978-3-642-53980-0_1,

1.1 Introduction

"Apatite" (Gr, to deceive) was the name given first by Werner in 1788 to describe a group of mineral crystals appearing with various tints (yellow, green, pink, etc.) that were often confused with more precious minerals or gems such as aquamarine, amethyst, topaz, etc. These minerals have the general formula $M_{10}(PO_4)_6X_2$, where M could be one of several metals (usually calcium, Ca), P is most commonly phosphorus (P), and X is commonly hydroxide (OH) or a halogen such as fluorine (F) or chlorine (Cl). Currently, the name "apatite" describes a family of compounds having similar structure (hexagonal system, space group, P63/m) in spite of a wide range of compositions [1, 2]. The unit cell of calcium hydroxyapatite (HAp) contains ten calcium (Ca), six PO_4, and two OH groups, arranged as shown in Fig. 1.1. The OH groups located in the corners of the unit cell are surrounded by two sets of Ca (II) atoms arranged in a triangular patterns at levels $z=0$ and $z=1/2$, by two sets of PO_4 tetrahedral also arranged in triangular patterns at levels $z=Y$ and %, and by a hexagonal array of Ca (I) atoms at a distance [3]. Critical to

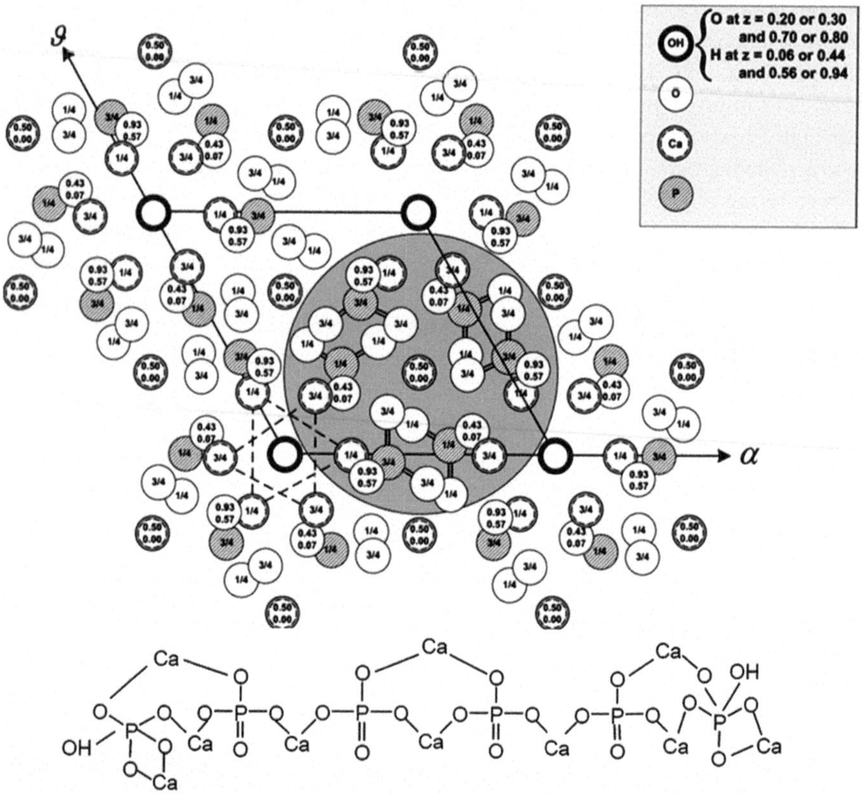

Fig. 1.1 The unit cell and simplified arrangement of hydroxyapatite, $Ca_{10}(PO_4)_6(OH)_2$

the apatite structure is the network of PO_4 groups in tightly packed arrangements [2]. Substitutions in the apatite structure affect lattice parameters (*a*- and *c*-axis dimensions, infrared absorption characteristics, morphology, dissolution properties, and thermal stabilities).

Biologic apatites are the inorganic phases of calcified tissues (teeth and bones). Similarity in composition of calcined bone to the apatite mineral was proposed by Proust and Klaproth in 1788 [4], and similarity in the X-ray diffraction patterns of bone and mineral apatites (HAp and fluorapatite (FA)) and similarity in composition (principally calcium and phosphate ions) led to the conclusion that the inorganic phases of bones and teeth are basically calcium hydroxyapatite [5–7]. Detection of carbonate associated with biologic apatites led to the speculation that these mineral phases are carbonate-containing apatites similar to the minerals dahllite (carbonate-containing apatite) or staffellite (carbonate- and fluoridecontaining apatite) [8]. Studies on synthetic carbonate-substituted apatites demonstrated that carbonate substitution in the apatite structure can proceed in two ways: CO_3-for-OH or type A [9, 10] and CO_3-for-PO_4 or type B, coupled with Na-for-Ca [11, 12], and combined analyses of synthetic and biologic apatites using X-ray diffraction, infrared spectroscopy, and chemical analyses demonstrated that biologic apatites are carbonate apatites approximated by the formula $(Ca,Mg,Na)_{10}(PO_4,CO_3,HPO_4)_6(CO_3,OH)_2$ [12–14]. For example, the following formula $Ca_{8.856}Mg_{0.088}Na_{0.292}K_{0.010}(PO_4)_{5.312}(HPO_4)_{0.280}(CO_3)_{0.407}(OH)_{0.702}Cl_{0.078}(CO_3)_{0.050}$ was proposed to describe the chemical composition of the inorganic part of dental enamel.

Early studies on synthetic apatites and related calcium phosphates were made to gain a better understanding of the structure, composition, and properties of biologic apatites, especially of human enamel apatites. However, studies on synthetic apatites in the last 30 years had focused on their preparation, their applications in medicine and dentistry, and their use as scaffolds for bone and teeth regeneration. Current commercial synthetic calcium phosphate biomaterials classified on the basis of composition include HAp, $Ca_{10}(PO_4)_6(OH)_2$; α- and β-tricalcium phosphates (α-TCP, β-TCP), $Ca_3(PO_4)_2$; and biphasic calcium phosphate (BCP), an intimate mixture of HAp and β-TCP with varying HAp/β-TCP ratios [15–19]. Other commercial HAp biomaterials are derived from biologic materials (e.g., processed human bone, bovine bone derived, hydrothermally converted coral or derived from marine algae) [20–22].

This chapter is a brief review of biologic and synthetic apatites used as biomaterials, updating reviews published earlier by the authors [13, 20, 23, 24].

1.2 Biogenic Apatites

Normal and pathologic calcified tissues are composites of organic and inorganic phases. For bone, dentin, and cementum, the organic phase is principally collagen (about 25 % by weight) with smaller amounts of non-collageneous proteins [25].

On the other hand, the main organic phase in enamel is a non-collageneous protein (amelogenin) comprising about 1 % by weight of the enamel. In normal calcified tissues, such as in teeth and bones, in fish enameloids (teeth or calcified scales of some species), and in some species of shells, only carbonate (carbonate hydroxyapatite, CHA)- or carbonate- and fluoridecontaining apatite (CFA) occurs as the principal inorganic phase [13, 24, 26, 27]. In pathologic calcifications (dental calculus, urinary stones, vascular calcification, and other soft-tissue calcifications), biologic apatite may occur as one of the mineral phases that include other calcium phosphates, e.g., amorphous calcium phosphate (ACP), $Ca_x(PO_4)_y$; dicalcium phosphate dehydrate (DCPD), $CaHPO_4{\bullet}2H_2O$; octacalcium phosphate (OCP), $Ca_8H_2(PO_4)_6{\bullet}5H_2O$; magnesium-substituted tricalcium phosphate (β-TCMP, $(Ca,Mg)_3(PO_4)_2$); and calcium pyrophosphate dihydrate (CPPD), $Ca_2P_2O_7{\bullet}2H_2O$ [24, 28].

1.3 Enamel, Dentin, and Bone Apatite

Enamel, dentin, and bone apatite differ in crystallinity, reflecting crystal size (Fig. 1.2) and concentrations of minor constituents, mainly Mg and CO_3 (Fig. 1.3a, Table 1.1) [13, 24, 29]. Enamel apatite contains the lowest concentrations of these ions and the highest crystallinity (larger crystals) compared to either dentin or bone apatite that shows much lower crystallinity (smaller crystals) or greater concentrations of Mg and CO_3 (Table 1.1). These apatites also differ in solubility, decreasing in the order bone > dentin >> enamel.

These differences in crystallinity (crystal size) and solubility may be attributed to the differences in the concentrations of the minor constituents (e.g., Mg, N, CO_3, HPO_4). Studies on the effect of Mg and CO_3 ions on the properties of synthetic apatites demonstrated that incorporation of these ions independently and

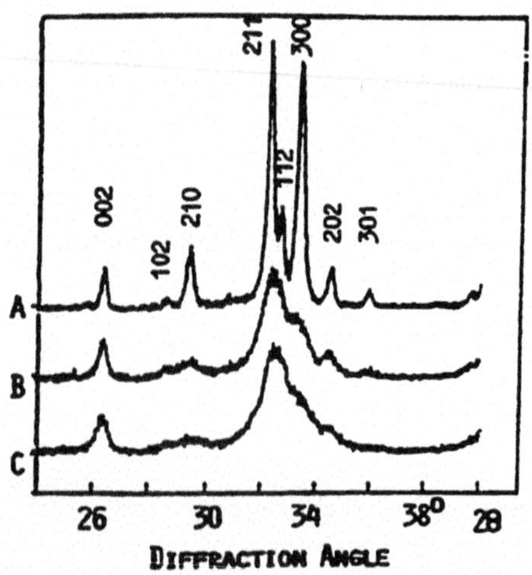

Fig. 1.2 X-ray diffraction profiles of biologic apatites from adult human enamel (**a**), dentin (**b**), and bone (**c**)

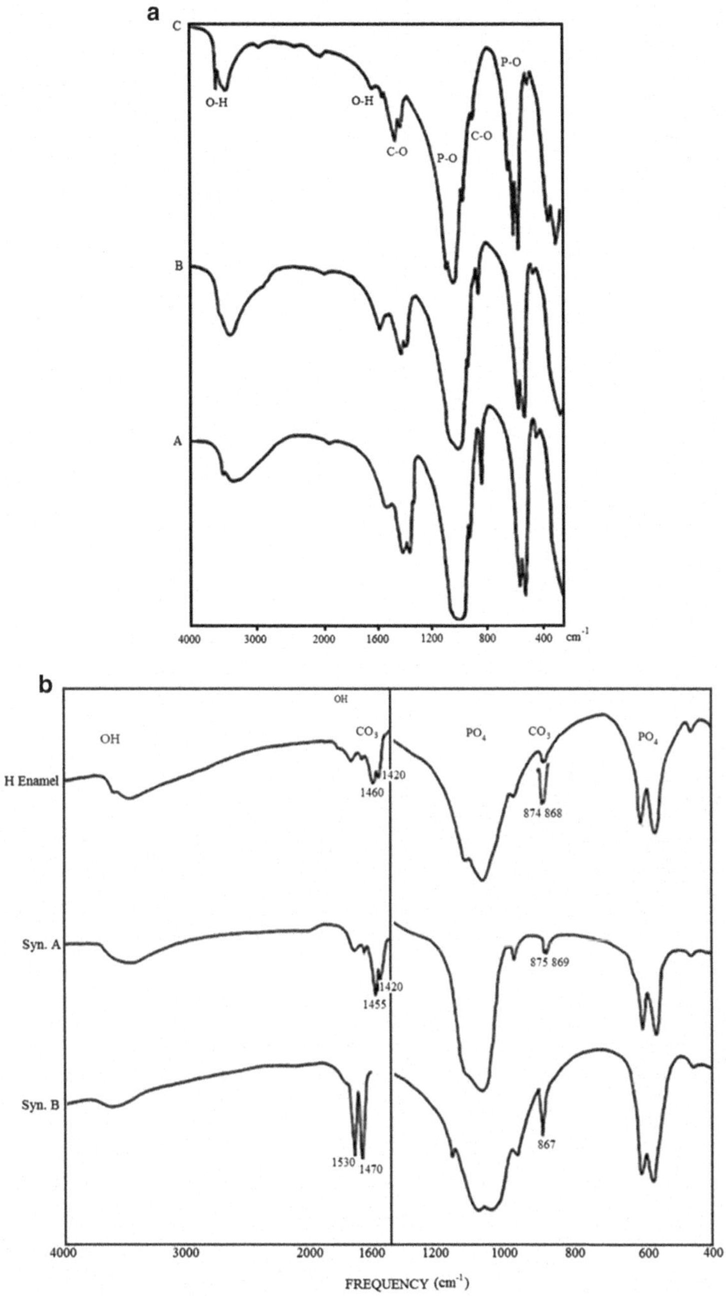

Fig. 1.3 (**a**) FTIR spectra of biologic apatites from adult human enamel, dentin, and bone. Note the higher resolution of the P–O (for PO_4 groups) absorption spectra of enamel (*C*), compared to those of dentin (*B*) and bone (*A*) apatites. (**b**) FTIR spectra comparing the characteristic C–O (for CO_3 groups) absorption bands in human enamel apatite compared to those in synthetic apatite with type A (CO_3-for-OH) substitution (syn A) and with type B (CO_3-for-PO_4) substitution (syn B)

Table 1.1 Composition (%) and physical properties of apatites in adult human enamel, dentin, and bone

	Enamel	Dentin	Bone
Composition			
Calcium, Ca^{2+}	36.5	35.1	34.8
Phosphorus, P	17.7	16.2	15.6
Ca/P (molar)	1.63	1.63	1.71
Sodium, Na^{+}	0.5	0.6	0.9
Magnesium, Mg^{2+}	0.34	1.23	0.72
Potassium, K^{+}	0.06	0.05	0.03
Carbonate, $CO_3{}^{2-}$	3.5	5.6	7.4
Fluoride, F^{-}	0.01	0.06	0.03
Chloride, Cl	0.30	0.01	0.13
Pyrophosphate	0.02	0.10	0.07
Total inorganic (mineral)	97.0	70.0	65.0
Total organic	1.5	20.0	25.5
Absorbed H_2O %	1.5	10.0	10.0
Trace elements: Zn, Cu, Fe, Sr, etc.			
Crystallographic properties			
Lattice parameters			
a-axis (+ 0.0003 nm)	0.9441		
c-axis (+ 0.0003 nm)	0.6880		
Crystallite size (nm, avg.)	33 × 3	2 × 0.4	2.5 × 0.3
Crystallinity index, *b*	70–75	33–37	33–37
Ignition products (800 °C)	HAp + β-TCMP	HAp + β-TCMP	HAp
HAp, $Ca_{10}(PO_4)_6(OH)_2$			
a-axis = 0.9422 nm,			
c-axis = 0.6882 nm			
Crystallinity index = 100			
Composition: Ca, P, OH			

synergistically causes the growth of smaller and more soluble apatite crystals [13, 24, 29–32]. The effects of CO_3 incorporation on apatite crystal size and morphology and on dissolution properties are much more pronounced than that of Mg [13, 24, 32]. Proteins [25] and/or other ions (e.g., pyrophosphate, citrate) [12, 24] may also inhibit the crystal growth of biologic apatites.

Biologic apatites are usually calcium-deficient (i.e., with Ca/P molar ratio less than the stoichiometric value of 1.67 obtained for pure HAp, $Ca_{10}(PO_4)_6(OH)_2$). Calcining above 900 °C of human enamel and dentin apatite results in the loss of the CO_3 constituent and formation of HAp and β-TCMP [13, 24]. Calcining of bone (human or bovine) above 900 °C results in the loss of CO_3 and formation of mostly HAp with small amounts of calcium oxide, CaO [13, 24].

Partial dissolution of biologic apatites and precipitation of other calcium phosphates (DCPD, OCP, β-TCMP) are believed to occur in human enamel and dentin caries, characterized by the dissolution of the tooth mineral (carbonate apatite) by acids produced by oral bacteria [33, 34]. The non-apatitic calcium phosphates (e.g., DCPD, OCP) may, in turn, transform to apatites by hydrolysis or by dissolution and reprecipitation processes [13, 24, 34].

Biologic apatites have been idealized as calcium HAp, $Ca_{10}(PO_4)_6(OH)_2$ [5–8]. However, the difference in lattice parameters: *a*-axis for enamel, 0.9442 nm vs. 0.9422 nm for HAp. Ca/P stoichiometry (e.g., about 1.63 for enamel or dentin apatite vs. 1.67 for HAp) and the association of other ions, notably magnesium (Mg) and carbonate (CO_3) with biologic apatites (Table 1.1), have caused many years of disagreements and research on the structure and composition of biologic apatites [8, 9, 13, 35].

The nature of CO_3 incorporation in biologic apatites, especially in human enamel apatite, had been a preoccupation of several researchers. The larger *a*-axis dimension of human enamel apatite compared to pure or mineral HAp was first attributed to the CO_3-for-OH substitution (type A) in these apatites [9]. Such type of substitution was observed in synthetic carbonate apatites prepared by diffusing CO_2 into HAp at 1,000 °C under very dry conditions, resulting in an expanded *a*-axis and contracted *c*-axis dimension B compared to pure HAp [9, 10]. However, studies on synthetic apatites prepared at much lower temperatures (60–95 °C) by precipitation or hydrolysis methods showed a partial CO_3-for-PO_4 substitution (type B) coupled with a partial Na-for-Ca substitution, resulting in a contracted *a*-axis and expanded *c*-axis dimension compared to CO_3-free apatites [11–13]. The observed expanded *a*-axis of enamel apatite may be attributed to partial Cl-for-OH substitution [36] and HPO_4-for-PO_4 substitution [37] rather than the CO_3-for-OH substitution in the apatite.

A possible H_3O-for-OH was also offered as a possible cause for the expanded *a*-axis dimension [8]. Additional evidence for the dominant partial CO_3-for-PO_4 substitution in enamel and all biologic apatites is the similarity of the characteristic CO_3 absorption bands between the IR spectra of enamel apatite with those of synthetic apatites exhibiting CO_3-for- PO_4 substitution as shown in Fig. 1.3b [13, 24, 38].

Studies in synthetic systems also showed that F incorporation (F-for-OH substitution) has the following effects: contraction in the *a*-axis dimension and no significant effect on the *c*-axis dimension compared to F-free apatites [13, 24], growth of larger and less soluble apatite crystals [13, 24, 39], and greater structural stability [3]. Such studies elucidated the nature of fluoride (F) incorporation in some biologic apatites (from modern and fossil teeth and bones). For example, the smaller *a*-axis dimension of shark enameloid compared to HAp or human enamel apatite is due to the high fluoride (F) concentration in shark enameloid (Table 1.1) [13, 27, 40]. The therapeutic use of fluoride in dentistry (sealants, topical gels, tablets) was based on the observation of low caries in areas of fluoridated water (1 ppm F) [41]. Fluoride treatment (topically or by the use of fluoridated dentifrices) of enamel and dentin leads to the formation of partially substituted (F, OH) apatite that is more resistant to acid dissolution, i.e., dental caries [29, 33, 34, 39]. Administration of F in the drinking water was shown to increase the crystal size and decrease the extent of dissolution of rat bones [42] and increase crystal thickness of enamel apatite [43]. Fluoride therapy (as NaF) has been recommended for the management of osteoporosis to increase bone density [44, 45].

1.4 Synthetic Apatites

Earlier extensive studies on synthetic apatites were made to gain a better understanding of biologic apatites and their properties. Because biologic apatite was idealized as HAp, most of the studies centered on HAp preparation and evaluation of HAp properties. Studies on synthetic apatites in the last 30 years were motivated by development of calcium phosphate-based biomaterials (principally HAp, TCP, or biphasic) for bone repair, substitution, and augmentation and as scaffolds for tissue engineering in bone and teeth regeneration. The rationale for developing HAp biomaterials was their similarity in composition to the bone mineral.

Synthetic HAp can be made by solid-state reactions or by precipitation or hydrolysis methods and subsequent sintering at high temperatures, usually 1,000 °C and above. Synthetic apatites can also be prepared using hydrothermal [46, 47], microwave [48, 49] or sol-gel [50, 51] methods. Apatite nanocrystals are obtained when prepared by precipitation or hydrolysis at lower temperatures (25–60 °C). Synthetic apatite crystals approximating the size of human enamel apatite may be obtained by precipitation or hydrolysis methods with reaction temperature, 80–95 °C (Fig. 1.4). Apatites may also be prepared in sol-gel systems [52], by electrodeposition [53, 54] or biomimetic precipitation on metallic or polymeric [55, 56] substrates.

Apatites obtained by precipitation involve the reaction of calcium salts (e.g., $CaNO_3$, $Ca(OH)_2$, $CaCl_2$, $Ca(Ac)_2$) and phosphate salts (Na^-, NH^{4-}, or K^- phosphates) [24, 57]. Hydrolysis of non-apatitic calcium phosphates (e.g., ACP,

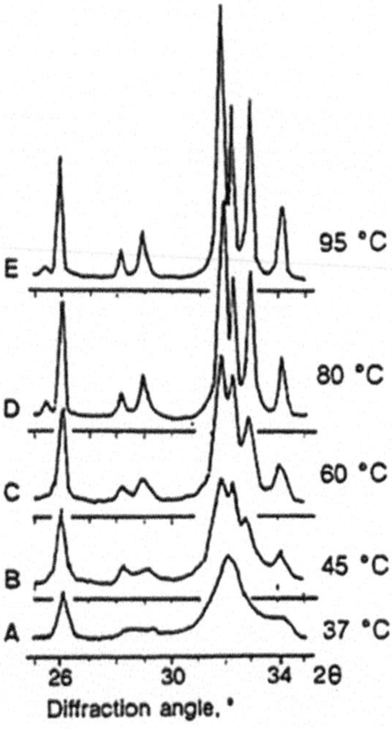

Fig. 1.4 X-ray diffraction profiles of precipitated apatites obtained at different reaction temperatures. The nanoapatite crystals similar to bone apatite are prepared at 37 °C (**a**) or at room temperature. The narrowing of diffraction peaks reflects increased crystallinity; the broader the diffraction peak, the smaller the crystals

DCPD, DCPA, OCP, β-TCP, α-TCP) or calcium compounds (e.g., $CaCO_3$, $CaMg(CO_3)_2$, CaF_2) in solutions containing OH, CO_3, or F results in the formation of apatite, CO^{3-} or F^- containing apatites [24, 32, 36, 58]. Apatites prepared by precipitation or hydrolysis methods when prepared at pH between 5 and 9 are calcium-deficient apatites (CDA), and subsequent sintering results in the formation of BCP [59]. Sintering or firing of synthetic apatites results in an increase in crystal size and decrease in microporosity.

Sintering of HAp at temperatures above 1,200 °C results in thermal decomposition of apatite forming other calcium phosphates such as β-TCP and α-TCP and possibly even mixed with ACP. The combination of calcium phosphates (e.g., ACP, DCPA, DCPD, CDA, α-TCP, β-TCP) with other calcium compounds (CaO, $Ca(OH)_2$, $CaCO_3$), mixed with phosphate solutions or organic acids, results in the formation of apatitic calcium phosphate cements [60, 61].

Studies on synthetic apatites showed that substitutions for Ca, PO_4, or OH ions in the apatite structure result in changes in lattice parameters (Table 1.2) and crystallinity (reflecting crystal size and/or strain) and dissolution properties. For example, CO_3-for-PO_4 coupled with Na-for-Ca substitution has the following effects on apatite properties:

(a) Smaller *a*- and larger *c*-axis dimensions compared to CO_3-free apatites
(b) Change from needlelike to rodlike to platelike with increasing CO_3 incorporation
(c) Lower resolution of the P-O (for PO_4) absorption bands in the IR spectra
(d) Higher solubility
(e) Lower thermal stability [11–13, 24, 31, 32, 38]

Such studies helped explain the contributions of some ions associated with biologic apatites as well as led to the development of some therapies and manufacture of calcium phosphate-based biomaterials.

1.5 Synthetic Apatites as Bone-Substitute Materials

The first successful use of a calcium phosphate reagent in bone repair was reported by Albee in 1920 [62], followed more than 50 years later by the first clinical study by Nery et al. [63] on periodontal bony defects using porous calcium phosphate identified by the authors as "TCP." X-ray diffraction analysis of Nery's material years later revealed that the "TCP" consisted of a mixture of HAp and β-TCP with a β-TCP/HAp ratio of 20/80 [20] and was thus renamed "BCP" [64]. Similarity in composition of the synthetic apatite to biologic apatite was the rationale for the development of calcium-phosphate-based biomaterials for bone repair, substitution, and augmentation and as scaffolds for bone and tooth regeneration. These calcium phosphate bioceramics include HAp, β-TCP, BCP, bovine bone-derived apatites (unsintered and sintered), and coral-transformed apatite (Fig. 1.5). Commercialization of HAp as bone graft materials was largely

Table 1.2 Lattice parameters of mineral and synthetic apatites compared to biologic apatite

		Lattice parameters	(+0.0003 nm)
Apatite	Substituent	*a*-axis	*c*-axis
Mineral			
OH apatite (Holly Springs)	–	0.9422	0.6880
F apatite (Durango, Mexico)	F-for-OH	0.9375	0.6880
Dahllite (Wyoming, USA)	CO_3-for-PO_4	0.9380	0.6885
Staffelite (Staffel, Germany)	CO_3-for-PO_4 and F-for-OH	0.9345	0.6880
Marine phosphorite (USA)	CO_3-for-PO_4 and F-for-OH	0.9322	0.6882
Synthetic (nonaqueous)[a]			
OH apatite	–	0.9422	0.6882
F apatite	F-for-OH	0.9375	0.6880
Cl apatite	Cl-for-OH	0.9646	0.6771
CO_3 apatite	CO_3-for-OH	0.9544	0.6859
Synthetic (aqueous)[b]			
OH apatite	–	0.9438	0.6882
OH apatite	HPO_4-for-PO_4	0.9462	0.6879
F apatite	F-for-OH	0.9382	0.6880
(Cl, OH) apatite	*Cl-for-OH	0.9515	0.6858
CO_3-OH apatite	*CO_3-for-PO_4	0.9298	0.6924
CO_3-F apatite	*CO_3-for-PO_4 and F-for-OH	0.9268	0.6924
Sr apatite	Sr-for-Ca	0.9739	0.6913
Pb apatite	Pb-for-Ca	0.9894	0.7422
Ba apatite	Ba-for-Ca	1.0161	0.7722
Biologic apatite			
Human enamel	(CO_3,HPO_4)-for-PO_4, (Na,Mg)-for-Ca, and Cl-for-OH	0.9441	0.6882
Shark enameloid	F-for-OH, Mg-for-Ca, and (CO_3,HPO_4)-for-PO_4	0.9382	0.6880

[a]Prepared at high temperature (1,000 °C) by solid-state reaction or diffusion [3, 9]
[b]Prepared at 95 °C either by precipitation or by hydrolysis of $CaHPO_4$ in solutions containing the desired substituent [13, 24, 58]

due to the independent efforts of Jarcho [15], deGroot [16], and Aoki [17]. Basic studies on BCP led to its commercialization and popularity as bone graft materials and as scaffolds for tissue engineering [18, 59, 64–69].

Commercial HA biomaterials are usually prepared by precipitation at high pH and subsequent sintering at about 1,000–1,100 °C [15–17]. Coral-derived HAp or coralline HAp is prepared by the hydrothermal reaction of coral ($CaCO_3$) with ammonium phosphate [70]. Bovine bone-derived HAp is prepared by removing the organic phase (resulting in bone apatite) or removing the organic phase and sintering at high temperatures. These different preparations and origin (synthetic vs. biologic) are reflected in the difference in their initial crystallinity reflecting crystal size (Fig. 1.6) and their dissolution rates [71], increasing in the order

HAp $<<$ coralline HAp $<$ bovine bone apatite (sintered) $<<$ bovine bone apatite (unsintered) HAp $<<$ BCP $<<$ β-TCP.

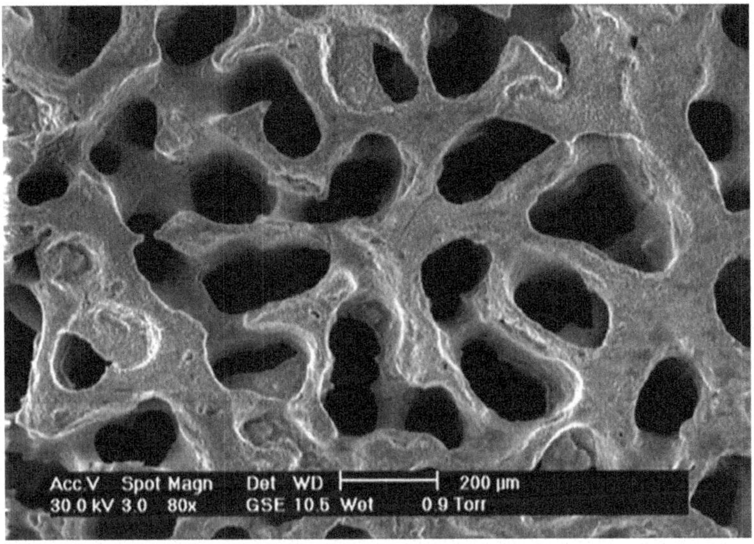

Fig. 1.5 Scanning electron micrograph of coralline apatite

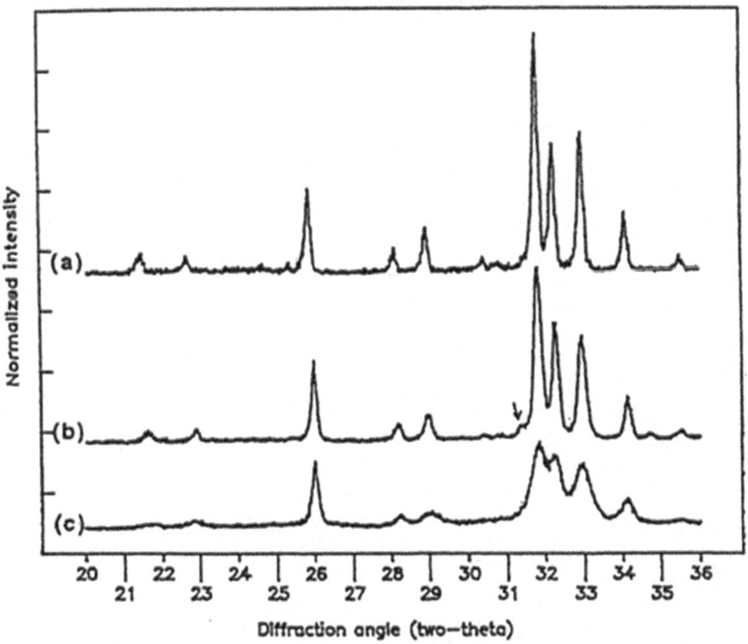

Fig. 1.6 X-ray diffraction profiles of apatite biomaterials (*A*, *B*, *C*). (*A*) Ceramic HAp (Calcite™), (*B*) coralline HAp (Interpore™), (*C*) unsintered apatite, calcium deficient (Osteogen™). The *arrow* on (*b*) indicates presence of β-TCMP

1.6 Synthetic HAp in Implant Surfaces and Coatings

Porous HAp and related calcium phosphates, in spite of their many desirable properties, are not strong enough to be used in load-bearing areas [15, 16]. The rationale for the development of "HAp"-coated orthopedic and dental implants is to combine the strength of the metal (usually titanium or titanium alloy) and the bioactive properties of HAp and other calcium phosphates. Dense HAp particles are used as the source material for depositing implant coating by the plasma-spray technique [15, 16, 72]. The high temperatures and other variable parameters involved in the plasma-spray process (e.g., velocity of feeding the HAp powder, distance of the gun from the metal substrate) result in the partial transformation of the original HAp into ACP and minor amounts of α-TCP, β-TCP, and tetracalcium phosphate (TTCP, $Ca_4P_2O_9$) [73]. Plasma-sprayed "HAp" coatings have nonhomogenous composition (principally ACP/HAp ratio), varying from the layer closest to the metal substrate to the outermost layer and varying from one manufacturer to another [73]. Alternatives to the plasma-spray method are nanocoating, electrochemical deposition [53, 54], and precipitation or chemical deposition [55, 56], the latter method being also applicable to nonmetallic substrates [56]. These other methods provide homogenous implant coating of the desired composition, e.g., HAp, FA, CHA, and OCP [53–56, 74], and allow coating deposition at much lower temperatures, thus permitting the incorporation of bioactive molecules and growth factors.

During the last decade, HAp or BCP has been used as an abrasive material for grit blasting to roughen the surface and provide a more bioactive surface (compared to alumina or silica abrasive), thus enhancing osseointegration of the implant [75].

1.7 Synthetic HAp in Composites

HAp and related calcium phosphates are used as the inorganic component in composites with natural (e.g., collagen, chitosan) or synthetic (polylactic acid or polylacticglycolic acid, PLA or PLGA, high-molecular-weight polyethylene) polymers [76, 77]. The rationale for developing composite biomaterials is the fact that bone is a composite of a biologic polymer (collagen) and inorganic phase (carbonate apatite).

1.8 Synthetic HAp and BCP as Scaffolds for Tissue Engineering

Several investigators have reported that mesenchymal stem cells (MSC) from bone marrow can be cultured in porous calcium phosphate biomaterials (ceramic HAp, coralline HAp, BCP ceramic) in vitro and implanted as a tissue-engineered material for bone regeneration [78, 79].

1.8.1 *Critical Properties of Synthetic HAp and Related Calcium Phosphates*

Porosity (interconnecting macroporosity) is an important property of biomaterials to allow bony ingrowth and vascularization [80, 81]. Macroporosity is introduced in HAp and other calcium phosphates by the incorporation of porogens such as naphthalene [82], H_2O_2, or sugar molecules. Biocompatibility of a material is determined in vitro from the cell response (proliferation, attachment, phenotypic expression) to the material. Material surface composition and surface roughness or topography influence cell response [83]. Bioactivity is defined as the property of the material to develop a direct, adherent, and strong bonding and interface with the bone tissue [84, 85]. Bioactivity is demonstrated in vitro and in vivo by the ability of the material to form carbonate apatite on the surface from the simulated body fluid in vitro [56] or biologic fluid in vivo in osseous or non-osseous sites [65, 66, 86, 87].

Osteoconductivity is the property of the material that allows attachment, proliferation, migration, and phenotypic expression of bone cells leading to the formation of new bone in direct opposition to the biomaterial [84]. Osteoinductivity is the property of the material that allows osteoprogenitor cell growth and development for bone formation to occur [88] and is usually determined by the formation of bone in non-bone-forming sites, e.g., under the skin or in the muscle. HAp and related calcium phosphates are generally considered to have all the above properties except osteoinductivity. However, although controversial, it has been reported that with the appropriate composition, geometry, and architecture, osteoinductive properties can be promoted [89, 90].

1.9 Conclusions

The total analysis of the results obtained over four decades of research in this fascinating field of science suggests that with newer scientific tools and with further refinement, we will succeed to address problems relating to the structure, morphology, and analysis of the biologic materials and produce synthetic apatites or composites that will emulate the structure and characteristics of natural soft and hard tissues.

References

1. Naray-Szabo S (1930) The structure of apatite $(CaF)Ca_4(PO_4)_3$. Z Kristallogr 75:387–398
2. Beevers CA, Mcintyre DB (1956) The atomic structure of fluorapatite and its relation to that of tooth and bone mineral. Miner Mater 27:254–259
3. Young RA, Elliott JC (1966) Atomic scale bases for several properties of apatites. Arch Oral Biol 11:699–707

4. Deer WA, Howie RA, Zussman J (1985) An introduction to the rock forming mineral. Longman, Hong Kong, pp 504–509
5. de Jong WF (1926) La Substance Minérale Dans les Os. Rec Trav Chim Pays-Bas 45:445–448
6. Kay M, Young RA, Posner AS (1964) The crystal structure of hydroxyapatite. Nature 204:1050–1052
7. Carlstroem D (1955) X-ray crystallographic studies on apatite and calcified tissues. Acta Radiol Suppl 121:1–59
8. McConnell D (1952) The crystal chemistry of carbonate apatites and their relationship to the composition of calcified tissue. J Dent Res 31:53–63
9. Elliott JC (1964) The crystallographic structure of dental enamel and related apatites. PhD thesis, University of London
10. Bonel G, Montel G (1964) Surune nouvelle apatite carbonatée synthétique. C R Acad Sci Paris 258:923–926
11. Zapanta-LeGeros R (1965) Effect of carbonate on the lattice parameters of apatite. Nature 206:403
12. LeGeros RZ, Trautz OR, LeGeros JP (1961) Apatite crystallites: effect of carbonate on morphology. Science 155:1409–1411
13. LeGeros RZ (1981) Apatites in biological systems. Prog Cryst Growth Character 4:1–45
14. Rey C, Renugopalakrishnan V, Collins B (1991) Fourier transform infrared spectroscopic study of the carbonate ions in bone mineral during aging. Calcif Tissue Int 49:251–258
15. Jarcho M (1981) Calcium phosphate ceramics as hard tissue prosthetics. Clin Orthop Relat Res 157:259–278
16. de Groot K (1983) Bioceramics of calcium phosphates. CRC Press, Boca Raton
17. Aoki H, Kato K, Ogiso M (1971) Studies on the application of apatite to dental materials. J Dent Eng 18:86–89
18. Daculsi G, Passuti N, Martin S, LeGeros RZ (1990) Macroporous biphasic calcium phosphate ceramic for long bone surgery in human and dogs: clinical and histological study. J Biomed Mater Res 4:379–396
19. Metsger DS, Driskell TD, Paulsrud JR (1982) Tricalcium phosphate ceramic–a resorbable bone implant: review and current status. J Am Dent Assoc 105(6):1035–1038
20. LeGeros RZ (1988) Calcium phosphate materials in restorative dentistry: review. Adv Dent Res 2:164–180
21. Schopper C, Moser D, Sabbas A, Lagogiannis G, Spassova E, König F, Donath K, Ewers R (2003) The fluorohydroxyapatite (FHA) FRIOS Algipore is a suitable biomaterial for the reconstruction of severely atrophic human maxillae. Clin Oral Implants Res 14(6):743–749
22. Holmes RE (1979) Bone regeneration within a coralline hydroxyapatite implant. Plast Reconstr Surg 63:626–633
23. Ben-Nissan B, Chai C, Evans L (1995) Crystallographic, and spectroscopic characterization and morphology of biogenic and synthetic apatites. In: Wise DL (ed) Encyclopedic handbook of biomaterials and bioengineering: Part B Applications, vol 1. Marcel Dekker, New York, pp 191–221
24. LeGeros RZ (1991) Calcium phosphates in oral biology and medicine. In: Myers H, Karger S (eds) Monographs in oral sciences, vol 15. Karger, Basel
25. Boskey AL (1985) Overview of cellular elements and macromolecules implicated in the initiation of mineralization. In: Butler WT (ed) The chemistry and biology of mineralized tissues. EBSCO Media, Birmingham, pp 335–343
26. LeGeros RZ, Pan CM, Suga S, Watabe N (1985) Crystallochemical properties of apatites in atremate brachiopod shells. Calcif Tissue Int 37:651–658
27. LeGeros RZ, Bautista C, Wong JL, LeGeros A, LeGeros JP (1994) Biological apatites in modern and fossil shark teeth and in calcified fish scales. Bull de l'Institut Oceanographique 14:229–236
28. LeGeros RZ (2001) Formation and transformation of calcium phosphates: relevance to vascular calcification. Z Kardiol 90(Suppl 3):116–124

29. LeGeros RZ, Salcae T, Bautista C (1996) Magnesium and carbonate in enamel and synthetic apatites. Adv Dent Res 10:225–231
30. Okazaki M, LeGeros RZ (1992) Crystallographic and chemical properties of Mg-containing apatites before and after suspension in solutions. Magnes Res 5:103–108
31. LeGeros RZ, Tung MS (1983) Chemical stability of carbonate and fluoride containing apatites. Caries Res 17:419–429
32. LeGeros RZ, LeGeros JP, Trautz OR, Klein E (1971) Conversion of monetite, $CaHPO_4$, to carbonate apatite: effect on crystallinity. Adv X-ray Appl 14:57–66
33. Margolis HC, Moreno EC (1985) Kinetic and thermodynamic aspects of enamel demineralization. Caries Res 19:22–35
34. LeGeros RZ (1982) Chemical and crystallographic events in caries. J Dent Res 69:567–574
35. Driessens FCM (1982) In moral aspects of dentistry. In: Myers HM (ed) Monographs in oral sciences, vol 10. Karger, Basel
36. LeGeros RZ (1975) The unit-cell dimensions of human enamel apatite: effect of chloride incorporation. Arch Oral Biol 20:63–71
37. LeGeros RZ, LeGeros JP, Bonel G (1979) Types of 'H_2O' in human enamel and in precipitated apatites. Calcif Tissue Res 26:111–116
38. LeGeros RZ, LeGeros JP, Trautz OR, Klein E (1970) Spectral properties of carbonate in carbonate-containing apatites. Dev Appl Spectrosc 7:3–12
39. Moreno EG, Kresak M, Zahradnik RT (1977) Physicochemical aspects of fluoride-apatite systems relevant to the study of dental caries. Caries Res 11(1):142–171
40. LeGeros RZ, Silverstone LM, Daculsi G, Kerebel LM (1983) In vitro caries-like lesion formation in F-containing tooth enamel. J Dent Res 62:138–144
41. Dean HT, Arnold FA Jr, Elvove E (1942) Domestic water and dental caries. V. Additional studies of the relations of fluoride domestic waters to dental caries experience in 4,425 white children aged 12 to 14 year, of 13 cities in 4 states. Public Health Rep 57:115–125
42. LeGeros RZ, Singer L, Ophaug R, Qujrolgico G, LeGeros JP (1982) The effect of fluoride on the stability of synthetic and biological (bone mineral) apatites. In: Menczel J, Robin GC, Makin M (eds) Osteoporosis. Wiley, New York, pp 327–341
43. Robinson C, Kirkham J (1990) The effect of fluoride on the developing mineralized tissues. J Dent Res 69(Spec No: 685–691):184–185
44. Pak CYC, Sakhaee K, Bell NK, Licata A, Johnson C, Rubine B (1996) Comparison of non-randomized trials with slow-release sodium fluoride with a randomized placebo controlled trial in postmenopausal osteoporosis. J Bone Miner Res 11:160–168
45. Kleerkoper M (1996) Auoride and the skeleton. In: Bilezlkian JP, Raisz LG, Rodan FA (eds) Principles of bone biology. Academic, San Diego, pp 1053–1062
46. Ito A, Nakamura S, Aoki H, Akao M, Traoka K, Tsutsumi S, Qnuma K, Tateishi T (1990) Hydrothermal growth of carbonate containing hydroxyapatite single crystals. J Cryst Growth 163:311–317
47. Hattori T, Iwadate Y (1990) Hydrothermal preparation of calcium hydroxyapatite powders. J Am Ceram Soc 73:1803–1805
48. Pena J, LeGeros RZ, Rohanizadeh R, LeGeros JP (2001) $CaCO_3$-biphasic materials prepared by microwave processing of natural aragonite and calcite. Key Eng Mater 192–195:267–270
49. Lerner E, Sarig S, Azoury R (1991) Enhance maturation of hydroxyapatite from aqueous solutions using microwave irradiation. J Mater Sci Mater Med 2:138–141
50. Milev AS (2002) Chemistry, synthesis and morphological stability of sol-gel derived carbonate substituted platelike hydroxyapatite. PhD thesis, University of Technology, Sydney
51. Deptula A, Lada W, Olczak T, Sarowska S, LeGeros RZ, LeGeros JP (1998) Complex Sol-gel process (CSGP) preparation of calcium phosphate biomaterials (powders, monoliths, fibers). In: Bioceramics, vol II. World Scientific Publishing, Singapore, pp 743–746
52. LeGeros RZ, Morales P (1973) Renal stone crystals grown in gel systems. Invest Urol 11:12–20
53. Vijayragbavan TV, Bensalem A (1994) Electrodeposition of apatite coating on pure titanium and titanium alloys. J Mater Sci Lett 13(24):1782–1785

54. LeGeros JP, Lin S, LeGeros RZ, Legeros JP (2000) Chemically deposited CaP coating on titanium alloy. J Dent Res 79:560–572
55. Rohanizadeh R, LeGeros RZ, Harsono M, Ben-David A (2004) Adherent apatite coating on titanium substrate using chemical deposition. J Biomed Mater Res 72A:428–438
56. Kokubo T (1996) Formation of biologically active bone-like apatite on metals and polymers by a biomimetic process. Thermochim Acta 280–281:479–490
57. Hayek E, Newesely H, Rumpel ML (1963) Pentacalcium monohydroxyorthophosphate. In: Kleinberg J (ed) Inorganic syntheses, vol 7. Wiley, Hoboken, pp 63–69
58. LeGeros RZ, Go P, Vandemaele KH, Quirolgico GB, LeGeros DJ (1980) Transformation of calcium carbonates and calcium phosphates to carbonate apatites: possible mechanism for phosphorite formation. In: Proceedings 2nd international congress on phosphorous compounds, Morocco Institut de Mondial de Phosphate, Boston, 21–25 Apr 1980, pp 41–54
59. LeGeros RZ, Lin S, Rohanizadeh R, Mijares D, LeGeros JP (2003) Biphasic calcium phosphate bioceramics: preparation, properties and applications. J Mater Sci Mater Med 14:201–210
60. Brown WE, Chow LC (1987) A new calcium phosphate water setting cement. In: Brown PW (ed) Cements research progress. American Ceramic Society, Westerville
61. Niwa S, LeGeros RZ (2002) Injectable calcium phosphate cements for repair of bone defects. In: Lewandrowski KU, Wise DL, Trantolo DJ, Gresser JD (eds) Tissue engineering and biodegradable equivalents: scientific and clinical applications. Marcel Dekker Inc., New York, pp 385–500
62. Albee FH (1920) Studies in bone growth: triple calcium phosphate as a stimulus to osteogenesis. Ann Surg 71:32–36
63. Nery EB, Lynch KL, Hirtbe WM, Mueller KH (1978) Preliminary clinical studies of bioceramics in periodontal osseous defects. J Periodontal 49:523–527
64. Ellinger RF, Mery EG, Lynch KL (1986) Histological assessment of periodontal osseous defects following implantation of hydroxyapatite and biphasic calcium phosphate ceramics: a case report. J Periodontics Restor Dent 3:223–233
65. LeGeros RZ, Daculsi G, Nery E, Lynch K, Kerebel B (1988) In vivo transformation of biphasic calcium phosphates of varying β-TCP:HA ratios: ultrastructural characterization. In: Proceedings of the 3rd world biomaterials congress. Business Center for Academic Societies Japan, Tokyo
66. LeGeros RZ, Daculsi D (1997) In vivo transformation of biphasic calcium phosphate ceramics: ultrastructural and physico-chemical characterizations. In: Yamamuro T, Wilson J, Hench LL (eds) Handbook of bioactive ceramics, vol 11. CRC Press, Boca Raton, pp 17–28
67. Daculsi G, Passuti N (1990) Bioactive ceramics fundamental properties and clinical applications: the Osseo-coalescence process. In: Heimcke G, Oonishi H (eds) Bioceramics, vol 2. Butterworth-Heinemann, Cologne, pp 3–10
68. Wykrota LL, Garrido CA, Wykrota FH (1998) Clinical evaluation of biphasic calcium phosphate ceramic used in orthopaedic lesions. In: LeGeros RZ, LeGeros JP (eds) Bioceramics, vol 11. World Scientific Publishing, Singapore, p 64
69. Nery E, LeGeros RZ, Lynch KL, Lee K (1992) Tissue response to biphasic calcium phosphate ceramic with different ratios of HA/β-TCP in periodontal osseous defects. J Periodontol 63:729–735
70. Roy DL, Linnehan SK (1974) Hydroxyapatite formed from coral skeletal carbonate by hydrothermal exchange. Nature 247:220–222
71. LeGeros RZ, Bautista C, LeGeros JP, Vijaragbavan TV, Retino M (1995) Comparative properties of bioactive bone graft materials. In: Sedel L (ed) Bioceramics, vol 8. Pergamon Press, London, pp 1–7
72. Berndt CC, Haddad GN, Farmer AJD, Gross KA (1990) Review: thermal spraying for bioceramic applications. Mater Forum 14:161–173
73. LeGeros RZ, LeGeros JP, Kim Y, Kijkowska R, Zheng R, Bautista C, Wong JL (1995) Calcium phosphates in plasma-sprayed HA coatings. Ceram Trans 48:173–189
74. Lin S, LeGeros RZ, LeGeros JP (2003) Adherent octacalcium phosphate coating on titanium alloy using a modulated electrochemical deposition method. J Biomed Mater Res 66A:8228

75. Salgado T, LeGeros JP, Wang J (1998) Effect of alumina and apatitic abrasives on TI alloy substrate S. In: Ohgushi H (ed) Bioceramics, vol 11. World Scientific Publishing, Singapore, p 686
76. Doyle C (1990) Bioactive composites in orthopaedics. In: Yamamuro T, Hench LL, Hench LL, Wilson-Hench J (eds) Handbook of bioactive ceramics, vol 2. CRC Press, Boca Raton, pp 195–207
77. Okazaki M, Ohmae H, Hino T (1989) Insolubilization of apatite-collagen composites by UV irradiation. Biomaterials 10:564–568
78. Ohgushi H, Caplan AI (1999) Stem cell technology and bioceramics: from cell to gene engineering. J Biomed Mater Res Appl Biomater 48:913–927
79. Toquet J, Rohanizadeh R, Guicheux J, Daculsi G (1999) Osteogenic potential in vitro of human bone marrow cells cultured on macroporous biphasic calcium phosphate ceramic. J Biomed Mater Res 44:98–109
80. LeGeros RZ (2002) Properties of osteoconductive biomaterials: calcium phosphates. Clin Orthopaed Relat Res 395:81–98
81. Klawitter JJ (1979) A basic investigation of bone growth in porous materials. PhD thesis Clemson University, Clemson
82. Hubbard W (1974) Physiological calcium phosphate as orthopaedic implant material. PhD thesis, Marquette University, Milwaukee
83. Harada Y, Want JT, Doppalppudi VA, Willis AA, Goldring SR (1996) Differential effects of different forms of hydroxyapatite and hydroxyapatite tricalcium phosphate particles on human monocyte/macrophages in vitro. J Biomed Mater Res 31:19–26
84. Hench LL (1994) Bioceramics: from concept to clinic. J Am Ceram Soc 74:1487–11510
85. Osborn JF, Newesely H (1980) The material science of calcium phosphate ceramic. Biomaterials 1:108–111
86. Heogbebaert M, LeGeros RZ, Gineste M, Guilhern M, Bonel G (1988) Physico-chemical characterization of deposits associated with HA ceramics implanted in non-osseous sites. J Biomed Mater Res 22:257–268
87. LeGeros RZ, Daculsi G, Orly I (1991) Substrate surface dissolution and interfacial biological mineralization. In: Davies JE (ed) The BoM biomaterials interface. University of Toronto Press, Toronto, pp 76–88
88. Urist MR (1965) Bone formation by autoinduction. Science 150:893–898
89. Ripamonti U, Ma S, Reddi AH (1992) The critical role of geometry of porous hydroxyapatite delivery system induction of bone by osteogenin, a bone morphogenetic protein. Matrix 12(3):202–212
90. Le Nihouannen D, Daculsi G, Saffarzadeh A, Gauthier O, Delplace S, Pilet P, Layrolle P (2005) Ectopic bone formation by microporous calcium phosphate ceramic particles in sheep muscles. Bone 36(6):1086–1093

Chapter 2
Clinical Applications of Hydroxyapatite in Orthopedics

Hiroyuki Oonishi Jr., Hironobu Oonishi, Hirotsugu Ohashi, Ikuo Kawahara, Yoshifumi Hanaoka, Ryoko Iwata, and Larry L. Hench

Abstract This chapter describes since 1982 the use of porous synthetic hydroxyapatite (HA) granules (0.1 to approximately 1.5 mm) interposed at the cement-bone interface to enhance bone bonding, a surgical procedure labeled interface bioactive bone cement (IBBC). HA granules were smeared on the bone surface just before cementing. Because the HA granules used in IBBC were pure polycrystalline HA, they were scarcely absorbed and their osteoconductive activity can continue indefinitely even after the onset of osteoporosis due to aging and even in conditions of extremely low pathological activity of bone. The appearance rate of radiolucent lines and osteolysis was extremely low even over 30 years when IBBC was used. Since 1986, in an attempt to fill the massive bony defect in the acetabulum at revision surgery of total hip arthroplasty, a mixture of HA granules with a size between 0.9~1.2 mm and 3.0~5.0 mm was placed densely and firmly into the bone defects. Bone ingrowth was measured to be over 2.5 cm in full depth and the new bone was very stable. Long-term clinical results over 26 years were excellent. On the weight-bearing area, bone ingrowth over 2.5 cm in full depth can be expected. However, on non-weight-bearing area, bone ingrowth is only 0.5 cm in depth. In large cavities

H. Oonishi Jr., M.D. • H. Oonishi, M.D., Ph.D. (✉) • I. Kawahara, M.D. • Y. Hanaoka, M.D.
H. Oonishi Memorial Joint Replacement Institute, Tominaga Hospital, 1-4-48, Mintatomachi, Naniwa-ku, Osaka 556-0017, Japan
e-mail: oons-h@os.rim.or.jp

H. Ohashi, M.D., Ph.D.
Department of Orthopaedic Surgery, Saiseikai Nakatsu Hospital, 2-10-39, Shibata, Kita-ku, Osaka 530-0012, Japan

R. Iwata, Ph.D.
Olympus Terumo Biomaterials Corporation, Shinjuku Monolith, 3-1, Nishi-Shinjuku 2-chome, Shinjuku-ku, Tokyo 163-0941, Japan

L.L. Hench, Ph.D.
Department of Biomedical Engineering, Florida Institute of Technology, Melbourne, FL 32901, USA

B. Ben-Nissan (ed.), *Advances in Calcium Phosphate Biomaterials*, Springer Series in Biomaterials Science and Engineering 2, DOI 10.1007/978-3-642-53980-0_2,

after resection of bone tumors, or after removal of pathological fatty bone marrow at joint replacements, excellent stability to provide long-term strong bony support was obtained by filling HA granules firmly into the defects.

Keywords Bioceramics • Hydroxyapatite • Orthopedics • Rheumatoid arthritis • Total hip arthroplasty • Osteoconduction • Interface bioactive bone cement (IBBC)

2.1 Introduction

Bioceramics have been widely used as bone replacement materials in orthopedic surgery. In particular, calcium phosphate ceramics such as synthetic hydroxyapatite (HA) have been applied as bioactive ceramics with bone-bonding capacities. Since 1982, we have used HA in the bony defect area at total hip and knee arthroplasty, sometimes in extremely progressed atrophic cancellous bone area of rheumatoid arthritis at joint replacement to get firm bony support. HA has also been used as bone filler in the area of bone deficiency after resection of bone tumors. In order to obtain physicochemical bonding between bone and implant, HA coatings on implants had been used for about 15 years. However, HA coatings were absorbed within 15 years after implantation due to the amorphous HA present in the HA coatings.

In order to protect from loosening of prostheses, osteoconduction has to be maintained at the interface between bone and implant even after onset of osteoporosis. Therefore, non-resorbable polycrystalline HA has to be used to obtain long-term stability. For this reason, we have been using the interface bioactive bone cement (IBBC) technique which involves interposing non-resorbable crystalline HA granules at the interface between bone and bone cement at the time of cementing during surgery.

2.2 Clinical Applications in Orthopedic Surgery: Interface Bioactive Bone Cement (IBBC)

Cemented total hip arthroplasty (THA) has been one of the most successful procedures in orthopedic surgery, since J. Charnley applied polymethylmethacrylate (PMMA) to fix the components [1–11]. Efforts to improve the mechanical bonding at the bone-bone cement interface have been pursued for many years by many teams or researchers. Even with these contemporary techniques, cement fixation is often limited with respect to long-term stability of the bone-cement interface. Furthermore, the physicochemical bonding cannot be expected in addition to the mechanical bonding for traditional cement fixation, since the bone cement is not osteoconductive [1–11].

To augment the bone-bone cement bonding, we investigated a new cementing technique to achieve the long-lasting physicochemical bonding at the bone-bone cement interface by interposing osteoconductive crystalline HA granules. In this technique, bone cement is covered by polycrystalline porous HA granules at the interface, thereby achieving essentially custom-made HA-coated cemented implants. HA granules for our technique were pure polycrystalline HA; thus they were scarcely absorbed and their osteoconductive activity continued indefinitely even after the onset of osteoporosis due to aging. We call this technique interface bioactive bone cement (IBBC) [7–28].

2.2.1 Materials and Methods

The IBBC method involves placing less than 2–3 layers of porous polycrystalline HA granules 0.3–1.5 mm in diameter with a porosity of 35–48 % (average 42 %) between the bone and cement (Fig. 2.1a). Although HA granules of 0.3–0.5 mm in diameter were used initially, they were later reduced to 0.1–0.3 mm, as it was found those sizes adhere to bone more easily. HA must be used on the surface of completely hemostatic bone. On the areas with slight bleeding, HA particles larger than 0.6 mm are more appropriate, as granules smaller than 0.3 mm will be covered by the blood. As a result, blood will be present between the HA and bone cement. Additionally, low-viscosity bone cements should not be used with HA granules, because the HA granules will sink into it. We used CMW-type I as the PMMA bone cement.

2.2.2 Experimental Studies

2.2.2.1 Histological Studies

Holes with a diameter of 6 and 10 mm in depth were made in both femoral condyles of mature rabbits, and HA granules of 300–500 μm in diameter were smeared in less than two layers over the bone surface of the hole, and the hole was filled with bone cement (Fig. 2.1b). In groups of three, rabbits were sacrificed at 2, 3, 4, 6, 12, and 24 weeks and at 3 years after implantation. Non-decalcified hard tissue specimens were prepared and examined by optical microscopy, scanning electron microscopy (SEM), and backscattered electron imaging.

One week after surgery, new bone began entering the first to second layer and adhering to the HA granules (Fig. 2.1c). At 2–3 weeks after surgery, new bone had entered a majority of the spaces in the second layer (Fig. 2.1d). After 6 weeks or more, all spaces were filled with new bone, thus forming a unified body, as illustrated in Fig. 2.1e at 8 months postsurgery. Three years after surgery (Fig. 2.1f),

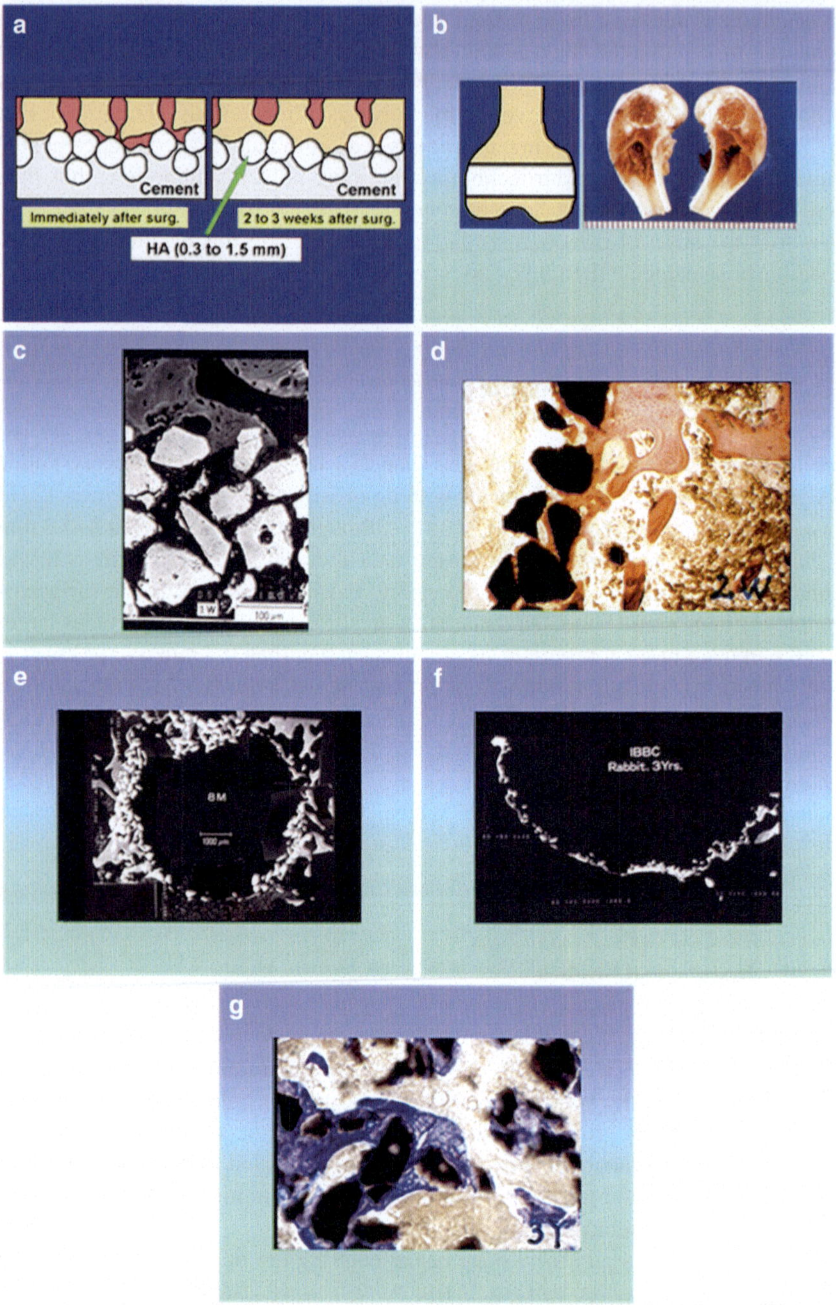

Fig. 2.1 (**a**) Scheme of IBBC at immediately after surgery and 2–3 weeks after surgery. (**b**) Animal experiment of IBBC cross section of femoral condyle of the rabbit performed with IBBC. (**c**) Animal experiment of IBBC 1 week after surgery. (**d**) Animal experiment of IBBC 2 weeks after surgery. (**e**) Animal experiment of IBBC 8 months after surgery. (**f**) Animal experiment of IBBC 3 years after surgery. (**g**) Higher magnification of Figure (**f**)

bone ingrowth into the spaces of HA granules was the same as that seen at 6 weeks and 8 months (Fig. 2.1e). The bone was retained only in the place where HA granules were smeared. There was no bony tissue in other place due to aging (Fig. 2.1f, g).

2.2.2.2 Bonding Strength of the HA Granule Layer to Bone

IBBC was tested on mature rabbits. Holes with a 6 mm diameter and a depth of 10 mm were made in both femoral condyles. The rabbits were sacrificed in groups of three at 2, 4, 6, 12, and 24 weeks after implantation, and a push-out test was performed. HA coating applied to a smooth titanium surface was used as a control.

A relatively strong initial fixation was obtained immediately after implantation using the IBBC technique. Two weeks after implantation, the bonding strength of IBBC was higher than that of the HA coating, but at 6 weeks after implantation, the bonding strength of IBBC became similar to that of HA coating. The fractures resulting from the push-out test occurred in the HA granule layer from 2 to 6 weeks after implantation and occurred in both the HA granule layer and the surrounding bone layer after 12 weeks. These results indicated that the strength of the HA granule layer gradually increased after surgery and reached almost the same level as the bone around the HA granule layer after 12 weeks. In these experiments, the bonding strength of bone cement to bone by interposing HA granules was found to be adequate (Fig. 2.2).

Stress shielding was not found in subsequent clinical trials. When cement fixation using PMMA bone cement was performed, excellent initial fixation can be obtained. However, after a period of time, a connective tissue membrane may form between the bone and bone cement, particularly in the acetabulum. This may lead to component loosening.

When cementless fixation with a HA-coated component was performed, micromotion of the component may occur if the initial fixation is insufficient. Therefore, we are confident that IBBC combines the fixation advantages of both conventional PMMA bone cement and HA coating in early stage.

2.2.3 Clinical Studies

2.2.3.1 Surgical Technique

A cobalt-chromium alloy femoral component (KC, Kyocera Co. Ltd. Kyoto, Japan) with a 28 mm alumina head was used in combination with an all-polyethylene acetabular component. All operations were performed by the senior author (H.O.) through an anterolateral approach in supine position.

HA granules were manufactured by sintering at 1,200 °C in Sumitomo Osaka Cement Co. Ltd., Chiba, Japan. Porous HA granules with 300–500 μm in diameter were used. For acetabular side, several small anchor holes for initial fixation were

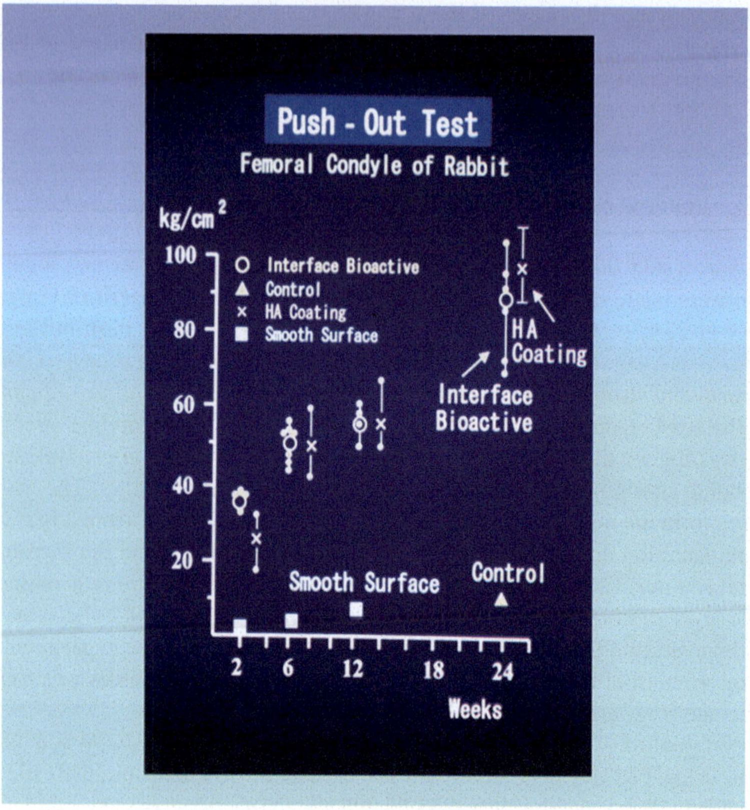

Fig. 2.2 Push-out test: Comparison of adhesive strength to the bone of IBBC and HA coating

made and intensive care was taken for sufficient hemostasis by means of hypotensive anesthesia (approximately 90 mmHg), temporal compress at the bleeding points with bone paste obtained by acetabular reaming, and a rinse with hydrogen peroxide followed by compressive gauze packing. HA granules (2–3 g) were smeared on the bone surface just before cementing of the acetabular component. CMW-I bone cement (C.M.W. Laboratories Ltd., Blackpool, UK) was used in all cases. Porous HA granules could easily adhere on the wet bone surface (Fig. 2.3a, b). For the femoral side, hemostasis was achieved in the same manner and HA granules (2–3 g) were smeared on the inner surface of the prepared femoral canal using a half-tube silicone rubber (3–5 cm in length) clamped by a long-straight Kocher's hemostatic clamp (Fig. 2.3c, d). The femoral component was fixed with second-generation cementing technique using an intramedullary bone plug and cement gun. These procedures resulted in the presence of less than 2–3 layers of HA granules in most of the bone-bone cement interface, while bone cement directly contacted with bone without interposition in some part. The same cementing technique was applied for the conventional THA procedures except for using HA granules.

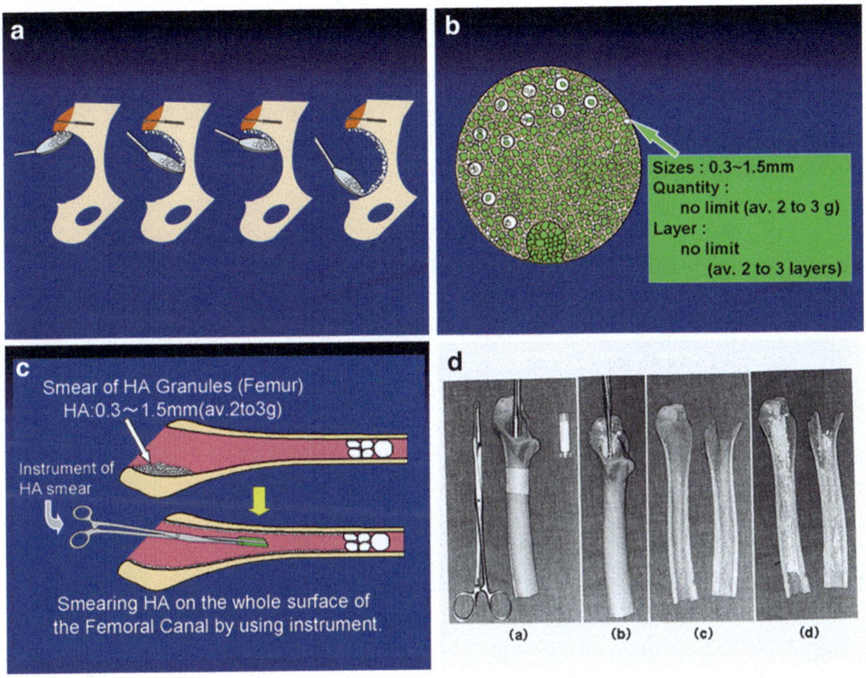

Fig. 2.3 (**a**) Smearing procedures of HA granules on the acetabulum. (**b**) After smearing of HA granules on the acetabulum. (**c**) Smearing procedures of HA granules on the inner surface of the femur. (**d**) Experimental studies of smearing of HA granules on the inner surface of the femur. (**d**–[*a*]) Homemade instrument to smear HA granules. (**d**–[*b*]) Smearing HA granules by using the instrument. (**d**–[*c*]) Inner surface of the femur before smearing HA granules. (**d**–[*d*]) Inner surface of the femur after smearing HA granules

The key points of surgical procedures were as follows:

1. Hemostasis immediately before cementing is very important.
2. Several small anchoring holes for initial fixation are necessary.
3. HA impregnated by antibiotics as a drug delivery system is very effective for prevention of infection.

2.2.3.2 Changes of IBBC Technique

In the first generation, from 1982 to 1988, HA granule size of 0.3–0.5 mm in diameter was used, and several small anchoring holes of 3 mm in diameter were made. In the second generation, from 1989 to 1997, HA granules of 0.1–0.3 mm were used because a smaller size of HA granules adhered more easily to the interface. However, as a smaller size of HA was covered easily by blood in the bleeding area, the connection of the bone cement with HA was prevented. As the result, a space appeared between bone cement and HA.

Consequently, in the third generation, from 1998 to 2001, HA granules of 0.3–0.5 mm were used again and several numbers of anchoring holes of 6 mm in diameter were made for stronger initial fixation. In the fourth generation, since 2001, HA granules of 0.3–0.5 mm with 1.0–1.5 mm were used and several layers of anchoring holes more than 6 mm in diameter were made, thereby enhancing safety even if IBBC was performed in the bleeding area.

2.2.3.3 Long-Term Clinical Results for 24–31 Years

Long-term clinical cases were classified into three groups. In group (1), 1982–1985, IBBC was performed in 12 joints as trials and conventional bone cement (non-IBBC) in 79 joints. In group (2), 1985–1986, IBBC was performed on one hip joint and non-IBBC was performed on the other hip joint in the same patient. These were performed in 25 patients. In group (3), 1986–1989, IBBC was performed in all cases in 285 joints (212 patients) (Fig. 2.4).

2.2.3.4 Group (2): (1985–1986, 25–26 Years After Surgery)

Group 2 has 16 patients with survival in both hips. In non-IBBC hips, the prostheses were loosened in five hips in the acetabulum and in two hips in the femur within 20 years. The radiolucent line and the osteolysis increased gradually and their appearance time was indefinite. Seven hips were revised within 15–20 years.

In IBBC hips, the radiolucent line and the osteolysis appeared in only small limited areas and did no progress. The rich new bone formation was maintained at the interface of bone and bone cement by interposing HA granules (Fig. 2.5a–c). In the survival cases of hips with both IBBC and non-IBBC, wide radiolucent lines and osteolysis and loosening were seen in non-IBBC cases; however, only few radiolucent lines and osteolysis were seen in the small limited areas in IBBC hip replacements (Fig. 2.5d, e).

2.2.3.5 Group (3): (1986–1989, 22–25 Years After Surgery)

In this group, IBBC technique was used in all cases in 285 joints (212 patients). The radiolucent line and osteolysis appeared in only small limited areas and did no progress (Fig. 2.6a). Extensive new bone formation was seen at the interface of bone and bone cement by interposing HA granules (Fig. 2.6b, c). In groups 1–3, when IBBC was performed in the bleeding area, the spaces appeared between bone cement and HA several months after surgery on the X-ray figure (Fig. 2.6d). However, the spaces did no progress (Fig. 2.6e). When the space appeared in the large area, the partial separation of bone cement from HA at the interface of HA and bone cement occurred in two cases (Fig. 2.6f). HA incorporated with the bone at the interface

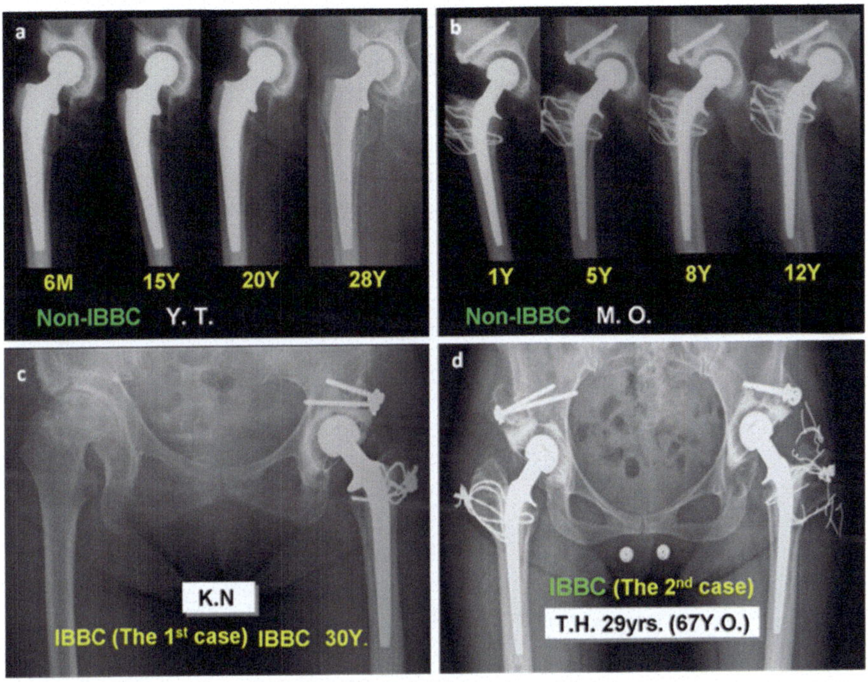

Fig. 2.4 (**a**) Clinical course of X-ray figure after THA with conventional bone cement (non-IBBC). Osteolysis was seen in the femur 15 years after THA. Osteolysis and radiolucent line were seen in the acetabulum and the femur 20 years after THA, and they progressed 28 years after THA. (**b**) Clinical course of X-ray figure after THA with non-IBBC radiolucent line was seen in the acetabulum 5 years after THA. Stem loosening was seen 8 years after THA and it progressed and radiolucent line progressed in the acetabulum and stem loosening progressed 12 years after THA. (**c**) This is the first case of THA with IBBC. Thirty years after THA, polyethylene socket wear increased in high degree. However, neither radiolucent line nor osteolysis was seen. (**d**) This is the second case of THA with IBBC in bilateral hips 29 years after THA. She has worked as a dancer for 28 years. Radiolucent line and osteolysis were seen in only small limited area

(Fig. 2.6g). In non-IBBC cases with only conventional bone cement, when wear particles of polyethylene increased, phagocytosis occurred and osteolysis appeared on the radiograph.

From the long-term clinical results of IBBC, the rate of formation of space or voids between HA and bone cement was less than 2 %. They appeared at the limited areas in both the acetabulum and the femur for the first- and second-generation IBBC procedures. The spaces were not radiolucent lines. They appeared at a rather higher rate in the second generation than in the first generation because the HA granule size in the first generation was bigger than that in the second generation.

The appearance rate of osteolysis was extremely low, less than 1.5 %, appearing in few restricted areas. The separation between bone cement and HA occurred in the acetabulum in the second generation in two joints that is 0.8 %. There was

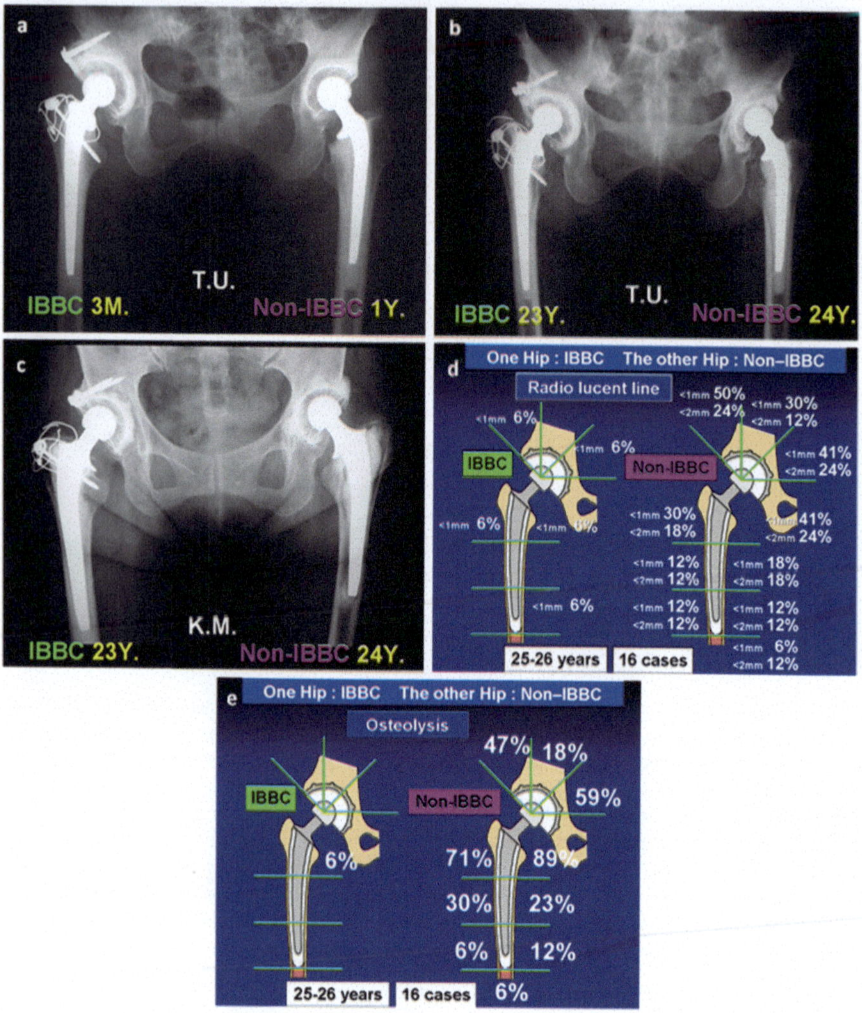

Fig. 2.5 (**a**) One year after THA with non-IBBC in the left hip and 3 months after THA with IBBC in the right hip. (**b**) In the right hip with IBBC, neither radiolucent line nor osteolysis was seen 23 years after THA in spite of progress of polyethylene wear. In the left hip with non-IBBC, both radiolucent line and osteolysis progressed in both acetabulum and femur 24 years after THA. (**c**) In the right hip with IBBC, neither radiolucent line nor osteolysis was seen 23 years after THA. In the left hip with non-IBBC, 24 years after THA, both radiolucent line and osteolysis were seen in the acetabulum, and osteolysis and stem loosening were seen in the femur. (**d**) Comparative appearance rate of radiolucent line 25–26 years after THA with IBBC and non-IBBC performed in the same patient. (**e**) Comparative appearance rate of osteolysis 25–26 years after THA with IBBC and non-IBBC performed in the same patient

no loosening between bone and bone cement. Since 2001, in order to prevent the occurrence of the spaces and the separation between bone cement and HA, several anchoring holes over 6 mm in diameter were made in the acetabulum and HA granules of 0.3–0.6 mm and 1.0–1.5 mm were smeared on the bone surface.

In the IBBC procedure, there was no loosening between bone and bone cement in groups 1, 2, and 3 for 27 years. However, in non-IBBC hip replacements, loosening occurred in over 80 % of cases, a high rate, for 31 years (Table 2.1).

2.2.4 Histological Studies on Retrieval Cases

2.2.4.1 Materials and Methods

In 14 patients, specimens containing a well-fixed bone-cement interface were retrieved during revision surgery. The diagnosis was degenerative osteoarthritis in ten hips and in one knee, rheumatoid arthritis (RA) in two, and osteonecrosis after radiation therapy for portio cancer in one. The causes of revision were dissociation of the metal-back socket from the bone cement in nine hips, aseptic loosening of the socket in one, and late infection in four.

At the revision surgery, the specimens were carefully cut out using a surgical osteotome or oscillating bone saw to retrieve the bone-cement composites without breaking the bone-cement interface. In the acetabulum, six specimens were retrieved from the superior wall, which was considered to be the principal weight-bearing site, and ten specimens were retrieved from the inferomedial wall, which was considered to be the auxiliary weight-bearing site. Three specimens were retrieved from sites where the HA granules failed to be smeared. In the femur, two specimens were retrieved from the greater trochanter and femoral neck. In the femoral condyle, two specimens were retrieved.

The retrieved tissues were immediately fixed with neutral buffered formalin (10 %) and dehydrated in increasing concentration of ethanol up to 100 % at room temperature. A polyester resin solution (Rigolac; Mixture of resin no. 2004 and resin no. 70 °F, 80/20 (wt.%/wt.%); Showa Highpolymer Co., Ltd., Tokyo, Japan) was used for embedding. To prevent complete loss of the bone cement, the treatment in the first resin solution was minimized. Finally, the resin solution was kept in a chamber at 60 °C for 8 h and polymerized. The cured blocks were cut into slices 300–500 μm thick using a metal cutting saw and then ground down to sections 50–80 μm thick. Sections were examined by backscattered electron microscopy (SEM) and conventional light microscopy after staining with methylene blue or toluidine blue.

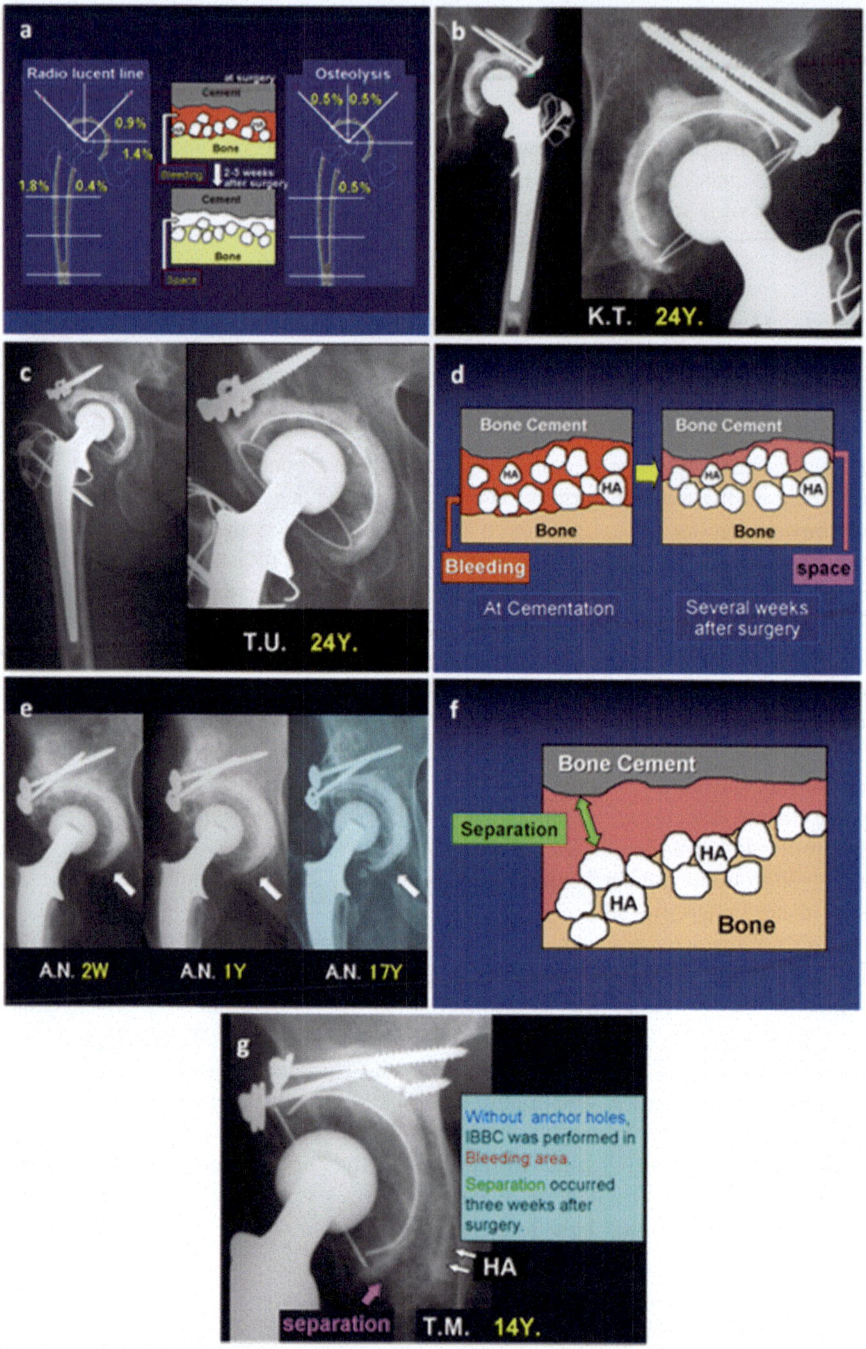
a
Radio lucent line
0.9%
1.4%
1.8%
0.4%
Cement
Bone
2-3 weeks after surgery
Cement
Bone
Osteolysis
0.5%
0.5%
0.5%
b
K.T. 24Y.
c
T.U. 24Y.
d
Bone Cement
HA
HA
Bone
Bone Cement
HA
HA
Bone
Bleeding
space
At Cementation
Several weeks after surgery
e
A.N. 2W
A.N. 1Y
A.N. 17Y
f
Bone Cement
Separation
HA
HA
Bone
g
Without anchor holes, IBBC was performed in Bleeding area.
Separation occurred three weeks after surgery.
HA
separation
T.M. 14Y.

Table 2.1 Summary of results of loosening rate between bone and bone cement in groups 1, 2, and 3

	Non-IBBC		IBBC	
	79 Joints		**12 Joints**	
G. 1	R.L.L.	7 Joints not loosened	R.L.L.	Extremely low rate no progress
	O.L.		O.L.	
	L.	6 Joints not revised	L.	0
	Revision, death, and lost	65	Death	3 Joints
			Lost	3 Joints
G. 2	Total: 25			
	Survival in both hips for 25–26 years: 16 patients			
	Loosening within 20 years	Acetabulum: 5 hips	L.	0 (except for separation between HA and cement)
		Femur: 2 hips		
G. 3				285 Joints
			R.L.L.	Extremely low rate no progress
			O.L.	
			L.	0

2.2.4.2 Results

Bone ingrowth was observed in all interfaces where the HA granules were interposed on the living bone. Dense bone ingrowth was present in all specimens retrieved from the superior wall of the acetabulum. Among specimens from the inferomedial wall of the acetabulum, cancellous bone ingrowth was recognized in nine specimens and dense bone ingrowth was recognized in one (Fig. 2.7a). Cancellous bone ingrowth was also recognized in specimens from the femur. On the

Fig. 2.6 (**a**) Clinical results of THA with IBBC 22 to 25 years after THA. Appearance rate of radiolucent line and osteolysis was extremely low. Radiolucent line appeared between bone cement and HA, because the cementation was performed in the bleeding area. This line was not a radiolucent line but a space in correct. (**b**) THA with IBBC was performed in dysplastic acetabulum 24 years after THA. Neither radiolucent line nor osteolysis was seen in both acetabulum and femur. Rich new bone formation was seen on the hole around the bone cement. (**c**) THA with IBBC was performed in dysplastic acetabulum 24 years after THA. Wear of polyethylene socket highly increased; nevertheless, neither radiolucent line nor osteolysis was seen. (**d**) Scheme of the condition performed IBBC in the bleeding area. Spaces appeared between bone cement and HA several weeks after THA on the radiograph. It did no progress. (**e**) IBBC was performed in the bleeding area. A *space* appeared several weeks after THA. It did no progress. (**f**) Separation between bone cement and HA after THA with IBBC in the bleeding area and without sufficient anchor holes. (**g**) IBBC was performed in the bleeding area without sufficient anchor holes. Separation occurred between bone cement and HA 3 weeks after THA. However, fixation of bone to the bone cement was continued by interposing HA granules (IBBC) at the laterosuperior area

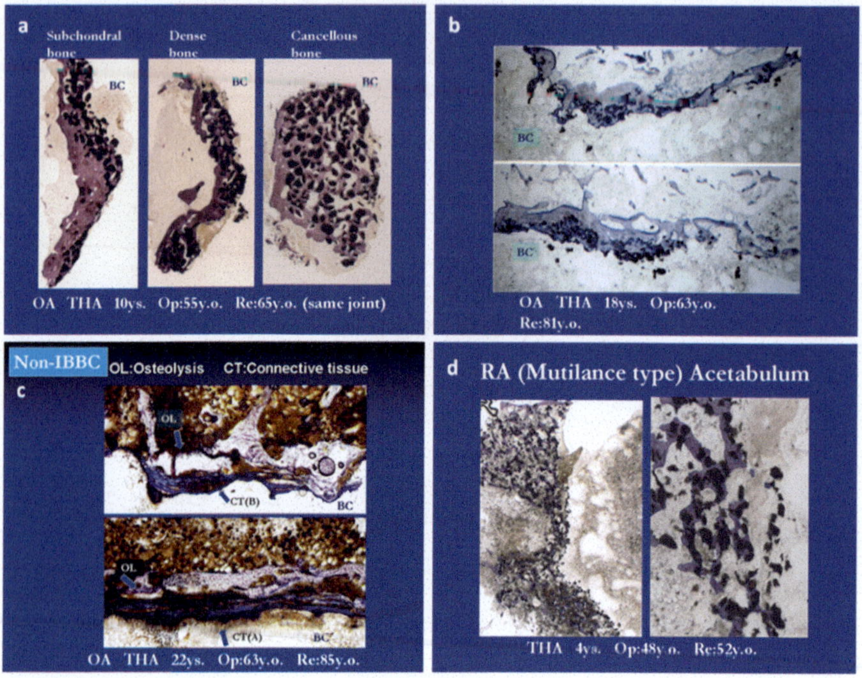

Fig. 2.7 (**a**) Photomicrographs of bone-cement interfaces. These three specimens were retrieved from the same joint. THA was performed on an OA hip joint at 55 years old and retrieved 10 years after surgery at 65 years old. Dense bone ingrowth is observed in superior wall of the acetabulum and cancellous bone ingrowth is observed in inferomedial wall of the acetabulum. (**b**) Photomicrographs of bone-cement interfaces. These two specimens were retrieved from the same joint. THA was performed for an OA hip joint at 63 years old and retrieved 18 years after surgery at 81 years old. This was implanted for 18 years. These were retrieved from the acetabular superior wall. (**c**) Photographs of interface without the HA granules. THA was performed for an OA hip joint at 63 years old and retrieved 22 years after surgery at 85 years old. These specimens were retrieved from acetabular inferior medial wall. Connective tissue (*CT*) interposition and osteolysis (*OL*) are observed at the interface (*BC* bone cement, *CT* connective tissue). (**d**) THA was performed for an RA hip joint at 48 years old and the specimen was retrieved 4 years after surgery at the age of 52 years old from the inferomedial wall of the acetabulum. New bone ingrowth around and between HA granules was formed and cancellous bone was made with HA granules only in the area where HA granules were smeared relatively sparsely

area in which thick layers of HA granules were smeared on the bone, thick and rich bone layer with HA granules was present. On the area in which even one layer of HA granules was smeared sparsely on the bone, a very thin new bone layer was formed (Fig. 2.7b).

In contrast, connective tissue interposition and osteolysis were observed at the sites where HA granules were not present (Fig. 2.7c). No foreign body reaction or proliferative granuloma formation was observed in any specimen.

The specimens were retrieved from 13 hips over 1–22 years, as well as 5 months in one knee after the initial operation. Considering the interval between the

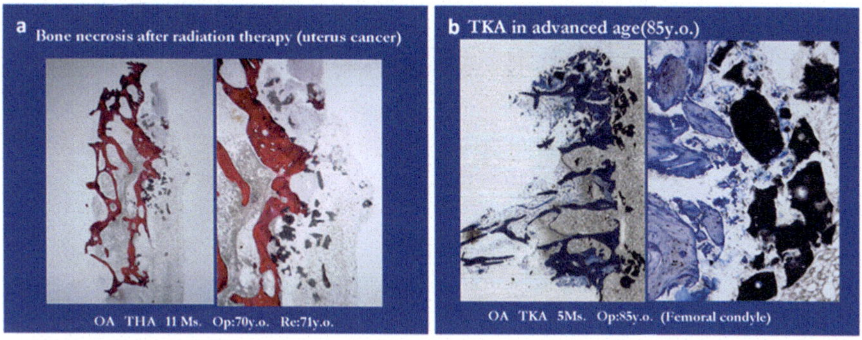

Fig. 2.8 (**a**) THA was performed for patient with bone necrosis after radiation therapy to portio cancer. Bone necrosis was found in iliac bone and hip joint. The joint replacement was performed at 71 years old and the specimens were retrieved 11 months after surgery from the inferomedial wall of the acetabulum at the age of 71 years old. IBBC was performed in scanty bleeding area due to bone necrosis. However, new bone formation was found to be relatively rich. (**b**) TKA was performed for an OA knee at the great age of 85 and the specimen was retrieved due to infection 5 months after surgery from the femoral condyle. New bone ingrowth was found around HA granules and between HA granules. However, speed of bone formation is rather slow

initial operation and revision, there was no difference in bone ingrowth except for the specimen from the knee joint. All specimens were retrieved from female patients, except for knee specimens, over 50 years of age. Although postmenopausal osteoporosis was observed in the host bone of the hip joint for the female patients, the findings of bone ingrowth around the HA granules were similar (Fig. 2.7b).

Considering patients with RA, new bone ingrowth around and between HA granules was formed and cancellous bone was formed in low density with HA granules only in the area where HA granules were smeared.

In this type of RA, cancellous bone was extremely atrophic and contained a large quantity of fatty marrow; thus, it was inevitable that HA granules were smeared in a thick layer in low density of bone (Fig. 2.7d). However, there was no new bone formation where host bone was observed necrotic.

On bone with extremely low osteoconductive ability, and scanty bleeding due to bone necrosis after radiation therapy for cancer, new bone formation was found (Fig. 2.8a). TKA was performed in an osteoarthritic (OA) knee at the great age of 85. The specimen was retrieved from the femoral condyle. New bone ingrowth around HA granules was found. However, speed of bone formation is rather slow due to the advanced age of the patient (Fig. 2.8b).

2.2.5 Discussion

In the IBBC technique, HA granules exist on the surface of cement mantle. This seems to be an HA-coated prosthesis-bone cement composite. In cementless

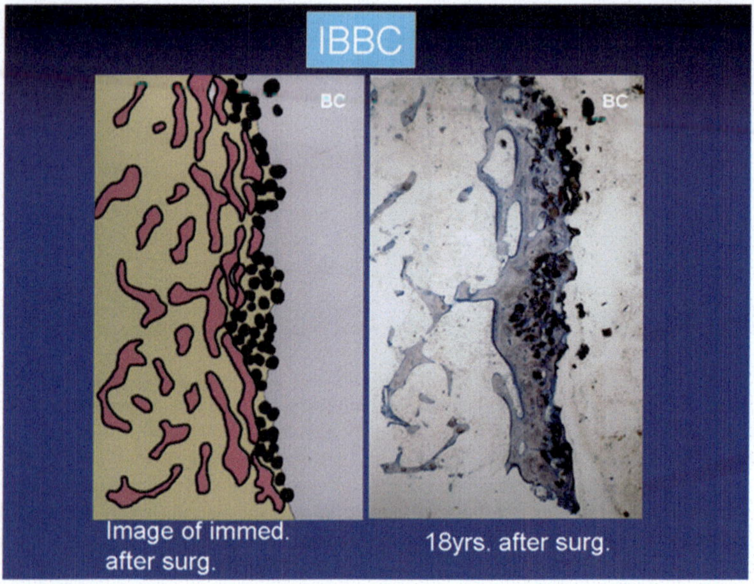

Fig. 2.9 Hypothetical time course of periprosthetic bone condition: immediately after THA (*left figure*) and 18 years after THA (*right figure*)

stems, it was reported that HA coating increases the amount of bone ingrowth and attachment leads to better bone fixation and enhanced the stability of the stem. The same effects can be expected for the cemented stem when the bone cement is coated with HA using IBBC technique. The clinical results using the IBBC technique were reported to be excellent. The characteristics of HA coated on a cementless prosthesis and HA granules for IBBC technique are different. As HA coated on prosthesis contains amorphous HA, HA resorbs with time.

In contrast, HA granules in our technique were pure polycrystalline HA phase and thus they were scarcely absorbed. We could not detect any sign of HA resorption in the retrieved specimens. It is expected that osteoconductive activity can continue indefinitely even after the onset of osteoporosis due to aging. Figure 2.9 shows our hypothetic time course of periprosthetic bone conditions; pre-osteoporotic bone smeared by HA granules at immediately after surgery and thick bone layer around HA granules surrounded by osteoporotic bone at 18 years after surgery.

In histological studies, dense bone ingrowth was observed in all specimens retrieved from the superior wall of the acetabulum, which was considered to be the principal weight-bearing site. Cancellous bone ingrowth was observed in specimens retrieved from the inferomedial wall, which was considered to be the auxiliary weight-bearing site. Connective tissue interposition and osteolysis were observed at the sites where HA granules failed to be smeared. The findings of bone ingrowth in the hip joints were similar regardless of the interval between the initial operation and revision or patient age at retrieval. New bone ingrowth was found around HA

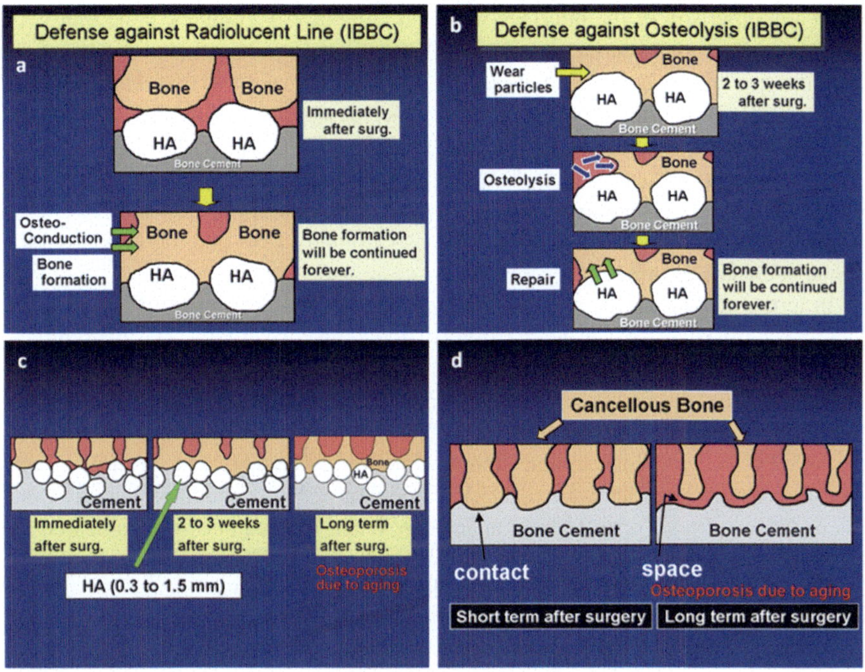

Fig. 2.10 (**a**) Scheme of effect of crystalline HA endures osteoconduction in IBBC. No radiolucent line appeared enduringly on radiograph due to osteoconductive effect of HA. (**b**) Scheme of effect of crystalline HA enduring osteoconduction in IBBC. Immediately before occurrence of osteolysis due to reaction of wear particles, it will be repaired by the osteoconductive effect of HA. (**c**) Scheme of the conditions cemented by IBBC at immediately after THA, 2–3 weeks after THA and long term after THA shifting to osteoporosis due to aging. (**d**) Scheme of the condition cemented using conventional cementation (non-IBBC) at short term after THA and long term after THA shifting to osteoporosis due to aging

granules and between HA granules, even when IBBC was performed at the great age of 85. However, speed of bone formation was understandably slow for this patient.

On the area in which thick layers of HA granules were smeared on the bone, thick and rich bone layers over the HA granule layer were formed. This bone layer with HA granules formed new bone around the HA granules that was fixed to the bone cement providing steady support to the prosthesis. Even on the area in which one layer of HA granules was spread sparsely, thin layer of new bone formation was found. However, at an interface where the bone was completely dead, there was no new bone formation.

At the sites where HA granules failed to be smeared, connective tissue interposition and osteolysis were observed. From these results, it can be concluded that the osteoconductive ability of HA prevents the occurrence of unmineralized connective tissue and osteolysis (Fig. 2.10a, b).

In a comparison of the interface with and without HA granules, bone ingrowth was observed at the interface with the HA granules (Fig. 2.10c), and the interface was interposed by connective tissue at the interface without the HA granules (Fig. 2.10d). Thus, the longevity of the bone-cement bonding for all these patients was attributed more to the interposed HA granules.

We retrieved the specimens between 5 months to 22 years after the initial operation. The HA granules were still present in the specimens after this long-term follow-up as the resorption of crystal HA is extremely slow and the bone directly contacts the HA granules.

In terms of patient age and postmenopausal osteoporosis, most of the patients were over 60 years of age at the time of the revision surgery. The histological findings were similar between elderly patients and patients less than 60 years of age. In addition, the specimens from the patients with rheumatoid arthritis and post-radiation osteonecrosis, conditions in which bone formation activity is considered to be very low, showed similar findings in the area where HA granules were smeared. These results indicate that HA granules have osteoconductive activity even in conditions of poor bone formation activity. When HA granules were smeared on the bone of a patient at the age of 85, the activity of osteoconduction was relatively low. However, relatively slow new bone formation was found in this patient.

In general, dense bone ingrowth was observed when HA granules were smeared on the dense bone and cortical bone. Cancellous bone ingrowth was observed when HA granules were smeared on the cancellous bone.

Further in the acetabulum, dense bone ingrowth was observed in specimens retrieved from the superior wall of the acetabulum, and cancellous bone ingrowth was observed in specimens retrieved from the inferomedial wall of the acetabulum; in both locations, the HA granules were evenly smeared. Assuming that the superior wall is the principal weight-bearing site and the inferomedial wall is the auxiliary weight-bearing site in the acetabulum, bone formation around the HA granules may be affected by mechanical conditions as an additional factor.

The use of HA granules in THA has some possible drawbacks, including loss of interdigitation of cement with bone, foreign body reaction, and third-body wear. For cement fixation, the strength of the cement-bone interface depends on the physical properties of the bony surface, the contact area, and the extent of penetration of cement into the bony trabeculae. In the IBBC technique, the HA granules cover the trabecular bony structure and prevent cement penetration following loss of interdigitation of cement. Consequently, the creation of small anchor holes in the acetabulum is recommended for initial fixation. No foreign body reaction was present at the interfaces with and without interposition of the HA granules. Although it has been reported that HA granules with a diameter of less than 10 mm cannot be incorporated, the HA granules used in the present study were 0.1–1.5 mm in diameter. Third-body wear is another potential risk. The retrieved polyethylene cups were not investigated for wear measurement and surface observation.

In a previously reported radiological study using an alumina head with IBBC technique in 111 hips, the linear wear rate depended on the thickness of the polyethylene and was compatible with other reported results. There were no untoward clinical complications attributed to the use of the HA granules.

Histological examination of the specimens containing well-fixed bone-cement interface 5 months to 22 years after THA and TKA with the IBBC technique showed bone ingrowth between the HA granules. Because bone ingrowth between the HA granules was observed in the specimens retrieved more than 20 years after the initial operation, the longevity of the bone-cement bonding was attributed more to the interposed HA granules. The histological findings were not affected by the pathological bony conditions associated with aging, postmenopausal osteoporosis, and diseases that lead to extremely low osteoconductive ability.

The histology showed there was no connective tissue interposition and no osteolysis in the area interposed by HA granules (Fig. 2.10a, b); however, they were found in the area without HA granules (Fig. 2.10c). From these results, there was long-term direct contact between the bones and HA granules and long-term longevity could be expected in patients receiving implants with IBBC (Fig. 2.10b).

2.3 Clinical Application: Reconstruction Surgery of the Acetabular Huge Bone Deficiency by Filling HA Granules at Revision Total Hip Arthroplasty

2.3.1 The First Generation

Before 1985, in the bony defect even in the massive bony defect at revision THA, the bony wall defect was covered by metal mesh and the bony defect was filled by bone cement (Fig. 2.11a, b). On the other hand, freeze-preserved, non-pathological allografts of the bone have been used in cases of massive bone deficiencies during revision total hip arthroplasty (THA) for more than 25 years in Europe and in the USA, and excellent results have been reported [1–4]. Cases using allografts have also been reported in Japan [5], although in Japan, materials other than femoral heads, partial femoral condyles, and partial tibial plateaus from patients undergoing arthroplasty are still very difficult to obtain. On the other hand, increasing interest in bioactive ceramics, particularly in HA over the past 30 years, has resulted in a significant increase in its clinical application during this period [6–32]. Under these circumstances, we began to use sintered HA granules clinically.

As a material, sintered HA is not resorbable, binds to the bone physicochemically, and is strong enough as bone defect filler. We obtained good results in three revision cases by placing fine HA granules (300–500 μm) between the bone cement and the bone graft on the deficiencies of the femur in 1984. In addition, since 1985, massive bone deficiencies have been filled with HA granules [26–28].

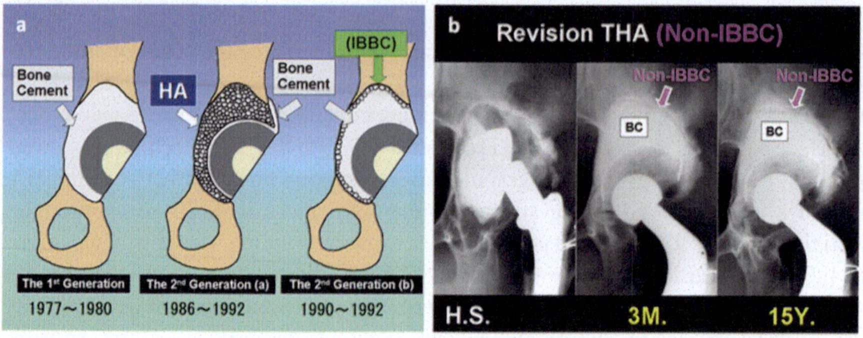

Fig. 2.11 (**a**) Revision THA in the acetabulum with massive bone deficiency. The 1st generation: deficiency was filled only by bone cement. The 2nd generation (a–a): deficiency was filled by HA granules. The 2nd generation (a–b): deficiency was filled by bone cement with IBBC. (**b**) Revision THA in the acetabulum with massive bone deficiency. Deficiency was filled only by bone cement (non-IBBC). *Left figure* is before revision THA. Radiolucent line was seen immediately after revision THA (*center figure*), and the component with bone cement was moving little by little superiorly (*right figure*: 15 years after revision THA)

2.3.2 *The Second Generation (a) (1986–1992)*

2.3.2.1 Materials and Methods

HA granules of 0.3–0.6 mm (G-2), 0.9–1.2 mm (G-4), and 3.0–5.0 mm (G-6) are mixed at a ratio of 10:45:45. Physiological saline is added to the mixture to increase the mixing density and to facilitate the adhesion of granules with each other due to the porous characteristic of the granules. This results in firmer adhesion and more stable shape formation. The acetabulum is filled with the mixture. If the same size of HA granules is used, the mixing density decreases, a firmer and more stable filling cannot be obtained, and the shape easily breaks.

A hemispherical compressor 2 mm larger than the outer diameter of the socket is then inserted successively into the previously determined space for the socket installation and firmly struck into the acetabulum using a plastic hammer while continuously making adjustments to determine the best socket location (Fig. 2.11a).

When cementing the socket, a 2–3 mm thickness of cement of paste-like condition is placed on the entire surface of the acetabulum and compressed with a compressor 2 mm larger than the outer socket diameter until the cement hardened. When a bone defect extended over a large area on the superior periphery of the acetabulum and it was not possible to fill the defect sufficiently with HA granules, additional HA granules were placed in this region and fixed using a 1–2 mm thickness of cement.

Before the socket was cemented, the hardened cement surface was dried, and the socket fixed with cement in a sticky condition on the hardened cement. This procedure facilitates binding the cements together.

2.3.2.2 Clinical Case

Between 1986 and 1992, we carried out this procedure on 40 hips. Whole peripheral segmental and cavitary deficiencies with medial walls intact were found in 13 joints (33 %), and peripheral cavitary deficiencies over the whole area with the medial wall absent were found in 18 joints (45 %). They were very unstable cases after revision surgery. There were 2 men and 38 women, and their ages at operation ranged from 35 to 81 years. The follow-up period was from 18 to 24 years. Our original revision THR was performed in osteoarthritis in 33 patients, rheumatoid arthritis in 5, avascular necrosis in 1, and systemic lupus erythematosus in 1. In 36 joints, this was the first revision, in 3 it was the second, and in 1 it was the third.

2.3.2.3 Results: X-Ray Evaluation

When HA granules are firmly packed, a stable filling is attained, similar to a stone wall. Although narrow spaces were observed in areas at the interface between HA granules and bone immediately after surgery, these spaces gradually disappeared within 3 months following surgery. This was probably due to new bone formation into the space between the HA granules and the subsequent binding with HA granules. Sclerotic bone surrounding loose components changed to cancellous bone over a period of 1–3 years following revision surgery.

Our radiographic evaluation showed neither morphological changes nor decreases in volume (Fig. 2.12a) except for some cases with very specific complications. In a case with a considerable cavitary and peripheral deficiency and a medial wall defect, HA granules were overfilled in the medial area of the acetabulum, and the socket settled laterally. Not only was there no detrimental effect radiographically or clinically, but the filled HA granules were also very stable following surgery.

In two cases, spaces were observed between HA granules near the bone at the laterosuperior lesion. If the superior peripheral deficiencies had been covered with an allograft plate, such as tibial plateau, HA granules could have been filled sufficiently in the superior peripheral region and, as a result, the appearance of the spaces could be avoided.

In two patients after the second revision and in one patient after third revision, the large part of the medial wall was absent and the overall deficiency was too great to allow stable filling of the granules. The packed HA granules broke and the prostheses migrated (Fig. 2.12b).

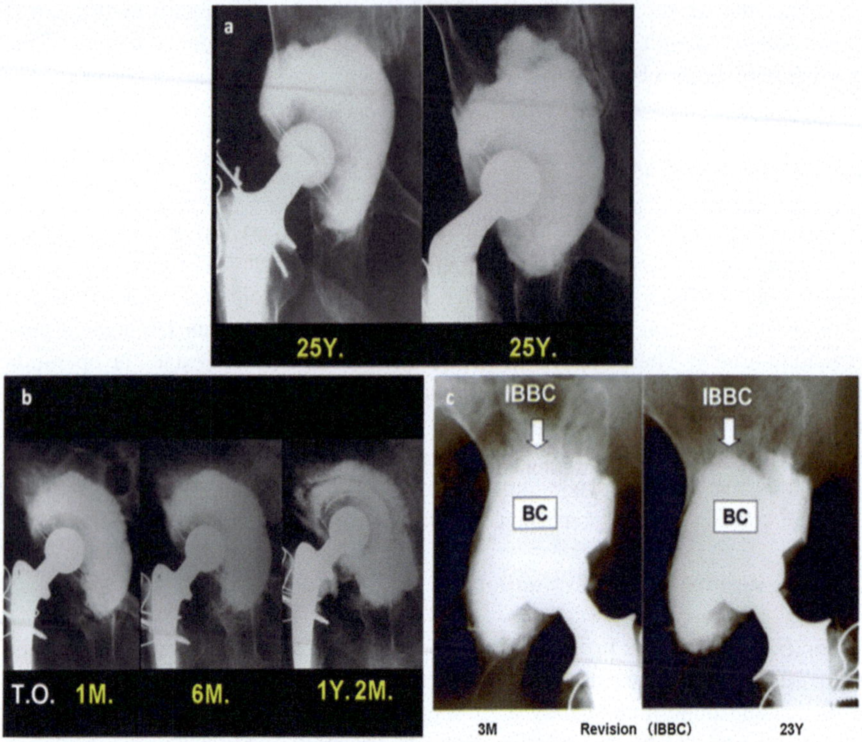

Fig. 2.12 (**a**) Revision of THA in the acetabulum with massive bone deficiency. Deficiency was filled by HA granules. Both *left* and *right* figures are 25 years after surgery. (**b**) Packed HA granules mass disintegrated after 1-year and 2-month revision THA. (**c**) IBBC was applied in a follow-up revision. The *left* figure shows 3 months and the *right* 23 years after revision surgery showing neither radiolucent line nor osteolysis

In these cases, peripheral bony wall deficiency should be covered by allograft bone to obtain stable HA granule filling [27, 28].

2.3.3 The Second Generation (b) (1990–1992)

In the old-age patients over 70 years old, bone cement was filled by using the IBBC technique in the huge cavity. In this case, a thicker layer of HA granules (3–5 layers) was smeared on the surface of the bone and soft tissue in the area of bone defect (Fig. 2.12). A very stable condition could be obtained immediately after surgery by using this technique (Fig. 2.12b, c). On the radiograph over 23 years after surgery, there was neither radiolucent line nor osteolysis (Fig. 2.12c).

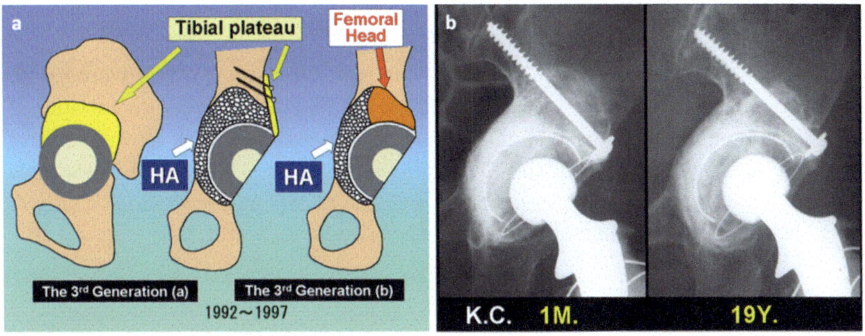

Fig. 2.13 (**a**) Scheme of the revision THA in the third (a) (b) generation. (**b**) Revision THA was performed by the third (**b**) generation. One month (*left figure*) and 19 years (*right figure*) after revision THA

2.3.4 The Third Generation (a) (Since 1992)

2.3.4.1 Materials and Methods

In the third generation, since 1992, peripheral segmental deficiencies were covered with allograft bone from the femoral head of patients undergoing arthroplasty to allow stable filling of HA granules. In some cases with a large cavitary deficiency combined with a large peripheral segmental deficiency, a large block of the femoral head was used. Since 1995, laterosuperior large peripheral deficiencies were covered with an allograft plate from the tibial plateau (Fig. 2.13a).

As a filler in the cavitary deficiency, mixtures of G-4 (0.9–1.2 mm) and G-6 (3.0–5.0 mm) HA granules were filled as in the first generation, and in some cases, mixtures of HA granules of 0.9–1.2 mm (G-4) and small bone chips at a ratio of 30:70 or 50:50 were filled. From 1995 to 1997, the Kerboull metallic cross-plate was used. However, after the Kerboull cross-plate had broken at the hook in 30 % of cases, it was discontinued.

2.3.4.2 Clinical Cases

In 1992–1997, 48 hips have been operated on using the procedure. The follow-up period was 14–19 years. Of the 48 hips, it was the first revision for 43, in 4 hips it was the second revision, and in 1 hip it was the third revision. They were very unstable cases, with great peripheral segmental and cavitary deficiencies, as in the first generation.

2.3.4.3 Results and Complications

In general, when the whole peripheral segmental deficiency was covered with allografts, filled HA granules were very stable. In one case filled with mixture of HA granules and bone chips, a slight volume change was observed. However, there were no clinical symptoms, and the change did not increase. There was no difference radiographically between HA alone and a mixture of HA and bone chips as fillers when the peripheral segmental deficiency was covered with allografts (Fig. 2.13b).

2.3.5 The Third Generation (b) (2002–Present)

In patients over 70 years of age, bony defects at the superolateral area were covered by using allograft of tibial plateau and huge bone defect was filled by bone cement by using IBBC technique. In these IBBC cases thicker layers of HA granules (3–5 layer) were smeared. This technique was the same as the first generation (b). A very stable condition was obtained immediately after surgery by using this technique. Clinical results were excellent with neither radiolucent lines nor osteolysis appearing.

2.3.6 Comparative Histological Studies of Retrieved Specimens Under a Loaded Condition and the Specimens from Animal Experiment Under an Unloaded Condition

2.3.6.1 Retrieved Specimens Under Loaded Condition

As Kerboull cross-plates as cup supporters broke in many cases, in two cases HA granule masses of approximately 2.0 and 2.5 cm in thickness were retrieved at 2 and 2.5 years after revision THA, respectively. They contained whole thickness of HA granules. Non-decalcified ground thin specimens stained by toluidine blue were observed by optical microscopy, and non-decalcified ground blocks were observed by backscattered electron image.

In clinical cases, in the weight-bearing condition, at the second revision THA, it was very difficult to drill into the HA granule mass and to cut the mass with a chisel. In histological studies, a large amount of dense bone ingrowth from the base of dense bone (Fig. 2.14a) and a large amount of cancellous bone ingrowth from the base of cancellous bone (Fig. 2.14b) were found in the whole spaces between HA granules into the whole depth, respectively. New bone adhered to HA directly.

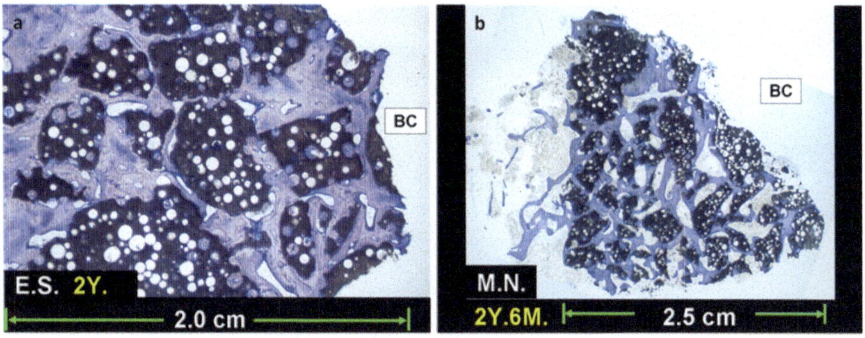

Fig. 2.14 (**a**) Retrieved specimen. Two years after revision THA. (**b**) Retrieved specimen. Two and a half years after revision THA

2.3.6.2 Animal Experiment in Bone Defect Cavity Under Unloaded Condition

Mixtures of G-4 (0.9–1.2 mm) and G-6 (3.0–5.0) HA granules as in clinical cases were filled into the cavity of 2 cm in diameter and 10 cm in length made at the proximal end of the tibia of goat (Fig. 2.15a). The proximal part of the tibia was cancellous bone and the distal part was cortical bone. Eighteen months after implantation, the animal was sacrificed, and radiographs by X-ray of A-P view and lateral view and the cross section of several levels were taken (Fig. 2.15b). From these specimens non-decalcified hard sections were made. A small amount of the new bone had entered from the periphery (Fig. 2.15c, d). As the quantity of bone ingrowth was small, some HA granules that filled the cavity dropped out while making non-decalcified hard tissue specimens and some HA granules dislodged from the specimens.

In a clinical case, HA granules were filled in the weight-bearing area. However, in experimental studies HA granules were filled in non-weight-bearing areas. From these results, it can be assumed that in the weight-bearing area, a great amount of new bone entered into the spaces of the HA granules and moved to the deep area. However, in the non-weight-bearing area in animal experiment, bone ingrowth could be expected only at the peripheral area of the cavity to approximately 5 mm in depth and not dense.

2.3.6.3 Discussion

The advantages of HA are as follows: (1) HA is osteoconductive and bonds to the bone physicochemically; (2) immunoreactions can be completely ignored; (3) postoperative morphological changes and volume decreases do not occur if a

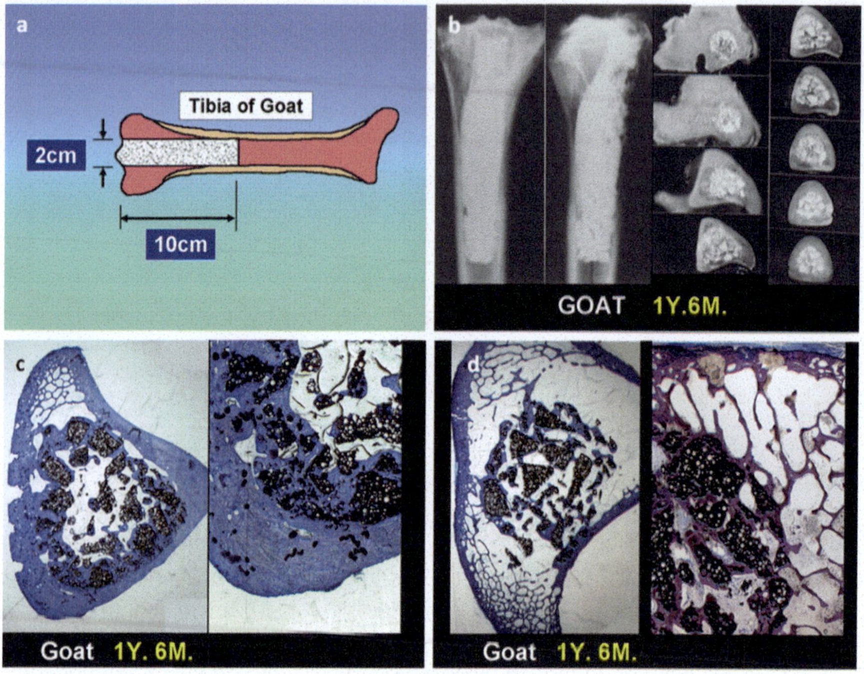

Fig. 2.15 (**a**) Scheme of animal experiment under unloaded condition as a control. (**b**) Radiograph. A-P view and lateral view (on the *left*) and cross sections (on the *right*). (**c**) HA granules were impacted into the cortical bone area. (**d**) HA granules were impacted into the cancellous bone area

mixture of adequate granule sizes is packed densely and firmly during surgery; (4) postoperative HA absorption, if any, is extremely small in amount and extremely slow; consequently, osteoconductivity can be continued; and (5) the occurrence of osteolysis by polyethylene wear particles at the interface of the bone is extremely few, because osteolysis can be recovered by osteoconduction of HA. We suggest that the reason for the marked pain-relieving effect is that there were neither changes in the shape of packed HA granules nor movement of the component, as HA granules were packed firmly and stably, bonded to the bone physicochemically, and fixed with bone cement mechanically.

The empty space or void at the interface between HA granules and bone immediately after surgery gradually disappeared within 3 months because new bone tissues entered into the space between the HA granules from the surface of the bony cavity. After filling HA granules into the cavitary deficiency, the sclerotic bone around the loosened socket changed to cancellous bone over a period of 1–3 years following revision surgery. This could be explained by the fact that bone ingrowth into the spaces of HA granules from the surrounding sclerotic bone was obtained, and the HA granules may have physicochemically bonded to the entire surface of the sclerotic bone wall. This phenomenon was very similar to bone union after nonunion of fracture.

On the retrieved studies, HA granules had formed a homogeneous mass, which was difficult to make a drill hole in or to cut with a chisel, and it adhered to the bone very firmly. Histologically, bone ingrowth was obtained 2 years and 2.5 years after surgery in the majority of the spaces between HA granules to the entire depth of about 2 cm and 2.5 cm, respectively. Consequently, if HA granules were filled very firmly and stably, a very strong new acetabulum could be reconstructed.

In the retrieved case, HA granules were filled in the weight-bearing area. However, in an animal experiment using a tibia of a goat, HA granules were filled in the non-weight-bearing area, and much less bone ingrowth into the spaces of HA granules was obtained. Consequently, excellent results can be expected when a mixture of several grain sizes of HA is packed densely and firmly during surgery into the massive defect of the bone in the weight-bearing area.

In conclusion, bone ingrowth over 2.5 cm in depth could be expected in weight-bearing area. However, it could not be expected over 5 mm in non-weight-bearing area.

As one of the complications, spaces between HA granules at nearby bone at the laterosuperior lesion (zone I) appeared. In this case the filling of HA granules may not have been dense near the bone base at the laterosuperior lesion (zone I), because the superior peripheral deficiency was covered with bone cement after filling with HA granules. As a result, continuous micromotion probably caused occurrences of the gaps before sufficient bone growth could provide bonding. If the superior peripheral deficiency had been covered by an allograft plate, such as tibial plateau, the HA granules would probably have filled the spaces more satisfactorily.

In the second generation, complications due to spaces between granules and the neighboring bony base at the laterosuperior lesion of the acetabulum have not been observed, and there was no socket migration, although breakage of the hook of Kerboull cross-plate was observed.

2.4 Other Clinical Applications

2.4.1 Bony Defect After Resection or Curettage of Bone Tumor

Bone ingrowth behaviors into the spaces of HA granules filled in the massive bony cavity are different in the weight-bearing area and in the non-weight-bearing area.

In the weight-bearing area, as shown in the clinical cases of massive bony defect of the pelvis at revision surgery, bone ingrowth could attain into the deep area. However, as shown in animal experiment of the massive bony defect of the tibia of the goat, bone ingrowth could not attain into the deep area in the non-weight-bearing area. Firm and stable filling of HA granules into the cavity is indispensable in both weight-bearing area and non-weight-bearing area. Otherwise, bone ingrowth could not be expected.

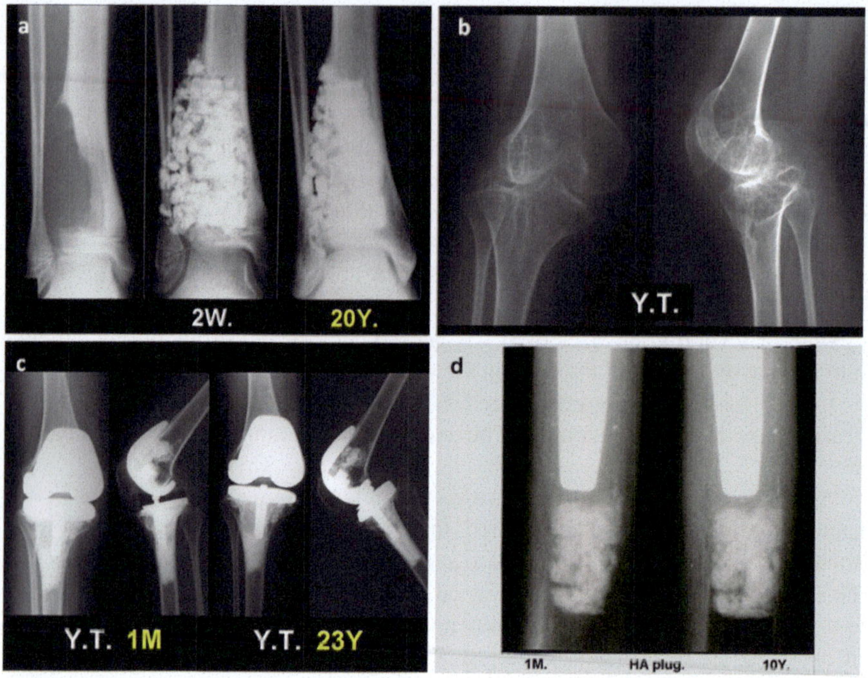

Fig. 2.16 (**a**) HA granules were filled into the cavity after resection of bone tumor in the tibia (*left*) before surgery, (*middle*) 2 weeks after surgery, and (*right*) 20 years after surgery. (**b**) Juvenile rheumatoid arthritis (*JRA*). 8 years old. Before surgery. (**c**) JRA. One month after surgery (*left figure*) and 23 years after surgery (*right figure*). A-P view and lateral view. (**d**) HA blocks were used as plugs at the distal end of the stem at THA. One month (*left figure*) and 10 years (*right figure*) after THA

2.4.1.1 Clinical Case 1: Giant Cell Tumor at the Distal End of the Tibia

This patient was operated on at 14 years old. HA granules were filled into the bony cavity and overfilled into the outside of the tibia, 20 years after surgery; on the radiograph in the weight-bearing area, bone ingrowth could be obtained densely into the whole spaces of HA granules. However, in the outside area of the tibia, which was non-weight-bearing area, dense bone ingrowth could not be obtained into the spaces of HA granules and the HA granules were retained (Fig. 2.16a).

2.4.1.2 Clinical Case 2: Juvenile Rheumatoid Arthritis (JRA)

This patient suffered from JRA since 8 years old. The multiple joints were destroyed, especially hip and knee bilaterally. This patient could not walk over 10 years due to flexion contracture of the knee bilaterally. This patient was operated on with total knee arthroplasty bilaterally. At surgery, cortical dense bone changed to very thin and cancellous bone changed to fatty marrow bone completely in both femur and tibia, especially in tibia (Fig. 2.16b). At surgery, HA granules were filled steady after removing fatty marrow, and HA granules were filled firmly into the bony cavity and atrophic bone marrow.

In this case, HA granules were filled into the weight-bearing area. Twenty-three years after surgery, bone ingrowth was obtained into the whole spaces of HA granules and very stable condition was continued on the radiograph (Fig. 2.16c). This patient could walk in the room after surgery.

2.4.1.3 Clinical Case 3: Bone Plug at the Distal End of the Stem in Cemented Total Hip Arthroplasty

In order to fill the bone cement strongly into the femoral canal, a bone plug is used at the end of the stem. For bone plug, bone block or plastic plugs are used, but a plastic plug is not stable. When we have no bone block, HA blocks are used. When a few number of small HA blocks are used, a very stable condition can be obtained.

In this case, as the HA blocks are filled in the weight-bearing area, bone ingrowth into the whole spaces of HA granules can be obtained (Fig. 2.16d).

2.4.2 Discussion

Stable bone condition could be made and continued, after HA granules were filled into the bone base even after bone marrow changing to fatty marrow due to degeneration by disease. Because crystalline HA exhibits excellent osteoconduction and is not resorbable, when used in the IBBC technique, osteoconductivity develops and continues for the lifetime of the patient. Such an excellent function was found in only the crystalline HA-based IBBC technique.

References

1. Denissen HW, de Groot K, Makkes PC, Van den Hooff A, Klopper PJ (1980) Tissue response to dense apatite implants in rats. J Biomed Mater Res 14:713–721
2. Hoogendoorn HA, Renooij W, Akkermans LMA, Visser W, Wittebol P (1984) Long-term study of large ceramic implants (porous hydroxyapatite) in dog femora. Clin Orthop Relat Res 187:281–288
3. Borja FJ, Mmaymneh W (1985) Bone allografts in salvage of difficult hip arthroplasties. Clin Orthop Relat Res 197:123–130
4. Gross AE, Laboie MV, McDermott P, Marks P (1985) The use of allograft bone in revision of total hip arthroplasty. Clin Orthop 197:115–122
5. Itoman M, Sunabe S (1988) Revision total hip replacement supplemented with allogenic bone grafting. J Joint Surg (Jpn) 7(3):83–93

Chapter 3
Bioactive Glass: Chronology, Characterization, and Genetic Control of Tissue Regeneration

Larry L. Hench

Abstract This chapter reviews the discovery and chronology of the development of bioactive glasses and the recent findings that controlled release of biologically active Ca and Si ions from bioactive glasses leads to the upregulation and activation of seven families of genes in osteoprogenitor cells leading to rapid bone regeneration. This finding offers the possibility of creating a new generation of gene-activating glasses designed for patient-specific in situ regeneration of tissues. Studies also indicate that controlled release of lower concentrations of ionic dissolution products from bioactive glasses can be used to induce angiogenesis and thereby offer potential for design of gene-activating glasses for soft tissue and cardiovascular system regeneration.

Keywords Bioactive glass • Bioglass • Gene expression • Osteogenesis • Osteoconduction • Osteostimulation • Regenerative medicine • Tissue engineering • Mineralization • Angiogenesis

3.1 Introduction

All biomaterials in use today are a compromise compared to the natural tissues they replace. Mismatches in elastic moduli, breakdown of the tissue-material interface, fatigue, wear, or other factors lead to 15–50 % failures of prostheses over a 15–30-year lifetime. An alternative approach to the present emphasis on replacement of body parts and tissues is now possible: *regeneration of tissues*. In order to regenerate tissues, it is essential to activate the body's own repair processes. To stimulate

L.L. Hench (✉)
Department of Biomedical Engineering, Florida Institute of Technology,
Melbourne, FL 32901, USA
e-mail: larryhench@embarqmail.com

B. Ben-Nissan (ed.), *Advances in Calcium Phosphate Biomaterials*, Springer Series in Biomaterials Science and Engineering 2, DOI 10.1007/978-3-642-53980-0_3,

self-repair it is necessary to control *both* the proliferation and the differentiation of progenitor stem cells towards mature cells capable of generating proper types and quantities of extracellular matrix that are present in nearly all tissues.

Controlled release of ionic dissolution products of soluble Ca and Si ions from bioactive glasses can provide this stimulus for enhanced osteogenesis. This chapter reviews the chronology of the development of bioactive glasses and the evidence of genetic control of bone regeneration that underlies development of a new approach to maintain quality of life in an aging population.

3.2 Development of Bioactive Glasses

For millennia it was accepted that any man-made material in the body would result in a foreign body reaction and formation of nonadherent scar tissue at the interface with the material. Thus, initial emphasis on biomaterials for use in the body was on materials that were as inert as possible when exposed to a physiological environment. Prevention of corrosion of metals or degradation of polymers was the primary design objective of first-generation biomaterials. A second generation of biomaterials to replace tissues was achieved when a special composition of soda-lime-phosphate-silicate glass was made by the author and implanted in the femurs of rats in 1969 [1–3]. The calcium phosphate-containing silicate glass composition had 45 % SiO_2, in weight % with network modifiers of 24.5 % Na_2O and 24.5 % CaO. In addition, 6 % P_2O_5 was added to the glass composition to simulate the Ca/P constituents of hydroxyapatite (HA), the inorganic mineral phase of bone, Table 3.1, with a nomenclature of 45S5 Bioglass.

The glass implants bonded to the living bone (rat femora) within 6 weeks and could not be removed from their implant site [1–3]. This discovery led to the development of a new class of biomaterials, called bioactive materials, for use in implants or prostheses and repair or replacement of bones, joints, and

Table 3.1 Composition of bioactive glasses and glass-ceramics used for medical and dental applications

Composition (wt%)	45S5 Bioglass (NovaBone, PerioGlas)	S53P4 (AbminDent1)	A-W glass-ceramic (Cerabone)
Na_2O	24.5	23	0
CaO	24.5	20	44.7
CaF_2	0	0	0.5
MgO	0	0	4.6
P_2O_5	6	4	16.2
SiO_2	45	53	34
Phases	Glass	Glass	Apatite beta-wollastonite glass
Class of bioactivity	A	B	B

Table 3.2 Chronology of science and clinical product development of 45S5 Bioglass

Discovery of bone bonding to 45S5 Bioglass at the University of Florida	
1971	First peer-reviewed publications of bonding of bone to bioactive glasses and glass-ceramics [1–3]
1972	Bonding of Bioglass bone segments and coated femoral stems in monkeys
1975	Bioglass-coated alumina bone bonding to sheep hip implants (in Germany)
1975	Bioglass dental implants bonded in baboon jaws
1977	Bonding of Bioglass implant in guinea pig middle ear
1977	Patent applications filed for Bioglass coatings on metals and alumina ceramics
1981	Discovery of soft connective tissue bonding to 45S5 Bioglass
1981	Toxicology and biocompatibility studies (20 in vitro and in vivo) published to establish safety for FDA clearance of Bioglass products
1985	First medical product (Bioglass Ossicular Reconstruction Prosthesis) (MEP) cleared by FDA via the 510 (k) process
1987	Discovery of osteoproduction (osteostimulation) in use of Bioglass particulate in repair of periodontal defects
1988	Bioglass endosseous ridge maintenance implant (ERMI) cleared by FDA via the 510 (k) process
1991	Development of sol-gel processing method for making bioactive gel-glasses extending the bioactive compositional range of bioactivity
1993	Bioglass particulate for use in bone grafting to restore bone loss from periodontal disease in infrabony defects (PerioGlas) cleared by FDA via the 510 (k) process
1995	PerioGlas obtained CE Mark in Europe
1996	Use of PerioGlas for bone grafts in tooth extraction sites and alveolar ridge augmentation cleared by FDA via the 510 (k) process
1999	European use of 45S5 particulate for orthopedic bone grafting (NovaBone)
2000	FDA clearance for use of NovaBone in general orthopedic bone grafting in non-load-bearing sites
2000	Quantitative comparison of rate of trabecular bone formation in the presence of Bioglass granules versus synthetic HA and A/W glass-ceramic
2000	Analysis of use of 45S5 Bioglass ionic dissolution products to control osteoblast cell cycles
2001	Gene expression profiling of 45S5 Bioglass ionic dissolution products to enhance osteogenesis
2004	FDA clearance of 45S5 particulate for use in dentinal hypersensitivity treatment (NovaMin)
2005	Development of variety of dental maintenance products (NovaMin)
2009	Anniversary of one million doses of NovaBone bone graft product and one million tubes of NovaMin toothpaste
2011	Acquisition of NovaMin technology by GlaxoSmithKline and world launch of Sensodyne Repair and Protect toothpaste for prevention of dentinal hypersensitivity and gingivitis

teeth. Table 3.2 summarizes the chronology of the development of bioactive glasses as a second generation of biomaterials. The seminal paper describes the composition of the glass and the evidence of bonding to bone by use of transmission electron microscopy (TEM) that reveals the bonded interface as a layer of growing Ca-P-based bone mineral that has interdigitated with collagen fibrils generated by osteoblasts growing at the interface [1]. An acellular in vitro model of soaking the glass samples in a 37 °C calcium phosphate-rich solution showed by X-ray diffraction (XRD) the steps of growth of a biologically active hydroxyapatite crystal phase on the surface of the glass that mimics the XRD pattern of the HA phase in living bone. Details of the bone-bonded interface are described in additional papers in 1971–1972 [1, 2].

3.2.1 *Compositions of Bioactive Glasses*

Bioactive materials, including bioactive glasses [1–3] and glass-ceramics [4–6], are special compositions made typically from the Na_2O-CaO-MgO-P_2O_5-SiO_2 system (Table 3.1). All of the compositions in Table 3.1 form a mechanically strong bond with bone within weeks or months. Details are described in references [7–15]. The rate of bone bonding depends upon composition of the material. Glass compositions with lower contents of SiO_2 (<52 % by weight) have the fastest rates of bone bonding and also bond to soft tissues [16]. Compositions such as 45S5 Bioglass with high rates of bioactivity produce rapid regeneration of trabecular bone with an amount, architecture, and biomechanical quality of bone that match that originally present in the site [14, 17–19]. The rapid regeneration of bone is due to a combination of processes called osteostimulation and osteoconduction [16–19]. Large differences in rates of in vivo bone regeneration and extent of bone repair indicate that there are two classes of bioactive materials (Table 3.1) [16–19].

3.2.2 *Classes of Bioactivity*

Class A bioactivity leads to osteoconduction, growth of new bone along the bioactive interface, and osteostimulation, growth of new bone throughout the defect to regenerate the architecture of bone natural to the site, as a consequence of rapid reactions on the bioactive glass surface [16–19]. The surface reactions involve dissolution of critical concentrations of soluble Si and Ca ions that give rise to both intracellular and extracellular responses at the interface of the glass with its physiological environment. The intracellular and extracellular response of osteoprogenitor cells results in rapid formation of osteoid bridges between particles, followed by mineralization to produce mature bone structures. This process is termed osteostimulation or osteoproduction. Rates of osteostimulation of various types of bioactive particulates have been quantified by Oonishi et al. that provide the fundamental in vivo comparisons of Class A versus Class B bioactive materials [14–19].

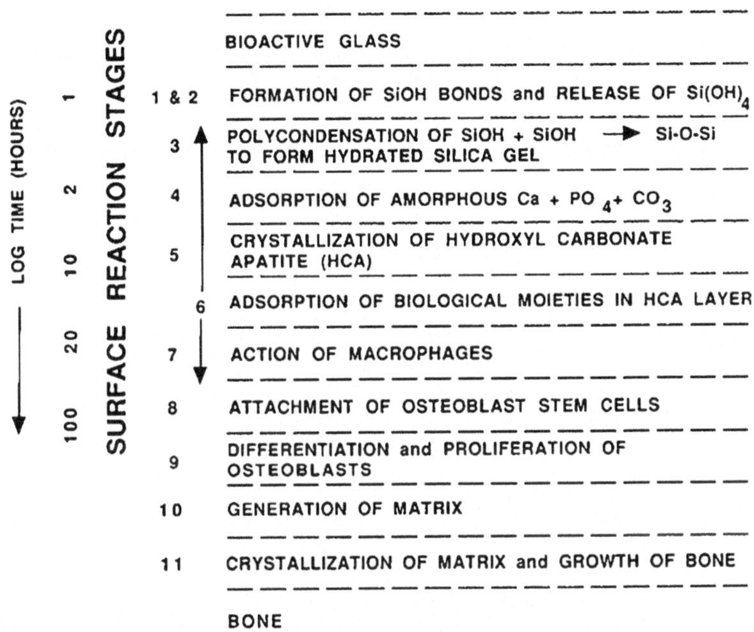

Fig. 3.1 Sequence and kinetics of interfacial reactions between bones and a Class A bioactive glass or glass-ceramic (Reprinted with permission from Hench [19], American Ceramic Society)

3.2.2.1 Characterization of Bioactivity Reaction Stages

New surface and interfacial analyses techniques were developed to understand the mechanisms and kinetics of bioactive reactions in vitro and in vivo [1, 13, 20–23]. These methods showed that there is a sequence of 11 reaction stages that occur at the surface of a Class A bioactive glass. Figure 3.1 indicates in the log time axis that the first five stages of surface reactions occur very rapidly and go to completion within 24 h for the bioactive glasses with highest levels of Class A bioactivity, e.g., 45S5 Bioglass. The effect of the surface reactions is rapid release of soluble ionic species from the glass into the interfacial solution. A high surface area composed of hydrated silica and polycrystalline hydroxyl carbonate apatite (HCA) as a bilayer is formed on the glass surface within hours (Stages 1–5) [23]. The reaction layers enhance adsorption and desorption of growth factors (Stage 6) and decrease the length of time macrophages prepare the implant site for tissue repair (Stage 7).

Attachment of stem cells (Stage 8) and synchronized proliferation and differentiation of the progenitor cells (Stage 9) rapidly occur on the surface of Class A bioactive materials [10, 14–16, 24]. Several weeks or months are required for similar cellular events to occur on the surface of Class B bioactive materials.

Differentiation of progenitor cells into a mature osteoblast phenotype does not occur on bio-inert materials and is rare on Class B bioactive materials because of the lack of ionic stimuli. In contrast, osteoprogenitor cells colonize the surface of Class A bioactive materials within 24–48 h and begin production of various growth factors which stimulate cell division, mitosis, and production of extracellular matrix proteins (Stage 10). Mineralization of the matrix follows soon thereafter, and mature osteocytes, encased in a collagen-HCA matrix, are the final product by 6–12 days in vitro and in vivo (Stage 11) [14–16, 24–30].

3.3 Genetic Control of Bone Regeneration by Bioactive Glasses

The original discovery of bioactive glasses and emphasis of research were on the mechanisms of interfacial bonding of bone to bioactive glasses [1–3, 7–22]. The seminal step to shift thinking from bioactive bonding to bone regeneration was the reporting by June Wilson et al. for the first time that new bone had colonized the surface of an array of 45S5 Bioglass particulate placed in a surgically created site in the jaw of monkeys that mimicked the loss of bone from periodontal disease [31]. New bone formed around the particles and created a regenerated architecture of bone that bridged the bioactive glass particles (Fig. 3.2). The new phenomenon was designated as osteoproduction, now generally called osteostimulation. The concept of osteostimulation was quantified by Oonishi et al. a few years later

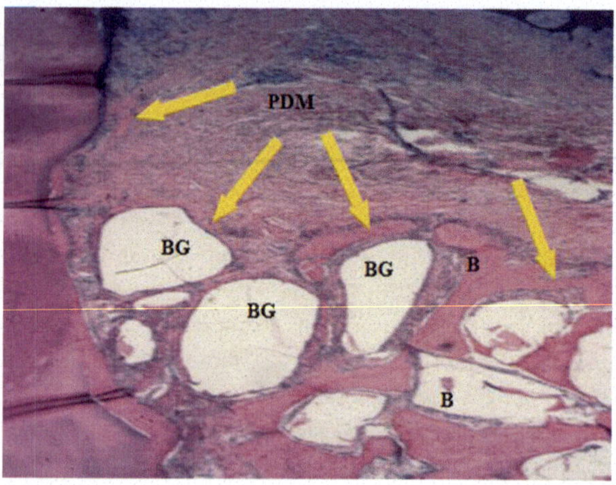

Fig. 3.2 Bioactive glass BG particulate used to enhance bone [*B*] formation around the tooth [*T*] and thereby restores its function following treatment of periodontal, gum, disease in a patas monkey periodontal defect model. Note the mineralized collagen that surrounds the bioactive glass particles forming a regenerated bone structure. Also note the periodontal ligament labeled PDM that is stable above the regenerated bone. (Magnification 20x). (Photo courtesy of Dr. June Wilson)

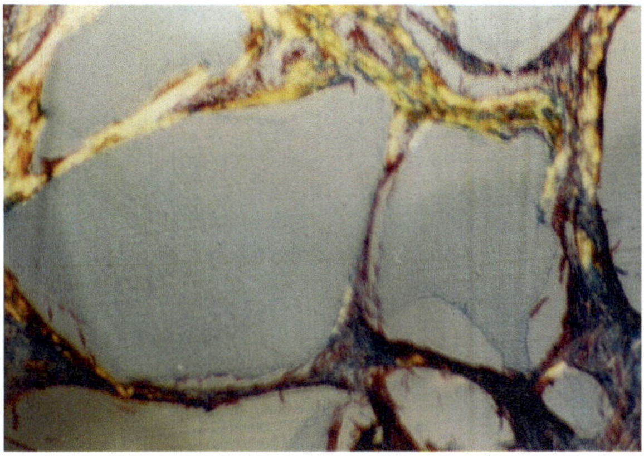

Fig. 3.3 Higher magnification of collagen fibrils that have been formed and adherent to bioactive glass particles in a regenerated periodontal defect model equivalent to that shown in Fig. 3.2. (Magnification 100x). (Photo courtesy of June Wilson)

[14, 32]. The second key finding to develop a genetic basis for bone regeneration was the finding of Xynos et al. that it was not only the glass but it was the ionic dissolution products released from 45S5 Bioglass that influenced and controlled the cell cycle of osteogenic precursor cells and ultimately controlled the differentiated cell population [26, 27]. Cells that were not capable of achieving a fully differentiated phenotype characteristic of mature osteocytes were eliminated from the in vitro cultures by programmed cell death, apoptosis. The shift in cell population towards mature osteoblasts occurred rapidly, in hours, and led to mineralized bone nodules in culture, without addition of organic bone growth factors, such as bone morphogenetic proteins (BMP). Another key finding from the work of Xynos et al. was that the effective ionic dissolution products released at slow rates from 45S5 Bioglass were biologically active soluble Si and Ca ions. Both ions are necessary for osteostimulation. Osteostimulation occurs only when the ions are present at a particular ratio of ions and at a particular concentration range of 15–30 ppm Si and 60–90 ppm Ca.

These findings provide an understanding of the clinical success of use of 45S5 Bioglass particles, NovaBone and PerioGlas, in a wide range of dental and orthopedic applications in use for nearly 20 years, as discussed in [17–19]. When used as a synthetic bone graft, the bioactive glass particles dissolve slowly and release the critical concentrations of Si and Ca over many weeks, as needed for progressive regeneration of bone to fill the defect. The initial effect is proliferation of osteogenic precursor cells at the periphery of the particles. These cells undergo mitosis and lead to an expanded population of mature osteoblasts that generate extracellular matrix proteins, especially Type I collagen that mineralizes to form regenerated bone (Fig. 3.3).

Oonishi et al. used a critical size defect model in a rabbit femoral condyle model to quantify the histological sequence of osteostimulation by 45S5 Bioglass particulate [14, 32]. The studies show that there is both more rapid bone formation in the presence of the osteostimulation particles and regeneration of a more highly mineralized quality of bone in the defect, in comparison with synthetic

Table 3.3 Cell and organ culture models used to establish genetic basis for osteostimulation by bioactive glass ionic dissolution products [26–30, 33–36]

Cell and organ culture	
Model # 1	Primary human osteoblasts (pHOBs)
Model # 2	Fetal human osteoblasts (fHOBs)
Model # 3	Murine embryonic stem cells (mES)
Model # 4	Human embryonic stem cells (hES)
Model # 5	Murine fetal long bones (metatarsals) (mFLBs)

hydroxyapatite (HA) particles or bioactive A/W glass-ceramic particles. The rate of bone regeneration in the Oonishi model is related to the rate of release of the soluble Si and Ca ions from the particulates tested. A rapid rate of release, as depicted in Fig. 3.1 Stages 1–5, is necessary for rapid bone regeneration and optimal fill of the defect by regenerated trabecular bone.

The third critical step in developing a genetic basis for tissue regeneration was the discovery that critical concentrations of ionic dissolution products (soluble Si and Ca ions) activate or upregulate seven families of genes in osteogenic precursor cells [27–30]. The genes encode transcription of numerous proteins that control the cell cycle, proliferation, and ultimately the differentiation of the cells towards the mature osteoblastic phenotype. The seminal paper leading to identification of the genetic response to bioactive dissolution products was published by Xynos et al. in 2001 resulting from a collaboration at Imperial College London of biomaterials investigators (the author's group) and the cell and molecular biology groups of Professor Dame Julia Polak [27].

3.3.1 Confirmation of Genetic Control of Bone Regeneration

Numerous studies have confirmed the results of the early Xynos et al. research and extended the generality to include several types of precursor cells and differing sources of ionic stimuli. Gene array analyses of five different in vitro models using five different sources of inorganic ions provide the experimental evidence for a genetic theory of osteogenic stimulation [26–30, 33–36]. The cell and organ culture models are summarized in Table 3.3. Sources of the ionic stimuli are given in Table 3.4.

In Table 3.4 the composition of the melt-derived 45S5 bioactive glass culture discs (A) and particulate (B) was 45 % (by weight) SiO_2, 24.5 % CaO, 24.5 % Na_20, and 6 % P_2O_5 [1]. Samples of (A) were obtained from US Biomaterials Corp., Alachua, FL, from a certified batch. Commercial powders of (B) with a particle size of 90–710 pm were obtained from NovaBone Products, Alachua, FL. The 58S sol-gel-derived particulate (C) composition (58 % SiO_2, 36 % CaO, 6 % P_20_5) and the 70/30 sol-gel sample (D) composition (70 % SiO_2, 30 % CaO) were made by the Dept. of Materials, Imperial College London [27, 37]. Sample (E) and the ionic

Table 3.4 Source of ionic dissolution products used in studies of osteostimulation by gene activation [26–30, 33–36]

Source of ionic dissolution products	
Source A	45S5 bioactive glass culture discs
Source B	4555 bioactive glass particulate (NovaBone)
Source C	58S bioactive gel-glass
Source D	70/30 bioactive gel-glass 3D porous tissue engineering scaffolds
Source E	Ionic dissolution products of B, C, D.

dissolution products of (B), (C), and (D) were obtained by immersing particulates of (B), (C), and (D) in simulated body fluid solution at 37 °C for various times to achieve concentrations of 15–30 ppm of soluble Si ions and 60–90 ppm of soluble Ca ions [38–40].

A study of dose dependence of ionic dissolution products showed this range of concentrations led to enhanced proliferation of osteoblasts [33–41]. Human primary osteoblasts (Table 3.3 Model #1) were obtained from excised femoral heads of total hip arthroplasty patients aged 50–70 years [24]. The first cell cycle and gene array experiments compared samples (A) with Thermanox plastic controls; the 2nd experiment compared ionic dissolution products of (B) with Thermanox controls; and experiment 3 used PCR methods to confirm effects of the ionic dissolution products of (B) on expression of specific genes from osteoblasts obtained from excised femoral heads of five individual patients [26]. Student's t tests were used to determine statistical significance of the results. The 4th and 5th experiments tested the effects of sample (E) on fHOBS and hES cells. The 6th and 7th experiments confirmed the findings of experiments 1–5 by comparing dosage effects of samples A and E on murine fetal metatarsals grown for 4 days in organ culture post-day 14 gestation [28] and growth of primary hOBs within three-dimensional scaffolds (Source D) [21].

All seven experiments showed enhanced proliferation and differentiation of osteoblasts towards a mature, mineralizing phenotype without the presence of any added bone growth proteins, such as dexamethasone or BMP. Shifts in osteoblast cell cycles were observed as early as 6 h, with elimination (by apoptosis) of cells incapable of differentiation. The remaining cells exhibited enhanced synthesis and mitosis. The cells quickly committed to generation of extracellular matrix (ECM) proteins and mineralization of the matrix. Gene array analyses at 48 h showed early upregulation or activation of seven families of genes that favored both proliferation and differentiation of the mature osteoblast phenotypes, including transcription factors and cell cycle regulators (six with increases of 200–500 %); apoptosis regulators (three at 160–450 % increases); DNA synthesis, repair, and recombination (four at 200–300 %); growth factors (four at 200–300 %) including IGF-I1 and VEG F); cell surface antigens and receptors (four at 200–700 %, especially CD44); signal transduction molecules (three at 200–600 %); and ECM compounds (five at 200–370 %). A summary of the seven families of genes activated or upregulated from the experiments listed above is given in Table 3.5.

the G_2 phase, then the cell proceeds to programmed cell death, apoptosis. Apoptosis is essential to prevent proliferation of cells that are an incorrect phenotype for bone repair. The chemical environment surrounding bio-inert implants does not stimulate apoptosis. Instead, on bio-inert materials there is rapid proliferation of cell types that are characteristic of nonadherent and non-mineralizing scar tissues. Bio-inert materials or Class B bioactive materials seldom enable the few osteoprogenitor cells present at their interface to pass through these cell cycle checkpoints and become fully differentiated osteoblasts. Only Class A bioactive materials that provide the biologically active ionic stimuli give rise to growth of mineralized bone nodules in vitro and rapid new bone formation in vivo. Details of differences in surface chemistry and cellular interactions between Class A and Class B bioactive materials are given elsewhere [17, 25]. Scanning electron microscopy (SEM) analysis of the human osteoblast cultures showed in the Xynos et al. studies that osteoblasts growing on the Class A bioactive substrate as early as 6 days had already organized, in a process called self-assembly, into a three-dimensional structure composed of cells and mineralized extracellular matrix [24]. This three-dimensional structure is called a bone nodule with an organizational complexity similar to natural bone grown in vivo, although without a blood supply. The time for formation of collagen on bioactive substrates in vitro is similar to the kinetics of collagen formation in vivo, as discussed elsewhere [42]. The rate of formation of mineralized bone nodules in vitro is also similar to the kinetics of bone growth in vivo, as reported by Oonishi et al. using a critical size defect model in the rabbit femoral condyle [14, 32].

Confirmation of the three-dimensional structure of the bone nodules was obtained by Xynos et al. using confocal scanning laser microscopy [24]. The three-dimensional structure of the nodule was mapped to show the presence and organization of the Type I collagenous matrix and calcium deposition within the bone nodules. The results confirm that human osteoblasts growing in culture in the presence of a bioactive glass self-assemble into a three-dimensional architecture and create a mineralized matrix that is characteristic of mature osteocytes in living bone. When the checkpoints in the osteoblast cell cycle described above have been satisfied, cell mitosis and formation of two daughter cells occur. The nuclei of both daughter cells each receive a complete and equivalent complement of genetic material. However, the checkpoints in the cell cycle also result in fewer and fewer progenitor cells that can enter into the M phase unscathed. The built-in protective mechanism from multiplication of damaged genes means that fewer osteoprogenitor cells are available to replace diseased, damaged, or dying bone cells of older people. The cumulative effect is a progressive decrease in bone density with age. Bone regeneration is much slower. In order for bone regeneration to occur at all, it is also necessary for a large fraction of the daughter cells to undergo differentiation into the mature osteoblast phenotype capable of undergoing mineralization and formation of osteocytes. These findings have been confirmed and extended to include other progenitor cell types by Bielby, Christodoulou, and the authors, as summarized in the experiments listed in Tables 3.3 and 3.4.

As discussed above, activation and completion of the osteoblast cell cycle do not merely provide the framework for cell proliferation but also determine to some extent cell commitment and differentiation. Bone cells cover a broad spectrum of phenotypes that include predominately the osteoblast, a cell capable of proliferating and synthesizing bone cell-specific products such as Type I collagen. However, in order for bone to be regenerated and repaired, there must be a vital cellular population consisting of osteocytes. Osteocytes are terminally differentiated osteoblasts that are usually postmitotic and are not capable of cell division. Osteocytes are capable of synthesizing and maintaining the mineralized bone matrix wherein they reside but subsequently do not divide. Thus, osteocytes represent the cell population responsible for extracellular matrix production and mineralization, the final step in bone development and probably the most crucial one given the importance of collagen-hydroxycarbonate-apatite (HCA) bonding in determining the biomechanical properties of bone. Therefore, it is important to observe that the end result of the cell cycle activated by the ionic products of bioactive glass dissolution was the upregulation of numerous genes that express growth factors and cytokines and extracellular matrix components (Table 3.5). An important finding was the 700 % increase in the expression of CD44 (Table 3.5), a specific phenotypic marker of osteocytic differentiation.

The cDNA microarray analysis showed that expression of the potent osteoblast mitogenic growth factor, insulin-like growth factor II (IGF-II), was increased to 320 % by exposure of the osteoblasts to the bioactive glass stimuli (Table 3.5). This is also an important finding because IGF-II is the most abundant growth factor in bone and is a known inducer of osteoblast proliferation in vitro. These results demonstrate that biogenic stimulation of IGF-II by the ionic dissolution products is a key factor in enhanced osteogenesis.

Xynos et al. confirmed the IGF-II mRNA upregulation using quantitative real-time PCR and also showed that the unbound IGF-II protein concentration was increased [26]. The results indicate that the ionic dissolution products of Bioglass 45S5 may increase IGF-II availability in osteoblasts by inducing the transcription of the growth factor as well as its carrier protein and also by regulating the dissociation of this factor from its binding protein. Bioactive induction of the transcription of extracellular matrix components and their secretion and self-organization into a mineralized matrix appears to be responsible for the rapid formation and growth of bone nodules and differentiation of the mature osteocyte phenotype.

3.4 Tissue Engineering of Bone Regeneration

Use of sol-gel processing of bioactive glasses to achieve additional control of the rates of ionic release of biologically active stimuli has led to production of an ideal scaffold for tissue engineering of bone. Compositions and textures of sol-gel-derived glasses can be varied over wide ranges and thereby be used to control the rates and concentrations of soluble Si and Ca released into the physiological solutions. Details of sol-gel processing of bioactive gel-glasses, textural analyses, and bioactivity studies are presented in an extensive series of papers [37–59].

Sol-gel processing makes it possible to produce hierarchical microstructures with nanometer-scale pores in the solid webs of three-dimensional scaffolds while creating an interconnected pore network with greater than 100 μm passages between macropores of 100–300 μm in diameter [41, 46].

Jones et al. demonstrated that such bioactive three-dimensional scaffolds support osteoblast growth and induced differentiation of the cells without use of supplementary organic growth factors [38–41]. Primary human osteoblasts (HOBs) were grown on 70S/30 (70 mol % SiO_2, 30 mol % CaO) foam scaffolds made by the sol-gel process [43]. The scaffolds had a modal interconnected pore diameter of 120 μm and a total porosity of 91 %. Prior studies showed that these unique materials resulted in a controlled release of soluble Si and Ca ions when exposed to simulated body fluids at 37°C. Jones et al. monitored cell viability and growth over a 3-week time period, and the osteoblast marker of alkaline phosphatase enzymatic activity was measured at 4, 7, 14, and 21 days. Production of collagen Type I, the extracellular matrix protein of fully differentiated osteoblasts, was measured at 7 and 14 days using an ELISA technique. The results showed that the bioactive scaffolds stimulated formation of mineralized bone nodules within 2 weeks of in vitro culture of the primary HOBs without the presence of supplementary growth factors in the medium. Evidence of the complete sequence of bone formation occurs by growth of the osteoblasts on the bioactive three-dimensional scaffolds, including cell attachment, cell growth, cell differentiation, extracellular matrix formation, and matrix mineralization. This study shows that the cells completed differentiation into the mature osteoblast phenotype and proceeded towards self-organization of bone architecture without the need of external organic supplements. All of these investigations [15–18, 21, 24] show that the sol-gel-derived bioactive gel-glasses provide controlled release of the ionic stimuli needed to control both proliferation and differentiation of cells of the osteoblast lineage [38–59].

The Bielby et al. study [33, 34] was especially significant because the cell source was embryonic stem (ES) cells. Soluble Si and Ca ions released from 58S sol-gel-derived glasses stimulated gene expression in the murine ES cells characteristic of a mature phenotype in primary osteoblasts. Differentiation of the ES cells into osteogenic cells was characterized by alkaline phosphatase (ALP) activity and the formation of multilayered, mineralized bone nodules. The nodules contained cells expressing the transcription factor runx2/cbfa-1. Deposition of osteocalcin in the extracellular matrix was detected by use of immunostaining. The osteogenic effect of the bioactive gel-glass extracts was dose dependent. The conclusion was that the bioactive gel-glass material was capable of stimulating differentiation of ES cells towards a lineage with therapeutic potential in tissue engineering. This conclusion extends the implications of the therapeutic use of the genetic findings of the studies of Xynos et al. described above (Table 3.5) where the cells were primary human osteoblasts from older people.

The study by Christodoulou et al. [35, 36] expanded even further the scientific basis for understanding the genetic effect of the dissolution products of bioactive gel-glasses on osteogenesis (Table 3.5). The material studied was 58S bioactive gel-glass [47–51]. The soluble Si and Ca dissolution products from the gel-glass were added to cultures of primary osteoblasts derived from human fetal long bone explants cultures (hFOBs). U133A human GeneChip oligonucleotide arrays were used to examine 22,283 transcripts and variants, which represent over 18,000 well-substantiated human genes. A 24-h treatment with a single dosage of ionic products induced the differential expression of a number of genes important to differentiation of the osteoblast phenotype, including IL-6 signal transducer/gp130, ISGF-3/STAQT1, HF-1-responsive RTP801, ERK1 p44 MAPK (MAPK3), MAP-KAPK2, IGF-I, and IGFBP-5. The over 200 % upregulation of gp130 and MAPK3 and downregulation of IGF-1 were confirmed by real-time RT-PCR analysis. These data suggest that 58S ionic dissolution products, Ca and Si, possibly mediate the bioactive effect of the gel-glass through components of the IGF system and MAPK signaling pathways. The results from human fetal osteoblasts also confirm many of the findings reviewed above (Table 3.5) using primary human osteoblast cultures derived from excised femoral heads of elderly patients and thereby demonstrate the generality of the findings of genetic stimulation by the ionic dissolution products of bioactive glasses and gel-glasses. The findings are also consistent with prior investigations of the role of ionic dissolution products in stimulation of growth and especially mineralization of fetal long bones, mouse fetal metatarsals, as reported by Maroothynaden and Hench [60].

The implication of the above studies is that it is now feasible to design the dissolution rates and architecture of bioactive, resorbable inorganic scaffolds to achieve specific biological effects in vivo that synchronize with the progenitor cell population present in situ, as discussed previously by the author [61]. This offers for the first time the potential to design biomaterials for specific patients and their clinical needs.

3.4.1 Control of Vascularization of Tissues by Bioactive Glass Ionic Dissolution Products

Clinical use of bioactive glass particulate for dental, maxillofacial, and orthopedic applications has been successful in part because fully vascularized bone is regenerated in situ (Fig. 3.4). The gene array studies summarized above show that VEGF (vascular endothelial growth factor) is one of the important growth factors upregulated (Table 3.5). Healing of wounds in soft tissues and soft tissue engineering also require establishment of a viable blood supply, i.e., vascularization. Recent studies show that ionic dissolution products released from 45S5 Bioglass particulate are effective in promoting angiogenesis in numerous in vitro and in vivo models [62–75]. The experiments confirm that there is upregulation of VEGF production from human microvascular endothelial cells (HMVEC) and other cells involved in the repair and maintenance of the circulatory system. The stimulation of angiogenesis depends upon the concentration of ions present in the cultures which can be controlled by using differing quantities of 45S5 Bioglass in collagen sponges

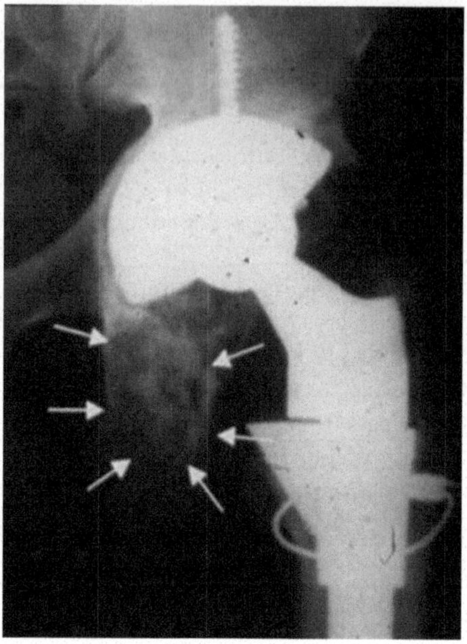

Fig. 3.4 The X-radiograph shows the use of bioactive glass, 45S5 Bioglass, after repair of bone following removal of a large unicameral cyst in the ischium of a patient prior to revision of hip arthroplasty due to implant loosening. The existing hardware was removed and replaced, and the cyst was debrided. The residual cavity (denoted by the *arrows*) then was grafted with a 50:50 mixture of autogenous bone and bioactive glass (NovaBone®). Three years after implantation, the graft site is stable with no recurrence of the cyst, the site being filled with dense bony tissue. There has been no recurrence of the cyst (Photo courtesy of Dr. Dave Gaisser, NovaBone Products, Alachua, FL, USA)

or other multiphase delivery systems. The findings are that when there are too few ions, there is no angiogenic stimulatory effect; too many ions also have no effect. Leu and Leach showed that larger concentrations of the ionic dissolution products led to osteogenesis [66], as described in the seven osteogenic experiments reviewed above. Thus, controlled release of a critical concentration of Si and Ca ions is required for the proangiogenic effect.

There are important implications from these findings. At present most treatment modalities for damage to the small intestine or many soft tissue defects, including chronic wounds, are at best palliative. There is great need for bioactive wound dressings that can counter the negative stimuli that prevent healing of chronic wounds. Combining the anti-inflammatory characteristics of 45S5 Bioglass particles with their proangiogenic potential, described above, offers great promise for design of wound dressings that stimulate keratinogenesis and angiogenesis required to achieve a rapid regeneration of the skin.

3.5 Conclusions

The molecular biological mechanisms involved in the behavior of bioactive glasses are now understood with sufficient confidence that the results can be used to design a new generation of bioactive materials for tissue regeneration and tissue engineering. The bioactive response appears to be under genetic control. Bioactive glasses that are osteostimulative enhance osteogenesis through a direct control over genes that regulate cell cycle induction and progression towards a mature osteoblast phenotype. This process is termed osteostimulation. Cells that are not capable of forming new bone are eliminated from the cell population, a characteristic that is missing when osteoblasts are exposed to bio-inert or Class B bioactive materials. The biological consequence of genetic control of the cell cycle of osteoblast progenitor cells is the rapid proliferation and differentiation of osteoblasts. The result is rapid regeneration of bone. The clinical consequence is rapid fill of bone defects with regenerated bone that is structurally and mechanically equivalent to normal, healthy bone. The use of bioactive glass particulate to release smaller concentrations of ionic dissolution products from a polymer sponge offers the possibility of designing a new generation of wound-care dressings and soft tissue engineering constructs.

Perhaps of even more importance in the long term is the possibility that bioactive ionic dissolution products can be used to activate genes in a preventative treatment to maintain the health of our bones as we age. Only a few years ago, this concept of using bioactive materials for preventative therapeutics would have seemed to be impossible. We need to remember that it was only 40 years ago that the concept of a material that would not be rejected by living tissues was considered to be impossible. If we can activate genes by use of glasses to grow bone and stimulate repair of soft connective tissues, it is certainly possible that we may one day be able to use glasses to control genes to prevent the loss of tissues.

References

1. Hench LL, Splinter RJ, Allen WC, Greenlee TK (1971) Bonding mechanisms at the interface of ceramic prosthetic materials. J Biomed Mater Res 2:117–141
2. Beckham CA, Greenlee TK, Crebo AR (1971) Bone formation at a ceramic implant interface. Calcif Tissue Res 8:165
3. Greenlee TK, Beckham CA, Crebo AR, Malmborg JC (1972) Glass ceramic bone implants. J Biomed Mater Res 6:235–244
4. Kokubo T, Ito S, Sakka S, Yamamuro T (1986) Formation of a high-strength bioactive glass-ceramic in the system MgO-CaO-SiO_2-P_2O_5. J Mater Sci 21:536
5. Gross U, Strunz V (1985) The interface of various glasses and glass-ceramics with a bony implantation bed. J Biomed Mater Res 19:251
6. Yamamuro T, Hench LL, Wilson J (1990) Handbook on bioactive ceramics: bioactive glasses and glass-ceramics. CRC Press, Boca Raton

7. Hench LL, Paschall HA (1973) Direct chemical bonding of bioactive glass-ceramic materials and bone. J Biomed Mater Res Symp 4:25–42
8. Hench LL, Paschall HA (1974) Histochemical responses at a biomaterials interface. J Biomed Mater Res 5:49–64
9. Piotrowski G, Hench LL, Allen WC, Miller GJ (1975) Mechanical studies of the bone- bioglass interfacial bond. J Biomed Mater Res 9:47–61
10. Hench LL, Paschall HA, Allen WC, Piotrowski G (1975) Interfacial behavior of ceramics implants. Natl Bur Stand Spec Publ 415:19–35
11. Griss P, Greenspan DC, Heimke G, Krempien B, Buchinger R, Hench LL et al (1976) Evaluation of a bioglass coated Al_2O_3 total hip prosthesis in sheep. J Biomed Mater Res 10:511–518
12. Clark AE, Hench LL, Paschall HA (1976) The influence of surface chemistry on implant interface histology: a theoretical basis for implant materials selection. J Biomed Mater Res 10:161–174
13. Hren JJ, Johnson PF, Bates SR, Hench LL (1976) STEM/EDX analysis of bone-bioglass interface. EMSA 290–291
14. Oonishi H, Hench LL, Wilson J, Sugihara F, Tsuji E, Matsuura M, Kin S et al (2000) Quantitative comparison of bone growth behaviour in granules of bioglass®, A-W glass-ceramic, and hydroxyapatite. J Biomed Mater Res 51:37–46
15. Hench LL, Clark AE (1982) Adhesion to bone. In: Williams DF, Winter GD (eds) Biocompatibility of orthopaedic implants. CRC Press, Boca Raton
16. Wilson J, Pigott GH, Schoen FJ, Hench LL (1981) Toxicology and biocompatibility of bioglass. J Biomed Mater Res 15:805
17. Hench LL, Hench JW, Greenspan DC (2004) Bioglass: a short history and bibliography. J Aust Ceram Soc 40:1–42
18. Hench LL (1991) Bioceramics: from concept to clinic. J Am Ceram Soc 74:1487–1510
19. Hench LL (1998) Bioceramics. J Am Ceram Soc 81:1705–1728
20. Hench LL (1975) Characterization of glass corrosion and durability. J Non-Cryst Solids 19:27–39
21. Clark AE, Pantano CG, Hench LL (1976) Auger spectroscopic analysis of bioglass corrosion films. J Am Ceram Soc 59:37–39
22. Kim CY, Clark AE, Hench LL (1989) Early stages of calcium-phosphate layer formation in bioglass. J Non-Cryst Solids 113:195–202
23. Hench LL, Clark DE (1978) Physical chemistry of glass surfaces. J Non-Cryst Solids 28:83–105
24. Xynos ID, Hukkanen MVJ, Batten JJ, Buttery ID, Hench LL, Polak JM (2000) Bioglass® 45S5 stimulates osteoblast turnover and enhances bone formation *in vitro*: implications and applications for bone tissue engineering. Calcif Tissue Int 67:321–329
25. Hench LL, Polak JM, Xynos ID, Buttery LDK (2000) Bioactive materials to control cell cycle. Mater Res Innov 3:313–323
26. Xynos ID, Edgar AJ, Buttery LD, Hench LL, Polak JM (2000) Ionic dissolution products of bioactive glass increase proliferation of human osteoblasts and induce insulin-like growth factor II mRNA expression and protein synthesis. Biochem Biophys Res Commun 276:461–465
27. Xynos ID, Edgar AJ, Buttery LDK, Hench LL, Polak JM (2001) Gene expression profiling of human osteoblasts following treatment with the ionic dissolution products of bioglass® 45S5 dissolution. J Biomed Mater Res 55:151–157
28. Hench LL, Xynos ID, Edgar AJ, Buttery LDK, Polak JM, Zhong JP et al (2002) Gene activating glasses. J Inorg Mater 17:897–909
29. Hench LL (2003) Glass and genes: the 2001 W. E. S. Turner memorial lecture. Glass Technol 44:1–10
30. Hench LL (2013) Bioactive glasses: gene activation. In: Hench LL (ed) An introduction to bioceramics, 2nd edn. Imperial College Press, London
31. Wilson J, Low SB (1992) Bioactive ceramics for periodontal treatment: comparative studies in the Patus monkey. J Appl Biomater 3:123–169

32. Oonishi H, Hench LL, Wilson J, Sugihara F, Tsuji E, Kushitani S et al (1999) Comparative bone growth behaviour in granules of bioceramic materials of different particle sizes. J Biomed Mater Res 44:31–43
33. Bielby RC, Christodoulou IS, Pryce RS, Radford WJP, Hench LL, Polak JM (2004) Time- and concentration-dependent effects of dissolution products of 58S sol-gel bioactive glass on proliferation and differentiation of murine and human osteoblasts. Tissue Eng 10:1018–1026
34. Bielby RC, Pryce RS, Hench LL, Polak JM (2005) Enhanced derivation of osteogenic cells from murine embryonic stem cells after treatment with ionic dissolution products of 58S bioactive sol-gel glass. Tissue Eng 11:479–488
35. Christodoulou I, Buttery LDK, Saravanapavan P, Tai GP, Hench LL, Polak JM (2005) Dose- and time-dependent effect of bioactive gel-glass ionic-dissolution products on human fetal osteoblast-specific gene expression. J Biomed Mater Res B 74B:529–537
36. Christodoulou I, Buttery LDK, Saravanapavan P, Tai GP, Hench LL, Polak JM (2005) Characterization of human fetal osteoblasts by microarray analysis following stimulation with 58S bioactive gel-glass ionic dissolution products. J Biomed Mater Res B 77B:431–446
37. Saravanapavan P, Jones JR, Pryce RS, Hench LL (2003) Bioactivity of gel-glass powders in the CaO-SiO_2 system: a comparison with ternary (CaO-P_2O_5-SiO_2) and quaternary glasses (SiO_2-CaO-P_2 O_5-Na_2O). J Biomed Mater Res A 66A:110–119
38. Jones JR, Hench LL (2004) Factors affecting the structure and properties of bioactive foam scaffolds for tissue engineering. J Biomed Mater Res B 68B:36–44
39. Gough JE, Jones JR, Hench LL (2004) Nodule formation and mineralisation of human primary osteoblasts cultured on a porous bioactive glass scaffold. Biomaterials 25:2039–2046
40. Jones JR, Ehrenfried LM, Hench LL (2006) Optimising bioactive glass scaffolds for bone tissue engineering. Biomaterials 27:964–973
41. Jones JR, Lee PD, Hench LL (2006) Hierarchical porous materials for tissue engineering. Phil Trans R Soc A 364:263–281
42. Hench LL, West JK (1996) Biological applications of bioactive glasses. Life Chem Rep 13:187–241
43. Saravanapavan P, Hench LL (2000) Low temperature synthesis, structure and bioactivity of gel-derived glasses in the binary CaO-SiO_2 system. J Biomed Mater Res 54:608–618
44. Saravanapavan P, Hench LL (2003) Mesoporous calcium silicate glasses. I. Synthesis. J Non-Cryst Solids 318:1–13
45. Saravanapavan P, Hench LL (2003) Mesoporous calcium silicate glasses. II. Textural characterisation. J Non-Cryst Solids 318:14–26
46. Atwood RC, Jones JR, Lee PD, Hench LL (2004) Analysis of pore interconnectivity in bioactive glass foams using X-Ray microtomography. Scr Mater 51:1029–1033
47. Li R, Clark AE, Hench LL (1991) An investigation of bioactive glass powders by sol-gel processing. J Appl Biomater 2:231–239
48. Sepulveda P, Jones JR, Hench LL (2002) Synthesis of sol-gel derived bio-active foams. Key Eng Mater 218–220:287–290
49. Sepulveda P, Jones JR, Hench LL (2002) Bioactive sol-gel foams for tissue repair. J Biomed Mater Res 59:340–348
50. Sepulveda P, Jones JR, Hench LL (2002) The effect of temperature on the processing and properties of macroporous bioactive glass foams. Key Eng Mater 218–220:299–302
51. Sepulveda P, Jones JR, Hench LL (2002) *In vitro* dissolution of melt-derived 45S5 and sol-gel derived 58S bioactive glasses. J Biomed Mater Res 61:301–311
52. Sepulveda P, Jones JR, Hench LL (2002) Bioactive materials for tissue engineering scaffolds. Imperial College Press, London
53. Lenza RFS, Jones JR, Vasconcelos WL, Hench LL (2002) Surface modified 3D scaffolds for tissue engineering. J Mater Sci Mater Med 13:837–842
54. Jones JR, Lenza RFS, Vasconcelos W, Hench LL (2002) Bio-molecular design of 3-D tissue engineering constructs. In: Banner N, Polak J, Yacoub M (eds) Lung transplantation and pulmonary disease. Cambridge University Press, Cambridge

55. Stamboulis AG, Boccaccini AR, Hench LL (2002) Novel biodegradable polymer/bioactive glass composites for tissue engineering applications. Adv Eng Mater 4:105–109
56. Boccaccini AR, Roether JA, Hench LL, Maquet V, Jérôme R (2002) A composites approach to tissue engineering. J Ceram Eng Sci Proc 23:805–816
57. Roether JA, Gough J, Boccaccini AR, Maquet V, Hench LL (2002) Novel bioresorbable and bioactive composites based on bioactive glass and polylactide foams for bone tissue engineering. J Mater Mater Med 13:1207–1214
58. Sepulveda P, Jones JR, Hench LL (2002) Bioactive sol-gel foams for tissue repair. J Biomed Mater Res 59:340–348
59. Jones JR (2004) Review of bioactive glass: from Hench to hybrids. Acta Biomater 9:4457–4486
60. Maroothynaden J, Hench LL (2006) The effect of micro-gravity and bioactive surfaces on the mineralization of bone. J Mater 58:57–63
61. Hench LL (2009) Genetic design of bioactive glass. J Eur Ceram Soc 29:1257–1265
62. Day RM (2005) Bioactive glass stimulates the secretion of angiogenic growth factors and angiogenesis *in vitro*. Tissue Eng 11:768–777
63. Gorustovich A, Roether JA (2004) Effect of bioactive glasses on angiogenesis: a review of in-vitro and in-vivo evidences. Tissue Eng Part B Rev 16:199–207
64. Day RM, Boccaccini AR, Shurey S, Roether JA, Forbes A, Hench LL et al (2004) Assessment of polyglycolic acid mesh and bioactive glass for soft-tissue engineering scaffolds. Biomaterials 25:5857–5866
65. Keshaw H, Forbes A, Day RM (2005) Release of angiogenic growth factors from cells encapsulated in alginate beads with bioactive glass. Biomaterials 26:4171–4179
66. Leu A, Leach JK (2008) Proangiogenic potential of a collagen/bioactive glass substrate. Pharm Res 25:1222–1229
67. Leach JK, Kaigler D, Wang Z, Krebsbach PH, Mooney DJ (2006) Coating of VEGF-releasing scaffolds with bioactive glass for angiogenesis and bone regeneration. Biomaterials 27:3249–3255
68. Moosvi SR, Day RM (2009) Bioactive glass modulation of intestinal epithelial cell restitution. Acta Biomater 5:76–83
69. Day RM, Maquet V, Boccaccini AR, Jérôme R, Forbes A (2005) *In vitro* and *in vivo* analysis of macroporous biodegradable poly(D, L-lactide-co-glycolide) scaffolds containing bioactive glass. J Biomed Mater Res 75A:778–787
70. Gerhardt LC, Widdows KL, Erol MM, Burch CW, Sanz-Herrera JA, Ochoa I et al (2011) The proangiogenic properties of multi-functional bioactive glass composite scaffolds. Biomaterials 32:4096–4108
71. Leu A, Stieger SM, Dayton P, Ferrara KW, Leach JK (2009) Angiogenic response to bioactive glass promotes bone healing in an irradiated calvarial defect. Tissue Eng Part A 15:877–883
72. Zhai W, Lu H, Chen L, Lin X, Huang Y, Dai K et al (2012) Silicate bioceramics induce angiogenesis during bone regeneration. Acta Biomater 8:341–349
73. Rahaman MN, Day DE, Bal BS, Fu Q, Jung SB, Bonewald LF et al (2011) Bio-active glass in tissue engineering. Acta Biomater 7:2355–2373
74. Hoppe A, Güldal NS, Boccaccini AR (2011) A review of the biological response to ionic dissolution products from bioactive glasses and glass-ceramics. Biomaterials 32:2757–2774
75. Boccaccini AR, Erol M, Stark WJ, Mohn D, Hong Z, Mano J (2010) Polymer/bioactive glass nanocomposites for biomedical applications: a review. Compos Sci Technol 70:1764–1776

Chapter 4
The Essential Role of Calcium Phosphate Bioceramics in Bone Regeneration

Guy Daculsi, Borhane Hakim Fellah, and Thomas Miramond

Abstract Various bioceramics or xenograft has been used to avoid autograft. However, there are large differences in the chemistry, the micro- and macrostructure, and consequently the performance in terms of resorption, absorption, and regeneration of physiological bone. The differences in such available bioceramics were reported and critical data presented. Recent developments related to CaP scaffolds including improvements in terms of engineering chemistry, surface properties, microstructure, and porosities, which lead them to be considered as being bioinstructive rather than osteoconductive scaffolds, have opened up new opportunities for bone regenerative technologies. Not only are some of these CaP bioceramics scaffolds osteoinductive in their own right, but evidence also supports the hypothesis that specific engineering bioceramics have a direct influence on the differentiation and proliferation of human mesenchymal stem cells (hMSCs). Tissue engineering, new bioactive molecules, and new surgical technologies increase the potential application of CaP bioceramics as carriers of these cells and also as scaffolds capable of guiding the behavior of these cells and the efficiency of bone regeneration. If the smart bioinstructive CaP scaffold technology led to a higher efficacy of CaP scaffolds, it would allow further surgical applications in bone

G. Daculsi (✉)
Inserm U791, University of Nantes and Inserm CIC-IT 802, Hospital of Bordeaux LIOAD Inserm Université de Nantes UMR U791, Faculté de Chirurgie Dentaire Pl A. Ricordeau, 44042 Nantes cedex, France
e-mail: guy.daculsi@univ-nantes.fr

B.H. Fellah
Oniris, National Veterinary School, Nantes, France
e-mail: borhane.fellah@oniris-nantes.fr

T. Miramond
LIOAD Inserm Université de Nantes UMR U791, Faculté de Chirurgie Dentaire Pl A. Ricordeau, 44042 Nantes cedex, France
e-mail: thomas.miramond@univ-nantes.fr

B. Ben-Nissan (ed.), *Advances in Calcium Phosphate Biomaterials*, Springer Series in Biomaterials Science and Engineering 2, DOI 10.1007/978-3-642-53980-0_4,

tissue regeneration. The mechanical properties required for bone ingrowth and bone remodeling and mechanotransduction must be explored to allow for development of new generation scaffolds.

Keywords Bone substitutes • Bone regeneration • Calcium phosphate bioceramics • Injectable calcium phosphate • Scaffolds • Tissue engineering

4.1 Introduction

Although bone tissue possesses the capacity for regenerative growth, the repair process is impaired in many clinical and pathological situations. Large bone loss caused by trauma and tumor resection and/or aging requires reconstructive surgery and/or bone regeneration. At present, bone surgeons have three different possibilities for replacing bone:

- *Autogenous bone grafts* are primarily used for bone replacement, despite the pain, septic complications, and the limited amount of bone harvested from the iliac crest or other sites.
- *Allogenic bone grafts* are obtained from tissue banks. These grafts have limitations because of the possible transmission of nonconventional agents or viruses and the risk of immunological incompatibility.
- *Alloplastic bone substitutes* are produced in various compositions and shapes. These biomaterials can be used to fill bone cavities, serving as a scaffold for bone regeneration from the peri-implant region. Bone substitutes can also be used to supplement autogenous bone, or in combination with bone marrow aspirates. The ideal biomaterial should have a variety of forms and sizes, all with sufficient strength for use in load-bearing sites. It should also be biocompatible, biodegradable, and able to be substituted by newly formed bone.

Numerous synthetic bone graft materials are currently available as alternatives to autogenous bone for repair, substitution, or augmentation. Synthetic biomaterials include special glass ceramics described as bioactive glasses and calcium phosphates (CaPs) (e.g., calcium hydroxyapatite, HA; tricalcium phosphate, TCP; and biphasic calcium phosphate, BCP). The review of Dorozhkin [1] reported the important historical data for CaP bioceramics. In 1920, Albee [2] reported the first successful use of a calcium phosphate reagent for the repair of a bone defect in a human. More than 50 years later, the clinical use of a TCP preparation was reported in surgically created periodontal defects in animals and the use of dense HA as immediate tooth root replacements. In the early 1980s, synthetic HA and β-TCP became commercially available as bone substitute materials for dental and medical applications [3].

The term BCP describes a bioceramic that consists of a mixture of HA and β-TCP. The first studies on BCP showed that the bioactivity of these ceramics might be controlled by manipulating the HA to β-TCP ratios [4]. Subsequently,

Table 4.1 Abbreviations, chemical compositions, Ca/P, and solubility product constants of some synthetic and biological calcium phosphates

Abbreviation	Chemical formula	Ca/P	Solubility K_{sp} at 25 °C
MCPM	$Ca(H_2PO_4)_2.H_2O$	0.5	18 g/L
MCPA	$Ca(H_2PO4)_2$	0.5	
DCPD	$CaHPO_4.2H_2O$	1.00	0.32 g/L 2.39×10^{-7}
DCPA	$CaHPO_4$	1.00	
OCP	$Ca_8(HPO_4)_2(PO_4)_4.5H_2O$	1.33	1.05×10^{-47}
TCPa	$Ca_9[]_1(HPO_4)(PO_4)_5(OH)[]_1$	1.50	
CDA	$Ca_{9.5}[]_{0.5}(HPO_4)_{0.5}(PO_4)_{5.5}(OH)_{0.5}[]_{1.5}$	1.58	
β-TCP	$Ca_3(PO_4)_2$	1.50	2.83×10^{-30}
HA	$Ca_{10}(PO_4)_6(OH)_2$	1.67	3.37×10^{-58}
Human bone[a]	$Ca_{8.3}[]_{1.7}(PO_4)_{4.3}(HPO_4,CO_3)_{1.7}$ $(OH,1/2CO3)_{0.3}[]_{1.7}$	1.55 – 1.75	$7.2 \times 10^{-53} - 6.4 \times 10^{-58}$

[] represents a lacuna in the crystal lattice of hydroxyapatite
[a] A possible chemical composition of bone mineral as it is constantly evolving

studies focused on BCP led to the significant increase in manufacture and use of commercial BCP bioceramics as bone substitute materials for dental and orthopedic applications [5].

Then, many studies were performed on CaP and especially calcium orthophosphate (Table 4.1). A large review of the chemical processing, manufacturing, biological properties, and applications of calcium orthophosphate was recently published [6]. CaP of pure HA, pure β-TCP, or BCP is achieved after sintering biological apatite or synthetic apatite obtained either by precipitation or hydrolysis. The BCP composition (HA to β-TCP ratio) obtained after sintering depends on the calcium deficiency of the unsintered biological or synthetic apatite and temperature [7]. The presence of other ions during the preparation of the unsintered calcium-deficient apatite (CDA) can also affect the HA and β-TCP or BCP sintering.

The sintering of commercial CaP reagents (labeled as "hydroxyapatite" or "calcium phosphate, tribasic" or "tricalcium phosphate") above 900 °C was shown to result in pure HA, pure β-TCP, or BCP (Table 4.1).

Recent developments related to CaP scaffolds including improvements in terms of engineering chemistry, surface properties, microstructure, and porosities, which lead them to be considered as being bioinstructive rather than osteoconductive scaffolds, have opened up new opportunities for bone regenerative technologies [8]. Not only are some of these CaP bioceramics scaffolds osteoinductive in their own right, but evidence also supports the hypothesis that specific engineering bioceramics have a direct influence on the differentiation and proliferation of human mesenchymal stem cells (hMSCs). Tissue engineering, new bioactive molecules, and new surgical technologies increase the potential application of CaP bioceramics as carriers of these cells and also as scaffolds capable of guiding the behavior of these cells and the efficiency of bone regeneration [8].

4.2 Definitions

4.2.1 Calcium Phosphate Bioceramics

For over 30 years, HA and related CaPs have been widely used in the field of biomaterials as bone graft substitutes [3, 6, 7, 9, 10]. These materials have clinical applications in orthopedic, spinal, and maxillofacial surgery. They are currently used in various forms, but macro-/microporous bioceramics are the most advanced products [11]. Bioceramics are manufactured from well-characterized CaP powders that are mixed with pore makers and sintered at elevated temperatures (e.g., 1,000–1,300 °C). Research has primarily focused on both the formulation of appropriate bioceramic chemistry and the optimization of the physical pore structure. Mastering the chemistry of CaP bioceramics is clearly crucial for reproducible and controlled production processes but also for ensuring the adequate biological response upon implantation in bone tissue. These materials have been considered as bioactive and osteoconductive as they bond directly to bone tissue without an interstitial fibrous tissue layer. Their bioactivity is related to the solubility of CaP in physiological media. Several groups have shown that biphasic CaP bioceramics composed of HA and β-TCP represented the optimal formulation in terms of bioactivity. The TCP phase is soluble and leads to a release of calcium and phosphate ions which saturate local body fluids and precipitate a biological apatite onto the less soluble HA crystals [6, 12, 13].

4.2.2 Injectable Calcium Phosphate Bioceramics and Putties

CaP bioceramic granules associated with hydrosoluble polymers are at present extensively used [14]. Different combinations have been proposed with polymers such as gelatine, collagen, fibrin, demineralized bone matrix, hyaluronic acid or synthetic polymers such as poloxamer, and cellulose derivatives. To date, several injectable biomaterials have been developed. Some of these injectable bone substitutes are made of CaP hydraulic cements that harden in the bone defect [15–17]. Others are composed of CaP granules suspended in hydrogel, as they are the most interesting carriers used for the development of injectable bone substitute.

MBCP Gel is a non-self-hardening injectable biomaterial. It is composed of BCP granules associated with a hydrosoluble polymer. These materials have been shown to be perfectly biocompatible and potentially resorbable, and thanks to their initial plasticity, they assume the shape of bone defects very easily, eliminating the need to shape the material to adjust it to the implantation site [14, 18]. MBCP Gel does not have the mechanical properties of hydraulic bone cements. However, bone cells are able to invade the spaces created by the disappearance of the polymer carrier.

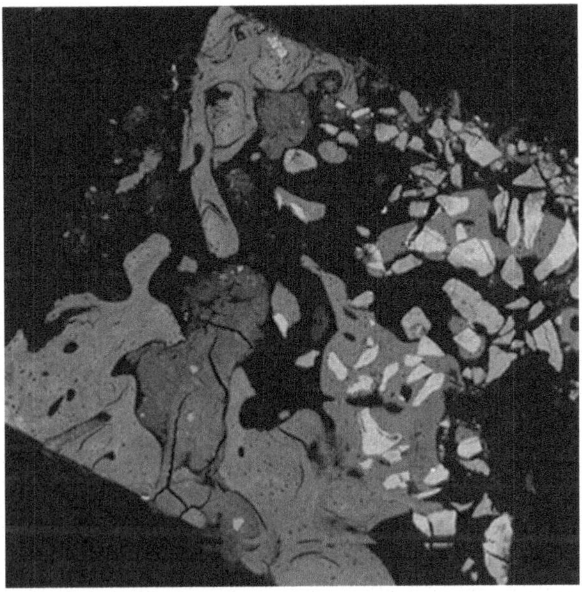

Fig. 4.1 MBCP Gel (In'Oss™). Human bone regeneration after revision surgery of nonintegrated dental implant, 8 months. SEM showing in *grey* the newly formed bone and in *light grey* the residual bioceramics particles integrated in the regenerated bone

Bone ingrowth takes place all around the granules at the expense of the resorption of the BCP granules (Fig. 4.1). In time, the mechanical properties are increased due to the presence of the newly formed bone. Numerous reports both in vitro and in vivo have confirmed the efficacy and performance of this concept for an injectable bone substitute used in bone reconstruction [14, 18–20].

IBS2 [21, 22] is a self-hardening composite. The BCP granules are associated with silanized HPMC-Si hydrogel. The guiding principles of silanized HPMC-Si hydrogel are its hydrophilic and liquid properties (it is viscous before being mixed with the CaP load and injection) and its pH-controlled reticulation process [23, 24]. The silanized hydrogel/CaP composite presents self-reticulation properties, due to the change in pH as a catalyst and without an exothermic effect. Once in the implantation site, in contact with the biological buffer liquids, a chemical reaction without additive and without any catalyst allows bridging and reticulation between the various macromolecular chains.

Prior to cross-linking, the composite is an injectable viscous liquid that hardens in the bone defect forming a gel loaded with BCP ceramic particles. IBS2 can entirely fill and remain in the bone defects. The BCP particles provide bioactivity supporting the bone healing process by osteoconduction. The cross-linked HPMC-Si hydrogel provides intergranular spaces for bone ingrowth. However, the jellification before blood diffusion delays osteoconduction of the BCP particles, and cells and tissue colonization at the expense of the composite.

Jellification is an important property of this material. It prevents the material from being washed out from the bleeding transplant site, after implantation. For an injectable bone substitute to maintain the bioceramic granules in unclosed cavities, the reticulation must increase the density of the material, reduce the dissolution or degradation of the polymer, and delay diffusion of the biological fluid and cell colonization [24].

The advantage of ready-to-use mixtures is their easiness of use and the reproducibility of the final material. Their kinetics for osseous reconstruction can be fast because of the many intergranular paths. These materials have relatively few intrinsic primary mechanical properties, even if the vehicles used harden by reticulation. Achieving mechanical properties is secondary to rapid physiological bone ingrowth.

BCP/fibrin glue: The association of bioceramics (TricOs®) and fibrin sealants may be interesting for the clinical applications of composite bone substitutes [25, 26]. Indeed, CaP granules are not easy to handle, are limited to filling bone cavities, and are not available for bone apposition. In addition, adding bioactive factors can improve the performance of bioceramics. In this regard, the adjunction of a binding agent, such as fibrin glue, improves the stability of the granules at the site of implantation and provides the scaffold effect of bioceramics with the additional osteogenic property. Fibrin-CaP composite could be obtained by mixing Baxter's fibrinogen, the thrombin components of fibrin sealant (Tisseel® Baxter BioSciences BioSurgery), and TricOs® granules [27]. Macroporous Biphasic Calcium Phosphate TricOs® is a mixture of HA/β-TCP in a 60:40 ratio. Granules of 1–2 mm in diameter presenting both macroporosity (50–55 %) and microporosity (30–35 %) are used. To enhance the working time, a low thrombin concentration (4 U) is used. The Tisseel/TricOs volume ratio is 1 to 2. Numerous preclinical studies have been performed in rabbits and goats, both for biocompatibility and biofunctionality, using, for example, sinus lift augmentation and bone filling in long bone. Histology, histomorphometry, and X-ray microtomography have demonstrated the osteogenic properties of the composite [27].

Calcium phosphate cements: The need for a material for minimally invasive surgery (MIS) prompted the development of a concept for self-setting injectable CaP cement (CPC) as bone substitute. Currently, several CPCs are commercially available and more are being investigated. LeGeros et al. first introduced the concept in 1982 [15], and the first patent was obtained by Brown and Chow in 1986 [16]. All current CPCs are reported to have good mechanical properties and reasonable setting times. However, after setting, these materials remain dense and do not provide rapid bone substitution because of the lack of macroporosity. Numerous studies have reported the applications of currently available commercial CPCs [1, 17]. New BCP-based CPCs have recently been developed [28]. The MCPC consists of multiphasic CaP phases, including BCP. In vivo, the components of the cement resorb at different rates, allowing the formation of interconnecting macroporosity, thus facilitating bone ingrowth and substitution of the cement with the newly forming bone [28].

The powder component is essentially made of a settable and resorbable matrix (which includes α-TCP, stabilized amorphous CaP (s-ACP), and monocalcium phosphate monohydrate (MCPM)). A sieved fraction of macroporous BCP granules ranging between 80 and 200 μm in diameter are incorporated into the matrix. The cement liquid is an aqueous solution of Na_2HPO_4.

After setting MCPC in distilled water at 20 °C, the mechanical properties in compression of such materials were 10 ± 2 MPa at 24 h and 15 ± 2 MPa after 48 h. The cohesion time for injectability was reached after 20 min. Animal models of critical size defects in rabbit epiphyses or goat vertebral bodies demonstrated the performance and efficacy of CPC. MBCP granules act as a scaffold for bone osteoconduction, and resorption of the ACP content of the cement allowed macroporosity and bone ingrowth between and at the surface of the BCP granules, extending to the core of the implanted site. The cement matrix dissolved as expected, forming an open structure for cell colonization and bone ingrowth at the expense of the self-setting bone void filler [7, 28].

4.2.3 Fundamental Physicochemical Properties

4.2.3.1 Resorption

CaP bioceramic resorption [29] is the process by which resorption cells such as macrophages and osteoclasts break down the biomaterials and release the ions, resulting in a transfer of calcium and phosphate from the bioceramic to the blood [30]. This active process undertaken by the cells is equivalent to bone remodeling. The process is largely associated with the degradation of the bioceramic [6, 31] by biological fluids, the mechanical stress of the implantation site, releasing smaller particles. In the inflammation process, the size of the particles has a strong influence on dissolution [32], leading to the conclusion that resorption is dependent on the dissolution.

4.2.3.2 Dissolution

The solubility of CaP phases is mainly related to their chemical composition and crystal properties [3, 6, 29, 33, 34]. Different solubility product constants (K_{sp}) have been reported for synthetic or biological CaP compounds, as shown in Table 4.1 [6]. The solubility is affected by cationic or anionic substitutions in the apatite lattice. For instance, carbonated or CDA are more soluble than fluoroapatite (FAP). Comparative dissolution in acetate buffer provided the following order of solubility: bone >> enamel >> β-TCP > HA. β-TCP has been found to dissolve faster in physiological solutions, as well as exhibiting a greater rate of dissolution or degradation than HA, when implanted in heterotopic or ectopic sites. Depending on the HA to β-TCP weight ratios, the solubility of BCP ceramics will be more similar to that of β-TCP or HA. The dissolution of CaP ceramics is also affected by its porosity and particle size. Increasing the porosity greatly enhances the surface

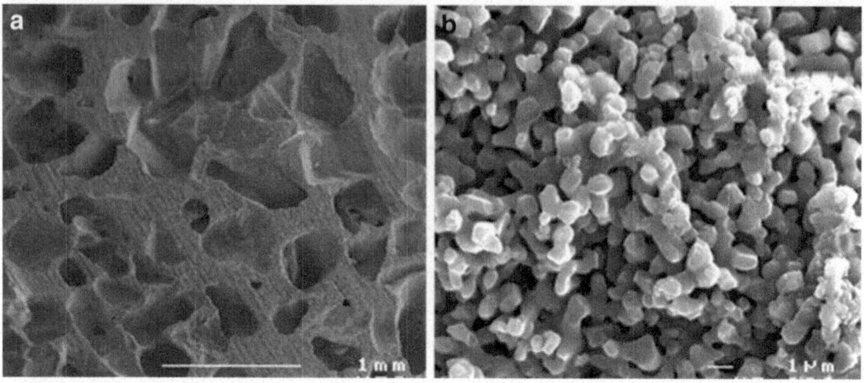

Fig. 4.2 (**a**) MBCP+, Micro- and Macroporous Biphasic Calcium Phosphate, macropores. (**b**) MBCP+, Micro- and Macroporous Biphasic Calcium Phosphate, micropores

area in contact with fluids and, thus, leads to a faster dissolution rate. As shown in Fig. 4.2, CaP ceramics exhibit macropores with diameter sizes ranging from 200 to 600 μm. While macropores are well interconnected, they permit the percolation of fluids, cells, and tissues within their structure. As illustrated in Fig. 4.2b, some ceramics may also exhibit a microporous surface. Spherical CaP grains appear bounded by necks leaving tiny pores approximately 0.1–1 μm in size. This remaining microporosity results from incomplete sintering of ceramics, especially when poorly crystalline precursor CaP powders and low sintering temperature and time (e.g., 1,000–1,200 °C for 1–10 h) are used. The lower temperature of sintering has a significant role in the formation in lattice defect. The lattice defect is particularly involved in the process of dissolution [32] explaining the large difference in the solubility of different HA scaffolds. According to the crystal size, lattice defect, and active cell resorption, the entire CaP can be resorbable. Only the kinetics differs according to time. A small-sized HA crystal with lattice defect is more resorbable than large, high crystalline TCP for example.

4.2.3.3 Absorption

The degradation and dissolution processes release high levels of calcium and phosphate ions into the extracellular fluid as the osteoclasts tunnel into the mineralized bone. Contrarily to degradation and elimination of some biomaterials, CaP ceramics elements released are absorbed during the physiopathological processes during bone regeneration. The released Ca and PO_4 ions are precipitated at the surface of the residual crystals, and secondary nucleation and hetero epitaxic growing processes have been reported [11, 13]. This process has also been observed in Bioglass by Larry Hench [33], and the basis of bioactivity has been well documented by Kokubo using simulated body fluid incubation [34].

4.2.4 Fundamental Biological Properties

4.2.4.1 Osteointegration and Osteocoalescence

All CaP ceramics have been found to be biocompatible. HA ceramics are considered as non-resorbable, while β-TCP is resorbable based on the amount of implant left as a function of time. It is now generally accepted that CaP ceramics are bioactive and osteoconductive. Bioactivity is a property of the ceramic surface that induces biological integration of soft and hard living tissues. The core mechanism of bioactivity is the partial dissolution and release of ionic products in vivo, elevating local concentrations of calcium and phosphate and precipitating a biological apatite on the surface of the ceramics. This process of dissolution/precipitation has been studied in detail using transmission electron microscopy (TEM) of ceramics implanted in ectopic or heterotopic sites. The BCP grains partly dissolve in body fluids leading to the precipitation of tiny apatite crystals on their surface or between the grains. TEM studies have shown that these apatite crystals were similar to bone apatite in size, shape, and electron diffraction patterns [11]. The abundance of the apatite microcrystals associated with large grains of ceramics appeared to be directly related to the HA to β-TCP ratio of BCP ceramic implants. A higher amount of β-TCP gave a greater amount of precipitated apatite crystals. These microcrystals were identified as carbonate-containing apatites that are associated with an organic matrix similar to bone.

This surface precipitation may incorporate various proteins and growth factors present in the microenvironment, which may subsequently promote cell attachment and function. The bioactive ceramics are assumed to have a surface phase biologically equivalent to bone mineral. It suggests that osteoblasts are attracted to this layer and produce bone extracellular matrix leading to bone apposition (osteoconduction), rather than fibrous tissue encapsulation of ceramics. This "bone bonding" has also been called osseocoalescence [35], a better definition to explain the chemical bonding between CaP bioceramics and bony crystals.

4.2.4.2 Osteoconduction

In 1991, Damien described osteoconduction as the ability of a substitute (graft or material) to promote development of vascular and osteoprogenitor cells from the recipient site [36]. In 1998, Davies described osteoconduction as the process by which the bone is directed into the material structure, pore channels, from the surface of materials by an invasion of differentiated oestogenic cells [37]. This specific integration of the surface of a substitute in direct contact with the bone, without the interposition of fibrous tissue, is called osteogenesis link [37]. In 1999, Cornell defined osteoconduction as the passive ability of a material to promote bone growth, and which supports continuity or cellular and vascular invasion [38].

In 2001, Albrektsson described osteoconduction as bone growth on a surface. An osteoconductive surface allows bone ingrowth into the pore channels and on its surface [39].

4.2.4.3 Osteogenicity and Osteoinduction

Osteoinductivity is the ability of a material to induce osteogenesis and is demonstrated by bone formation in non-osseous (heterotopic) sites. Osteoinductive factors have previously been associated only with bone morphogenetic proteins (BMPs) present in bone matrix. However, many studies have reported osteoinductive properties associated with biomaterials. Several factors that contribute to the osteoinductive property of a material include the animal model, implantation sites, and biomaterial properties [40–44]. Biomaterial properties include composition, surface roughness, and geometry (concavities, porosities). To improve the biological properties of biomaterials and bone substitute in order to optimize the healing of bone critical size defects, it is necessary to evaluate their ability to induce osteogenesis in ectopic sites and to have a complete physicochemical characterization. For example, the specific surface area of the bioceramics crystals is generally not evaluated or reported in the articles in relation with CaP scaffolds associated with MSCs, as reported by Gibson [8]. The lack of information, the controversial studies, and the semantic aspect of osteogenicity or osteoinduction hamper the correct evaluation of intrinsic osteoinductive properties of CaP bioceramics.

In 1889, Senn reported that the implantation of decalcified dog bone promoted healing of large-bone defects [45], but the work was difficult to reproduce [46]. In 1931, Huggins observed an ectopic ossification after implantation of soft tissue (bladder wall) in the superficial muscle of the abdomen (rectus abdominis) of adult dogs [47]. He found an osteoid tissue 16 days after implantation, but did not find a mineralized bone tissue. From day 18 to 26 post implantation, he observed a characteristic bone tissue (tissue and cell components), formed by intramembranous ossification. This type of structure is generally present in the bones of the skull, shoulder blades, and the ilium [48]. During the past 30 years, Levander found ossification in muscle tissue after injection of extract of pure alcohol [49, 50]. In 1958, Bridges observed formation of bone and cartilage in nonskeletal tissue (kidney capsule, subcutaneous) after implantation of devitalized tissue or tissue extracts (epiphyseal cartilage, bone fragments) [51]. Urist and McLean in 1952, training in ectopic anterior chamber of the eye, described ectopic bone formation [52]. Urist described induced bone formation in ectopic sites using decalcified bone matrix in several species [53].

In 1968, Friedenstein defined osteoinduction as the "induction of undifferentiated inducible osteoprogenitor cells that are not yet committed to the osteogenic lineage to form osteoprogenitor cells" [54]. In 1987, Wilson-Hench described osteoinduction as the process by which osteogenesis is induced [55]. In 2001, Albrektsson described the term "osteoinduction" by undifferentiated pluripotent primary cells that are stimulated in one way or another to grow in an osteoprogenitor lineage [39].

4.3 Smart Scaffolds

4.3.1 Scaffolds and Cells Combination

CaP in bone mineral is not a pure HA but a carbonate-substituted apatite with other minor constituents. Current commercial CaP-based biomaterials consist of HA, β-TCP, biphasic CaP, BCP (an intimate mixture of HA and β-TCP), and polymer/CaP composites. Physical forms include granules, blocks, scaffolds, cements, and coatings on orthopedic and dental implants. Numerous CaP scaffolds have received the CE mark, or FDA approval. Given that the physicochemical characteristics impact directly or indirectly on the bioactive properties of biomaterials, it is essential to correlate them with their effect in vivo. A panel of biomaterials available on the market (based on HA and β-TCP) have been studied in terms of surface area, hydrophilicity, porosity, zeta potential, crystalline phases, and density. We have performed total chemical and structural characterization of 12 commercial products (granules). The characterization was assessed by:

- Scanning electron microscopy (SEM) to characterize the surface morphology and check the homogeneity and the presence of both micropores and macropores
- Specific surface area (SSA) (by BET method) to evaluate the available surface for protein
- Mercury porosimetry to measure the porosity
- X-ray diffraction (XRD) in order to check the nature and the proportion of the crystalline phases as mentioned by the manufacturer
- Permeability qualitatively evaluated by methylene blue absorption

The results (Tables 4.2, 4.3, and 4.4) highlight the differences in the properties of commercial CaPs and demonstrate how the quality criteria required for such bone substitutes are based on biomimicry. Pores distribution may be a more relevant quality criterion and it is often not discussed in the literature, even at times concerning incorrect HA to TCP ratio. Only 4 products of the 12 tested are constituted with both essential macropores and micropores: MBCP, MBCP+, Calciresorb 35, and BCP Bicalphos. These chemical differences in micro- and macrostructure provided controversial results in terms of resorption/absorption, osteogenic/osteoinductive properties, and finally performance in bone regeneration [56].

Osteoinductivity in CaP biomaterials can be introduced in one of two ways:

- First, by designing the CaPs with appropriate geometry and topography (combined macroporosity, microporosity, and concavities) that will entrap and concentrate the circulating growth factors (e.g., BMPs)
- Second, by combining the CaP biomaterials with growth factors (BMPs, mesenchymal cells) and bioactive proteins (collagen, OPs, peptides based on osteonectin) or by seeding chondrocytes

Table 4.2 Differences in the properties of commercial CaPs

Products	Macropores	Micropores	SSA m^2/g
MBCP™	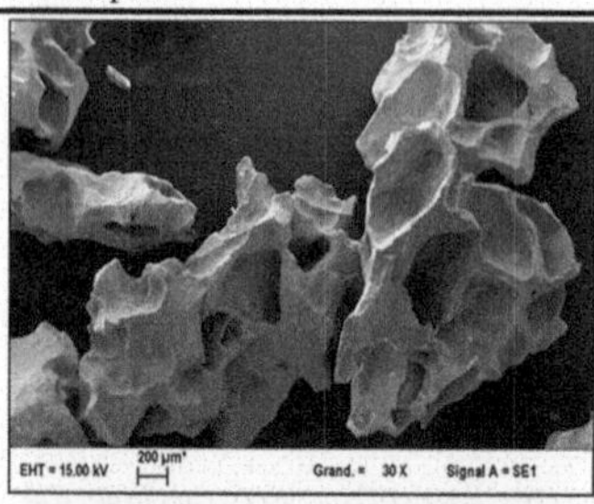	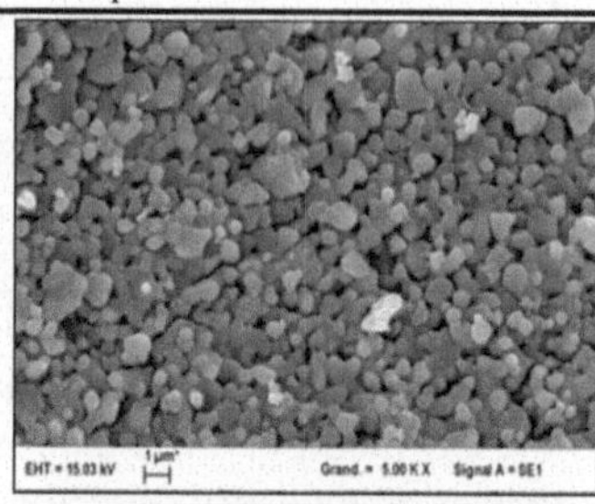	5
MBCP+™	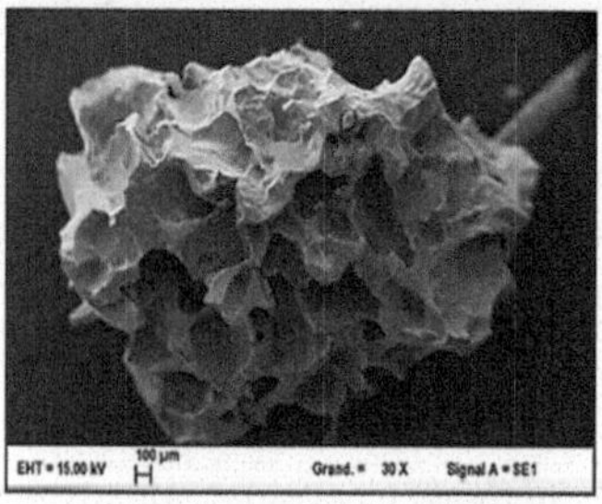	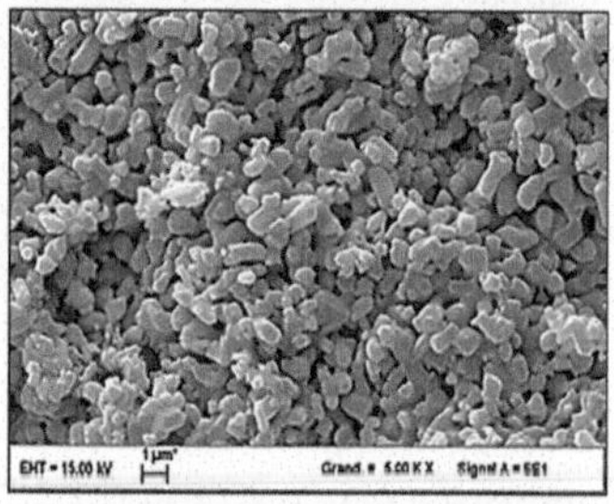	6
Sinbone HT	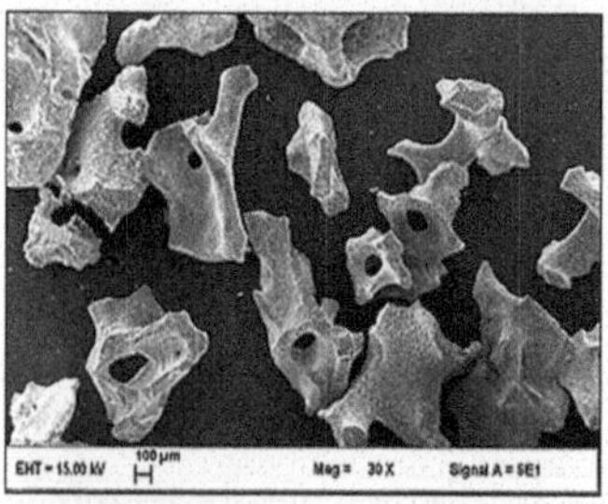	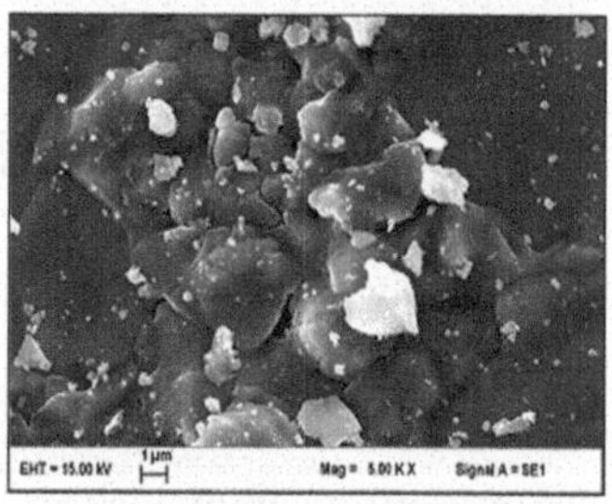	4
BCP Bicalphos	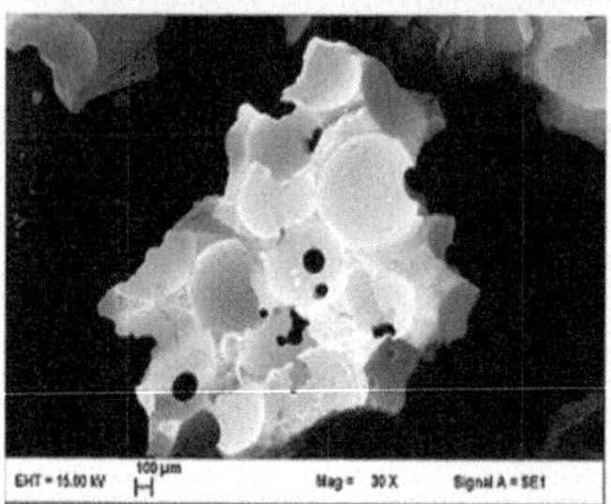	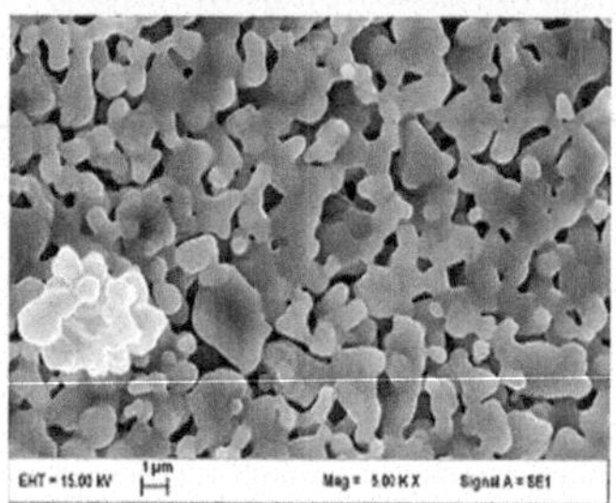	4

(continued)

Table 4.2 (continued)

Products	Macropores	Micropores	SSA m^2/g
Calciresorb 35	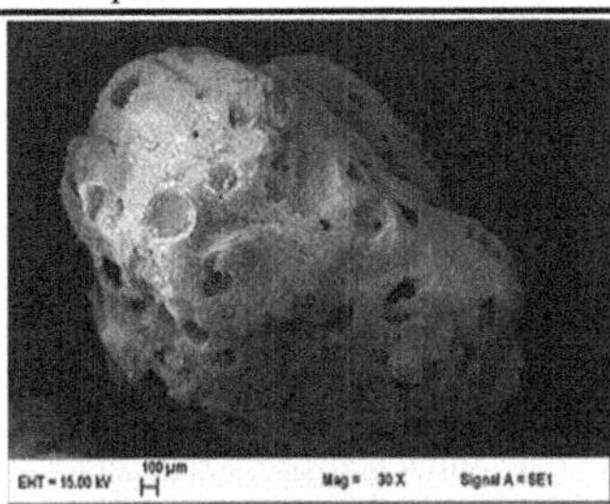	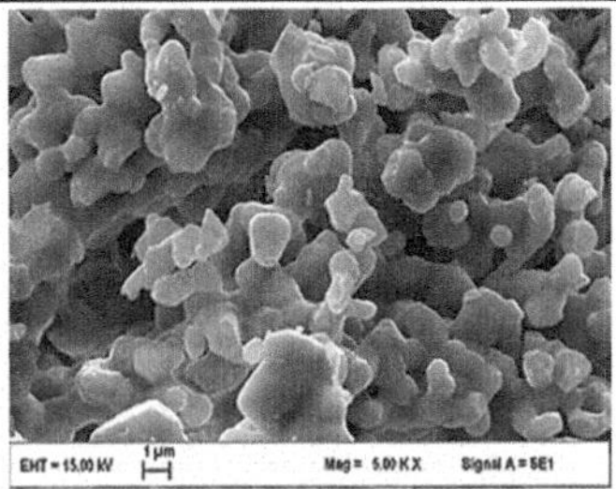	6
Granulado Keramedic	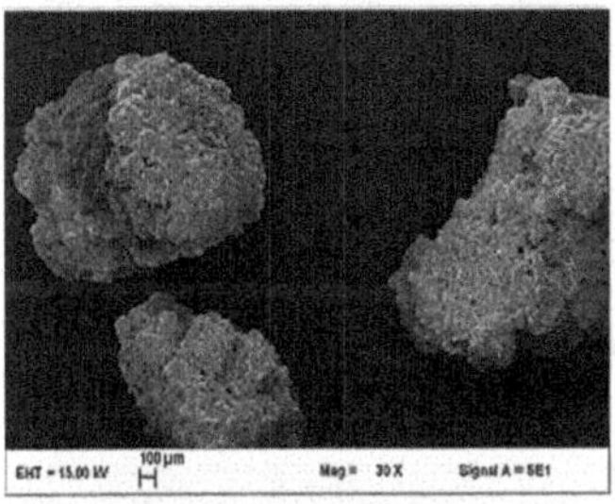	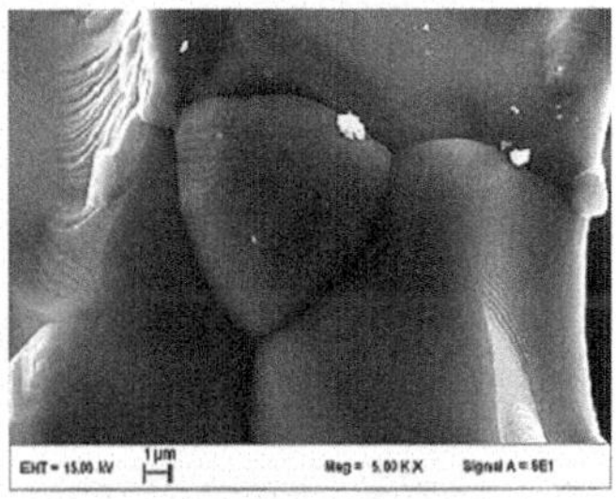	<1
Syncera	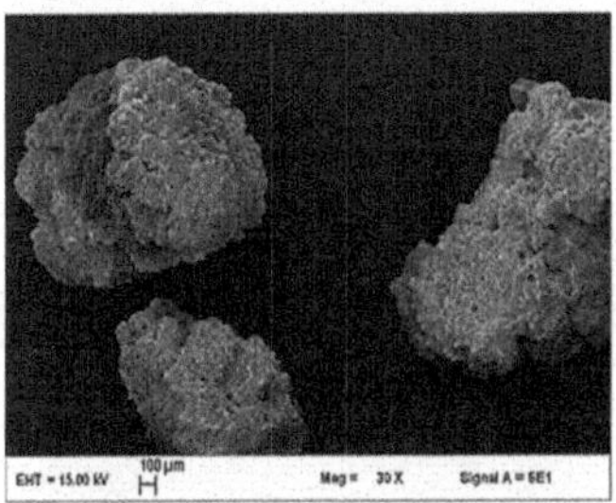	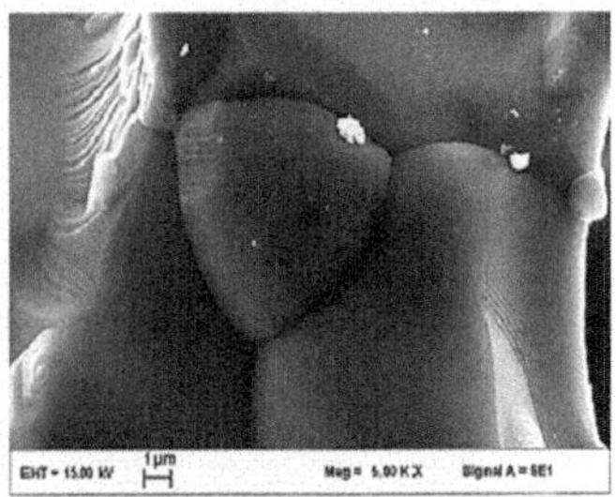	3
Bonit Matrix	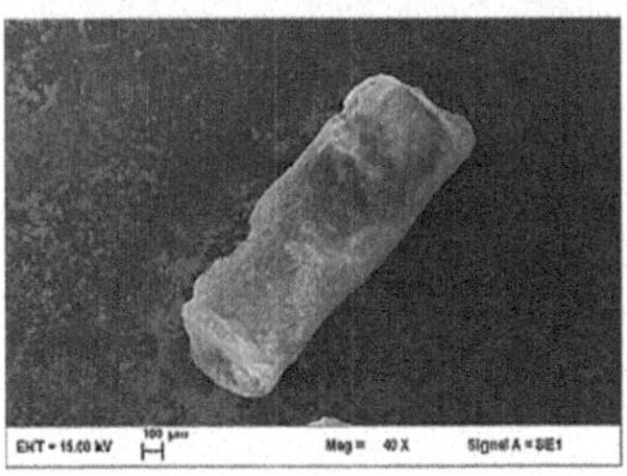	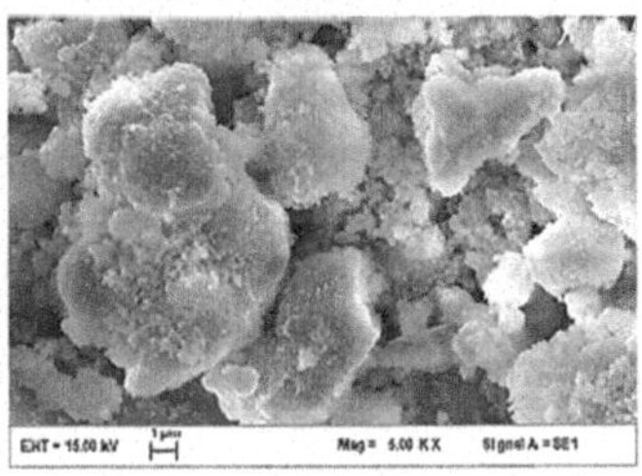	64

(continued)

Table 4.2 (continued)

Products	Macropores	Micropores	SSA m^2/g
Ceraform	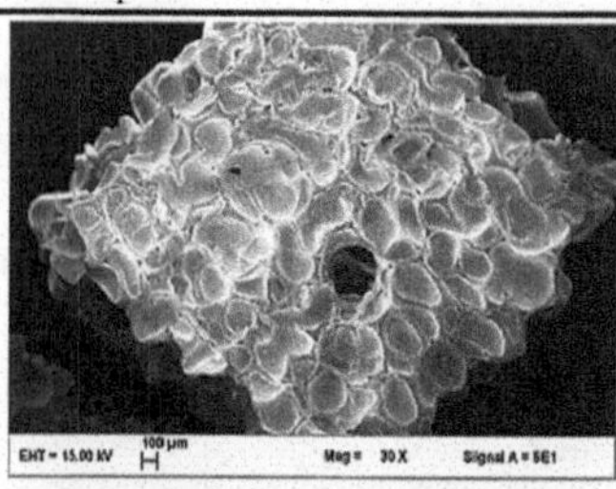	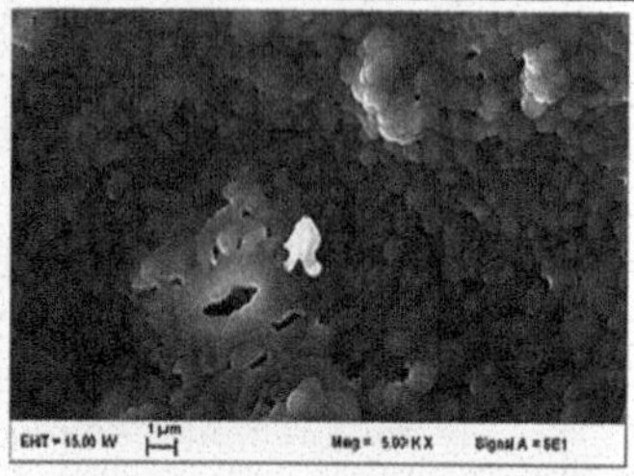	6
Interpore 200	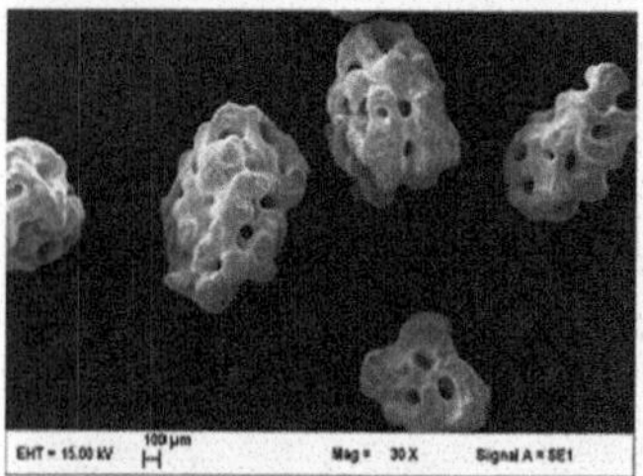	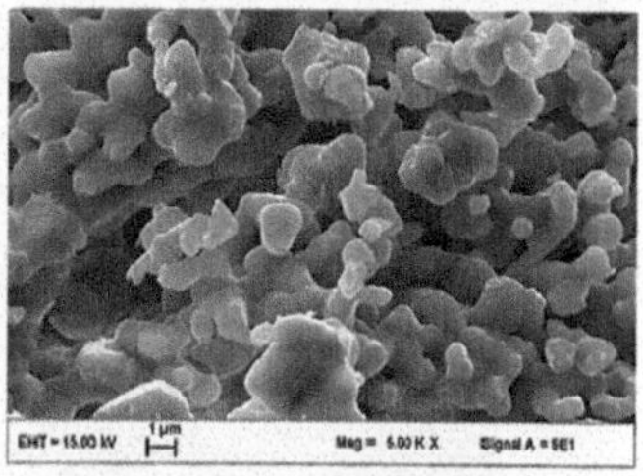	4
Bone Medik	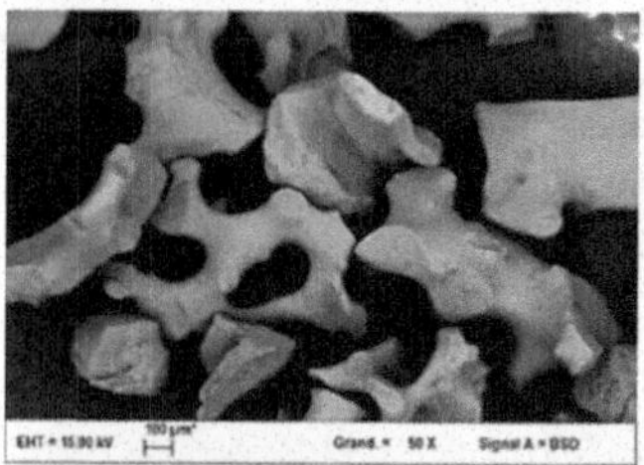	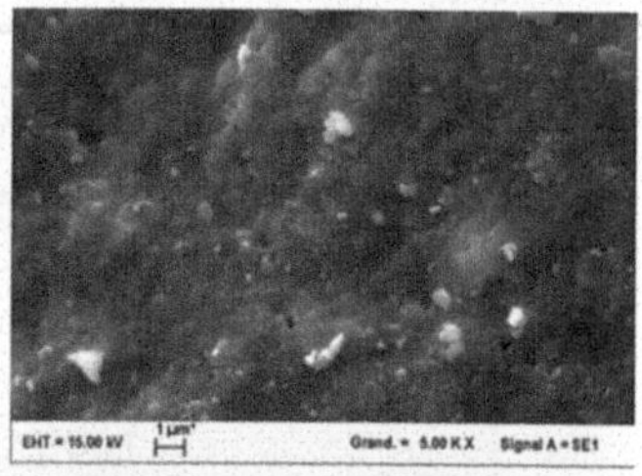	<1
Actifuse	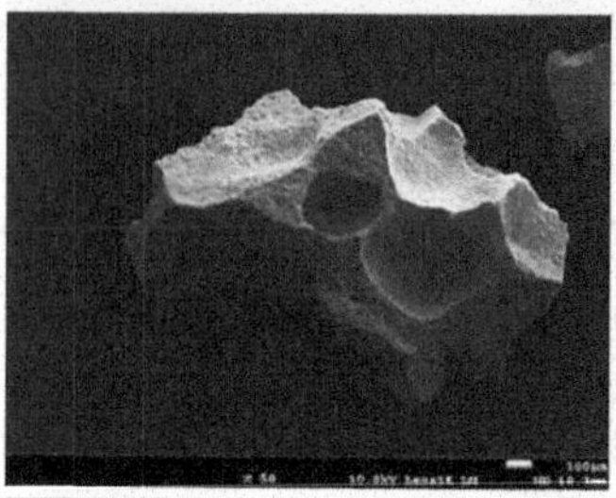	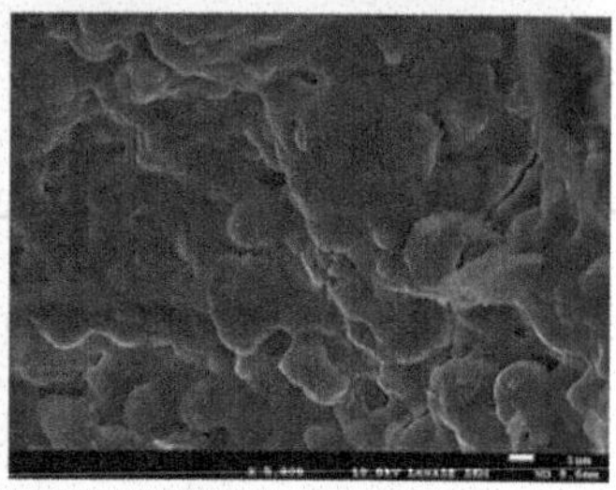	3

Table 4.3 Correlation between density and porosity measurements for some representative commercial scaffolds

	Bulk density g/cm^3	Total porosity
Actifuse	1.25	60.4
Ceraform	1.89	39.8
Interpore 200	1.05	66.7
MBCP	0.79	74.7
MBCP+	0.77	75.1

Table 4.4 Essential criteria for smart scaffolds in tissue engineering

	Permeability	Homogeneity	Micro-/macroporosity	SSA > 3
MBCP	Yes	Yes	Yes	Yes
MBCP+	Yes	Yes	Yes	Yes
Bonit Matrix	No	Partially	Partially	Yes
Syncera	Partially	No	Partially	No
Sinbone HT	Partially	Partially	No	Yes
Actifuse	No	No	Yes	No
Interpore 200	Yes	No	Partially	Yes
Bone Medik	Yes	No	Partially	No
Calciresorb 35	Yes	Yes	Yes	Yes
BCP Bicalphos	No	Yes	Yes	Yes
Granulado	Partially	No	Partially	No
Ceraform	Partially	Partially	Partially	Yes

The exact geometrical factors and the way to reproducibly obtain them are still unknown. The appropriate dosage of growth factors, mode of incorporation, and timed release remain to be determined.

The concept of introducing osteoinductive CaP biomaterials is an exciting one. Such materials will eventually replace the use of autografts and allografts with their attendant shortcomings. Numerous pieces of evidence indicate that the intrinsic MSC capacity to activate endogenous regenerative mechanisms and to recruit host cells in an ectopic bone formation model is critically dependent on MSC technology but also the physicochemical and structural properties of the scaffolds [57]. Nonetheless, for the success of the MSC transplant, the nature and the structure of scaffolds onto which cells are seeded are very critical. In addition to being a three-dimensional carrier for the cells, and a matrix with the correct shape for new tissue to form within, scaffolds are crucial in determining the optimal microenvironment for the cells to fully express their regenerative potential. A large collaborative project of the seventh framework program (topic HEALTH-2009-1.4.2 on Regenerative Bone defects using New biomedical Engineering approaches, REBORNE) [58] explores these scientific and clinical fields. The main objective is to develop smart scaffolds that stimulate bone tissue formation in combination with adult stem cells for regenerating bone defects in orthopedic and maxillofacial surgery.

We have optimized the new scaffolds based on a micro-/macroporous concept of MBCP, with a microstructure highly suitable for tissue engineering techniques and showing improved osteogenic properties. In different animal models, a mixture of MBCP granules and total bone marrow appeared to be the most efficient, amongst all the materials tested for bone substitution in difficult circumstances like irradiated areas and radionecrosis [59, 60].

The development of CaP ceramics for use in bone grafts involves a better control of the process of biomaterials resorption and bone substitution. Bone graft biomaterials are largely represented by CaP HA, TCP, and biphasic CaP, MBCP. The concept based on biphasic CaP ceramics is achieved by an optimum balance of the more stable phase of HA and more soluble TCP. The material is soluble and gradually dissolves in the body, leading to the formation of new bone as it releases calcium and phosphate ions into the biological medium [5]. These bioceramics are largely used for bone reconstruction and will be optimized for combination marrow during surgery or for bone tissue engineering using stem cells. We have optimized matrices in terms of their physicochemical and crystal properties, in order to improve cell colonization and to increase the kinetics of bone ingrowth. The fast cell colonization and resorption of the material are associated with the interconnected macropore structure, which enhances the bone resorption substitution process. The micropore content involves diffusion of biological fluids and suitable absorption surfaces for circulating growth factors. A difference of only 10 % of the amount of micropores into the CaP bioceramics improves the permeability and adsorption of proteins of more than 40 %.

Our work developing smart scaffolds for tissue engineering [12, 41] was based on the concept of MBCP technology. Interconnected Micro- and Macroporous Biphasic CaP ceramic (MBCP+, CE mark, and FDA 510k, Biomatlante SA France) was an improvement in the microporous and macroporous CaP bioceramic developed 20 years ago [5]. Briefly, CDA was associated to a mixture of selected particles of porogen. After isostatic compaction, the block was sintered according to a specific process of sublimation/calcination at low temperature. The low sintering temperature has the advantage of preserving the high micropore content and smaller crystal size, in addition to a higher sintering temperature. The bioceramics were then characterized using X-rays, FTIR, X-ray microtomography, permeability, Hg porosimetry, BET specific surface area, mechanical testing, and SEM. The crystal structure at the nanoscale was observed and analyzed using high-resolution transmission electron microscopy (hrTEM) and electronic diffraction (ED). The granules of MBCP+ have been tested in several preclinical studies in goats, rabbits, and rats, with or without cell addition (total bone marrow, MSCs), in critical size defects of femoral epiphysis and non-bony sites to test osteogenicity/osteoinductive properties.

X-ray diffraction identified the HA and β-TCP content despite the molecular mixture in the single crystal (MBCP technology used the mechanical combination HA and TCP crystals separately). The HA to TCP ratio was 20:80 (Fig. 4.3a, b). No trace of other sources of CaP or foreign species could be observed by FTIR. Using hrTEM of a single crystal of HA/TCP, we were unable to observe separate crystals of HA or TCP. The single crystal observed was a molecular mixture (nano-crystallographic domains) consisting of the biphasic compound (Fig. 4.4). Convergent Beam Electron Diffraction had insufficient resolution to characterize the precise HA or β-TCP domains, but the two crystallographic parts were intimately associated into single crystals.

The combination of chemistry and microstructure has also been studied by Yuan [44]. The study confirmed the essential role of the microstructure, that the smaller crystals displayed high microporosity, and that there was greater bone formation when combined with MSCs. The data were obtained with TCP and BCP; the best results related to the higher content of TCP. In this study, the pure TCP contained 5–10 % HA, corresponding to a BCP with a low HA ratio.

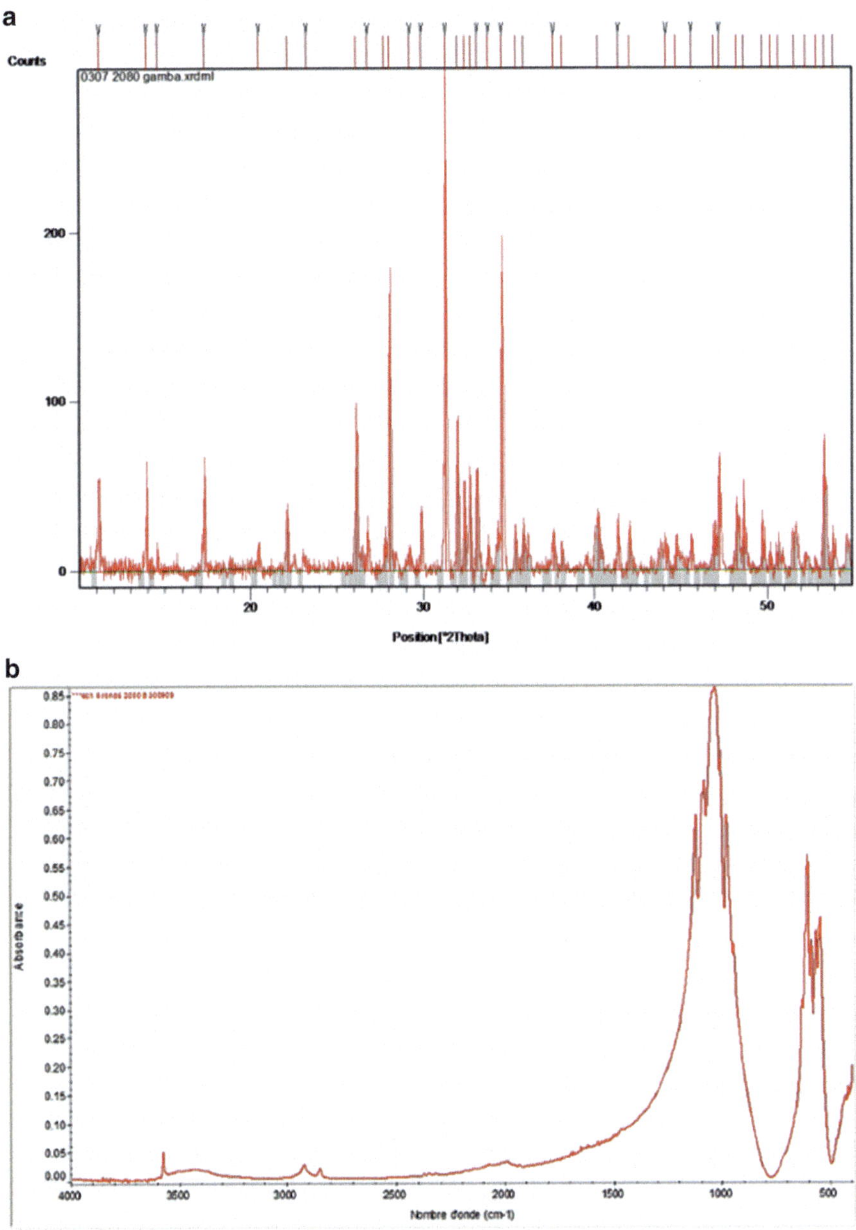

Fig. 4.3 MBCP+, Micro- and Macroporous Biphasic Calcium Phosphate. (**a**) *XRD*, (**b**) *FTIR*. FTIR confirms high purity of HA and TCP without any carbonate

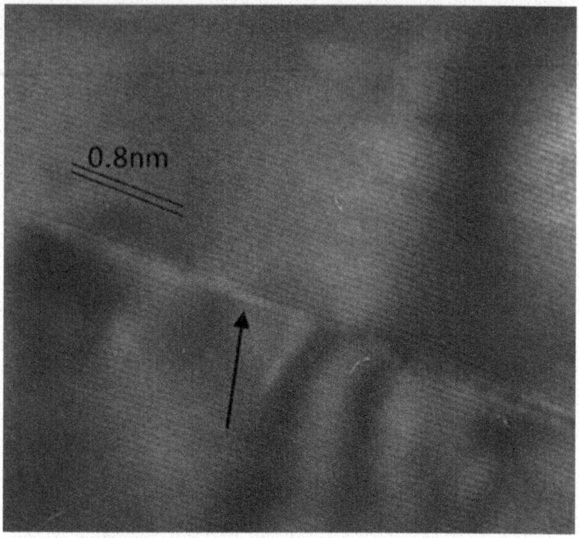

Fig. 4.4 hrTEM showing lattice place plane of HA/TCP. Numerous grain boundaries are observed between BCP crystals (*arrow*)

The smart scaffold we developed for tissue engineering (MBCP+ ™) has the following characteristics: the crystal size is 0.5 μm and the SSA (specific surface area) 6 m^2/g for MBCP+. The SSA difference in bioceramics (sintered CaP) (Table 4.2) showed a large range, from less 1 to 6 m^2/g. This involved high difference in the adsorption capacity of non-collagenic proteins, growth factors, adhesion molecules, etc. For example, with SSA of 6 m^2/g, the adsorption capacity was six times higher than SSA of 1 m^2/g, or >1,000 % comparing to SSA <0.5 m^2/g.

The compression test result is 4 MPa. The porosity consists of 19.6 ± 2.4 % macropores (>100 μm), 39.8 ± 3.1 % mesopores (5–100 μm), and 40.6 ± 3.2 % micropores <5 μm, for a total porosity of 73 %.

Numerous concavities on the granules increased the developed surface for cell colonization and seem to support higher osteogenic cell differentiation and spreading. The larger amount of newly formed bone appearing in the concavities was demonstrated by human alveolar pocket filling after 4 months of implantation (Fig. 4.5).

The advantage of a smart scaffold includes faster bone ingrowth into the macropores and the concavities, as observed in short-term implantation of MBCP+, relative to classical MBCP. However, after 12 weeks of implant in rabbit preclinical models, no statistical difference was observed between the two implant types. The rate of resorption was higher for MBCP+, 17 % versus 12 % at 6 weeks and 19 % versus 17 % after 12 weeks (no significant difference). These properties can be advantageous for tissue engineering scaffold technologies.

This higher permeability and absorption ability were mainly due to the distribution of pore size, particularly mesopores, with the high micropore content representing around 40 % of the total porosity. After implantation, bone ingrowth

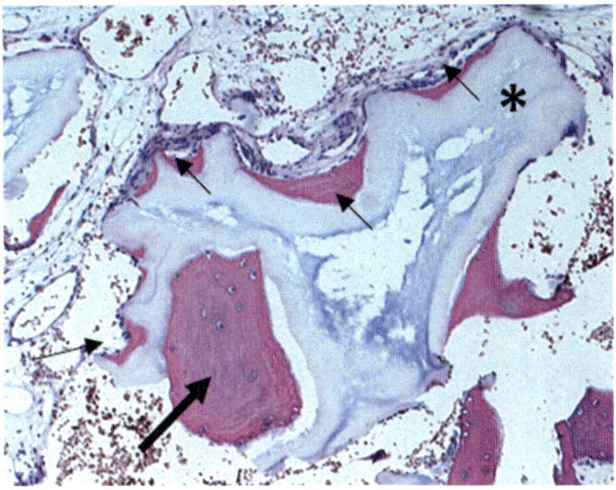

Fig. 4.5 Light microscopy, sinus lift after 4 months of implantation showing newly formed bone (*large arrow, pink*) formed at the expense of the MBCP+ granules (*) particularly into the concavity of them (*light arrow*)

was observed at the expense of the bioceramic, and newly formed bone progressively replaced the bioactive material, followed by Haversian bone remodeling [5]. In vitro 3D MSCs/BCP constructs were formed after a few days of culturing the BCP particles and MSCs. In the proliferative medium, we measured higher BSP and BMP-2 expression than the cells on TCP plates alone, demonstrating the importance of the 3D scaffold for osteogenic expression [39].

The in vivo experiments indicated that the high cell colonization by osteogenic cells is due to the interconnected and microporous structure associated with higher solubility and 3D environment [61]. Moreover, a previous study comparing the equivalent macro- and microstructures of different calcium phosphate bioceramics (HA, TCP, or BCP 60/40 and BCP 20/80) showed that the best scaffold for tissue engineering was a 20:80, thanks to the combination of stem cells cultivation and expansion, followed by implantation in a non-bony site [62]. Osteogenic or osteoinductive properties of CaP ceramics with an optimal micro- and macroporosity have also been demonstrated without cell combination, after implantation in a non-bony site (muscular area) [40, 41, 43]. Ripamonti has also postulated that the geometry of the material (concavity) is a critical parameter in bone induction [42, 63]. The events and the origin of these important osteoinductive properties are the dissolution of the most soluble phase and the release of calcium and phosphate ions, followed by the precipitation of biological apatite leading to concentration of local growth factors [41]. The osteoprogenitor cells may in turn recognize the bone-like apatite layer formed in vivo by dissolution-reprecipitation on the material, leading to production of mineralized bone.

The kinetics of bone ingrowth by osteogenic cell differentiation needs to develop inside the macropores. Without macropores and mesopores, these processes are unable to occur within the implants. The association of dissolution at the crystal level, the diffusion of the biological fluid into the micropores, and the resorption by macrophages and osteoclastic cells of the materials at the surface and inside the macropores involve a progressive bone substitution of the materials by physiological well-vascularized bone. This is the common process of resorption-absorption/bone substitution of the Micro- and Macroporous Biphasic Calcium Phosphate ceramics. The intimate mixture of the process developed for smart scaffold MBCP+ gave a unique and original property, contrarily to some others BCP described in the literature using a mechanical mixture of HA on one side and β-TCP on the other [6].

4.3.2 *Scaffold for Drug Delivery*

CaP bioceramics have frequently been proposed for the adsorption of bioactive factors and for drug delivery systems. A recent study by Smucker et al. [64] was the first to demonstrate enhanced posterolateral spinal fusion rates in rabbits, using a synthetic peptide (B2A2-K-NS) coated on to microporous granules of BCP, with a 60:40 HA to TCP ratio. Different concentrations of the peptide (a synthetic receptor-targeted peptide that appears to amplify the biological response to *rh*BMP-2) were tested. This study provided more evidence of mature/immature bone ingrowth across the inter-transverse process spaces than the controls did. Microporous and macroporous biphasic CaP granule bioceramics for peptide adsorption and local delivery seem to be a good compromise for future associations of osteoconductive/osteogenic properties for such bioceramics and for the osteoinductive properties of peptides and growth factors.

Antibiotics may also be candidates to be delivered by this technology. It is common practice for surgeons to mix antibiotics with bone grafts when treating infected bone defects or for preventing infection after surgery [65]. Local delivery of antibiotics is both pharmacologically more effective and safer. If properly formulated, bioactive cements have been shown to be an ideal carrier for local delivery of antibiotics [66, 67]. New CPC has been specifically engineered to have microporosity, macroporosity, and resorbability for optimal cell adhesion, cell migration, and bone formation. Recently, the MCPC® reported in this paper was associated with delivery of gentamicin [68].

The gentamicin release profiles from the cement samples with different setting times were quite similar. Both cement groups showed an initial burst of gentamicin release in the first 24 h. After the initial burst, the release rate slowed significantly and stayed relatively constant between day 7 and day 28 (the endpoint). The amount and rate of the initial burst release were affected by the cement setting time. The release of gentamicin from the cement allowed to set for 1 h showed greater variation than the cement allowed to set for 24 h. Within the first 24 h, approximately 72 % of the gentamicin was released from the cement with 1 h, compared to the slower release of the gentamicin from the cement with a 24-h set time (approximately 51 %). By 28 days, around 87 and 76 % of the gentamicin had been released from the cements that had set for either 1 h or 24 h, respectively. The gentamicin release rates from both the 1-h and 24-h set-time samples were almost constant after day 7, averaging 59 μg/day for the cement with a 1-h set time and

87 μg/day for the 24-h set time. Therefore, in our release system, these constructs are capable of releasing gentamicin concentrations of 12 and 17 μg/ml on a daily basis for the 1-h and 24-h set-time cement samples, respectively. This is more than one order of magnitude greater than the minimum inhibitory concentration (MIC) for reference strains of *S. aureus*, which is in the range of 0.12–0.25 μg/ml [69].

It was interesting to note that the cement without gentamicin showed a decrease in ultimate compressive strength during setting, from 24 to 48 h in phosphate-buffered saline at 37 °C. The ultimate compressive strength dropped from 5.5 to 3.87 MPa indicating that the cement had dissolved. When the gentamicin was present, the cement showed an increase in both the strength and modulus, when the set time was extended from 24 to 48 h. It appeared that the addition of gentamicin might have delayed the dissolution of the cement, while allowing it to continue to set and thus further increase its mechanical strength.

Due to its unique preparation method and bioresorbability, the bioactive cement employed in this study may be effective as both a bone graft substitute and a carrier for the local delivery of antibiotics to prevent or treat infections. Ideal bioactive cement will initially release a clinically effective amount of antibiotics, maintain a steady release of a safe dose over an extended period, and retain no residual amount of antibiotics at the end of the desired treatment time. As demonstrated in this study, the MCPC™ bioactive cement released over 50 % of the loaded gentamicin per cylinder, that is, 7.5 mg in the first 24 h. A steady release of a therapeutically significant amount of 60–90 μg of gentamicin per day was maintained up to 28 days. As the MCPC™ is engineered to bioresorb and quickly develops a macroporous structure, the remaining amount of 2–4 mg of gentamicin per set-time sample is expected to discharge completely as the bioactive cement resorbs. The MCPC™ resorbable bone substitute has demonstrated its potential to be used as a carrier for the local delivery of gentamicin. Future studies will expand the investigation to evaluate the release profile and mechanical properties of this bioactive cement when loaded with other antibiotics, such as tobramycin and vancomycin.

4.4 Conclusions and Future Prospects for Calcium Phosphate Materials as Bone Substitutes

Advanced technologies for developing smart osteogenic scaffold bioceramics for tissue engineering involve focusing on improving the efficacy of such matrices for further relevant surgical technologies, such as the combination with bone marrow for surgery or expanded stem cell in vitro for bone tissue engineering.

It has recently been shown that some porous CaP bioceramics induce ectopic bone formation after implantation into the muscles of large animals. These biomaterials have demonstrated the ability to induce bone formation after 6–12 weeks in muscular sites, without the addition of osteogenic cells or bone growth factors prior to implantation. Ectopic bone formation with Haversian structures was observed in close contact with the MBCP granules. Well-mineralized bone with mature osteocytes had formed on or between the granules. The ectopic bone showed trabeculae bridging the granules, restoring the bone architecture.

Although many groups have described induction of ectopic bone by biomaterials, it remains a subject of controversy because the mechanisms are poorly understood. In vivo studies have shown that materials should exhibit two features in order to induce ectopic bone: (1) a microporous surface and (2) a macroporous structure. Osteoinduction does not seem to be related to the chemistry of the material, as various types of bioceramic compositions have demonstrated ectopic bone formation. Osteoinduction by biomaterials also seems to be animal dependent and has so far only been observed in the muscles of large animals such as dogs, baboons, sheep, and goats. Several explanations have been proposed. First, CaP ceramics may concentrate bone growth factors from body fluids, which then trigger stem cells to form bone tissue. Second, the geometry of the material is a critical parameter in bone induction, and third, osteoprogenitor cells might in turn recognize the bone-like apatite layer formed in vivo by dissolution-reprecipitation on the material and produce mineralized bone. Other studies have proposed that low oxygen tension in the central region of the implants might provoke a dedifferentiation of pericytes from blood microvessels into osteoblasts. Microparticles released from low sintered ceramics might provoke a specific inflammatory reaction leading to osteogenesis, or the circulating progenitor cells might differentiate into osteoblasts following stimulation by the inflammatory cytokines released by macrophages. The process might be similar to the healing of bone fractures, where debris and fragments of bone are present. Nevertheless, the cascade of biological events leading to material osteogenesis remains unclear.

In the future, this intriguing property will benefit synthetic bone substitutes. Advanced CaP bioceramics with superior bone healing properties might replace biological bone grafting from materials such as autologous or demineralized bone. Much of the interest in the development and modification of the smart CaP bioceramics is based on improving the osteoconduction or the initial mechanical properties of bone substitutes. There is evidence to suggest that small-sized particles that are released into the microenvironment after implantation and degradation are then recognized as debris and promote an inflammatory reaction that recruits phagocytic macrophages and induces potential bone breakdown, a phenomena that can boost osteogenic cell differentiation [31]. Ongoing work is required to explore the modulation of inflammation, the optimization of the initial mechanical property for easy-to-use bioceramics, and expression of mechanotransduction, in order to develop more clinically relevant applications for synthetic bone graft.

If the smart bioinstructive CaP scaffold technology led to a higher efficacy of CaP scaffolds, it would allow further surgical applications in bone tissue regeneration. The mechanical properties required for bone ingrowth and bone remodeling and mechanotransduction must be explored to allow for development of new generation scaffolds [70].

Acknowledgments We would like to thank the 7th framework program HEALTH-2009-1.4.2 of the European Commission on Regenerative Bone defects using New biomedical Engineering approaches (REBORNE project).

References

1. Dorozhkin S (2013) A detailed history of calcium orthophosphates from 1770s till 1950. Mater Sci Eng C33:3085–3110
2. Albee FH, Morrison HF (1920) Studies in bone growth. Triple calcium phosphate as a stimulus to osteogenesis. Ann Surg 71:32–39
3. De Groot K (1983) Bioceramics of calcium phosphate. CRC Press Inc., Boca Raton
4. Legeros R, Guy D, John L (2009) Bioactive bioceramics, orthopaedic biology and medicine. In: Pietrzak WS (ed) Musculoskeletal regeneration, biological materials and methods. Humana Press, Totowa, pp 153–181
5. Guy D, Franck J, Pierre L (2009) The micro macroporous biphasic calcium phosphate concept for bone reconstruction and tissue engineering. In: Bikramjit B, Dhirendra SK, Ashok K (eds) Advanced biomaterials: fundamentals, processing, and applications. Wiley, Hoboken, pp 101–141
6. Dorozhkin S (2012) Calcium orthophosphates: applications in nature, biology, and medicine. Pan Stanford Publishing Pte Ltd., Singapore, pp 1–853
7. LeGeros RZ (1991) Calcium phosphates in oral biology and medicine, vol 15, Monographs in oral science. Karger, Basel
8. Gibson IR (2012) Calcium phosphate as scaffolds for mesenchymal stem cell. In: Ramalingam M, Ramakrishna S, Best S (eds) Biomaterials and stem cells in regenerative medicine. CRC Press, Boca Raton, pp 219–237
9. Bohner M (2000) Calcium orthophosphates in medicine: from ceramics to calcium phosphate cements. Injury 31:37–47
10. Hench LL, Thompson I (2010) Twenty first century challenges for biomaterials. J R Soc Interface 7(4):S379–S391
11. Daculsi G, Laboux O, Malard O, Weiss P (2003) Current state of the art of biphasic calcium phosphate bioceramics. J Mater Sci Mater Med 14(3):195–200
12. Daculsi G, LeGeros R, Nery E, Lynch K, Kerebel B (1989) Transformation of biphasic calcium phosphate ceramics in vivo. Ultrastructural and physicochemical characterization. J Biomed Mater Res 23:883–894
13. Daculsi G, LeGeros RZ, Heughebaert M, Barbieux I (1990) Formation of carbonate apatite crystals after implantation of calcium phosphate ceramics. Calcif Tissue Int 46:20–27
14. Daculsi G, Weiss P, Bouler JM, Gauthier O, Aguado E (1999) Biphasic calcium phosphate hydrosoluble polymer composites: a new concept for bone and dental substitution biomaterials. Bone 25:59–61
15. LeGeros RZ, Chohayeb A, Shulman A (1982) Apatitic calcium phosphates: possible restorative materials. J Dent Res 61:343
16. Brown WE, Chow LC (1987) A new calcium phosphate water-setting cement. In: Brown PW (ed) Cement research progress. American Ceramic Society, Westerville, pp 352–379
17. Niwa S, LeGeros RZ (2002) Injectable calcium phosphate cements for repair of bone defects. In: Lewandrowski K-U, Wise DL, Trantolo DJ, Gresser JD (eds) Tissue engineering and biodegradable equivalents. Scientific and clinical applications. Marcel Dekker, New York, pp 385–400
18. Daculsi G (2006) Biphasic calcium phosphate Granules concept for Injectable and Mouldable Bone Substitute. In: Vincenzini P, Giardino R (eds) Advances in science and technology, vol 49. Trans Tech Publications, Faenza, Italy, pp 9–13

19. Weiss P, Layrolle P, Clergeau LP, Enckel B, Pilet P, Amouriq Y, Daculsi G, Giumelli B (2007) The safety and efficacy of an injectable bone substitute in dental sockets demonstrated in a human clinical trial. Biomaterials 28:3295–3305
20. Daculsi G, Durand M, Fabre T, Vogt F, Uzel AP, Rouvillain JL (2012) Development and clinical cases of injectable bone void filler used in orthopaedic (Développement et cas cliniques d'un substitut osseux injectable en orthopédie). IRBM 33:253–261
21. Lapkowski M, Weiss P, Daculsi G, Dupraz A (1997) Composition pour biomatériau, procédé de préparation II Date de dépôt. CNRS Patent WO 97/059
22. Fellah BH, Weiss P, Gauthier O, Rouillon T, Pilet P, Daculsi G, Layrolle P (2006) Bone repair using a new injectable self-crosslinkable bone substitute. J Orthop Res 24(4):628–635
23. Fatimi A, Tassin JF, Quillard S, Axelo MAV, Weiss P (2008) The rheological properties of silated hydroxypropylmethylcellulose tissue engineering matrices. Biomaterials 29:533–543
24. Turczyn R, Weiss P, Lapkowski M, Daculsi G (2000) In situ self hardening bioactive composite for bone and dental surgery. J Biomater Sci Polym Ed 11(2):217–223
25. Le Guehennec L, Layrolle P, Daculsi G (2004) A review of bioceramics and fibrin sealant. Eur Cell Mater 13(8):1–11
26. Le Nihouannen D, Saffarzadeh A, Aguado E, Goyenvalle E, Gauthier O, Moreau F, Pilet P, Spaethe R, Daculsi G, Layrolle P (2007) Osteogenic properties of calcium phosphate ceramics and fibrin glue based composites. J Mater Sci Mater Med 18(2):225–235
27. Khairoun I, LeGeros RZ, Daculsi G, Bouler JM, Guicheux J, Gauthier O (2004) Macroporous, resorbable and injectable calcium phosphate-based cements (MCPC) for bone repair, augmentation, regeneration and osteoporosis treatment. Provisional patent 11/054 623
28. Daculsi G, Durand M, Hauger O, Seris E, Borget P, LeGeros R, LeHuec JC (2012) Self hardening macroporous biphasic calcium phosphate bone void filler for bone reconstruction. Animal study and human data. Key Eng Mater 493–494:703–713
29. Goyenvalle E, Aguado E, Legeros R, Daculsi G (2007) Effect of sintering process on microporosity, and bone growth on biphasic calcium phosphate ceramics. Key Eng Mater 333–334 (in press). Trans Tech Publication, Switzerland
30. Fellah BH, Delorme B, Sohier J, Magne D, Hardouin P, Layrolle P (2010) Macrophage and osteoblast responses to biphasic calcium phosphate microparticles. J Biomed Mater Res A 93(4):1588–1595
31. Basle MF, Chappard D, Grizon F, Filmon R, Delecrin J, Daculsi G, Rebel A (1993) Osteoclastic resorption of CaP biomaterials implanted in rabbit bone. Calcif Tissue Int 53:348–356
32. Daculsi G, Legeros RZ, Legeros J, Mitre D (1991) Lattice defects in calcium phosphate ceramics: high resolution TEM ultrastructural study. J Biomed Mater Res Appl Biomater 2:147–152
33. Hench LL (1994) Bioceramics: from concept to clinic. J Am Ceram Soc 74:1487–1510
34. Kokubo T, Takadama H (2006) How useful is SBF in predicting in vivo bone bioactivity? Biomaterials 27(15):2907–2915
35. Daculsi G, Passuti N (1990) Bioactive ceramics, fundamental properties and clinical applications the osteocoalescence process. In: Oonishi H, Heimcke G (eds) Ceramics in medicine, pp 3–10
36. Damien CJ, Parsons JR (1991) Bone graft and bone graft substitutes: a review of current technology and applications. J Appl Biomater 2(3):187–208
37. Davies JE (1998) Mechanisms of endosseous integration. Int J Prosthodont 11(5):391–401
38. Cornell CN (1999) Osteoconductive materials and their role as substitutes for autogenous bone grafts. Orthop Clin N Am 30:591–598
39. Albrektsson T, Johansson C (2001) Osteoinduction, osteoconduction and osseointegration. Eur Spine J 10(Suppl 2):S96–S101
40. Barradas Ana MC, Yuan H, van Blitterswijk CA, Habibovic P (2011) Osteoinductive biomaterials: current knowledge of properties, experimental models and biological mechanisms. Eur Cell Mater 21:407–429

41. Le Nihouannen D, Daculsi G, Saffarzadeh A, Gauthier O, Delplace S, Pilet P et al (2005) Ectopic bone formation by microporous calcium phosphate ceramic particles in sheep muscles. Bone 36(6):1086–1093
42. Ripamonti U, Crooks J, Kirbride A (1999) Sintered porous hydroxyapatites with intrinsic osteoinductive activity: geometric induction of bone formation. S Afr J Sci 95:335–343
43. Yuan H, Yang Z, De Bruijn JD, De Groot K, Zhang X (2001) Material-dependent bone induction by calcium phosphate ceramics: a 2.5-year study in dog. Biomaterials 22:2617–2623
44. Yuan H, Fernandes H, Habibovick P, de Boer J, Barrads AMC, de Ruiter A, Walsh WR, van Blitterswijk CA, de Bruijn JD (2010) Osteoinductive ceramics as a synthetic alternative to autologous bone grafting. Proc Natl Acad Sci 107:13614–13619
45. Senn NS (1889) On the healing of aseptic bone cavities by implantation of antiseptic decalcified bone. Am J Med Sci 98(3):219–243
46. Rengachary SS (2002) Bone morphogenetic proteins: basic concepts. Neurosurg Focus 13(6):e2
47. Huggins CB (1931) The phosphatase activity of transplants of the epithelium of the urinary bladder to the abdominal wall producing heterotopic ossification. Biochem J 25(3):728–732
48. Bronner ME, LeDouarin NM (2012) Development and evolution of the neural crest: an overview. Dev Biol 366(1):2–9
49. Levander G (1934) On the formation of new bone in bone transplantation. Acta Chir Scand 74:425–426
50. Levander G (1938) A study of bone regeneration. Surg Gynecol Obstet 67:705–714
51. Bridges JB, Pritchard JJ (1958) Bone and cartilage induction in the rabbit. J Anat 92(1):28–38
52. Urist MR, McLEAN FC (1952) Osteogenetic potency and new-bone formation by induction in transplants to the anterior chamber of the eye. J Bone Joint Surg Am 34-A(2):443–476
53. Urist MR (1965) Bone formation by autoinduction. J Sci 150(3698):893–899
54. Friedenstein AY (1968) Induction of bone tissue by transitional epithelium. Clin Orthop 59:21–37
55. Wilson-Hench J (1987) Osteoinduction. In: Williams D (ed) Progress in biomedical engineering. Elsevier, Amsterdam, p 29
56. Daculsi G, Fellah BH, Miramond T, Durand M (2013) Osteoconduction, Osteogenicity, Osteoinduction, what are the fundamental properties for a smart bone substitutes. IRBM 34(4):346–348
57. Ramalingam M, Ramakrishna S, Best S (eds) (2012) Biomaterials and stem cells in regenerative medicine. CRC Press/Taylor & Francis Group, Boca Raton, pp 1–546
58. Regenerative bone defects using new biomedical engineering approaches, REBORNE 2010–2014, 7th PCRD EC program. www.reborne.org
59. Espitalier F, Vinatier C, Lerouxel E, Guicheux J, Pilet P, Moreau F, Daculsi G, Weiss P, Malard O (2009) A comparison between bone reconstruction following the use of mesenchymal stem cells and total bone marrow in association with calcium phosphate scaffold in irradiated bone. Biomaterials 30(5):763–769
60. Lerouxel E, Moreau A, Bouler JM, Giumelli B, Daculsi G, Weiss P, Malard O (2009) Effects of high doses of ionising radiation on bone in rats: a new model for evaluation of bone engineering. Br J Oral Maxillofac Surg 47(8):602–607
61. Cordonnier T, Layrolle P, Gaillard J, Langonné A, Sensebé L, Rosset P, Sohier J (2010) 3D environment on human mesenchymal stem cells differentiation for bone tissue engineering. J Mater Sci Mater Med 21(3):981–987
62. Arinzeh TL, Tran T, McAlary J, Daculsi G (2005) A comparative study of biphasic calcium phosphate ceramics for human mesenchymal stem-cell-induced bone formation. Biomaterials 26(17):3631–3638
63. Ripamonti U (1996) Osteoinduction in porous hydroxyapatite implanted in heterotopic sites of different animal models. Biomaterials 17:31–35

64. Smucker JD, Aggarwal D, Zamora PO, Atkinson BL, Bobst JA, Nepola JV, Fredericks DC (2007) Assessment of B2A2-K-NS peptide coated on an osteoconductive granule in a rabbit postrolateral fusion model. In: Proceedings AAOS, San Diego, 12–14 Feb 2007
65. Hanssen AD (2005) Local antibiotic delivery vehicles in the treatment of musculoskeletal infection. Clin Orthop Relat Res 437:91–96
66. Sasaki T, Ishibashi T, Katano H, Nagumo A, Toh S (2005) In vitro elution of vancomycin from calcium phosphate cement. J Arthroplasty 20:1055–1059
67. Frutos P, Torrado S, Perez-Lorenzo ME, Frutos G (2000) A validated quantitative colorimetric assay for gentamicin. J Pharm Biomed Anal 21:1149–1159
68. McNally A, Sly K, Lin S, Bourges X, Daculsi G (2007) Release of antibiotics from macroporous injectable calcium phosphate cement. Key Eng Mater 333–334 (in press). Trans Tech Publication, Switzerland
69. Andrews JM (2001) Determination of minimum inhibitory concentrations. J Antimicrob Chemother 48(Suppl 1):5–16
70. Liedert A, Kaspar D, Blakytny R, Claes L, Ignatius A (2006) Signal transduction pathways involved in mechano transduction in bone cells. Biochem Biophys Res Commun 349:1–5

Chapter 5
Self-Assembly and Nano-layering of Apatitic Calcium Phosphates in Biomaterials

Akiyoshi Osaka

Abstract Among many calcium phosphates, apatitic ones are by far familiar because of their lattice structure similar to bone apatites. Yet, if one wants an apatite layer as a tool for improving tissue compatibility, regardless of hard or soft tissues, stoichiometric apatite is not necessary but nonstoichiometric apatite, e.g., with calcium ion deficiency or partial carbonate ion substitution, is preferable. Such apatite is easily provided on the surface of several materials when they are in contact with plasma; the materials include silicate glass and glass-ceramics and organic–inorganic hybrids with Si–O or Ti–O bonds as their skeleton, as well as some oxide gels derived via the sol-gel procedure. Moreover, proper water-soluble glass with specific compositions will be converted to apatite agglomerates or to rod- or needlelike apatite crystallites in array on their surface. The present chapter reviews deposition of apatitic calcium phosphates on such materials under body environment and their deposition mechanism in relation to constructing bone tissue as a hybrid between collagen fibrils and apatite crystallites.

Keywords Apatite • Nonstoichiometric • Apatite deposition • Tissue compatibility • Glass-ceramics • Titanium alloys • Oxide gels • Organic–inorganic hybrids

---

A. Osaka (✉)
Faculty of Engineering, Okayama University, Tsushima, Okayama-shi 700-8530, Japan
e-mail: a-osaka@cc.okayama-u.ac.jp

B. Ben-Nissan (ed.), *Advances in Calcium Phosphate Biomaterials*, Springer Series in Biomaterials Science and Engineering 2, DOI 10.1007/978-3-642-53980-0_5,

5.1 Introduction

5.1.1 Apatites and Their Deposition Under Body Environment

5.1.1.1 Apatites or Apatite Family

Self-assembling of the component ions in aqueous media to form calcium phosphates, especially apatitic ones (denoted hereafter as apatite(s)), on substrate materials has significant roles when they are employed as implants and scaffolds. pH controls the chemical states of the component ions in the medium from which an apatite phase is deposited, and it thus introduces imperfections in the apatite lattice, e.g., vacancies or ion substitutions, and hence complexity in the physiological properties. Apatites constitute a group or family in a super group with the general formula $M1_2M2_3(XO_4)_3Z$. In the apatite group, PO_4 groups occupy predominantly the XO_4 sites, while divalent or trivalent larger cations occupy the M1 and M2 sites. Among the apatite family, stoichiometric and nonstoichiometric calcium apatites with hydroxyl ions (OH–) as Z are the phases that have been the most extensively studied, predominantly because they are very similar in lattice structure and composition to the bone mineral, i.e., carbonated hydroxyapatite. Note here regarding the name of a calcium apatite phase with OH for the Z site: hydroxyl apatite may be considered appropriate in some fields of science, owing to the presence of hydroxyl ions, while hydroxyapatite is also acceptable for use in other fields of science where it is often and conventionally abbreviated as HA or HAp. Interestingly, smaller oxoanions like CO_3^{2-} can occupy both sites for XO_4 and Z, but larger ones like SiO_4 may substitute only XO_4. Crystallography distinguishes those sites as a-site (for Z) and b-site (for XO_4), and either of a- or b-site, or both sites, can partially or fully be occupied by CO_3^{2-} ions in hydroxy-carbonate apatites (HCAs). Moreover, the possibility of bicarbonate ion (HCO_3^-) substitution might not be ruled out due to its size. Similarly, hydrogen phosphate ion HPO_4^{3-} can occupy the b-site or replace XO_4 accompanying some imperfections associated with the decrease in the negative charge by one at the site. Thus, the apatite lattice is so unbiased toward the accommodation of ions, but not polymeric ions like condensed silicate or polyphosphate ions. Furthermore, if good biological activity is the target, one may control the nonstoichiometry of apatites.

Apatite Formation Under the Body Conditions

Stability of calcium phosphates and dissociation state of orthophosphate ions are closely related to the apatite formation under aqueous conditions. The chemical (dissociation) state of P(V) and C(IV) highly depends on pH of the medium in which they are present. According to the stability scheme of H_3PO_4 [1], $H_2PO_4^-$ and HPO_4^{2-} have the same activity at pH 7.19, while at pH 12.03 for the pair HPO_4^{2-} and PO_4^{3-}.

$$\log\ (HPO_4^{-}) / (H_2PO_4^{2-}) = -7.19 + pH, \tag{5.1a}$$

$$\log\ (PO_4^{-}) / (HPO_4^{3-}) = -12.03 + pH \tag{5.1b}$$

Under a physiological medium with pH ~7.2, like blood plasma, therefore, both $H_2PO_4^-$ and HPO_4^{2-} are not only the stable and predominant species but also present in a very similar content. The PO_4^{3-} content is marginal if the dissociation equilibrium should apply. Hydroxyapatite and its derivatives are precipitated via nucleation and crystal growth processes. Permitting orthophosphate ions of a form $H_nPO_4^{3-}$ (*n*: 0–2) to take part in the formation of stoichiometric HAp, Eq. 5.2 describes the overall precipitation reaction:

$$10Ca^{2+} + 6H_nPO_4^{3-n} + 2OH^- \rightarrow Ca_{10}(PO_4)_6\,(OH) + nH^+ \tag{5.2}$$

When two HPO_4^{2-} ions replace two PO_4^{3-} ions at the b-sites (XO_4), one vacant Ca site is created due to the charge compensation principle. Unfortunately, powder X-ray diffractometry cannot discern such substitution, but ^{31}P nuclear magnetic resonance (NMR) spectroscopy could distinguish PO_4 from HPO_4 owing to their different chemical shift values. The substitution of carbonate ions at either a- or b-site introduces further complexity. The atomic ratio Ca/P is a measure of the nonstoichiometry: it frequently happens that precipitated calcium phosphate crystallites give a set of X-ray diffraction lines assignable to HAp, but the ratio Ca/P is far below 1.67, even below the ratio (1.5) for TCP [2]. Appropriate imperfection should stabilize the lattice owing to entropy effects and hence reduces the solubility product Ksp. That is, when the imperfection is exceedingly high to cause strains in the lattice, the lattice will be destabilized and the crystallite size decreases to store the excess energy in a form of surface energy. Such smaller size and large specific surface area favor to stimulate dissolution of the calcium phosphates or the reverse reaction of Eq. 5.2. Dissolubility depends on the lattice energy itself and the energy of hydration: the net free energy $\Delta G = \Delta H_{hyd}$ (the sum of the heat of hydration) + U (lattice energy). Since the calcium orthophosphate family members, such as dicalcium phosphate ($CaHPO_4$; anhydrous form: DCPA, dihydrate: DCPD), octacalcium phosphate ($Ca_8H_2(PO_4)_6{\bullet}5H_2O$: OCP), tricalcium phosphate ($Ca_3(PO_4)$; α- and β-TCP), and HAp, consist of the same ions, i.e., Ca^{2+} and PO_4^{3-} or HPO_4^{2-}, dissolubility is mostly a function of the lattice energy, while the energy of hydration of the component ions primarily depends on the pH of the medium. The solubility phase diagram given by Chow [3, 4] shows that HAp is least soluble among those members in the whole pH range 4.4–13, in accordance with the smallest value of Ksp (−log Ksp = 116.8), followed by α-TCP (−log Ksp = 28.9).

Our blood plasma is supersaturated in calcium and orthophosphate ions with respect to apatite precipitation. In other words, our blood contains calcium and phosphate ions more than enough in concentration for apatite crystallization. Then, may a question arise why not apatite should be precipitated in blood in our ordinary life. At this moment, no clear explanation is provided: one can say that our blood vessels or their endothelial tissues would not allow heterogeneous nucleation. The nucleation process of this kind is thermodynamically much advantageous than its counterpart process: homogeneous nucleation. Consider diamond dust (homogeneous nucleation of water) will require a temperature range far below the freezing temperature, say −10 °C or at much lower temperature in highly clean atmosphere, but frosting (heterogeneous process), on the other hand, is observed when temperature is just below 0 °C. In either case above, thermodynamic significance is the activity of the relevant species, but not their concentration. The incredibly small value of the solubility product Ksp, aforementioned, indicates that free calcium and phosphate ions can never coexist under the physiological pH. Then, one may interpret the apparent stability of blood plasma with respect to the apatite precipitation as showing that the activity of those ions is kept below the level for crystallization for some reasons: chelation with blood proteins or other molecules is possible to depress the activity. Yet, any trigger, like sudden change in pH from defective homeostasis, puts such latent potential into action. Probably, that applies to spontaneous apatite deposition on a few kinds of materials to be described below.

5.1.2 Materials Inducing Apatite Deposition Under Physiological Conditions

5.1.2.1 Bioactive Materials

Materials are classified into many groups in terms of specific properties. For biomedical applications, physicochemical reactions such as apatite deposition, biodegradation or in vivo resorption, or protein adsorption at the material surface under the body environment are of vital importance as well as biological material–cell interactions. Apatite layer deposition is one of the most crucial reactions of bone substitutes, partly because it assures them to form direct bonds to bone tissues. They are sometimes denoted as being bioactive. Table 5.1 gives examples of bioactive, inert, and resorbable materials. The materials classified as bioactive will spontaneously deposit apatite on their surface when in contact with blood plasma or implanted in bone tissues. Note here that the term "bioactive" is also used in a very different meaning to represent literary "biologically active," e.g., to stimulate tissue regeneration, and hence, one should pay good attention on what the work really means.

The invention of Bioglass® and its family by Hench [5, 6] in the last days of the 1960s was epoch making: they were the first man-made *bioactive* materials that form a strong bond to living bone tissue. They are silicate glasses in a specific composition region A in Fig. 5.1 in the system Na_2O–CaO–SiO_2 with a small portion of P_2O_5. Discussions on the mechanism of bone material bonding have been originated from the analysis of the interactions between Bioglass® and bone tissues. Therefore, it is appropriate to describe some details about Bioglass® family.

Table 5.1 Some examples of ceramic biomaterials classified by interactions with living tissues

Interactions		Components, products	Applications
Bioinert	Oxides	Al_2O_3, ZrO_2, ZrO_2-toughened Al_2O_3	Hip-bone cup, head
		Glass-ceramics/leucite, $Li_2Si_2O_5$, F–(Na, K)$_2$O–CaO–SiO_2	Tooth crown, staining, layering
		F–Na_2O–Al_2O_3–SiO_2	Filler: glass ionomer cement
	Nonoxides	Colloidal SiO_2, ZrO_2	Filler: tooth cement
		Pyrolytic carbon	Heart valves
Bioactive (Non-resorbable)	Silicate glasses	Bioglass® and those with similar compositions	Ear ossicles, coatings
	Borosilicate glasses	13-93B1, 13-93B2	Bone regeneration scaffolds
	Silicate glass-ceramics	Ceravital®	Bone substitutes, defect filler
		BIOVERIT®	Bone substitutes
		A-W GC®	Bone substitutes
	Sol-gel glasses	Ca silicates	Gene stimulating
	Oxide gels	Mesoporous SiO_2 gel (Nakanishi's recipe)	Vehicle: gene, proteins
		Amino-modified SiO_2 gel particles Bone graft, filler	Bone graft, filler
		TiO_2 gel layers Ti surface modification	Ti surface modification
	Calcium phosphate	$Ca_5(PO_4)_3(OH)$	Bone defect and tooth cavity filler
Degradable, resorbable	Borate glass	13–93 cotton candy	Wound healing
	Calcium phosphate	$Ca_5(PO_4)_3(OH)$	Bone defect and tooth cavity filler
		$Ca_3(PO_4)_2$	Filler: tooth cement

The glasses in the region circled with a broken line inside of region A are so active as to form bonding with soft tissues like the eardrum membrane. A glass with an asterisk (⋆) in the center of region A which has a code name 45S5 consists of 45SiO_2, 24.5CaO, 24.5Na_2O, and 6P_2O_5 (in mass %) and exhibits the highest biological activity. It is frequently denoted as Bioglass without any notice. A layer of carbonated apatite (hydroxy-carbonate apatite, HCA), as well as a silica-rich layer, was found at the interface of a 45S5 implant and the bone tissue in which the glass implant was embedded [5, 6]. Other glasses, glass-ceramics, or oxide gels listed in Table 5.1 that are classified as bioactive deposit similar HCA layers on their surface when implanted in bone tissues. Several review papers have been published.

To name a few, Hench et al. [7] presented several examples of ceramic materials in clinical practices, including tooth crown application of inert glass-ceramics. Cormack and Tilocca stressed the importance of analyzing the correlation between the structure and biological activity of those active glasses and glass-ceramics [8].

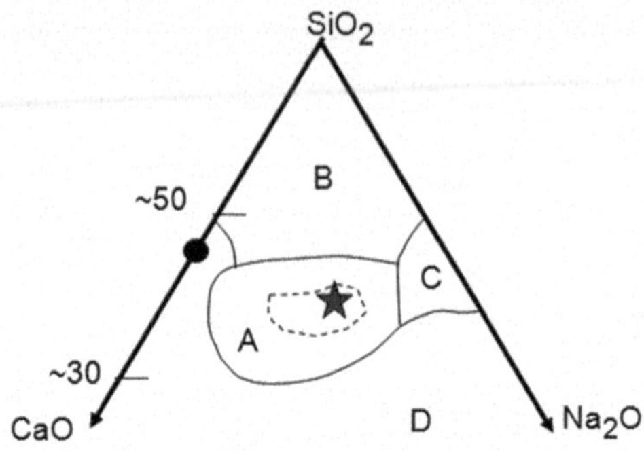

Fig. 5.1 The composition region (mass%) of Bioglass® family in the system Na_2O–CaO–SiO_2 that includes 6 mass% P_2O_5 (Modified and redrawn based on Ref. [3]). *The filled circle*, $CaSiO_3$. *A*, the region of Bioglass®. The glasses inside the broken line bond to soft tissues. *The asterisk*, 45S5 (45SiO_2–24.5CaO–24.5Na_2O–6.0P_2O_5 (mass%)). *B*, the region of inert glasses, like window glasses, for which no surface hydrolysis takes place under ordinary conditions. *C*, the region of water-soluble glasses. *D*, the region of no glass formation

In contrast, Hoppe et al. summarized dissolution of those ceramic materials from more biological viewpoints, i.e., biological response of our living cells to the ionic entities dissolved from those active glasses and ceramics [9]. Jones has brought up some problems that Bioglass® and bioceramics have to overcome, by proposing new materials like bioactive nanoparticles and organic–inorganic hybrids [10].

5.1.2.2 Zeroth Order Mechanism of In Vivo Apatite Layer Deposition on Classic Silicate Systems

A sequence of reactions proceed one after another at the interface and lead to the formation of apatite layers, as is widely accepted nowadays: (a) the surface of glass or glass-ceramics is hydrolyzed to release calcium ions, (b) leaving a silica-rich layer on the surface (Eq. 5.3a):

$$\text{Si–O–Ca}^{2+}\ (\text{in glass}) + \text{H}_2\text{O} \rightarrow \text{Si–OH (aq)} + \text{Ca}^{2+}\ (\text{aq}) + \text{OH}^- \quad (5.3\text{a})$$

$$\text{Si–O–Na}^{+}\ (\text{in glass}) + \text{H}_2\text{O} \rightarrow \text{Si–OH (aq)} + \text{Na}^{+}\ (\text{aq}) + \text{OH}^- \quad (5.3\text{b})$$

The hydration of Si–O–Na^+ releases more OH together with Na^+ ions (Eq. 5.3b). (c) The hydrated silica-rich layer serves the sites of heterogeneous nucleation of apatite. This layer may be protective of the glass surface from further corrosion under high pH ~9 which is attained by the hydroxyl ions due to the hydration processes (Eqs. 5.3a and 5.3b). The local high pH also drives the apatite formation (Eq. 5.2). Thus, the calcium ions released from Bioglass® as well as hydroxyl ions contribute greatly to further increasing supersaturation or (d) trigger the nucleation. Clark et al. [11] employed Auger electron spectroscopy to analyze the surface reactions in the earlier stages, while Hayakawa et al. used ^{29}Si magic angle spinning (MAS) NMR technique [12, 13] to confirm that recondensation of those resulted Si–OH back to Si–O–Si also takes place in the silica-rich layer. This reverse reaction would rationalize the protective activity of the layer.

Several years after the introduction of Bioglass®, another glass-ceramic bone substitute family Ceravital® was introduced in 1973 by Brömer, Pfeil, and Käs [14]. Gross and his co-workers refined the composition to improve mechanical strength [15]. A typical member in the Ceravital® family contains smaller fractions of Al_2O_3 and Ta_2O_5, in addition to $38SiO_2$, $13.5Ca_3(PO_4)_2$, 31CaO, and $4Na_2O$ as the primary components, while it contains 1 % TiO_2 (in mass %) as the crystallization initiator. It is capable of depositing an apatite layer at the material–bone interface. A decade later, another bone-bonding glass-ceramics, BIOVERIT® family [16, 17] and Cerabone A-W® (A-W GC®), were commercialized from Jena and Kyoto, respectively. A member of the BIOVERIT® family, BIOVERIT® II, is derived from an aluminosilicate mother glass with an approximate composition of $45SiO_2$, $30Al_2O_3$, 12MgO, $9(Na+K)_2O$, and 4F (in mass%). This mother glass experiences phase separation into two glass phases on heating, followed by crystallization to yield glass-ceramic that involves a mica phase (fluorophlogopite), which has a spherically arranged lamellae (cabbage-like) microstructure with cordierite precipitated between the mica platelets. Owing to this mica precipitation, the glass-ceramics is machinable with ordinary metal tools, enabling on-site modification during surgical procedure. It is common that the presence of Al or other oxides, known as intermediate oxides in glass science, suppresses apatite-depositing ability of glass, primarily because those metal oxides highly suppress the hydrolysis of the glass surface. The Al species is present in the cordierite phase and $AlPO^4$ in BIOVERIT® II and III, respectively. For this reason, the glass-ceramics are active to deposit apatite when implanted.

It was almost the same time that Kokubo, Yamamuro, and their group members fabricated Cerabone A-W® or A-W GC® [2, 18, 19] from a glass of the composition $46MgO–45CaO–34SiO_2–16P_2O_5–1CaF_2$ (mass%). Since surface crystallization, or heterogeneous nucleation and crystal growth, takes place in the mother glass, pulverization, heating, and sintering processes are inevitable to secure mechanical strength appropriate for load-bearing bone substitutes, like those for vertebra and iliac bones. Apatite and β-wallastonite (β-$CaSiO_3$) are the precipitated phases in the mass fractions ~38 % and 34 %, respectively, dispersed in the glass matrix of an approximate composition $17MgO–24CaO–59SiO_2$ (mass%). The name A-W is after those phases. Figure 5.2 demonstrates the presence of an apatite layer at the interface between A-W GC® and the tibia of a rat after implantation for 8 days [19]. A similar apatite layer was observed on pieces of A-W GC® in an in vitro experiment [2] where the samples were soaked in a simulated body fluid (SBF) [5, 6].

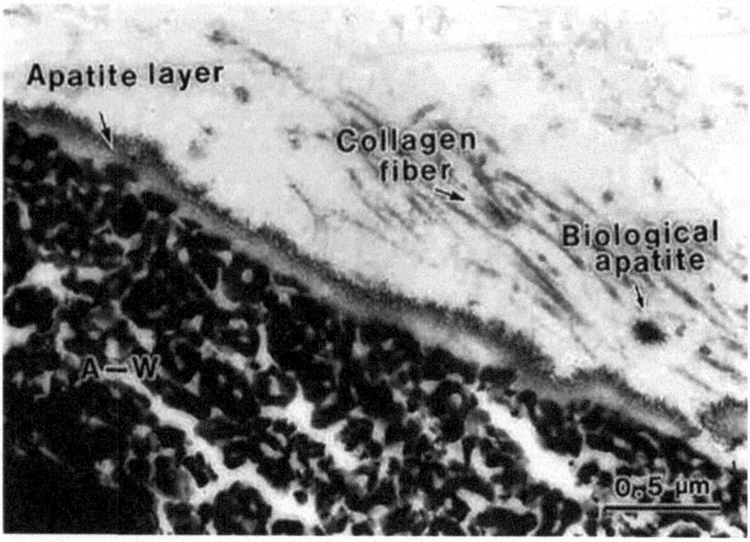

Fig. 5.2 A scanning electron micrograph of the interface between A-W GC® and a bone tissue (rat tibiae), indicating a newly deposited apatite layer (8 days after implant) (Reproduced from Ref. [19] by permission of John Wiley & Sons Ltd.)

5.1.3 Bioactivity as a Tool for Apatite Layer Coating Under In Vitro Conditions

5.1.3.1 Apatite Coating on Materials Provided with a Bioactive Surface

SBF or Kokubo's solution is an aqueous solution that contains the same inorganic ions as blood plasma in similar concentrations, whose recipe has been chosen as a result of extensive trials [5, 6]. Table 5.2 lists the concentrations of selected ions in blood plasma (HBP) and SBF (std-SBF). The in vitro (in SBF) deposition of a new apatite layer similar to that deposited in vivo is a strong piece of evidence that SBF well reproduces the in vivo apatite deposition under in vitro conditions [5, 20–22]. The recent worldwide round robin test confirmed this [23], even on Ca-free mesoporous silica gel [21, 24–26]. Yet, the interpretation of the material behavior in SBF needs some care, as Kokubo and Takadama warned [20]. Note here that those studies implicitly consider for the relevant single ions, or calcium, orthophosphate, and hydroxyl ions, to deposit to the active sites one after another before nucleating. At the end of the 1990s, Onuma and Ito reported [27] that SBF involves the Posner-type [28] calcium phosphate clusters ($Ca_9(PO_4)_6$), 0.7–1.0 nm in size. Betts and Posner proposed such clusters with water molecules within the interstices in 1974, when they conducted an X-ray radial distribution function analysis on amorphous

Table 5.2 The concentration of the ions[a], associated with apatite, in human blood plasma (BP), ordinary simulated body fluid (std-SBF), and three modified ones: P-, Ca-, and pH-SBF

	Ca^{2+}	HCO^{3-}	HPO_4^-	pH	log IAP[b]	Ind period
HBP	2.5	27.0	1.0	7.4	−117.26	–[c]
std-SBF	2.5	4.2	1.0	7.25	−96.35	>14 d[d]
Ca-SBF	3.7	4.2	1.0	7.25	−95.01	5.4 h
P-SBF	2.5	4.2	1.9	7.25	−95.04	16.1 h
pH-SBF	2.5	4.2	1.0	7.42	−95.02	58.6 h

The values of ion activity product (IAP; Eq. 5.5) and the induction period (Ind Period) of apatite deposition on mesoporous silica gel of Nakanishi type [21, 24, 25] are also indicated

[a]See Kokubo and Takadama [20] and Cho et al. [21] for the other component ions

[b]IAP derived from the measured concentration; the targeted log IAP was −95.0

[c]No data

[d]∼7 days after Cho et al. [21]

calcium phosphate and HAp, and a refined model was presented in 1975 by Posner and Betts [28]. Onuma et al. proposed [29] that the cluster is the growth unit of HAp because the HAp growth step is an integer times as large as the cluster size (∼0.89 nm) and the incorporation of the units into the lattice is the rate-determining step of the crystal growth. That is, the single relevant ions would not be attached on the step and diffuses themselves to the growing sites. Onuma and Ito pointed out that those clusters are present not only in an inorganic aqueous solution (2.5 mM $CaCl_2$, 1 mM $K_2HPO_4{\bullet}3H_2O$, 140 mM NaCl; buffered at pH 7.4 with HCl and tris(hydroxymethylaminomethane)), supersaturated with the ions relevant to apatite, but also in solutions undersaturated with those relevant to octacalcium phosphate or amorphous calcium phosphates [27]. Moreover, according to Hayakawa et al. [12], the orthophosphate ions originally present in SBF turned into pyrophosphate ones on the surface of inert glass or crystals. Thus, the atomic scale procedure of apatite precipitation on material surfaces needs some more detailed studies before any conclusive interpretation is elucidated. Yet, one can distinguish empirically the materials that can or cannot deposit apatite under body conditions.

On the basis of those preceding extensive studies, the spontaneous apatite deposition on a material now is a synonym to the bone-bonding ability. Yet, the hydrated silica layer was sometimes unable to be observed when bioactive silicates were in contact with plasma. This applies to A-W GC® [2], from which, as Kokubo et al. showed [22], an appreciable amount of Si(IV) was released into SBF. Ohtsuki et al. [2] attributed the released Si(IV) to the species for stimulating apatite deposition. If the amount of released S(IV) is an appreciable level, one cannot rule out another possible interpretation: the apatite crystallites in A-W GC®, got exposed to SBF by the dissolution, are the direct nucleation sites for new precipitation of apatite, as their transmission electron micrograph demonstrated [2].

Table 5.3 Bioactive glass coating[a]

Coating glass	Substrates	Coating technique	References
45S5 Bioglass®	SUS316L	Dipping into melt	[30]
Bioglass® type	SUS316L,Ti4Al6V, Co–Cr–Mo	Plasma spraying	[31]
52S4.6 ($52SiO_2$–$6P_2O_5$–21CaO–$21Na_2O$)	Co–Cr–Mo	Dip + sintering	[32]
Ceravital® (KG Cera)[b]	Ti particles	Hot isostatic press	[33]
$48.8SiO_2$•48.8CaO•$2.4B_2O_3$ (mol%) and that with 2.2 %TiO_2	Ti + glass particles on Ti4Al6V	Plasma spraying	[34]
Abo Akademi code 1–98	Ti	CO_2 laser sintering	[35]
Code 6P57, 6P68, 6P55, 6P61	Ti4Al6V	Enameling	[36, 37]
45S5 + HAp particle	Ti4Al6V	Enameling	[38]
$50SiO_2$–44CaO–$6K_2O$ (mol%)	Ti4Al6V, Al_2O_3	Enameling	[39]
Calcium borosilicate glass	Ti	Enameling	[40]

[a]See text for liquid phase deposition (LPD) of oxide (TiO_2, SiO_2) layers
[b]GC: $46.2SiO_2$, $25.5Ca(PO_3)_2$, $4.8Na_2O$, $0.4K_2O$, 2.9MgO, 20.2CaO (mass%)

5.1.3.2 Active Glass and Glass-Ceramic Coatings on Inert Metals

In consequence, it might be acceptable that the term bioactivity is employed to stand for such apatite deposition without confirmation of actual in vivo material–bone bonds. However, many people use this word these days to express different meaning. For the moment, "bioactive" is used in the classical way unless otherwise noted. Thus, when correlation is to be taken among bioactivity, apatite formation, and material–bone tissue bond formation for established, the first stage for assessment of bone implant candidates is simplified to soak them into SBF and watch the in vitro apatite deposition, and one can minimize the number of sacrificing animals. Current metallic bone implants are definitely inert in terms of apatite layer deposition, though titanium alloys like Ti6Al4V have better bone cell attachment than stainless steels. Providing those inert materials with bioactivity is an issue of importance. For metals and ceramics, coating with active layers is presumably the only way: layers of glass, gel-derived glass, oxide gels, or HAp ceramic. Table 5.3 lists a few examples for bioactive glass coatings on metallic materials [30–40].

5.1.3.3 Apatite Coating on Polymeric Materials: Intermediate Layers and Liquid Phase Oxide Coating

For polymer materials, hybridization and compositing are possible ways, in addition to the coating of an intermediate layer like titania. Table 5.4 summarizes several examples of attempts to vitalize inert substrates regarding apatite deposition.

Non-galvanic plating of metal on glass or polymers is a liquid phase deposition (LPD) process. In the long history of LPD, the most famous one may be the silver mirror reaction with Tollens' reagent. In contrast, a group in Nippon Sheet

Table 5.4 A few examples of intermediate layers or pretreatments for apatite coating on inert biomaterials

Substrates	Intermediate layer	Formation procedure	Reference
Liquid phase deposition of apatite			
Soda-lime glass	SiO_2	Liquid phase deposition (LPD)	[41, 42]
Quartz	TiO_2	LPD	[43]
PE, PMMA, PET, etc.	TiO_2, ZrO_2, SiO_2	LPD	[44–46]
PET, poly(ether sulfonate)	Hydrated silica	A-W GC® granules/SBF	[47]
PET, Nylon6®, EVOH[a]	Silane coupling agents + TiO_2	Soaking in titania sol	[48, 49]
PEEK, HDPE, UHMWPE[b]	(NaOH)	Soaking in 1.5SBF	[50]
PMMA	(NaOH) or (NaOH + EtOH)	Soaking in 2.38 mM Ca^{2+} and 4.80 mM PO_4^-	[51]
Chitin, chitin + chitosan	(H_3PO_4 + $Ca(OH)_2$)	Phosphorylation	[52, 53]
Carbon–carbon	Sodium silicate (water glass)	Soaking in SBF/exchanged	[54]
Direct coating of apatite nanocrystals			
PET fabric	(NaOH), MPTS[c]	Soaking in HAp suspension	[55]
Silk fabric	MPTS + 2-methacryloxyethyl isocyanate	Soaking in HAp suspension	[56]
Silk fabric	4-META[d]	Soaking in HAp suspension	[57]
Silicone rubber (PDMS)	PAA, γ-APTS[e]	Soaking in APTS-modified HAp suspension	[60]

[a]EVOH, ethylene-vinyl alcohol copolymer
[b]PEEK, poly(ether ether ketone); HDPE, high-density polyethylene; UHMWPE, ultrahigh molecular weight polyethylene
[c]MPTS, 3-methacryloxypropyltrimethoxysilane
[d]4-META, poly(4-methacryloyloxyethyl trimellitate anhydride)
[e]PDMS, poly(dimethylsiloxane); PAA, poly(acrylic acid); γ-APS, γ-aminopropyltriethoxysilane

Glass Company, lead by Kawahara, proposed an elegant silica layer formation LPD process [41, 42]. The principle of Kawahara's group is an anion (ligand) exchange between an oxide and a fluoride under a fluoride ion scavenger, for example, boric acid (Eqs. 5.4a and 5.4b):

$$SiF_6^{2-} + nH_2O \rightleftarrows SiO_2 + 6HF \tag{5.4a}$$

The resulted HF is scavenged with boric acid:

$$H_3BO_3 + 4HF \rightleftarrows BF_4^- + H_3O^+ + 2H_2O \tag{5.4b}$$

Yao et al. [43] applied a similar LPD process to fabricate ZrO_2 layer, while Deki et al. fabricated titania layers by the use of TiF_6^{2-} ions instead of SiF_6^{2-} [41].

Those oxide layers can be good intermediates for apatite deposition in SBF. Actually, Ozawa et al. [45] conducted preliminary studies on deposition of titania (anatase) on polymer substrates, such as polystyrene, poly(ethylene terephthalate) (PET), poly(methyl methacrylate) (PMMA), and poly(ethylene) (PE), via the same LPD procedure with TiF_6^{2-} as Deki et al. [43] and demonstrated that the anatase layers were active to deposit apatite. Sato et al. [46] deposited double oxide layer on PMMA and PE substrates: a mixed oxide layer of $SiO_2 + ZrO_2 + TiO_2$ beneath the top TiO_2 layer. When soaked in SBF or 1.5SBF (a solution 1.5 times as concentrated as SBF), the titania films deposited apatite within a couple of weeks.

Tanahashi et al. placed several polymer substrates on a bed of granular mother glass of A-W GC®, held in a container filled with SBF for a while, and then moved into another container filled with 1.5 SBF [47]. With these processes, apatite layers were deposited on the polymer substrates. Yet, the adhesive strength was fair for PET and poly(ether sulfonate), but marginal for PMMA, PE, Nylon6®, or PTFE. A speculation was presented [47] that at the first process of soaking in SBF, the silicate species from the mother glass should be redeposited on the substrate surface to form nuclei, and, in the second treatment with 1.5 SBF, the nuclei grew to form the apatite layers. In order to attain further increase in the bioactivity of polymer materials, Balas et al. [48] followed Oyane et al. [49] and took a two-step surface-modifying treatment on PET, ethylene-vinyl alcohol copolymer (EVOH), and Nylon6®. They modified the surface with silane coupling agents, i.e., isocyanatopropyl triethoxysilane for PET and EVOH, and 3-glycidoxypropyl trimethoxysilane for Nylon6®, and then soaked in titania sol, derived from a mixture of tetra2-propylorthotitanate, EtOH, HNO_3, and H_2O. Those surface-treated PET and Nylon6® substrates deposited hemispherical aggregation of apatite crystallites in SBF within 2 days, while EVOH took <7 days before the deposition. Though it seems a crude way to improve biocompatibility of the skirt of an artificial cornea, Pino et al. [50] treated candidate polymers, such as poly(ether ether ketone) (PEEK), high-density polyethylene (HDPE), and ultrahigh molecular weight polyethylene (UHMWPE), with 1–5 M NaOH prior to soaking those polymer substrates in 1.5SBF for up to 18 days and then incubating in SBF for 3–15 days. Although no X-ray diffraction profiles were given for any samples, based on the Raman and IR spectra, the deposition of calcium phosphate was concluded. Choi et al. conducted a similar experiment on biomimetic apatite deposition on PMMA [51]. They treated PMMA substrates with 0.1–10 M NaOH and mixture of EtOH and NaOH at room temperature before they soaked the samples in their own saturated solution containing 2.38 mM Ca^{2+} and 4.80 mM PO_4^- ions. Regretfully, they did not disclose the pH, the presence of other ionic species, or the stabilizing agent for the solution, but they found calcium phosphate deposition on the substrates with either treatment.

The above experiments utilize hydroxyl-related groups like Si–OH or –COOH to capture calcium ions onto material surface. In contrast, Yokogawa et al. applied phosphorylation of chitin fibrils [52]. Chitin fibers were phosphorylated using urea and H_3PO_4 and then soaked in saturated $Ca(OH)_2$ solution at ambient temperature, and a fraction of the grafted phosphoryl groups were hydrolyzed to form –P–O•Ca^{2+} groups, with which bioactivity was provided to the fibrils. Indeed, calcium phosphate was deposited on the surface within 12 h when they were soaked in 1.5SBF. The same procedure was applied to chitin–chitosan fibrils [53].

5.1.3.4 Direct Coating of Nanocrystallite Apatite on Polymeric Substrates

Considering longer induction periods or the period necessary by the detectable deposition, the NaOH treatment seems less effective. Furuzono's group has provided sophisticated and more promising technology [54–56, 58, 59]. They did not take a biomimetic way for coating polymers with apatite in the development of an artificial blood vessel material, but they employed sintered HAp nanocrystallites (50 nm in diameter). For coating apatite on PET, Furuzono et al. [54] chemically treated the substrate with NaOH first to introduce carboxylate groups (–COO–) on the surface and further modified by grafting γ-methacryloxypropyltrimethoxysilane (MPTS). With the surface modification of MPTS grafting, the HAp nanocrystallites are fixed to the substrate due to the interactions:

$$[\text{PET}] - (\text{the organic skeleton}) - \text{Si(OH)}_3 - [\text{OH of HAp nanocrystals}]$$

Here, MPTS is covalently bonded to PET, while ionic interactions control the bonding between the silanol groups of MPTS and the OH groups of HAp. They found the polyester fabric adhered human umbilical vein endothelial cells in the same amount as collagen-coated one, but in a shorter incubation period [54]. Silk fibers are also good candidates for scaffolds since long, though they sometimes cause inflammation. For suppressing such inflammation, Furuzono et al. employed similar grafting of an intermediate layer of MPTS and 2-methacryloxyethyl isocyanate for fabrication of silk fibroin–HAp composites [55]. Korematsu used 4-methacryloyloxyethyl trimellitate anhydride (4-META) [56]. The silk fabric was treated with 10 mM KOH to open up the anhydrous cyclic group on the grafting 4-META molecule into an active group that looks like phthalic acid. Here, the two –COOH groups were introduced to form a kind of chelate bond to HAp nanoparticle. The surface-modified silk fabric well supported the proliferation of fibroblast cell line cell L929. From a simply scientific viewpoint, silk fibroin is an interesting object to study, because it significantly influences the morphology and polymorphic state of calcium carbonate mineralization [57].

Nakamura et al. investigated the crystallographic orientation of HAp nanorods laid on PET substrate to which poly(acrylic acid) (PAA) was grafted beforehand [58]. They concluded that a prism plane of HAp with an index {1120} was the contact plane, i.e., the graft surface was ionically interacted with calcium ions on that surface of HAp. This suggests the importance of a periodic atomic arrangement on the prism plane for the bonding between the HAp and the carboxyl group of PAA graft molecules on the surface. For the fabrication of composites of poly(dimethylsiloxane) (PDMS) and HAp, Furuzono et al. used PAA and γ-aminopropyltriethoxysilane (γ-APS) for surface modification of the PDMS substrate and sintered HAp nanoparticles (2 μm in diameter) [59]. The HAp coating on PDMS exhibited human periodontal ligament fibroblast-like cells (HPLFs) and improved adhesion with living tissue according to percutaneous implanting tests with rats, as well as adhesion of human periodontal ligament fibroblast-like cells via living tissue.

The bonding strength at the material–coating layer interface is the most significant factor when the inert materials are introduced for load-bearing or shear stress-bearing sites. The presence of a distinct interface is itself disadvantageous since it would inevitably induce sharp difference in properties between the substrate and the coated layer. Crack generation and propagation in the coating layer even stimulates peeling off and spalling of the layer or introduces inflammation-causing substances into the implant site.

5.1.4 Ionic Activity or Concentration of the Ions in SBF

At implant surgery procedure, pH of plasma nearby is locally and temporarily lowered due to inflammation, which is unfavorable for the apatite deposition, although the homeostasis works to recover it soon to the ordinary conditions. Moreover, Eqs. 5.3a and 5.3b reveal that bioactive glasses and glass-ceramics are hydrolyzed to release not only mono- or divalent cations, e.g., Na^+ or Ca^{2+}, but also hydroxyl groups, with which increases pH in the vicinity of the contact surface. Although Posner-type clusters might be the growing units, we have no estimation of their activity in vivo. Moreover, pH and calcium concentration of plasma or SBF will be increased when it becomes in contact with Bioglass® or other materials active in stimulating spontaneous apatite deposition. Thus, it is significant to know the effects of individual ions in the media surrounding the implant materials. At this moment, therefore, a consideration on the ion activity of each component ion of HAp is introduced here.

Tsuru et al. studied the effects of the calcium and phosphate ion concentrations and pH of SBF on the rate of apatite deposition [26], where each of the ion concentrations and pH was controlled independently in order to keep the same ion activity product (IAP: Eq. 5.5) $-\log \mathrm{IAP} = 95.00$, while Ksp was equivalent to IAP at the equilibrium state, i.e., $-\log \mathrm{Ksp} = 117.26$. Tsuru et al. took the induction period (Ind Period in Table 5.2) as a measure of the ability of stimulating apatite deposition: the time for the deposited apatite crystallites to give detectably strong X-ray diffractions.

$$\log \mathrm{IAP} = 10 \log a\,(\mathrm{Ca\,(II)}) + 6 \log a\,(\mathrm{P\,(V)}) + 2 \log a\,(\mathrm{OH^-})\,. \qquad (5.5)$$

Here *a* like *a*(Ca(II)) represents the chemical activity of each species described in the parentheses. The ratio IAP/Ksp corresponds to the thermochemical driving force ($-\Delta G$) of apatite crystallization (Eq. 5.6) with *n* as the sum of the involved ions in mole: 18 for the present apatite deposition from Ca^{2+}, $PO_4{}^{3-}$, and OH^-.

$$-\Delta G\,(\mathrm{n/RT}) = \ln\,(\mathrm{IAP/Ksp}) \tag{5.6}$$

If the nucleation and growth are simply a function of IAP as Eq. 5.5 describes, the induction time should be the same for all those cases. In reality, it increases in the order: Ca-SBF < P-SBF ≪ pH-SBF ⋘ std-SBF. This might be reasonable, because, according to Eq. 5.5, an infinitesimal increment of *a*(Ca(II)) would cause five times as much effects as that of $a(OH^-)$. Moreover, the growth rate, in terms of the increasing rate for the X-ray diffraction intensity, was highest for pH-SBF, followed by Ca-SBF. In consequence, the calcium ions most favor the nucleation, while the hydroxyl ions most stimulate the growth. It means that when one wants to assess bone-bonding characteristics under in vitro experiments using SBF, or to biomimetically coat a layer of apatite for surface property control, one should take the highest care of the calcium ion concentration of SBF because the activity of Ca(II), or concentration of Ca(II) as a first-order approximation, affects most sensitively the apatite deposition. In addition, Gower and her co-workers proposed a growth model involving polymer-induced liquid-precursor (PILP) process [60, 61]. With such cluster growth models [27–29, 60, 61], the discussion with the activity of individual ions might be too simple.

5.2 Ca–P Formation on Silica Gels

5.2.1 Nakanishi's Mesoporous Silica Gel

5.2.1.1 Nakanishi's Silica Gels with Mesopores and Micropores

Hydrated silica layers have shown a critical role, as mentioned above, on the bioactivity or apatite formation on calcium silicate glasses and some inert materials. How about silica gel via the sol-gel route as they inevitably hold many silanol groups in the course of gelation? The silica gels from common systems consisting of tetraalkoxysilane $Si(OR)_4$, water, and solvent together with acid or alkali catalysts would never induce apatite nucleation in the Kokubo's simulated body fluid (SBF). Nakanishi was the first who fabricated a single oxide gel with proven bioactivity: it was pure silica gel with mesopore and micropores inside [24, 25]. Therefore, it is worthwhile to take a deeper look into the gels. Nakanishi elegantly employed phase separation phenomenon to fabricate mesoporous silica gels [24]. The systems consist of $Si(OR)_4$ ($R = CH_3$ (TMOS) and C_2H_5 (TEOS)); water as the solvent and hydrolyzer; organic additives such as formamide, polyethylene glycol (PEG), and poly(acrylic acid) (PAA); and nitric acid as the catalyst. As hydrolysis of Si–OR groups (Eq. 5.7a) and condensation polymerization of the resultant silanol groups (Si–OH) (Eq. 5.7b) proceed, silicate oligomers are produced, together with water and ROH as the by-products that are involved into the solvent.

$$\mathrm{Si(OR)_4 + H_2O \rightarrow (RO)_3Si{-}OH + ROH} \tag{5.7a}$$

$$\mathrm{2Si{-}OH \rightarrow Si{-}O{-}Si + H_2O} \tag{5.7b}$$

Miscibility among those silicate oligomers, solvent ($H_2O + ROH$ (= a reaction product), and organic additives controls the phase separation into two phases: silicate-rich and solvent-additive phases. As those reactions proceed, the composition of the solvent continuously changes, and the miscibility is also changed, accordingly. In conventional cases, the phase separation is caused by the decrease in miscibility due to reduced temperature, and it is the physical cooling. In the Nakanishi's case [24], the separation takes place under chemical cooling where the interactions among the species change with the growth in the molecular size of the silica oligomers and the solvent composition. Nakanishi interpreted those changes in a thermodynamic way. Regardless of the cooling principle, the change in the free energy of mixing ΔG (Eq. 5.8) controls the thermodynamic stability of the system.

$$\Delta G \sim \mathrm{RT}\left[\left(\frac{\phi_1}{P_1}\right)\ \ln\ P_1 + \left(\frac{\phi_2}{P_2}\right)\ \ln\ P_2 + \chi_{12}\phi_1\phi_2\right] Z \tag{5.8}$$

Here, ϕ and P stand for the volume fraction and degree of polymerization of the separating phases 1 and 2, respectively. Parameter χ represents the interactions between those phases and contributes either to destabilize or to stabilize the system. The first two terms represent the entropy contribution and the third the enthalpy one. Equation 5.8 indicates that the degree of polymerization of either phase destabilizes the system. Thus, proper selection of the starting materials in the precursor solution leads to appropriate phase morphology as well as the volume fraction of the silicate phase. When the system is metastable, $\partial\Delta G/\partial\phi^2 > 0$, certain level of density fluctuation is necessary prior to the separation, as a classic model of nucleation and growth postulates, where the droplet-type separation takes place to yield particle aggregates or gels with isolated pores. In contrast, when the system becomes unstable on the polymerization, $\partial\Delta G/\partial\phi^2 < 0$, any small fluctuation in density triggers the phase separation known as spinodal decomposition, leading to entangled microstructures. As the rate of polymerization is highly dependent on the temperature, and affinity among the atomic groups and molecular in the systems, as well, the temperature control and the period of reaction are critical to obtain the gels with desired microstructures.

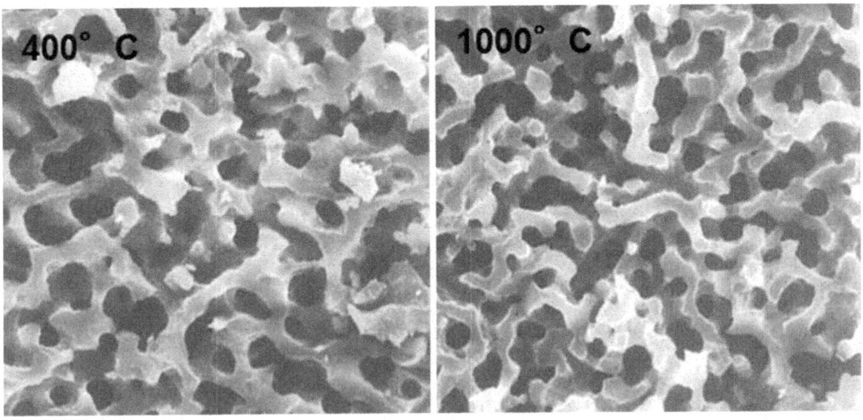

Fig. 5.3 Scanning electron micrographs of mesoporous silica gel (fracture surface) derived from Nakanishi's recipe [21, 25] $Si(OC_2H_5)_4$–H_2O–polyethyleneglycol under HNO_3 catalysis. Calcined at 400 and 1,000 °C for 2 h. Bar, 10 μm (Reproduced from Ref. [21] by permission of John Wiley & Sons Ltd.)

5.2.1.2 Attempts to Correlate the Silica Gel Structure and Apatite Deposition

The hydrated silica layers on glass or glass-ceramics, aforementioned, have presumably the same as or similar to the Nakanishi's mesoporous silica gel in atomic structure. Cho et al. examined the apatite formation on several mesoporous silica gels derived under different additives (polyethylene glycol: PEG and polyacrylic acid: PAA) [25] as well as the formation on those heated up to 1,000 °C [21]. Figure 5.3 shows scanning electron micrographs of the fracture surfaces of the PEG-derived mesoporous silica gels, calcined at 400 and 1,000 °C for 2 h. Entangled pores used to be filled with the solvent and PEG [25]: both have a very similar macroporous microstructure. Strangely enough, the gel from the PEG-containing precursor solution was able to induce the apatite deposition in SBF within 14 days but not the gel from the PAA-containing solution [25]. The PAA gel had a finer entangled microstructure than the PEG gel, while the former exhibited a type I N2 adsorption–desorption isotherms and the latter showed a type IV profile. No other obvious difference was noticed. Among the structural defects, those known as D1 and D2 defects, i.e., four- and three-Si–O-membered cyclic groups, respectively, were detected in both PAA- and PEG-involved gels by Raman spectroscopy, whereas the former defects remained even after soaking both gels in SBF but the latter disappeared on soaking. It was also found that dissolution of Si(IV) from both gels was at the same level, as well as both had almost the same amount of Si–OH groups regardless of being soaked in SBF or not. At this moment, therefore, no definite reasoning or correlation to the structure has been given for the apatite deposition on the mesoporous silica gels depending on the polymers in the precursor solutions. In contrast, the calcining temperature effects superficially seem more straightforward: according to the analyses by Fourier transform infrared spectroscopy and scanning electron microscopy, the gels calcined at 900 °C or above would not deposit any apatite in SBF within 14 days, but the gels calcined at 400 °C or above up to 800 °C deposited apatite. Since dissolution of Si(IV) in 14 days from the gels calcined above 800 °C was half as much as that from the gels calcined at 400–800 °C, such release of Si(IV) species is common among the sol-gel-derived silica and silicate systems. When they are dead-burned, the surface silanol groups are fully condensed. Again, it is the hydrated silica layer that is active to induce apatite deposition in SBF or plasma.

A simple question of knowing the mesoporous silica gels are bioactive is whether those gels are structurally very similar to the hydrated silica layers produced on those bioactive silicate glass or glass-ceramics. No known attempts were made to compare both in terms of their structures, partly because the silica layers are mostly too thin to deserve analyses and partly because the bioactivity of the silica layers is dependent on the calcium ions in the glasses and glass-ceramics.

5.2.2 *Apatite Layer Deposition on Ca-Containing Silica Gel Microparticles and Macrospheres*

The physiological pH conditions in SBF or blood plasma have greater effects on the apatite deposition or coating as have been discussed in the above sections. Suppose, as Fig. 5.4 schematically represents, that a piece of wet gel that contains calcium ions and is sustainable against severe water corrosion is in contact with a phosphate solution with pH 8–9. Since the gel network is rather open due to incomplete silica condensation with water, the gel provides good ion diffusion paths in all direction through which the calcium ions can migrate. The phosphate ions in the solution (denoted as P(V) in Fig. 5.4) are free to migrate in any direction. As soon as the gel gets contact with the phosphate solution, the calcium ions in the surface region find fellow HPO_4^{2-} and OH^- ions, idling in the vicinity of the interface, and hence, those three instantly get together to form apatite crystallites. Soon after this apatite formation procedure has started, the mobile or free Ca^{2+} ions will be exhausted because the rate of Ca^{2+} consumption due to apatite formation is far greater than the calcium ion diffusion rate through the gel surface region which is assumed stable. In contrast, the concentration of the phosphate and OH^- ions would not change, except at the very vicinity of the reaction zone, because they can migrate very fast in the aqueous solution. This is the case of glass–apatite conversion procedure that the Missouri group (Rahaman, Day, and their co-workers) has reported [62, 63]. This process is totally different from the previous classical Hench–Kokubo–Yamamuro one [2, 5, 6] where the presence of the stable silica layer is prerequisite.

Being inspired by the glass conversion procedure, Li et al. applied this procedure to apatite coating on silica gel macrospheres [64, 65]. Simple addition of Ca^{2+} ions into conventional silica gel systems like TEOS–EtOH–H_2O with HCl would not

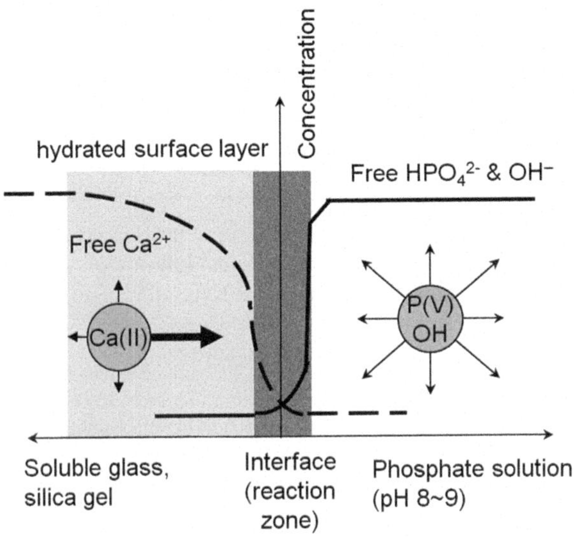

Fig. 5.4 Schematic representation of ion concentration profiles for Ca^{2+} in glass or gel body and for HPO_4^{2-} and OH^- in the phosphate solution. Apatite is formed at the interface (reaction zone) of the material and solution. The arrows show the concentration gradient for each ion soon after the formation reaction has started. The thick arrow for Ca^{2+} denotes a greater driving force, along the direction of the normal of the concentration profile that enables the preferred Ca diffusion into the surface region. The concentration gradient is established because the rate of calcium ion diffusion is much slower than the rate of Ca consumption due to apatite formation

yield an improvement in terms of the amount of the calcium ions held in the gel. Basically, the calcium ions are electrostatically interacted with $Si–O^-$ and hydrated. Thus, as gelation proceeds, Ca solubility in the gelling silica is reduced, that is, syneresis takes place with the gelation reaction, and the calcium ions are to be squeezed out of the silica body together with the solvent. Hence, it is very likely that almost all calcium ions are absent in the gel body. Li et al. took water glass solution whose pH was adjusted to 3 with HCl as the silica source, into which sodium alginate was added. The mixture was then added dropwisely to calcium chloride solution for the preparation of silica macrospheres. The calcium ions were held as Ca-alginate chelate molecules, and those molecules kept the gel spherical. The gel spheres were subsequently soaked in NH_4OH solution for neutralization, before they were soaked in a 1:1 (volume) mixture of 0.1 M Na_2HPO_4 and EtOH. They expected the reactions at the interface.

$$[\text{Ca in alginate chelates}] + HPO_4^{2-} + OH^- \rightarrow \text{HAp} + \text{alginate} \qquad (5.9)$$

Indeed, the X-ray diffraction analysis confirmed the apatite deposition on their surface. What was more, the mesopores in the original silica gel macrospheres disappeared when they were soaked in the phosphate solution [64]. Their energy dispersion X-ray (EDX) analysis, presented in Fig. 5.5, showed rather homogeneous Ca

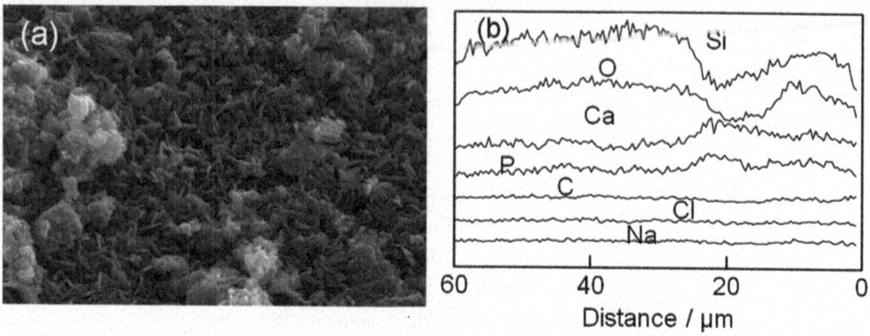

Fig. 5.5 (**a**) A scanning electron micrograph shows the surface microstructure of HAp-coated silica gel macrospheres. Flakey crystallites of HAp were observed. (**b**) Energy dispersion X-ray (EDX) line analysis of the atoms for the fracture surface of the macrosphere. A few humps in the profiles of Ca and P are observed at the surface region (0–30 μm). Ca and P are homogeneously distributed in the bulk region (<30 μm)

and P distribution in the bulk region, while a couple of humps for the Ca and P profiles in the surface region indicated that rigorous HAp deposition took place there.

Stöber-type silica gel microparticles may hold calcium ions owing to the alkaline moiety of the system. Chen et al. established a Stöber-type system TEOS–EtOH–$CaCl_2$–H_2O [66]. A ^{27}Si magic angle spinning (MAS) nuclear magnetic resonance (NMR) analysis indicated [67] both Ca-free and Ca-containing silica gel particles consisted only of Q^4, Q^3, and Q^2 units, and their fractions were ~70, 30, and ~1 (mol, %), respectively, regardless of the Ca incorporation. Interestingly, the ^{27}Si CP MAS NMR spectrum of the Ca–silica particles showed the greatly reduced signal intensity (~1/10) for those Q^n units in comparison to the MAS spectrum while the ratio Q^4/Q^3 remained constant. This simply means that very few protons were present near the Si nuclei, or one can say that the calcium ions pushed away the protons. The bioactivity in terms of apatite deposition in SBF was moderate as the particles gave weak but distinct apatite X-ray diffractions only after soaked in SBF for 5 days or longer. It is natural that the weaker intensity can partly be ascribed to the nano-sized particles: the absolute amount and volume of the apatite were too small.

5.2.3 *Self-Catalysis of Aminosilanes and Apatite Deposition*

Aminosilanes like aminopropyltriethoxysilane (APTS) and aminopropyldimethylmethoxysilane (APMS) compose a group of surface modifiers owing to their bifunctionality when an aqueous system is established:

$$RO{-}Si{-}(skeleton){-}NH_2 + 2H_2O \rightarrow HO{-}Si{-}(skeleton){-}NH_3{}^+ + OH^- + ROH \quad (5.10)$$

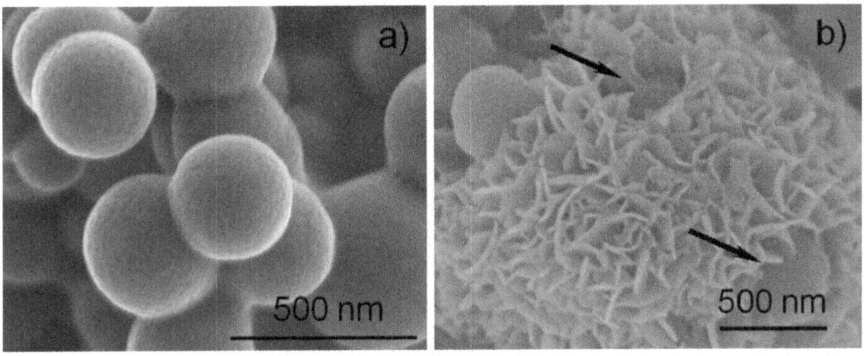

Fig. 5.6 Scanning electron micrographs of silica microparticles (300–400 nm) from the mixture 4.5TEOS-0.45APTS-280H_2O-440EtOH (mM). (**a**) As-prepared. (**b**) After soaked in Kokubo's simulated body fluid (*SBF*) for 7 days. Petallike entities are apatite crystals. One can see a part of the silica microparticles (*arrows*) (Reproduced from Ref. [72] by permission of John Wiley & Sons Ltd.)

This hydrolysis process produces 3 or 2 Si–OH groups and a $-NH_3^+$ group on APTS and APMS. Liu and Maciel reported that fuming silica derived from high-temperature (~660 °C) hydrolysis of $SiCl_4$ in a hydrogen–oxygen flame contains both isolated and hydrogen-bonded silanols on the surface while all silanols in the silica gel body are hydrogen bonded [68]. Therefore, conventional sol-gel-derived silica gels hold so many silanols, and they are susceptible to condensation with those on molecules nearby, that is, they deserve being grafted with such aminosilanes at the silanol end. In contrast, the amino group at the other end would remain associated with the surrounding medium to introduce positive charges on the host silica particles. Pham et al. employed APTS and APMS for surface modifiers to prevent colloidal silica from coagulation [69], while Manzano et al. considered using the amino group for capturing drugs [70]. Grafting onto dry and less reactive surfaces requires the use of piranha solution, like HF–HNO_3 [70] or H_2SO_4–H_2O_2. Reaction (Eq. 5.10) yields an alcohol molecule ROH as the by-product and releases a hydroxyl ion, as well. The OH ion will favor the condensation of the Si–OH group, that is, self-catalyzed gelation will proceed within the aminosilane system. In a preliminary study, Chen et al. employed this reaction sequence for preparing silica gel spheres coated with a HAp crystallite layer, using APTS as the self-catalyzing silane together with tetraethoxysilane (TEOS) [71].

They obtained only aggregates of component particles, whereas their size was reduced with increase in the mixing ratio TEOS: APTS [72]. Therefore, if an objective is to obtain discrete gel particles with amino-modified surface, postgrafting as Pham et al. [69] took is probably the best way. According to the gelling reaction schemes where the concept of acid and base catalyses works well, the protons favor hydrolysis of Si–OR and the hydroxyls favor condensation [73]; the results above should be interpreted as showing that a greater amount of APTS induces higher pH to stimulate condensation of the Si–OH leading so many nuclei of silica gel, but not showing that APS still disturbs the condensation to suppress size growth. Figure 5.6a shows the surface morphology of those silica microspheres, some of which are fused together to form aggregates. When they soaked those silica particles from the system TEOS-APTS in SBF, Chen et al. found deposition of petallike apatite crystallites agglomerated in hemispheres on the particle surface [72].

Figure 5.6b shows the morphology of the apatite crystallites that cover the surface of the silica microspheres. In consequence, active amino groups yield many –OH groups in SBF or surrounding medium to stimulate apatite deposition as far as calcium and orthophosphate ions are available.

5.3 Ca–P Formation and Contemporary Glass and Glass-Ceramics

5.3.1 Exploring New Glass and Glass-Ceramics with Apatite-Forming Ability

Bioglass® family has given so great an impact to the bioceramic field that the efforts of exploring new systems still continue. Several examples of glasses or glass-ceramics are listed in Table 5.5 [37, 38, 74–108]. Among those, Anderson et al. pointed out that Al_2O_3 was incorporated up to 1.5 mass%, without destroying the bioactivity, in their glasses in the 6-component oxide system [74]. The surface hydrolysis of 45S5 and other glasses is one of the key factors for achieving bioactivity. Moritz et al. [77] used a CO_2 laser to coat Ti implants with a thin layer (30–40 μm) of their glasses, taking advantage of local heating ability of laser irradiation in a line-scan mode. Zhang et al. reported antibacterial effects of the species dissolved from Ag-free multicomponent bioactive glasses [85]. The antibacterial glasses commonly involve Ag and Cu and sometimes Ce as the dopants [85]. The ability of the dopant-free glasses comes from the increase in local pH and a few ionic species dissolved from the glass granules or particles.

Hong et al. electrospun precursor sols containing poly(ethylene oxide) and a surfactant and calcined the spun fibers to fabricate amorphous nanotubes with thin walls consisting of nano-sized silicate glass particles [86]. Note here that the bioactive glasses from the melt-quenching route contain about 50 mol% SiO_2, while those from the sol-gel route have rather greater fractions (60 % or more) of SiO_2 [86–96]. Referring to a few examples of sol-gel-derived ternary glasses with bioactivity [91] and the parameters of the sol-gel syntheses, Lei et al. examined the effects of organic acids, such as citric, lactic, and acetic acids, instead of common HCl, on the morphology and dispersion of the silicate glass of a composition, $60SiO_2$, 36CaO, $4P_2O_5$ (in mol%), which was originally known as 58S [87]. Citric and lactic acids yielded more regular-shaped microspheres with better dispersion and smoother surfaces: those might be preferred in drug delivery applications. Recently, Vaid and Murugavel reported the behaviors of the sol-gel-derived ternary and quaternary Na–Ca silicate systems [94].

Table 5.5 Examples of exploring new biologically active or bone-bonding glass and glass-ceramics[a]

Description	Typical compositions	References
$+Al_2O_3$, B_2O_3[b]	$48SiO_2$–$28Na_2O$–19CaO–$2P_2O_5$–$1.5Al_2O_3$–$1.5B_2O_3$, etc. (mol %)	[74]
$+B_2O_3$, MgO, K_2O	(<59)SiO_2–(14–30)(Na + K)R_2O–30(Mg + Ca)O (mol%)	[75, 76]
Abo Akademi code 1–93	$53SiO_2$–22CaO–$6Na_2O$–$11K_2O$–$6P_2O_5$–5MgO–$1B_2O_3$ (mass%)	[77]
45S5 types[c]	$(94–2x)SiO_2$–xNa_2O–xCaO–$6P_2O5$; $x = 25.5$∽19.5 mol%	[78]
45S5 + P_2O_5	45S5 enriched with 0–12 mass % P_2O_5	[79]
+ MgO, K_2O	$57SiO_2$–$11Na_2O$–$3K_2O$–15CaO–9MgO–$6P_2O_5$, etc. (mass%)	[37, 38]
$+Na_2O$, MgO	$55SiO_2$•xNa_2O•$(45-x)$MgO (depositing TCP)	[80]
+MgO, tricalcium phosphate	3CaO · P_2O_5–SiO_2–MgO	[81]
$+Fe_2O_3$; hyperthermia	(FeO, Fe_2O_3)-CaO-SiO_2 glasses: magnetite, wallastonite	[82]
$+MnO_2$, Fe_2O_3; hyperthermia	CaO–P_2O_5–SiO_2–MgO–CaF_2–MnO_2–Fe_2O_3	[83]
+ZnO, Fe_2O_3; hyperthermia	x(ZnO, Fe_2O_3)$(65-x)SiO_2$•20(CaO,P_2O_5)•$15Na_2O$	[84]
Antibacterial activity[d]	$76SiO_2$–22CaO–$2P_2O_5$, code S53P4, 45S5	[85]
Electrospinning, precursor sol	$5P_2O_5$, 25CaO, $70SiO_2$	[86]
Sol-gel: CaO–SiO_2	58S ($60SiO_2$•36CaO•$4P_2O_5$) (mol%)	[87, 88]
	58S, acid (citric, acetic, lactic) catalysis on morphology and bioactivity	[89]
	60S ($60SiO_2$•35CaO•$5P_2O_5$) (mass%)	[90]
	$70SiO_2$, 30CaO (mol%)	[91]
Sol-gel silicates		[92–94]
Sol-gcl, $+Ag_2O$	AgBG (76 SiO_2–19CaO–$2P_2O_5$–$3Ag_2O$) (mass%),	[95]
	$(Ag,Na)_2O$–CaO–$2SiO_2$	[96]
MgO, K_2O: glass to HA conversion: code 13–93, 1393B1,1393B3	$53SiO_2$–$6Na_2O$–$12K_2O$–5MgO–20CaO–$4P_2O_5$ (mass %) and the derivatives	[97–99]
$+(Na,K)_2O$, B_2O_3; code: D-Alk-3B	$6Na_2O$–$8K_2O$–8MgO–22CaO–$54B_2O_3$–$2P_2O_5$ (mol%)	[100]
Ca-pyrophosphate glass + TiO_2	60CaO–$30P_2O_5$– $3TiO_2$–$7Na_2O$ (mol%)	[101, 102]
F-containing glass	Crystallization	[103]
F (as NaF) containing glass	Derivatives of 50CaO•$50SiO_2$	[104]
F(as CaF_2) containing glasses	(28–38)SiO_2, (4.7–6.3)P^2O^5, (19–50)CaO, (0, 22–30)Na_2O, (4–26)CaF_2	[105, 106]
F as CaF_2 and SrF_2, SrO, ZnO	(29–44)SiO_2–(3–5)P_2O_5–(20–30)(Ca,Sr)O–(4–33)(Ca,Sr)F_2–(13–20)$(Na,K)_2O$	[107]
F (as CaF_2)-containing glass	$46.2SiO_2$–$24.3Na_2O$–$(26.9–x)$CaO–$2.6P_2O_5$–$xCaF_2$ ($x = 0$–15)	[108]

[a]See also Table 5.3
[b]"+" stands for some additive oxides other than SiO_2, Na_2O, CaO, or P_2O_5
[c]Bioglass® 45S5: $45SiO_2$–24.5CaO–$24.5Na_2O$–$6.0P_2O_5$ (mass%) [4, 5]
[d]See also several references cited in this chapter

5.3.1.1 Effects of Fluoride Ions in Glass

The mother glass of Cerabone A-W® involves F as CaF_2 and is subjected to crystallization or devitrification procedure before solid and pore-free bone substitutes are produced. Calliano and Lopez conducted a similar study on crystallization and sintering of F-containing lime silicophosphate glasses [103]. While F can be involved in silicate glasses in two ways, the free ions (ionic F) are coordinated by the corresponding modifier ions, and the other (covalent F) is covalently bonded to Si and P (Si–F or P–F) [104, 109]. The former ones were predominant in the calcium silicate glasses [104]. When F remains ionic in glass, the network connectivity is determined only by the ratio CaO/SiO_2. That is, the connectivity is the same as that for the F-free glass. In contrast, the formation of Si–F bonds yields a degraded glass network, comparing with the F-free glass. This may lead to better susceptibility of hydrolysis when in contact with SBF or plasma. Moreover, the ionic F species, or the free fluoride ions, will be incorporated in the apatite lattice to form fluorapatite, which is chemically more stable than ordinary hydroxyapatite. An earlier work by Bauer et al. reported that an increase in the F content in the glass promoted the CaF_2 precipitation but suppressed the precipitation of apatite, in comparison to the F-free glass [105]. Bauer et al. [110] suggested that the phosphate content determined the CaF_2 and $CaCO_3$ (calcite) formations in the F-containing and F-free glasses, respectively. Lynch et al., in contrast, reported a seemingly contradicting result that a series of fluoride-containing glasses were so active to deposit apatite within 6 h. In consequence, it is surely accepted that we have varied factors to control, such as glass compositions (content of F, P_2O_5, SiO_2, CaO, or other components), the period of soaking the samples in solution, sample size, surface area to solution volume ratio, and solution itself (SBF or other buffer solution), to name a few. Therefore, as Coccihi et al. postulated [108], multivariate data analysis is necessary when one should elucidate reliable conclusions out of individual experiments.

5.3.1.2 Crystallization Yielding Magnetic Glass-Ceramics

Bioglass® 45S5 glass is liable to devitrification on shaping. Moreover, according to a differential thermal analysis to derive Johnson-Mehl-Avrami exponent conducted by Massera et al. [111], 45S5 glass strangely changed the crystallization mode from surface crystallization to bulk one when the grain size increases. Some efforts thus have been paid to fabricate "longer" glass, that is, glasses with better workability or a wider working temperature range [112]. Glass-ceramics involving magnetic phases can be applied to hyperthermia, where the heat evolved from the magnetic phases susceptive to microwave irradiation. A few groups attempted to provide such magnetic glass-ceramics with bioactivity [82–84]. For example, Ebisawa et al. [82] were the first who developed not only magnetic but also bioactive glass-ceramics involving ferrites. Here, the bioactivity was provided by the wallastonite phase precipitated in the course of crystallization. For the hyperthermia cancer therapy, various types of magnetic particles were proposed like hollow and mesoporous silica spheres [113, 114], cobalt ferrite (core)–apatite (shell), and magnetite–apatite composite nanoparticles [115, 116], while Maehara et al. [117] preferred magnesium ferrite ($MgFe_2O_4$) to the other ferrites of Cu, Fe (magnetite), Mn, Ni, Sr, or Co. Incidentally, Mother Nature gives us bacterial magnetic particles (BMPs) [118, 119], which are mostly 50–100 nm in size and nowadays are considered for gene therapy or other clinical treatments [120]. It is a key disadvantage in the hyperthermia with magnetized materials that microwave can only penetrate into shallow regions under the skin. In order to overcome this issue, some applicators like antenna or needles have been employed to raise the temperature at deeper region, but a good care is necessary for avoiding burning the skin.

5.3.1.3 Residues of Bioactive Glasses as Stimuli to Gene Activity

In 2001, Xynos et al. reported that the ionic species dissolved from 45S5 Bioglass® should stimulate expression of the genes relevant to human osteoblasts [121]. Then, a movement was emerged [88, 122, 123] to develop third-generation biomaterials that should stimulate the body to heal itself, i.e., cell- and gene-activating materials, in contrast to the previous generation materials that would simply be active only to replace the damaged tissues, to fill up the defects, or to protect from the invasion of cells or tissues harmful for swift recovery. A tendency is emerged to drive researches to develop biodegradable materials from the molecular biology aspect. The materials derived from the sol-gel procedure are advantageous in degradation compared to those via the high-temperature processes such as melt-quenching, sintering, and dead-calcining, since they commonly have many –OH groups due to incomplete calcination. Table 5.5 lists some examples of sol-gel-derived glasses. Unfortunately, against expectations, the sol-gel amorphous materials, like 58S [87], had not yielded statistically significant results in terms of osteoblastic marker gene expression. Note here that although most people praise apparent homogeneity of the sol-gel-derived amorphous materials, the truth is that the atomic distribution in the sol-gel-derived bodies is heterogeneous as far as the multicomponent ones are concerned. This would be justified by the consideration that on the derivation of the sol-gel materials, the alkoxides and inorganic salts are different in the rate of hydrolysis or condensation. In the classic sol-gel science, a few techniques for homogeneous gels were attempted such as prehydrolysis of the components, use of chelating agents, and application of ultrasound [124, 125].

5.3.2 Glass–Apatite Conversion

5.3.2.1 Borate and Borosilicate Glasses to Dense and Hollow Apatite Spheres

Classic model of bioactivity is based on the principle that the material surface should give a metastable hydrated gel layer to serve nucleation sites of apatite deposition [5, 6, 126]. As has been discussed in Sect. 5.2.2, the Missouri group [63, 64, 123, 127, 128] has proposed a method to convert glass into apatite, i.e., to obtain apatite hollow spheres and solid spheres, dependent on the glass composition, at the expense of glass itself. When dissolvable glass containing calcium ions is in contact with a phosphate solution of $pH > 8$, the chemical state of the glass–solution interface described in Fig. 5.4 will be established. At the beginning, the hydrolysis proceeds at the glass surface to leave a stable hydrated gel. When the surface layer is chemically unstable or dissolved, the calcium ions in the glass are supplied almost freely and ready to precipitate apatite particles. The borate glass derived by substituting B_2O_3 for SiO_2 in 45S5 glass is highly susceptible to the dissolution attack by the alkaline medium, according to the process similar to that described by Eqs. 5.3a and 5.3b, to form a less dense hydrated layer, in which the calcium ions can migrate in all directions to meet the phosphate ones from the solution. That is, calcium borate glass particles are fully converted to polycrystalline hydroxyapatite with random orientation [64] while the borosilicate glass particles are partially converted to yield apatite core–shell glass particles or hollow apatite particles depending on the compositions [123, 127, 128].

5.3.2.2 Conversion of Platelike Calcium Silicate Glasses to Apatite Rod Arrays

In contrast, when a piece of flat calcium silicate glass with moderate dissolvability is in contact with similar phosphate solution, the metastable hydrated layer is sustained as the surface hydrolysis and dissolution of cations proceed. In this situation, the Ca ion supply in the direction parallel to the surface is impractical, being different from the particle case. As a result, established is the Ca^{2+} ion concentration gradient within the interface region of the glass, the normal of which is perpendicular to the interface. If a large number of reaction sites are available to nucleate the crystallites, the nuclei, earlier produced or comparatively larger ones, will have a freedom to grow. Then nanometer-scale apatite rods will be formed in array perpendicular to the mother glass surface. Indeed, Hayakawa et al. [129] found for a series of soda-lime glasses with lower silica contents, $x Na_2O$–$(45-x)CaO$–$(54 \text{ or } 55)SiO_2$, $x = 0$, 10, 20 (mol%). Among a few glass compositions, a glass-coded G36 (containing 36 % CaO) yielded the most elegant self-assembled apatite nano-rod arrays that grew with an alignment in the direction of the c-axis of the apatite lattice when it was kept in contact with 0.01 M Na_2HPO_4 at 80 °C for 1 h. The degree of alignment is as high as 0.85, in terms of the measure proposed by Lotgering [130], which was almost equivalent to that of the dental enamel. They could not, unfortunately, detect the hydrated silica layer at the glass–apatite interface. Yet, longer soaking in the phosphate solution fully converted the glass substrates to a block of apatite nano-rod array. Interestingly, when soaked in SBF (Kokubo's solution), glass G36 gave hemispherical agglomerates of apatite crystallites for which the c-plane grew to give the same petallike morphology as the conventional bioactive silicate glasses or glass-ceramics [13, 18–22].

5.3.3 *Apatite Formation on Invert Phosphate Glasses and Glass-Ceramics*

5.3.3.1 Apatite Deposition in SBF on Phosphate Glass Surface

In addition to the silicate, borate, and borosilicate glasses and glass-ceramics, some phosphate glass-ceramics in the systems $CaO–P_2O_5–TiO_2$ deposited apatite in SBF. The commonly accepted glass formation region in the binary calcium phosphate system [131] is rather narrow and limited in the vicinity of the metaphosphate composition ($CaO/P_2O_5 = 1$): $\sim 0.8 < CaO/P_2O_5 < 1.3$. Kasuga and Abe expanded the glass-forming region by the addition of Na_2O and TiO_2 [132], while Kasuga et al. [101] later prepared a glass of the pyrophosphate ($2CaO•P_2O_5$) composition with a small amount of TiO_2, that is, $6CaO•3P_2O_5•TiO_2$. Their glass is far outside of the metaphosphate range, with a less glass-forming oxide P_2O_5 content than the glass-modifying oxide content, and it is an invert glass. Indeed, their ^{31}P NMR analysis confirmed the involvement of pyrophosphate (Q^1) and orthophosphate (Q^0) ions as constituents of glass of the composition $6CaO•3P_2O_5•TiO_2$ [102]. The glass gave the NMR peaks at ~ -2.5, ~ -7.5, and -23.5 ppm for those Q^0, Q^1, and Q^2 units, respectively, together with an unassigned peak at ~ -30 ppm [102]: this assignment for Q^2 is in fair accordance with that unit for calcium metaphosphate glass, given by Brow et al. [133]. The peak for Q^0 is in good agreement with that assigned by Yang et al. for the orthophosphate ions (2.6–2.8 ppm) in calcium silicophosphate glasses [134]. The invert glass particles deposited apatite in SBF within 20 days. The concentration of Ca(II) and P(V) in SBF, as well as pH, after in contact with the invert glass remained unchanged, whereas calcium metaphosphate glass released greater amounts of Ca(II) by an order of magnitude, and the concentration of P(V) kept increasing up to $\sim$80 mM, almost two orders of magnitude greater one within 6 days. An EDX analysis detected an intermediate thin layer (0.5–2 μm) at the invert glass–apatite interface, involving Ca, P, and Ti. Kasuga et al. interpreted this layer as being formed by the redeposition of once dissolved Ca(II) and P(V) and supposed that the layer should provide the apatite nucleation sites [101, 102]. Although the metaphosphate glass released a large amount of Ca(II) and P(V) into SBF, pH of SBF was decreased from the original value of 7.4 to 6.20, or the acid range. This might contribute to suppressing the apatite deposition.

5.3.3.2 Precipitation of Apatite in Glass-Ceramics as a Constituent

Later, Kasuga and colleagues derived a glass-ceramic of the composition $45CaO•30P_2O_5•25TiO_2$, which on heating precipitated a Nasicon-type stable $CaTi_4(PO_4)_6$ phase as well as some acid-soluble calcium phosphate phases. The mother glass was known to be susceptible to spinodal-type decomposition or phase separation [135]. When CaF_2 was replaced by a portion of CaO to yield a glass of the composition $35CaO–10CaF_2–30P_2O_5–25TiO_2$, F-containing oxyapatite

$Ca_{10}(PO_4)_6(O, F_2)$ particles were precipitated in the resulted glass-ceramic together with the Nasicon-type one [136]. Because of the water-insoluble oxyapatite, the glass-ceramic showed high water resistivity around the neutral pH region. Their F-containing glass-ceramic was different in inertness to deposit apatite in the aqueous systems (plasma or SBF) from A-W GC®, primarily because of the stability of the F-oxyapatite phase. A bioactive glass-ceramic from mother glass of the composition $60CaO–30P_2O_5–3TiO_2–7Na_2O$ [101, 102] is well machinable with conventional steel tools [101]: Kasuga attributed the machinability to the $2CaO{\bullet}P_2O_5$ phase that was precipitated in a large amount [101].

5.4 Apatite Deposition on Metal Oxide Gels and Oxide Layers on Ceramic and Metallic Substrates

5.4.1 *Sol-Gel-Derived Metal Oxide Gels: ZrO_2, Nb_2O_5, Ta_2O_5, and Al_2O_3*

5.4.1.1 Hydrated Oxide Gels

In the course of discussing the apatite deposition on the silicate glasses and glass-ceramics, the importance of hydrated silica layer has been emphasized [2, 5, 6, 123]. This stimulated the sol-gel synthesis of simple oxide gels, such as titania (TiO_2), zirconia (ZrO_2), niobium oxide, and tantalum oxide, and examination of their bioactivity in SBF. A key issue is the presence of metal–OH (M–OH) groups for the sol-gel-derived hydrated oxide species to exhibit bioactivity: the physical chemistry behind the activity is that the colloid or microparticles of oxide gels will be charged, and the amount of the charge is determined by the pKa of each M–OH (Eq. 5.11):

$$M - OH + H_2O \rightarrow M - O^- \, (aq) + H_3O^+ \tag{5.11}$$

and protonation (Eq. 5.12) and deprotonation (Eq. 5.13).

$$M - OH + H_3O^+ \rightarrow M - O\,H_2{}^+ \, (aq) + H_2O \tag{5.12}$$

$$M - OH + OH^- \rightarrow M - O^- \, (aq) + H_2O \tag{5.13}$$

As a result, an electric double layer is formed around the particles. The series of surface-chemical changes are the bases for the isoelectric point (IEP) or point of zero charge (pzc) [137, 138]. Since IEP for TiO_2 is around 6.9 [138], titania gels are negatively charged in total under the body conditions (pH ~7.2), which favors them to attract calcium ions and then to form apatite. Tengvall and Lundström presented a good review on such physicochemical aspects of titanium as a biomaterial [139].

5.4.1.2 Zirconia Gels and Those Prepared on Metal Substrates

Zirconia (ZrO_2), niobium oxide, and tantalum oxide (Nb_2O_5, Ta_2O_5 – niobia and tantala, though rarely called) are other examples of inert ceramics. Those gels are found to actively deposit apatite under aqueous solutions. Uchida et al prepared zirconia gels on silica glass slide with a dip coating process [140]. The precursor sol was derived from $Zr(OPr^n)_4$ (Pr^n:1-propyl group) via the hydrolysis with HNO_3 where the solution system was cooled with ice and water. They soaked the as-dried samples not only in conventional SBF (original Kokubo's solution) but also in the solutions enriched with OH^- ions (higher pH), calcium ions, and phosphate ions. It took 14 days for the gel films to exhibit the sign of apatite deposition (X-ray diffraction and scanning electron microscopy) in SBF but took 3 days in the ion-enriched solutions. Moreover, a year later, Uchida et al. greatly improved its bioactivity [141]: they calcined the same zirconia gel [140] at 600 and 800 °C for 10 min to transform into the mixture of tetragonal (t) and monoclinic (m) phases. The resultant crystalline zirconia films deposited apatite in conventional SBF within 3 days. They attributed this good activity to an epitaxial correlation between hydroxyapatite lattice and the t- and m-zirconia.

A similar zirconia layer may be formed on the surface of metallic Zr if it is properly corroded, and the layer is likely to deposit apatite in SBF. Uchida et al. exposed Zr substrates to 1, 5, and 15 M NaOH solutions at 95 °C for 24 h [142]. Each solution was equally corrosive enough to introduce amorphous layers, thin or thick, but those specimens were inferior in inducing biomimetic apatite deposition: they found that the treatment with 5 and 15 M NaOH was effective to the apatite deposition. Yet, it took ~28 days before the deposited apatite would cover most of the specimen surface. They interpreted this weak activity as showing the presence of small amount of Na on the treated surface: Uchida et al. [142] expected that the surface layer should contain numerous Zr–ONa groups where the sodium ions are loosely bonded due to the electrostatic interaction as the specimens are not calcined, and hence the hydrolysis with SBF should give Zr–OH and high pH in the vicinity, both of which should facilitate apatite deposition.

$$Zr - ONa + H_2O \rightarrow Zr - OH\ (aq) + Na^+ + OH^- \qquad (5.14)$$

As described in Sect. 5.4.3, the alkali treatment succeeded greatly in providing the bioactivity (apatite-depositing ability) to titanium and a few titanium alloys, as Kokubo et al. reviewed [143, 144]. Since zirconia ceramics stabilized with additives like Ce, Y, and Ca as well as composited with alumina are the stiffest ceramics, it would be advantageous if they could be provided with bioactivity. Uchida et al. also challenged this issue by taking nanocomposite ceramics, Ce-stabilized zirconia in which dispersed are alumina nanoparticles (10Ce-TZP/Al_2O_3), and by exposing those ceramics to (5 M and concentrated) H_3PO_4, (5 M and concentrated) H_2SO_4, concentrated HCl, and 15 M NaOH [145]. (They did not disclose the meaning of "concentrated," but it is commonly represented as ~15 M for H_3PO_4, ~18 M for H_2SO_4, and ~10 M for HCl, respectively.) They found that all of those chemically treated ceramics deposited apatite within 7 days in SBF, but the 5 M H_3PO_4 was the most effective as the sample deposited within 3 days. The scanning electron micrographs (SEM photos) indicate that the H_3PO_4-treated sample gave the largest number of hemispherical aggregates of apatite, showing that the treatment induced nucleation the most. On the basis of the stronger O1s peaks in the X-ray photoelectron spectra of the chemically treated samples than those of other samples, Uchida et al. [145] considered here that the Zr–OH group on the surface is the key for the bioactivity.

5.4.1.3 Niobium Oxide and Tantalum Oxide Gels

Niobium and tantalum oxide ceramics are inert in terms of apatite formation under body conditions, too. Yet, their gels can be active, as we have seen for ZrO_2 gel mentioned above. Miyazaki et al. [146] prepared niobium oxide (Nb_2O_5) gel via the hydrolysis and condensation of $Nb(OEt)_4$ (Et: ethyl group) in water–ethanol solution: the resultant as-dried gels were calcined at 600–1,000 °C for 30 min. When soaked in SBF, the as-dried gel and gels calcined at 600 °C (amorphous) and 800 °C (orthorhombic Nb_2O_5 was precipitated) exhibited in vitro bioactivity. One might attribute the bioactivity to certain amount of Nb–OH groups remaining on the surface. Niobium oxide gels might be introduced onto Nb metal substrate surface with the treatment with 0.5–2.0 M NaOH at 60 °C for 24 h and gentle rinsing. This treatment was similar to that taken by Uchida et al. to in one way or another and successfully provided metallic Zr specimen with apatite deposition ability [145]. The as-treated Nb substrates needed some sort of crystalline sodium niobates, and it was unfortunate that the oxide layers were inert, regardless of the concentration of the NaOH solution. On these bases, Miyazaki et al. speculated [146] that there might be some specific structure in which the Nb–OH groups from the hydrolysis of sodium niobates would be arranged, as well as specific porous microstructure for the surface oxide layer.

Tantalum metal is a rare case in that it induces apatite deposition in vitro though the induction time is ~4 weeks. High expectation is that the activity will be improved if the metal surface is covered with the hydrated tantalum oxide. Miyazaki et al. [147] proved this: the induction time was shortened to ~7 days when they treated Ta metal substrates with 0.2 and 0.5 M NaOH at 60 ° C for 24 h to form a hydrated sodium tantalite gel layer. Here, they considered that the Ta–OH groups as an ion exchange product are yielded according to Eq. 5.15:

$$\mathrm{Ta-ONa + H_3O^+ \rightarrow Ta-OH\,(aq) + Na^+ + H_2O} \tag{5.15}$$

which is equivalent to Eq. 5.14 under pH 7.4. They play a key role for the apatite nucleation, and the increase in the ion product for SBF by the released sodium ions favors it, too. It seems more adequate to assume Eq. 5.14 and to consider the resultant hydroxyl ions should stimulate the apatite formation. Miyazaki et al. further attempted to confirm the significance of the Ta–ONa on the tantalum oxide gel layer by controlling the atomic ratio Na/Ta in sol-gel-derived sodium tantalite gels [148]. The Na-free tantalum oxide gel was found to be bioactive, indicating that the Ta–OH in the pure oxide gel should stimulate the heterogeneous crystallization of apatite in SBF. Moreover, the increase in the ratio Na/K improved its bioactivity. Thus, they concluded that the hydrolysis of the Ta–ONa is one of the key reactions. Following a preliminary in vivo study by Miyazaki et al. [148], Kato et al. [149] conducted a detailed in vivo test: they prepared Ta metal plates with and without the alkali (NaOH) and subsequent heating treatment and implanted them transcortically into the proximal metaphyses of the bilateral rabbit tibiae, alkali- and heat-treated plates for one limb and untreated plates for the contralateral limb. The Ta implants without treatment showed almost no direct bond to bone even at 16 weeks after implantation, even leading to encapsulation. The treated implants, on the contrary, gave satisfactory results: they had a weaker bond to bone at 8 weeks, but the strength was found improved at 16 weeks. Their histological examination exhibited direct contact of bone tissue and the implant surface. It appears extraordinary that the Ta implants without the treatment behave like an inert material, despite that it was found active in vitro. Yet, it would be interpreted as showing that the tissue reactions against the implants with weak activity are so speedy that the encapsulation takes place before the implants demonstrate their true activity.

5.4.1.4 Inert Alumina Gel

Li et al. prepared alumina gels from a commercially available alumina sol [150] and examined its in vitro apatite deposition like the Nakanishi-type silica gel [25, 151] as well as niobium and tantalum oxide gels [146–149]. The result was totally unsatisfactory: their α-alumina, after calcination at 400 or 600 °C for 2 h, would not even adsorb the calcium and phosphate ions when soaked in SBF. Thus, the calcined alumina gels remain still inert in terms of apatite formation.

5.4.2 *Providing Bone-Bonding Activity to ZrO_2 Ceramics*

5.4.2.1 Chemical Procedure to Form an Intermediate Layer and Direct Coating of Apatite

Zirconia ceramics, especially stabilized zirconia ceramics, are of highest importance in the field of structural ceramics. In the previous section, introduced was the success of the direct surface modification of the ceramics, i.e., alkali treatment of stabilized zirconia/alumina ceramics to provide bioactivity. This section describes several layer coating treatments: coating of intermediate layers and direct apatite layer coating. Abe et al. proposed a biomimetic route of coating an active layer on yttria-stabilized zirconia ceramics (Y-TZP) [152]: It was similar to Tanahashi et al. [47]. Here, a piece of the ceramic plate was set parallel to a plate of the mother glass of A-W GC®, with distance 0.5 mm or less, and soaked in SBF held in a polystyrene bottle. The background concept is that the calcium and some silicate ions, dissolved from the mother glass, are transferred to the ceramic surface and redeposited there to form a hydrated silicate layer, and that the layer stimulates the apatite deposition [47].

In addition, Akashi and his colleagues developed a process of direct apatite formation on inert materials [153], where a target specimen piece was soaked alternatively in calcium and phosphate solutions. Takemoto et al. [154] applied this coating process to Ce-TZP/Al_2O_3 ceramics that Uchida et al. used previously [145]: they first etched the ceramic surface with HF and heated at 1,300 °C to introduce micropores. Conducting alternate soaking for those specimens yielded a sub-micrometer thick apatite layer. When they soaked this thin-layer coated specimen in SBF, they had ~4 μm thick apatite layer on the surface. Their in vivo test of those two samples using rabbits confirmed that both apatite pre-coatings were similarly effective on the bone–ceramic bonding in a long term, although the thicker layer secured the greater bonding strength until 4 weeks, but no difference in the bonding strength was found in longer implantation. The most significant issue in the coating of an inert substrate with any functional layer is the presence and behavior of the interface between the layers: the intermediate layer results in two interfaces. Thus, the adhesion between the ceramic substrate and the intermediate (silicate) layer should be improved by the HF treatment before the biomimetic processes that roughen the substrate surface to introduce micropores (expecting mechanical or chemical improvement) [154].

Fluorhydroxyapatite can also be obtained via a sol-gel process onto zirconia substrates. Kim et al. [155] slowly added calcium nitrate solution to solution containing triethylorthophosphate ($P(OEt)_3$; Et: ethyl group) and ammonium fluoride: the resulted solution was kept stirred at room temperature for 72 h. The ratio Ca/P and P/F was adjusted to be 1.67 and 4. Then, this precursor solution was spin-coated on partially stabilized zirconia (3Y-TZ), dried, and heated to a temperature between 400 and 800 °C for 1 h to form dense and uniform fluorapatite layers. Heating to above 500 °C drastically improved the apatite–ceramic surface adhesion. At the same time the treatment also decreases the release of calcium ions into physiological saline solution (0.9 % NaCl) by 30 %. The fluorapatite layer proliferated MG63 cells well, as comparably as to culture dish and HAp ceramic.

5.4.2.2 Physical Procedure to Assist the Formation of an Apatite Layer on ZrO_2 Ceramics

When a ceramic sample is poled under a DC electric filed between a pair of Pt electrodes, a positive and negative charge is evoked and accumulated at the surface (P- and N-surface) adjacent to cathode and anode, respectively, as Nakamura et al. described [156]. The poled HAp ceramics exhibited some interesting properties: enhanced tissue regeneration of bone [157] and soft tissue [158] or accelerated protein adsorption [159]. Then Nakamura et al. applied this polling treatment onto yttrium-stabilized zirconia (YSZ): 20 V/cm^{-1} for 30 min at 200 °C. The poled specimens were further corroded with 5 M NaOH at 60 °C for 3 h to induce Zr–OH groups on the surfaces and soaked in SBF [160]. They observed apatite deposition on all specimens regardless of the polling, while the scanning electron micrographs indicated that the ability of inducing apatite was larger in the order O-surface ~N-surface < P-surface (O surface, only with the NaOH treatment, no polling). The order was consistent with the OH content on the surface derived from the O1s X-ray photoelectron spectra. They explained such tendency in terms of the oxygen vacancies. The vacancies increased in number by the polling at the P-surface and attracted hydroxide ions during the chemical treatment. Such polling was found also effective to enhance bioactivity of 45S5 glass [161].

(NB: Ref. [162] was partly concerned with low-temperature-degradation or slow crack growth of stabilized zirconia ceramics. Refer also to Sato et al., J. Mat. Sci., 22, 882–886 (1987) or Benzaid et al., Biomaterials, 29, 3636–3641 (2008)).

5.4.3 Bioactive Titania Bulk Gels and Coatings via the Alkoxide Routes

5.4.3.1 Titania Ceramics and Gels

When Fujishima and Honda detected the electrochemical photolysis of water (water splitting) or photocatalytic activity of titania ceramics in 1972 [162], titania was suddenly in the spotlight for researchers working in the fields of solar energy, photocatalysis (oxidation of organic substances), and so forth, as Roy et al. reviewed [163]. Yoko et al. reported similar activity for their sol-gel-derived titania films [164], prepared via the route similar to that taken by Dislich and Hussman [165]. Titania was produced in a variety of shapes and morphologies such as nano-hollow fibrils [166], nanotube assemblies, or self-aligned nanopores [163]. Table 5.6 [167–172] lists only a few examples of titania (anatase) sol preparation via the alkoxide routes. Again, factors controlling the solution chemistry in the sol-gel route include the source materials, solvent, catalyst, temperature, reactant concentrations, and mixing ratio. In addition, the gelation environment can be modified by enclosing the system under a confined space or by exposing the system to atmospheres (open/closed) [174]. In the sol-gel reactions under a closed system, all of the additives can remain in the gel, but under open conditions, some products or even sources might be lost or the system absorbs humidity, and the resultant sols or gels would exhibit properties which are different from expectations. Countless works have been published, even nowadays, but this list mostly covers the wet-chemical routes, except the hydrolysis of titanium halides.

Table 5.6 Several examples of titania gels and titania on titanium alloys studied from the biomedical viewpoints later than 1988: Sol-gel preparation of titania sols and films from titanium alkoxides for non-biological purposes

$Ti(OR)_4$[a]	Solvent	Catalyst; pH	Temperature	Description	References
$Ti(OPr^i)_4$[a]	EtOH, H_2O	HNO_3;–[b]	20 °C; reflux 80°, 8 h	An[c]; dipcoat	[167]
	EtOH, H_2O	HNO_3; pH 1–2	100 °C; autoclave, 3–6 h	An; spin coat	[168]
	EtOH, H_2O	–; pH 1–2	–; 10 min	–; cotton knit	[169]
	EtOH	H_2O_2; –	75 °C; 0–120 h	An; closed[d]; NP[c]	[170]
				An; spin coat	[171]
$Ti(OBu^n)_4$	PrOH, H_2O	HNO_3; pH 2.5	Reflux 75 °C, 24	An; dipcoat	[172]
$Ti(OEt)_4$	EtOH, H_2O	HNO_3; pH 1–3	50–70 °C; 1–24 h	An sol; closed	[173]

[a] *Pr^i* isopropyl, *Bu^n* n-butyl, *Et* ethyl
[b] –, no explicit description available
[c] *An* anatase, *NP* nanoparticles
[d] Sol-gel reactions under a closed system

Due to the availability of the Ti compounds as the sources, it is synthesized via a few routes, such as:

(a) Sol-gel 1: Peptizing commercially available titania sol with an acid and drying the suspension.
(b) Sol-gel 2: Hydrolysis of titanium alkoxides under the acid catalysis (HCl or HNO_3). Titanium propoxides are common because of commercial availability.
(c) Sol-gel 3: Hydrolysis of titanium halides ($TiCl_4$ and TiF_4) with water. Some prepared via varied sol-gel routes, but would not focus their attention to the bone tissue compatibility aspects, like Uekawa et al. [170].
(d) Anode oxidation of metallic Ti: The redox potential of $Ti^{2+} + 2e^- \rightarrow Ti$ ($E = -1.63\ V + 0.0295\log\ (Ti^{2+})$ [1]) is out of the electrochemical window of water (reduction of H^+, $E = -0.059pH$ (V); reduction of O_2, $E = 1.229-0.059pH$ (V)). Moreover, necessity of breaking passivation requires a potential greater than ~2 V, and sometimes a high voltage (>100 V) enough to cause spark discharge is applied between the Ti (working electrode: anode) and the counter electrode (Pt or graphite, in common). Considerations are needed in the selection of electrolytes: the cations and anions must be chosen that would not be susceptible to reduction at the cathode (cations) and oxidation at anode (anions). In this regard, chloride salts sometimes are avoided because of possible oxidation to oxychloride ions.
(e) Chemical oxidation with hot alkali, H_2O_2, or oxidative acids like H_2SO_4.

Biocompatibility of titanium oxides is subjected to intensive studies since the oxides are formed on the surface of titanium and titanium alloy implants. Among many aspects of the compatibility, that with bone tissue became the most effortlessly examined in vitro after the use of SBF is mostly accepted to well reproduce the in vivo inorganic reactions under the in vitro conditions. Table 5.7 lists several examples of the works on the titania for the bone-bonding ability. The titania formation on metallic substrates via the routes (d) and (e) will be detailed in Sect. 5.4.4.

5.4.3.2 Titania Gels and Apatite Deposition In Vitro

In 1993, Li and de Groot conducted a pioneering study, in vitro and in vivo, on the bioactivity of titania [175]. They derived titania sol from the hydrolysis of $Ti(OPr^i)_4$ with HCl under the presence of ethylene glycol monoethylether. After dipcoating the sol onto commercially available pure Ti (cpTi) substrates, they calcined the films at 400–600 °C for 10 min. They found the calcined titania film deposit apatite within 2 weeks. They also applied the same procedure as above to coat Ti6Al4V implant pins with titania for an in vivo study to see if the gel layer should work expectedly. They implanted the titania coated pins into the femurs of mature goats for 12 weeks. An intermediate layer, composed of titania and calcium phosphate (CaP), was yielded between the titania layer and bone tissue, with which the CaP layer was directly and strongly bonded, that is, the push-out test broke the oxide layer. Therefore the sol-gel titania layer was concluded to play the expected role. Here, a wider intermediate layer was produced on the in vivo test piece than that on the in vitro piece. An energy-dispersive X-ray analysis showed smooth changes of the atomic concentration of Ti, Ca, and P in the implant–bone interface zone. This indicates that the CaP is formed within the titania layer [175]. Li et al. conducted a detailed study on the in vitro apatite deposition, using the same titania gel coated on cpTi substrates and calcined at 500 °C for 10 min [176]. The titania layer yielded apatite crystallite agglomerates within 3 days in SBF and was fully coated by a dense apatite layer within 7 days.

In addition, Li et al. prepared titania-fragmented gel (xero) pieces where they peptized commercially available titania sol with HCl and then evaporated the solvent at 80 °C out of the amorphous titania suspension. Then, they calcined those pieces at 450 °C for 2 h to obtain bulk titania [150]. Kumar et al. discussed the drying process leading to titania gel membrane [177], while Grosso et al. reviewed the evolution of self-assembled mesostructure due to evaporation [178]. Moreover, they developed the same titania suspension on silica glass substrates by dipcoating and calcined at 450 °C for 10 min to yield titania films. Both titania products deposited hemispherical agglomerates of apatite when soaked in SBF for 2 weeks. That is, they were bioactive [150]. Figure 5.7 shows the surface microstructure after soaked in SBF for 2 weeks. The hemispherical shape is common to the apatite agglomerates, but the number density seems larger for the titania film on the silica glass than for the bulk.

What causes those titania gels to become bioactive? In the calcium silicates [2, 5–7, 10], the sudden increase in the calcium ion concentration of SBF in the vicinity of the sample surface is one of the stimulating factors. Yet, this

Table 5.7 Several examples of titania gels and titania on titanium alloys studied from the biomedical viewpoints later than 1988: Titania sol films for tissue-bonding applications (AP: apatite deposition)

Titania types (coating tech, substrates, etc.)	Significance of the studies	References
Sol-gel layers and coatings		
Peptized titania sol; bulk, film	AP in SBFs	[150]
$Ti(OPr^i)_4$; dipcoat; 500 °C, 10 min	AP in SBF with cpTi; in vivo test with Ti6Al4V	[175]
$Ti(OPr^i)_4$; dipcoat; 500 °C, 10 min; cpTi	AP in SBF; local surface charges with affinity to Ca(II) or P(V)	[176]
$Ti(OPr^i)_4$; dipcoat; cpTi, silica glass	Pretreatment; substrate-gel bonding strength	[179]
$Ti(OPr^i)_4$; dipcoat; cpTi	Albumin and fibrinogen in SBF with retarded AP deposition	[180, 181]
$Ti(OPr^i)_4$; dipcoat; cpTi	AP in SBF; additives, heating	[184]
$Ti(OPr^i)_4$; dipcoat; cpTi	AP in SBF; aging	[186]
$(Ti, Si)O_2$, TiO_2; dipcoat; cpTi	AP in SBF; AFM surface topography	[185]
$Ti(OPr^i)_4$; HNO_3, AcAcH, DEA; dipcoat; SiO_2 glass	AP in SBF; An, An + Ru; topotaxy with HAp[a]	[187]
$Ti(OPr^i)_4$; dipcoat; cpTi	In vivo: subcutaneous implants; strong soft tissue attachment	[188]
$Ti(OPr^i)_4$; ethylene glycol: dipcoat; cpTi	An and Ru, Ap in 7 d/SBF; soft tissue attachment[b]	[189]
$Ti(OEt)_4$; dipcoat; cpTi	AP in SBF; DDS: anti-osteoporosis drug	[191]
Hydrolysis and condensation of titanium halides and sulfate		
Acid hydrolysis TiF_4; An on cpTi	Ap <5 days/SBF; 300–700 °C	[194]
Acid hydrolysis TiF_4; An on Ti, NiTi, SUS316L	Ap <5 days/SBF; 300 °C	[195]
$TiOSO_4/H_2O_2$ + hot water aging; cpTi	Ap <1 day/SBF	[196]
$TiOSO_4$; H_2O_2; cotton fibril	An and Ru, Ap <1day	[197]
$TiOSO_4$; HCl	Ru + trace An, Ap <1day	[190]
$TiCl_4$; cpTi, PTFE	Ru; Ap <2 days on Ru layer on PTFE; no difference in An and Ru	[198]
Titania on Ti with chemical treatments		
Okayama procedure: CHT		
H_2O_2 oxidation of Ti	•OH or O_2– radical scavenging	[125, 126]
H_2O_2; cpTi; $+TaCl_5$	AP in SBF	[239, 241]
H_2O_2, cpTi tibia pin	In vivo, shear and push-out force	[242]
H_2O_2/HCl, NaOH, air oxidation; cpTi	Comparing the treatments for in vitro bioactivity[c]	[250]
8.8 M H_2O_2 + 0.1 M HCl; 400–600 °C, 1h cpTi	Ap <3 days/SBF	[246]
30 mass% H_2O_2; natural oxide layer free cpTi	Ap 2 days/SBF; aging in H_2O at RT and 80 °C	[247]
H_2O_2/Ta; Ti mesh on rectangular Ti64 rod	In vivo (dog femoral implant)	[243]

(continued)

Table 5.7 (continued)

Titania types (coating tech, substrates, etc.)	Significance of the studies	References
8.8 MH_2O_2 + 0.1 MHCl; 80 °C, 30 min; 400 °C, 1 h: cpTi	Mechanical attrition provided nanopores	[244]
Autoclaving, in 3 % H_2O_2: Ti6Al4V/ abraded[d]	Improved cytochrome C adsorption and MC3T3-E1 proliferation	[245]
Toxicity: TiO_2 NPs		[192]
GRAPE®		
Air oxidation	Ap on contact surface, negative for anodized surface	[250, 251]
Kyoto procedure: NaOH + HT		
5 and 10 M NaOH or KOH on Ti and alloys[e]	AP in SBF	[199]
10 M NaOH, 60 °C, 24 h + 600 °C, 1 h; Ti and alloys	AP in SBF; effective for pure Ti, Ti–6Al–4V, Ti–6Al–2Nb–Ta, and Ti–15Mo–5Zr–3Al, not for SUS or Co–Cr–Mo	[200]
0.1–10 M NaOH; cpTi	AP in SBF; effects of NaOH conc. and period	[201]
5 M NaOH; cpTi	AP in SBF; heating temperature effects	[202]
Alkali and HT (5 M NaOH)[f]	XPS; TiO–Na to Ti–OH	[203]
	TEM-EDX; TiO–Na to Ti–OH	[204]
0.2 or 0.5 MNaOH, 60 °C, 24h; Ta	AP <7days in SBF; sodium tantalate gel	[147]
	In vivo: rat tibiae; weak bond at 8 weeks, strong bond at 16 weeks	[149]
5 M NaOH[f] + hot water aging; cpTi	In vivo; aging promoted bone-bonding than without aging	[205]
5 MNaOH[f] + aging in H_2O; cpTi	AP in SBF; improved by hot water aging; $NaTiO_3$–>An	[206]
HCl–alkali + HT; porous cpTi scaffolds	Highest osteoconduction among AH, water-AH, and HCl-AH[g]	[207]
	Dental applications	[214]
AH (5 M NaOH) + aging in H_2O, 0.5 mM HCl	Partial removal of Na stimulated Ap deposition in SBF: confirmed	[208]
5 MNaOH + aging in $CaCl_2$ + HT + aging in H_2O	Better in vitro bioactivity	[210]
5 M NaOH + (10 mM HCl, HNO_3, H_2SO_4) + HT	Better in vitro bioactivity; the surface positive charges	[209]
Ca-less (<5 ppm) 5 M NaOH; cpTi	AP in SBF; importance of Ca-less NaOH as the etchant	[218]
(1–5 M) NaOH (60 °C, 24 h) + aging in $CaCl_2$ + HT + aging in H_2O; Ti–36Nb–2Ta–3Zr–0.3O	$CaTi_2O_5$ induces Ap in SBF	[211]
5 M NaOH[f]; cpTi	HT under air, Ar flow, vacuum: Na sublime to decrease bioactivity	[215]
5 M NaOH[f]; Ti6Al4V	An appropriate surface topography and pore architecture[h]	[216]
5 M NaOH[f]; cpTi	Alumina and SiC blasting: alumina accelerates, SiC inhibits apatite deposition	[217]

(continued)

Table 5.7 (continued)

Titania types (coating tech, substrates, etc.)	Significance of the studies	References
Chubu–Kyoto procedure		
H_2SO_4 + HCl (1:1 mass); 70 °C; + heating[i]; cpTi	In vitro: bioactivity in SBF from the surface positive charges not from surface roughness or rutile; in vivo: bone contact	[219]
HCl/H_2SO_4; + heating[i]; porous cpTi scaffold	In vivo: highest bone ingrowth for the acid + heating treatment; Ap in vivo due to the positive surface charge	[220]
Electrochemical oxidation of Ti and alloys		
Anode oxidation + $Ca(OH)_2$; cpTi[j]	AP in SBF	[226]
Anode/155 V, 1 M H_2SO_4; + HT; cpTi[c]	In vivo; direct bond to bone; No diff. from Na-free alkali and HT	[228]
Anode/90, 155, 180 V; 0.5–3 M H_2SO_4; cpTi	Ap in 3 d/SBF; An and Ru; HT stimulated	[227]
Anode/30 V + 600 °C; Ti6A14V	Ru + An; SBF: no Ap on heat treated	[229]
Anode/65–100 V; varied solutes and pH (1–13); cpTi	In vivo; good bone contact for 20–55 °C H_2O-contact angle[k]	[230]
Anode/discharge: 416 mA/cm^2, 1 M NaCl; cpTi	Antimicrobial activity; better proliferation of primary osteoblasts	[234]
Combination		
5 M NaOH, 60 °C, 24 h + electrochemical	Electrodeposited HAp layer: $Ca(NO_3)_2$ + $NH_4H_2PO_4$, pH 6	[225]
HCl/H_2SO_4 + boiling 0.2 M NaOH (two steps)	CaP dep.; Ca-supersaturated solution	[222]
HCl/H_2SO_4 + 6 M NaOH (two steps); 10 M NaOH; 60 °C, 24h + 600 °C: cpTi foam[l]	Ap-coated implants; in vivo; no difference in osteoconduction and induction between the two treatments	[224]
30 % HNO_3, 30 min + 5 M NaOH, 60 °C, 24h + HT: 600 °C (two steps): Ti–6Al–7Nb	Alkali + HT or HNO_3 + alkali + HT were active. Unclear effects of Na	[221]
HCl + 10 M NaOH, 60 °C, 24 h	Better ability than the alkali treatment	[223]

[a] *AcAcH* acetyl acetone, *DEA* diethanolamine, *An* anatase, *Ru* rutile, *HAp* hydroxyapatite
[b] *An* anatase, *Ru* rutile
[c] Spark discharge happened at >105 V. HT, heating
[d] 121 °C, 0.2 MPa, 20 min
[e] Ti–6A1–4V, Ti–6A1–2Nb-Ta, and Ti–15Mo–5Zr–3A1
[f] Kyoto procedure: 5 M NaOH, 60 °C, 24 h before heating (HT) up to 600 °C at 5 °C/min, kept for 1 hcpTi (commercially available pure titanium)
[g] Porous Ti via the plasma-spray procedure; A, 5 M NaOH, 60 °C for 24 h; H, +600 °C, 1 h; water-AH, A + aging in H_2O at 40 °C for 48 h + H; HCl-AH, A + aging in 0.5 M HCl at 40 °C for 24 h + aging in H_2O at 40 °C for 24 h
[h] Appropriate roughness (alumina gritting): Ra 0.56 μm, and face-centered cubic type 3D glides with spatial gaps of 200–700 μm
[i] 66.6 % H_2SO_4, 10.6 % HCl (mass%)
[j] The electrode polarization change (sample = cathode)
[k] Not given: the cathode–anode distance
[l] cpTi foam, 74.3 % porous; 18 % HCl + 48 % H_2SO_4; Ap coating in SBF

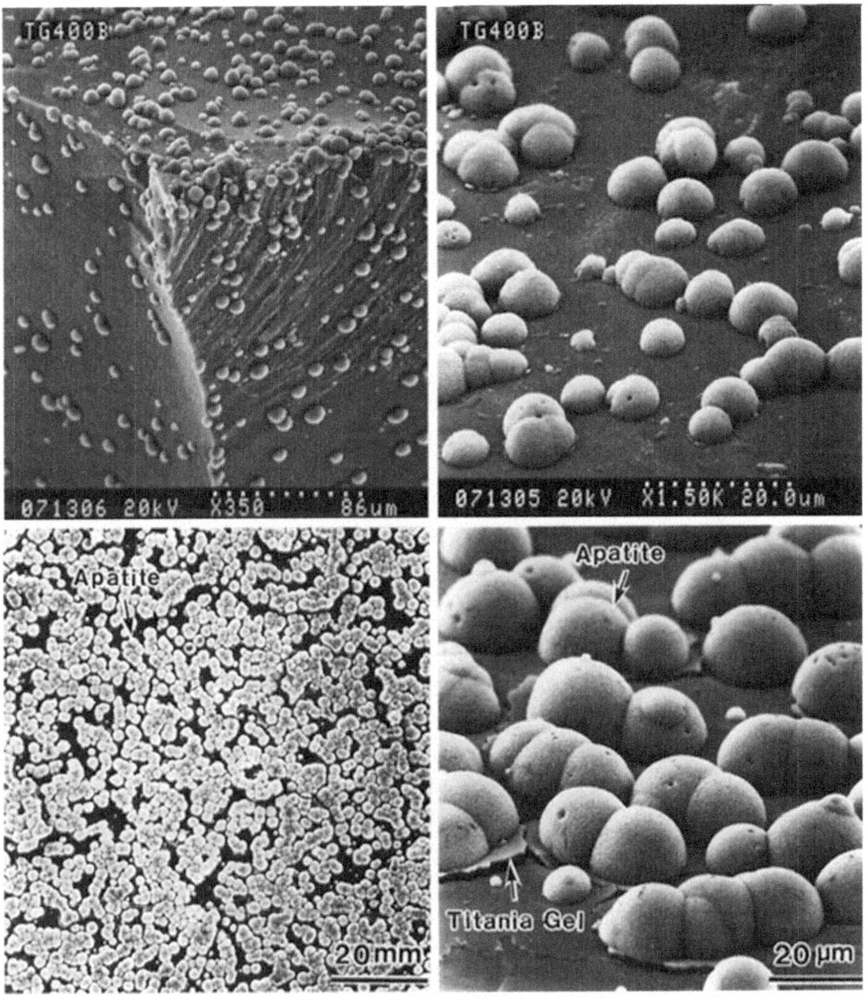

Fig. 5.7 Scanning electron micrographs of hemispherical agglomerates of apatite deposited on titania gel: (*top row*) bulk titania gel; (*bottom row*) titania layer developed on silica glass. See text for the sol and calcining conditions (Reproduced from Ref. [150] by permission of John Wiley & Sons Ltd.)

effect is never applicable to titania as it is a single oxide. Li et al. considered, though primitively, the hydrated surface of the titania bulk and films induced the heterogeneous nucleation of apatite [150] as in the cases of niobium and tantalum, and zirconium oxide gels, already described above in Sect. 5.4.2.

Significance of the bonding strength is never stressed too much. Patsi et al. compared the effects of pretreatments of cpTi on the substrate-titania gel bonding strength [179]. They found that pre-corrosion with NaOH, titanium nitride coating, or ground gave good adhesion and fracture took at the glue–coating interface. It seems reasonable that the alkali treatment was greatly successful in providing Ti and Ti alloys with apatite-forming ability, according to Kokubo et al. [143, 144], as described in Sect. 5.4.5.

5.4.3.3 Apatite-Depositing Ability Depends on the Sol-Gel Routes

Addition of some physiological substances to SBF or other test solution may lead to an improved evaluation of in vitro behavior of those oxide gels. In a preliminary study, Areva and Lindén [180] pretreated cpTi substrates with 5 M NaOH at 60 °C for 24 h and heated at 600 °C for 1 h, following Kokubo et al. [143, 144]. They then soaked those substrates for up to 14 days in SBF with 1,000 ppm bovine serum albumin (BSA) and fibrinogen (Fib) and examined the bioactivity. They found that the BSA addition completely inhibited apatite deposition, while the addition of Fib reduces the apatite deposition. Areva et al. [181] examined the effects of the BSA and Fib addition on the apatite deposition onto the sol-gel-derived titania-coating layer on cpTi substrates. They dipcoated the precursor sol from the system, consisting of $Ti(OPr^i)_4$ (Pr^i: 2-propyl group), HCl, ethanol, and H_2O, and then calcined the substrates at 500 °C for 10 min before soaking in SBF up to 14 days. The protein concentration in SBF was 1 mg/mL for BSA and 0.1 mg/mL for Fib. Areva et al. found that both serum proteins retarded the apatite deposition as evidenced by the X-ray diffraction and P(V) concentration of SBF. The results regarding the BSA addition seemed contradicting: the NaOH-corroded cpTi found inert in the BSA-added SBF. They did not touch upon the apparent discrepancy in the behavior of the titania gels, derived from the NaOH corrosion and from the sol-gel procedure. Yet, the situation seems similar to the different behaviors of tantalum metal implants in vitro and in vivo [148, 149].

It seems reasonable that the behavior of titania depends on how it is derived and in which solution or media it is examined. Actually, the presence of proteins may affect in a few different ways the apatite deposition. Both BSA and Fib are acid proteins and are negatively charged under the physiological pH. Thus, they are electrostatically interacted with the calcium ions if they form nuclei with the phosphate ions. That is, those proteins would not disturb Ca(II) to be captured at the nucleating sites, but might have a good chance to decrease the rate of growth of calcium phosphate phases. Approving a model that fibrinogen, though negatively charged, would be interacted with Ti–OH groups at the subdomains with positive charges [182, 183], one might interpret those results differently. Would the results suggest that such titania layers should have similar depressing effects in vivo or would they be limited to titania and not the case for silica layers? The implants surely encounter those physiological substances when implanted, and they are adsorbed on the surface. Would their in vitro results be pertinent to the behavior of the implants in vivo? None has given definite and proper answers to those questions.

Peltola et al. [184] examined the effects of an additive (valeric acid) in the titania sol from $Ti(OPr^i)_4$ and a few pretreatment of cpTi substrates following Pätsi et al. [179]. The highest ability was achieved by the titania layer derived from the sol with the valeric acid addition and calcined 600 °C, or the sol-gel coating from the precursor sol without valeric acid, and calcined at 450–550 °C. Further, Jokinen et al. pointed out the importance of roughness or topography of the (Si, Ti)O_2 and TiO_2 gel films [185]. Peltola et al. [186] dipcoated cpTi substrates with the titania sols from $Ti(OPr^i)_4$, different in both aging time and iteration of coating (five layers in maximum), while all samples were heated at 500 °C for 10 min. The aging time was recorded before the top layer was coated. Apatite deposited in SBF first with 3-layer coating and 24 h aging, followed by 5-layer coatings, regardless of the aging time. With atomic force microscopy analysis, they suggested that the topography of the outermost surface was an important factor for the activity. They also pointed out the importance of surface topography. Uchida et al. [187], in contrast, compared the lattice structure of the titania gels, derived by the hydrolysis and condensation of $Ti(OPr^i)_4$, under the presence of HNO_3 (Ti–NO), acetyl acetone (Ti–AC), and diethanolamine (Ti–DE). Both Ti–NO and Ti–AC consisted only of amorphous titania on calcination at 300 °C; when calcined at 500 °C or above, the anatase was precipitated. Ti–DE remained amorphous on calcination at 500 °C and consisted of amorphous titania and anatase at 600 °C and of amorphous phase and rutile when calcined at 700 and 800 °C. The tendency of apatite formation was very similar among Ti–DE (500 °C), Ti–NO (500–800 °C), and Ti–AC (500–800 °C), while Ti–DE (700, 800 °C) gave greater numbers of smaller agglomerates than the others. Amorphous gels were inert, regardless of the additives. Uchida et al. suggested that anatase is superior in stimulating apatite deposition because Ti–DE (500 °C), Ti–NO (500–800 °C), and Ti–AC (500–800 °C) all involve anatase and an amorphous phase. They attempted to interpret from the lattice matching (topotaxy) between the anatase and apatite lattices. According to their calculation, the anatase–apatite pair has slightly better matching (1.0 and 1.4 %) for the 110 plane of anatase and 0001 plane of apatite than the rutile–apatite pair (0.5 and 2.5 %) for rutile 101 plane and the 0001 one of apatite.

5.4.3.4 In Vivo Responses of Sol-Gel-Derived Titania Gels

Following seemingly standardized procedure of fabricating titania gel, Areva et al. [188] prepared the titania gel layer on cpTi via dipcoating the titania sol, derived from the hydrolysis and condensation of $Ti(OPr^i)_4$, under the presence of ethylene glycol monoethylether, and catalyzed by HCl [164]. When they implanted subcutaneously in the back of rats and under the periosteum in the skull area, they confirmed a direct attachment of soft tissues on to the substrates. Here, Areva et al. conclusively remarked that the titania coatings can initiate the reactions that lead to tissue bonding by directly adsorbing the useful physiological species from the plasma. In contrast, bioresorbable coatings may have good connections to the bone tissue, whereas the underlying inert substrate should be exposed in a long term, and the implant–tissue bonds will be deteriorated soon or later. Thus, they insist, better results can be obtained with non-resorbable coatings, but the coating should be reactive with the target tissue. Rossi et al. then compared the soft tissue adhesion on anatase and rutile layers [189]. The titania sol was prepared in the same way as employed by Jokinen [164, 185] and dipcoated on cpTi discs. Calcination of the discs gave anatase-coated implants, while CO_2 laser treatment yielded rutile-coated ones. However, histological analysis could not detect any difference in soft tissue attachment between the two kinds of implants. No difference in the in vitro bioactivity was observed either between the anatase- and rutile-coated specimens, as found by Zhao et al. [190]: this result is inconsistent with Uchida et al. [187]. Recently, Harmankaya et al. coated mesoporous titania file on bone screw and impregnated anti-osteoporosis drugs [191]. The titania sols, aforedescribed, are equally applicable to drug carriers, but Liu et al. warned about toxic aspects of titania nanoparticles (NPs) [192].

5.4.3.5 Hydrolysis–Condensation of Some Inorganic Salts of Titanium

Titanium tetrahalides TiX_4 yield TiO_2 and an associated acid as:

$$TiX_4 + 6H_2O \rightarrow TiO_2 + 4H_3O^+ + 4X^- \tag{5.16}$$

With partial hydrolysis,

$$TiX_4 + 6H_2O \rightarrow TiOX_2 + 4H_3O^+ + 2X^- \tag{5.17}$$

$$TiOSO_4 + 3H_2O \rightarrow TiO_2 + 2H_3O^+ + SO_4{}^{2-} \tag{5.18}$$

The by-product HX ($H_3O^+ + X^-$) may promote hydration of the depositing oxide, and if X = F, the fluoride ions should even corrode substrates assisted with H_3O^+. It might be suspected that the fluoride ions remaining in the oxide layer even after rinsing may retard the apatite formation by scavenging the calcium ions to precipitate CaF_2. Titanyl sulfate is subjected to similar hydrolysis procedure under the presence of HCl to form titania layers and release sulfate ions. If those acid by-products can fiercely corrode the surfaces of substrates or even deteriorate them, then the procedure will not be ideal for those substrates. However, those acids might favor the ion attachment and nucleation of apatite if the corrosive activity does not exceed a certain degree.

Shimizu et al. [193] coated not only borosilicate glass slide but also synthetic polymers, such as polyethylene, polypropylene, poly(vinyl alcohol), poly(methyl methacrylate), and so forth with anatase thin films, using TiF_4-based aqueous solutions. Wu et al. [194] followed them to prepare TiF_4–HCl solution, into which they soaked cpTi substrates, after removing surface natural oxide layer with HF–HNO_3. They found two anatase layers after calcination at 300–700 °C for 1 h: the bottom layer was dense and strongly adhered to the substrate, while the outer layer was porous and loosely bound to the bottom layer. The bimodal microstructure evolution is explainable from the concentration change in Ti(IV) in the solution:

high concentration of Ti(IV) at earlier stages enabled vigorous nucleation to result in the dense bottom layer, while lower concentrations in the later stages would not favor crystallization. Calcining at 800 °C yielded rutile and anatase, but the rutile was the result of air oxidation at high-temperature treatment. When soaked in SBF, those titania layers induced apatite deposition nicely, even heating to 800 °C showed apatite within 7 days. Interestingly, the apatite was discovered to crystallize at the bottom layer. This procedure was applicable to coat metallic substrates such as NiTi, Ta, and SUS 316 [195].

5.4.3.6 Hydrolysis of Titanyl Sulfate ($TiOSO_4$) and $TiCl_4$

Titanyl sulfate also yielded titania layers on hydrolysis under acidic conditions with HCl [190] or with H_2O_2 [196]. With weaker corrosive activity, $TiOSO_4$ is superior for titania coating on chemically fragile substrates. Cotton fibrils were coated with titania (anatase and rutile) in a dilute (30 mM) aqueous solution of $TiOSO_4$ and H_2O_2. The titania-cotton fibrils deposited apatite within 1 day to yield cotton–titania–apatite composites when soaked in SBF [197]. Moreover, Wu et al. demonstrated that the titania from the hydrolysis of $TiCl_4$ can coat poly(tetrafluorethylene) (PTFE) to provide with bioactivity [198].

5.4.4 Titania Surface Layers on Ti and Alloys via Chemical and Electrochemical Treatments

Oxidation of metals proceeds in air under the ambient conditions. Titanium and titanium alloys, like other heavy metals, experience passivation to form a chemically stable oxide thin layer. Corrosion by oxidative acids such as HNO_3, H_2SO_4, and H_2O_2 or by caustic alkali hydroxides yields hydrated titania gel layers, as well as anode oxidation in an electrochemical cell. When considering for implant applications, especially when the load-bearing implant ones are considered, any surface modification of the implants should be avoided if it reduces the mechanical strength causing too much corrosions with deeper roughness. This section introduces only a few kinds of procedure: the NaOH treatment with subsequent heating (Kyoto U procedure), $H_2SO_4 + HCl$ treatment (Chubu–Kyoto procedure), H_2O_2 treatment (Okayama U procedure), and GRAPE (GRoove and APatitE) treatment.

5.4.4.1 NaOH Treatment (AL–H Treatment; Kyoto U Procedure)

The group led by Kokubo and Nakamura at Kyoto University employed NaOH to provide surface titania layer on titanium and titanium alloys. In previous works carried out in 1996 and 1997, they tried NaOH and KOH aqueous solutions with various concentrations ranging between 0.1 and 10 M and different lengths of the treatment and temperature at chemical and heating treatments [199–202]. The alkali and heat treatment (hereafter denoted as A and H treatment) procedure was standardized: treating the substrates with 5 M NaOH solution at 60 °C for 24 h, and subsequent heating at 600 °C for 1 h. Using X-ray photoelectron spectroscopy (XPS) [203] and transmission electron microscopy with energy-dispersive X-ray analysis (TEN-EDX) [204], Takadama et al. analyzed the surface of the titanium substrate after the standard alkali and heating treatment and gave the following conclusive remarks:

1. The NaOH solution corroded the titanium/alloys to yield a Na-containing gel.
2. The layer was crystallized into $NaTiO_3$ and rutile when heat treated at 600 °C.
3. The ion exchange took place to yield Ti–OH and free sodium ions when the specimen is soaked in SBF or under plasma (see Eqs. 5.14 or 5.15 for Zr or Ta).
4. The Ti–OH groups interacted with the calcium ions in the vicinity to form a calcium titanate.
5. The calcium titanate incorporated the phosphate ions and calcium ions to form apatite nuclei. Those steps are vital until the nucleation takes place.
6. The nuclei grew into apatite crystallites of macroscopic sizes by consuming the component ions.

This treatment was also applicable to tantalum as described above [147–149]. It is common to try to remove the sodium ions out of the sodium titanate layer before implanting, because if the Ti–OH is the key species and should appear on the surface, it takes certain time for the removal of Na due to hydrolysis. Indeed, Fujibayashi et al. aged the alkali- and heat-treated titanium specimens before using them for an in vivo test [205]. Uchida et al. confirmed in vitro the effects of hot water aging to stimulate the apatite deposition [206]. A more effective way to remove Na is to expose the heat-treated samples to HCl [207, 208] or other acids, like HNO_3 and H_2SO_4 [209]. The removal of the sodium ions also reduces a concern, as Pattanayak described [209], that the sodium titanate formed by this treatment may have an undesirable effect on living cells in the narrow spaces of the porous material by releasing Na^+ ions. Additional aging in $CaCl_2$ solution and in water also boosted A and H procedure [210].

Furthermore, Yamaguchi et al. took multistep procedure, the alkali treatment, aging in $CaCl_2$ solution, heating, and aging in water for gum metal (Ti–36Nb–2Ta–3Zr–0.3O) [211], and reported that $CaTi_2O_5$ induced apatite deposition in SBF. Yamaguchi et al. [212] and Fukuda et al. [213] also pointed out the significance of the calcium ions on the metal surface oxide layer. The success of the alkali and heat treatment stimulated many researchers to verify the effects or to propose some improvements in the methodology. Fawzy et al. [214] attempted to apply this A and H treatment and Na-removing processes to dental materials. Ravelingien et al. [215] attempted to control the surface Na content due to sublimation of Na_2O, accompanying Ti_2O_3 formation, by heating the alkali-treated specimens under flowing Ar or under reduced pressure. They also assembled Ti6Al4V fibers into 3-dimensional lattice or grids with simple-tetragonal (st) and face-centered (fc) arrangements and treated them with the A and H procedure [216]. The coverage by apatite was greater for the fc arrangement than for the st one. When the alloy plate specimens with different surface roughness were subjected to soaking in SBF after the A and H treatment, the specimen with a proper roughness Ra $\sim$0.56 μm was found highly active in comparison to those with others. They concluded the importance of surface topography and pore architecture for the in vitro bioactivity. Another example of phenomenological examination on the surface roughness was reported by Aparicio et al. [217]. They compared the effects of blasting with alumina and with SiC before A and H treatment on the bioactivity: The alumina blasting accelerated apatite nucleation but the SiC blasting inhibited it. Even if different microroughness was introduced by the alumina and SiC blasting, the 5 M NaOH treatment at 60 °C for 24 h should level out the difference. Moreover, bombardments by alumina and SiC particles would not always yield the same mechanical effects on the metal surface, which may lead to different corrosive reactions by the NaOH treatment. Aparicio et al. considered the importance of the concave parts caused by the trace of the blasting. However, more experiments under much refined conditions seemed necessary before any definite conclusions might be elucidated because too many factors are hindered behind such mechanical treatments including sandpaper roughening or mirror polishing.

5.4.4.2 Two-Step Procedure: Acid and Alkali (Chubu–Kyoto Scheme) or Acid and Heating (Leiden Scheme)

Though the Kyoto U procedure has enjoyed great success in providing metallic implant (Ti and a few titanium alloys) bone-bonding ability, somewhat different opinions have been delivered these days. After Kizuki et al. [218], the ratio of solution volume to the specimen surface area was a factor to control the bioactivity of the substrates. That is, the optimum ratio was in the range 5 ml of 5 M NaOH and 20 ml versus $1 \times 1 \times 0.1$ cm^3 sample. Their study indicated that the calcium impurity in the NaOH source should be less than 1.5 ppm. They considered that the impurity calcium became concentrated to reduce the amount of active $NaTiO_3$. Admitting the apparent observation on the apatite deposition on the surface treated with Ca $<$ 1.5 ppm, it would contradict the fact that the $CaCl_2$ treatment favors the apatite deposition [210, 211].

Moreover, in a recent article [209], Pattanayak et al. stressed the importance of positively charged surfaces to induce the apatite nucleation. The efficacy of the Kyoto U procedure has been explained as the following: the titania layer first adsorbs calcium ions and then phosphate and calcium ions leading to nucleation and growth of apatite [203, 204]. A different way of explanation [209, 219, 220] is recently proposed for the effects of the A and H treatment, that is, the hydrated titania layers with many Ti–OH are positively charged, and the charges attract, in turn, phosphate ions first, then calcium ions in the vicinity of the oxide layers. In addition, the

Chubu–Kyoto group seems abandoning the traditional A and H treatment, partly because, as described in [219], the apatite-forming ability of titanium implants subjected to the A and H treatment is lost by the Ti–ONa and H_3O^+ ion exchange when they are stored for extended periods of time under humid environment. Thus, the group favors a newer acid and heat treatment technique. Kokubo et al. [219] soaked the cpTi specimen first in a mixed acid solution, containing 66.3 % H_2SO_4 and 10.6 % HCl (mass%) in 1:1 mass ratio, at 70 °C for 1 h, followed by heating the specimen at 400–800 °C for 1 h. The first treatment is basically an etching treatment to remove the surface natural oxide layer, to oxidize the fresh surface to yield a hydrated oxide layer. According to the microstructure observation under a scanning electron microscope and the X-ray diffraction profiles, the optimum heating temperature was in the range between 400 and 650 °C, while heating at 700 °C greatly reduced the activity. Since positive zeta potential values were detected for the acid-treated samples when they were subjected to heating, Kokubo et al. concluded that the positively charged titania surface should induce apatite nucleation and deposition. Kawai et al. [220] applied this acid and heating treatment to a porous titanium scaffold, and from their in vivo test, they confirmed that the scaffold subjected to this two-step treatment achieved the highest bone ingrowth.

In consequence, one has observed that the A and H treatment and the two-step treatment (acid and heating) both are equally effective to provide titanium implants with apatite-forming ability, although the bilateral explanations are proposed; the negatively or positively charged surface favors it. It should be emphasized here that the surface roughness or the types of the titania phases are not the primary factors [220].

Spriano et al. tried another multistep treatment [221] for Ti6Al7Nb alloy, involving the alkali treatment as the basis: (1) mechanical treatments (mirror polishing or sandblasting), combined with the alkali treatment (5 M NaOH at 60 °C, 24, 2), and heating at 600, 700, and 800 °C for 1 and 3 h), and (2) the polishing or sandblasting, forming passivation layer with 30 % HNO_3, and heating at 600 °C, 1 h. In short, they examined the mechanical pretreatments, but they have nothing to do with the bioactivity as far as the roughness remained moderate. Important was the passivation treatment between the mechanical and alkali treatments, according to the report.

Another combination of acid and alkali treatments was proposed from Leiden by Wen et al. [222], where a mixed acid treatment with HCl/H_2SO_4 was combined with 0.2 M NaOH at 140 °C. The two-step treatment induced apatite in 2 days in SBF. A similar study was conducted by Jonásová et al. [223] to confirm that a combination of acid etching with HCl (no concentration disclosed) and 10 M NaOH treatment at 60 °C for 24 h favored apatite deposition within 2 days in SBF in contrast to the single alkali treatment, for which apatite appeared in 10 days. Zhao et al. [224] compared two sets of treatments: acid–alkali (AA) and alkali–heat (AH); they used a mixture of 18 % HCl + 48 % H_2SO_4 for the acid treatment and 6 M NaOH for the alkali treatment at 70 °C for 5 h. For the alkali–heat treatment, they employed 10 M NaOH at 60 °C for 24 h, while heating was conducted at

Table 5.8 Examples of organic and inorganic components for hybridization

Components	Biodegradable hybrids	Sustainable hybrids
Polymers	Natural polymers	Synthetic polymers
	Chitosan, gelatin, collagen	PDMS, poly(lactic acid)
Inorganic	X–Z(OR)$_3$: Z = Si, Ti, etc.	
	OR: alkoxy groups	
	X: vinyl, glycidoxy, methacryloxy, or amino group	
Additives	Poly(ethylene oxide), poly(ethylene glycol), Copolymers like PEO–PPO–PEO	
Applications		
Solid bodies	Resorbable fillers	Tissue defect fillers
Porous bodies	Scaffolds	Scaffolds
	Tissue guides	Bioreactors
Beads, granules	Drug delivery	Fillers
Sheets, films	Protector of cell invasion	
Tubes, fibrils	Wound healing agents	Fillers
Coatings	Tissue guides	Tissue guides
Gelling sols, gels	Injectable sols	Injectable sols
	Carriers	Tissue defect fillers
	Tissue defect fillers	

600 °C for 1 h. Zhao et al. subjected those treatments onto porous titanium scaffolds. AA yielded greater apatite formation than AH. Yet, no histological difference was found in osteoconductivity between the two apatite-coated implants with A and AH pretreatments [224].

5.4.4.3 Electrochemical (Anode) Oxidation of Ti and Alloys

Many anode oxidation studies for bioactive surfaces were conducted. Table 5.8 lists only a few [225–232]. Electrodeposition is one of the direct apatite coatings. On the anode, hydrated titania deposited

$$\text{Anode}: Ti + 2H_2O \rightarrow TiO_2\,(aq) + 4H^+ + 4e^- \quad (5.19)$$

On the cathode water evolves hydrogen and hydroxyl groups (Eq. 5.20). If the reactions went under calm conditions, calcium hydroxide should be precipitated on the cathode (Eq. 5.21):

Cathode:

$$2H_2O + 2e^- \rightarrow H_2 + 2OH^-\,(aq) \quad (5.20)$$

$$Ca^{2+}\,(aq) + 2OH^-\,(aq) \rightarrow Ca(OH)_2 \quad (5.21)$$

That is, anode oxidation of Ti cannot be conducted without accompanying water decomposition. Adding Eqs. 5.19 and 5.20 yields the total electrode reaction:

$$Ti + 2H_2O \rightarrow TiO_2\,(aq)\,[anode] + 2\,H_2\,[cathode] \quad (5.22)$$

When a greater voltage was loaded, the hydrogen agitated the solution nearby and the hydroxide would not deposit on the electrode. Most of them [227–230] employed one-cell system with two electrodes in an electrolyte solution, just like that for simple electrolysis practiced in primary schools. Therefore, the actual anode potential over the electrolyte solution or any reference redox electrode remained uncertain. Moreover, they loaded high voltages between the working electrode (Ti and alloys) and counter electrode (Pt), say around 100 V or more. For example, Yang et al. [227] employed 90–180 V and 0.5–3 M H_2SO_4, combined with the heating at 600 °C, 1 h, and found spark discharge at loads >105 V, regardless of the electrolyte concentration. Yamamoto et al. [230] anodized cpTi at 65 to 100 V under various electrolytes. Yang et al. showed [227] that anatase and rutile layers from several combinations of voltage, heating (600 °C, 1 h), and concentration of the electrolyte (0.5–3 M) had good apatite deposition capability, and the 180 V treatment yielded active rutile layer, though the layer of anatase from the 90 V anodization was inert. The layer derived from the higher-voltage anodization was three-dimensionally microporous, and such morphology was suggested necessary for the bioactivity. Liang et al. [228] showed that the micropores in the rutile and anatase layer derived from anodizing cpTi at 155 V in 1 M H_2SO_4 penetrated the oxide layer down to the interface between the substrate and the oxide. From their in vivo test and histological analysis, the titania layer was as active as the alkali-free oxide layer from the A and H treatment [143, 144, 204–207]. They found little bone ingrowth into the micropores or apatite-like layer formation only on the oxide surface. Zhao et al. [229] applied 30 V electrolysis (1 M H_2SO_4) to Ti6Al4V together with subsequent heating at 600 °C for 1 h. The surface rutile and anatase layer showed a three-dimensional microporous structure, whose scanning electron micrographs seem very similar to those presented by Liang et al. [228]. Zhao et al. [229] found that heating reduced the in vitro bioactivity and attributed this reduction to a less number of Ti–OH on the surface oxide layer. Since the high voltages result in highly roughened anode surface, Yamamoto et al. [230] took note on the surface roughness of cpTi, introduced by several combinations of electrolysis factors: the electrolyzing voltage (70 to 150 V), electrolytes including inorganic and organic acids, inorganic salts like Na_2SO_4 and $NaHPO_4$, their concentration, and pH of the solution. They obtained only anatase layers on the cpTi substrates regardless of their electrolysis conditions. Their in vivo tests indicated that the optimum amount of bone-tissue was given by the layers with water-contact angle between 20° and 30° that were created by the electrolysis in 0.1 M H_2SO_4 and 0.1 M H_3PO_4 at 100 V. The second optimum amount was attained by the layers with the contact angle between 40° and 50°, derived from the electrolysis of 0.1 M NaOH and 0.1 M KOH at 80 V. Iwai-Yoshida et al. also reported the advantage of anode oxidation of cpTi under

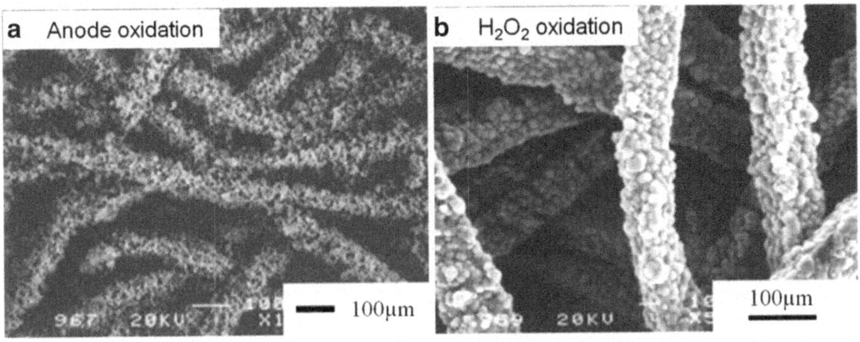

Fig. 5.8 Apatite deposition on Ti thin wire mat (50 μm fibrils) when soaked in Kokubo's SBF for 3 days. (**a**) Electrochemical treatment: 9.5 V, 1 h (anode); − 2.0 V, 0.5 h (cathode). (**b**) Chemically treated with 6 %H_2O_2/1 mM $TaCl_5$, 24 h, and subsequently heated at 400 °C 1 h

discharging in 1 M Na_2HPO_4 [231]. It is reasonable then that UV irradiation keeps the biological activity of the anode- or acid-oxidized titania with oxide layers from aging [232, 233].

In contrast, Osaka et al. [226] set up a standard system consisting of three electrodes in two cells and a salt bridge: Ti and Pt were the working electrode and the counter electrode in the main cell, respectively, and Ag/AgCl was the reference electrode in the subcell. Both cells held 1 M calcium nitrate as the electrolyte and are connected with a salt bridge. The Ti (working electrode) was positively polarized at +9.5 V versus the Ag/AgCl. Unfortunately, after Osaka et al. [224], the titania deposited on cathode was found too inert. Then they changed the polarity of the titanium electrode at –2.0 V versus Ag/AgCl to make it as an cathode, so that the calcium ions could be deposited on it as $Ca(OH)_2$ according to Eq. 5.21. However, the hydroxide soon changed to carbonate, to which the layer Osaka et al. attributed the highest bioactivity of their electrochemical treatment: the induction time of apatite deposition was ~12 h. The advantage of their electrodeposition of titania and calcium hydroxide at low voltages is that the treatment is applicable to titanium thin wire grids or thin wire mats, as indicated in Fig. 5.8.

Shibata et al. [234] focused their attention on retaining biological activities like osteoconduction on the surfaces of titania layer from degrading. They set an electrolysis cell with cpTi as the working electrode, SUS as the counter electrode, and 0.1 M Na_2HPO_4 and NaCl as the electrolytes, with spark discharge voltage. The anode-oxidized titanium substrates showed a high adhesion of primary calvarial osteoblasts and enhancement of the osteoblast phenotype, without time-dependent degradation of in vitro biological ability due to adsorbed organic impurities. Shibata et al. preferred NaCl as the electrolyte, because of its better antimicrobial activity, which they attributed to more reactive oxygen species to be generated on the surface. Att et al. [235] recognized this degradation by adsorption of hydrocarbons on titanium oxide surface, derived from acid etching with 67 % (w/w) sulfuric acid (H_2SO_4) at 120 °C for 75 s. Regarding the effects of nano- or microtopography on cell proliferation and osteointegration, Khang et al. conducted detailed experiments in terms of fibronectin adsorption, stem cell culture, and attachment, using titanium film developed on slide glass by the electron-beam evaporation technique [236]. They pointed out that nano- to submicron hybrid roughness was the one responsible for promoting osteoblast differentiation, initiating integrin activation and accelerating cyclin expression. In addition, they observed significant reorganization of cytoskeletons for surface height of 2–4 nm.

5.4.4.4 Hydrogen Peroxide Oxidation of Ti

Interactions of titanium and hydrogen peroxide had been long investigated before Tengvall et al. [237, 238] presented the effects of titanium oxide to quenching hydroxyl radicals from inflammation, and Walivaara et al. reported that the H_2O_2-treated titanium adsorbed not only plasma proteins and anti-fibrinogen but also calcium ions. Ohtsuki et al. [239] were inspired by those preceding works and studied the in vitro behavior of H_2O_2-oxidized cpTi substrates. They found the as-oxidized substrate with amorphous titania to be inert in terms of in vitro apatite deposition in SBF. Yet, a couple of additives improved the activity, i.e., Ta(V) and Sn(IV), in the order: $SnCl_2 < TaCl_5$. Unpublished data reveals $PbCl_2$ is the most effective [240]. Wang et al. [241] indicated that heating to 200 °C will cause anatase to precipitate first, followed by rutile at higher temperature ~400 °C, accompanying improved bioactivity: the scanning electron microscope observation showed hemispherical agglomerations of apatite crystals scattered at a frequency of 1 particle in 13 μm square after the sample was soaked in SBF for 12 h. Wang et al. pointed out the importance of the similarity of the lattices of apatite and anatase to explain the favoring effects of anatase, as Uchida et al. noticed this issue later [187]: the lattice matching between pairs of [001]an and [010]an of anatase and [010]ap and [001]ap, where the difference [001]an versus [010]ap is 1 % and [010]an versus [001]ap is 9 %. Kaneko et al. [242] conducted an in vivo study where they implanted the titanium bone pins, treated with the $TaCl_5$-doped H_2O_2 solution, in rabbit tibia. When they evaluated the bone pin bonding strength in terms of push-out stresses, the $H_2O_2/TaCl_5$-treated bone pins showed superior bonding within 4 weeks, but the increasing rate in the later period was the same as that for the pins without the treatment, as just observed by Takemoto et al. [157] for zirconia ceramics. Kim et al. [243] treated a Ti6Al4V implant with the $TaCl_5$-doped H_2O_2 solution: here the pieces have a quadratic prism shape with Ti-fiber mesh (0.2 mm in diameter) layer on each side. They confirmed the superiority of the treated implant species, in terms of bone ingrowth, to the implants without the treatment and attributed to better osteoconductive properties of the treated species. This H_2O_2 treatment was applicable to fragile titanium samples like mesh or thin grids. Figure 5.8b indicates the apatite microcrystallites deposited on the mesh fiber subjected to the treatment. When compared with the crystallites induced by the anode oxidation accompanied by calcium ion fixation [227], the chemical treatment yielded more round crystallites, while the anode-oxidized fiber gave those with sharper edges.

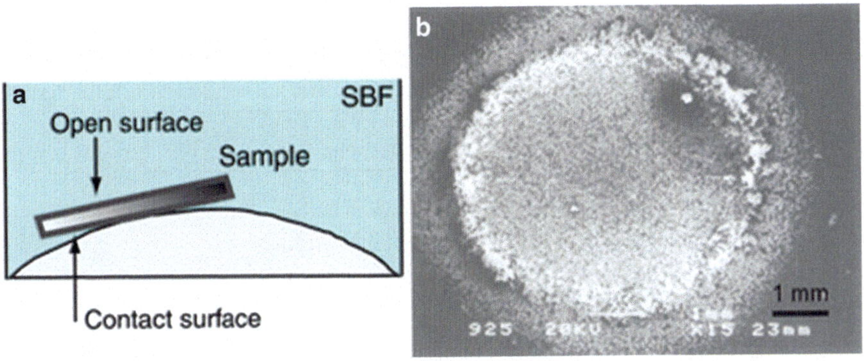

Fig. 5.9 Biomimetically deposited apatite crystallites on the contact surface (**a**) within 2 months in SBF, in a form of a volcano crater (**b**). No apatite on the open surface. Specimen, cpTi, heated in air at 400 °C for 1 h. Bar, 1 mm. (**b**) (Reproduced from Ref. [250] by permission of John Wiley & Sons Ltd.)

Apatite deposition on the anatase–rutile titania layers derived by the H_2O_2 oxidation of cpTi very much depends on the specimens, the oxidizing solution, temperature, and the SBF concentration. Titanium specimens from different companies and those fabricated in different days are definitely not equivalent in terms of corrosion. For example, mechanical attrition caused nanopores [244], while posttreatment can modify the properties of the oxide layer [245] and the same applies to the H_2O_2 solution itself. Thus, constant results seem hardly obtained. Wang et al. [246] and Wu et al. [247–249] tried to standardize the route of oxidizing cpTi to yield bioactive titania layers. The concentration of the H_2O_2 solution and the treating temperature are two important key factors as Ti forms chelate complexes and dissolves in H_2O_2.

5.4.4.5 GRAPE® Technology: Air Oxidation of Grooved Implants

In the course of examining the behavior of titanium substrates, Wang et al. noticed that a sample air-oxidized after polishing and deposited apatite in SBF. A cpTi square piece was placed on the upward concave bottom of a container filled with conventional SBF, and the surface in contact with the bottom deposited apatite: Fig. 5.9 demonstrates the crystallites form a shape like a volcano crater, though it took two months or so, whereas the surface open to SBF showed no signs of apatite deposition. Wang et al. [251] showed that the optimum heating temperature was around 400–500 °C, and no apatite was deposited when heated to 800 °C or higher for 1 h. The fact that apatite deposited on the heated specimen within a narrow area confined by the substrate suggests that thin grooves should yield similar environment and deposit apatite in SBF. In a preliminary study, Sugino et al. [252] machined microgrooves of 0.5 mm deep and 0.2–1 mm wide on a surface of a piece of cpTi block and placed it upside down on the flat bottom of a container filled with SBF, after heating at 400 °C for 1 h.

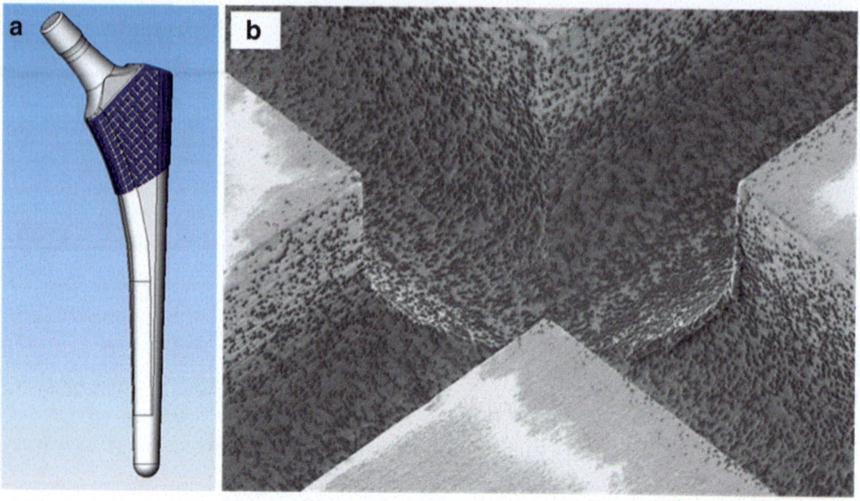

Fig. 5.10 An example of application of GRAPE® technology to hip-bone prosthesis. (**a**) A commercially available stem and (**b**) the apatite (*small grayish spots*) deposited in the grooves (0.5 mm in depth and width) on the surface of a test piece block of Ti15Zr4Nb4Ta alloy (Photos: courtesy of Nakashima Medical, Okayama, Japan). The alloy specimen was heated at 500 °C for 1 h and soaked in SBF for 7 days. Bar, 0.1 mm

Indeed, they found apatite deposition, as expected, on the wall of the grooves. The groove dimensions had an optimum range, after Sugino et al. [253, 254], depth of 0.2–1 mm, and width 0.8 mm or narrower: those grooves deposited many hemispherical agglomerates of apatite crystallites on every wall of the grooves. In this regard, the technique deserves a name GRAPE® technology, literally meaning: GRoove and APatitE. Figure 5.10 shows one potential application of this technique applied to hip-bone prostheses. The grooves are cut in a lattice with 0.5 mm in depth and width, showing small dots, which are apatite crystallites. It is unfortunate that this gap technology cannot be applied to Ti6Al4V, due to the poisonous activity of dissolved Al(III) to depress the oxide ability. Note that, according to Shozui et al. [255], UV irradiation on rutile layer on the cpTi specimen, mirror-polished and heated in air to 500 and 700 °C, provided the ability of in vitro apatite deposition: the rutile layer due to heating to 500 °C was found the most susceptible to UV activation.

Moreover, if the Ti–OH is the key species as has been emphasized so far, autoclaving should stimulate in vitro apatite deposition on the cpTi specimen heated in air, and indeed it enhanced the ability as expected [256]. Thus, the combination of the GRAPE® technology with those additional treatments would provide better bone implant fixation.

5.4.5 *Preferred Plain of Apatite Growth*

We have observed many hemispherical agglomerates of apatite, precipitated biomimetically in SBF, which crystallized via the heterogeneous nucleation and growth. The agglomerates consist of petallike crystallites, and the normal of the petallike crystallites is randomly oriented. On the other hand, the apatite crystallites in our bone tissue and tooth enamel or dentin have beautifully oriented in one direction, mostly aligned to the c-axis. However, Sato empirically proved [257, 258] that the petallike crystallites are formed by extending one of the three sets of equivalent {100} faces, using a Langmuir–Blodgett film of arachidic acid as a model of collagen fibrils. That is, the c-axis of the apatite crystallites was preferentially oriented to be parallel to the LB film–crystal interface. Recently, Wang et al. [259] indicated that type I collagen can initiate oriented growth of apatite in the absence of any other molecule except collagen fibrils. This result throws a doubt on a common concept that Ca-rich non-collagenous proteins are necessary for the mineralization of collagen in vivo. The basic experiment was a one-pot coprecipitation of apatite by exposing collagen monomers with calcium and phosphate ions to ammonia vapor [260]. Here, collagen showed a liquid crystalline behavior, and that ordered microstructure favored forming an apatite matrix hierarchy similar to that found in bone. Landis et al. [261, 262] considered that the gaps between single collagen fibrils and overlap zone of the collagen bundles in the assembled fibers would be the imitation zone of apatite crystallization. In recent days, Gower and her group propose a liquid-precursor-particles (PLP) model for biomineralization [263]. They hypothesized the presence of some organic–inorganic clusters that are the basis of crystal growth.

An intensity-enhanced dynamic light scattering technique revealed the presence of calcium phosphate clusters from 0.7 to 1.0 nm in size in a SBF. The clusters were also present in fluids undersaturated with respect to octacalcium and amorphous calcium phosphates and supersaturated with respect only to hydroxyapatite. These clusters are the growth unit of hydroxyapatite judging from the fact that hydroxyapatite grows by step flow 0.8 or 1.6 nm in height and that the probability of incorporation of the growth unit into the crystal is extremely low, as revealed previously. Onuma et al. proposed [27] a cluster growth model where hydroxyapatite grows by selective hexagonal packing of left- and right-handed chiral $Ca_9(PO_4)_6$ clusters 0.8 nm in size. They stressed that this cluster growth model well explains the twin crystals and dislocations frequently found in a few apatite systems.

Except the classic Posner clusters, those models aforementioned all involve collagen or other polymers or oligomers. For ceramics and metals, the oxide layers on those inorganic materials are charged either positively or negatively depending on the surrounding environment. We thus need assistance from the bone and soft tissue cells for the inorganic species to be integrated into the real tissues.

5.5 Biological Activity of Sol-Gel-Derived Organic–Inorganic Hybrids

5.5.1 *Organic–Inorganic Hybridization*

One of the advantages of sol-gel processes is the flexibility of the system to accommodate any organic and inorganic substances that are soluble in common solvent used for the procedure. Because of the controllability of hydrolysis and condensation reactions, silanes such as tetraethoxysilane (TEOS) or its derivatives like aminopropyltrimethoxysilane (APTMS) and 2-glycidoxypropyltrimethoxysilane (GPTMS) are the most widely utilized. In the latter two, one of the four -OEt (Et: ethyl) groups is substituted by an organic group that may demonstrate some definite role in the hybrids. Organotitanium and other similar compounds are seldom used unless no other compounds are present that match the demand. The organic counter parts are also countless, but for biomedical applications, the choices are not so few: biodegradable gelatin and chitosan, or lactic acid and its derivatives. Several additives can control the properties of the precursor systems. Table 5.8 lists some examples of the inorganic and organic components frequently employed in the sol-gel synthesis.

5.5.2 *Organically Modified Silicates: Ormosils*

5.5.2.1 Silicate Hybrids

Organic–inorganic hybrids commonly consist of inorganic skeletons and organic components as property modifiers. Ormosils can be the name for all of the silane hybrids, but it is commonly used to denote specifically the hybrids of poly(dimethylsiloxane) and silica nanoparticles derived from hydrolysis and condensation of TEOS. The properties can be controlled from rubber- [264] to brittle-like ceramics. Tsuru et al. were the first to provide the ormosils with the apatite-forming ability, by incorporating calcium ions in the precursor solution [265]. Such Ca-containing ormosils may be applied to bone fillers or protect the invasion of unnecessary cells. With an advantage of the biocompatibility enhanced by the calcium ions, several cells well proliferated in the porous ormosils, such as keratinocyte (HaCaT), osteoblast (HuO–3N1), or hepatocyte (OUMS-29). Thus, those are applicable to fabricate porous hybrids [266] for bioreactors or artificial organs as far as those human cells are retained in the pores. Kataoka et al. cultured human hepatocellular carcinoma cells in the porous scaffolds and detected albumin production [267].

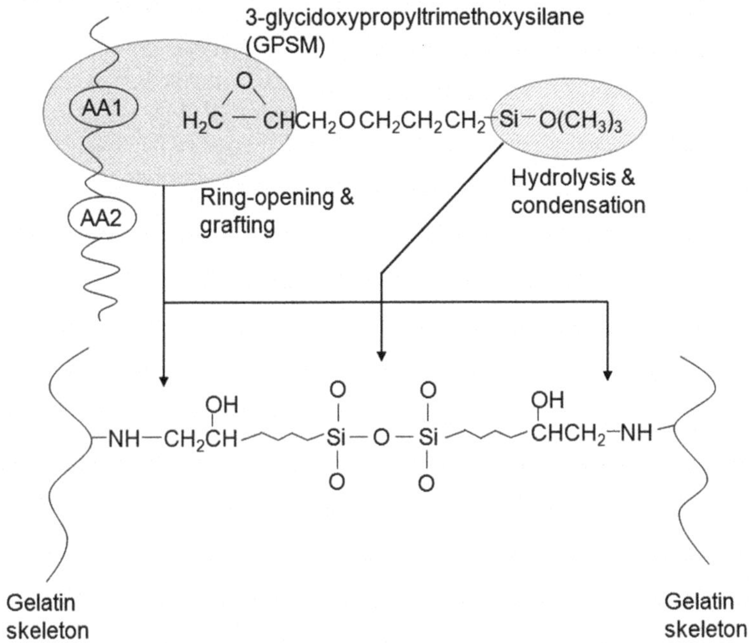

Fig. 5.11 A structure model of gelatin–GPTMS hybrids. AAn stands for an amino acid residue. After the amino acid analysis, lysine and histidine residues are the primary grafting sites

5.5.2.2 Titanate Hybrids with PDMS

Combination of PDMS and titanium tetraisopropoxide ($Ti(OPr^1)_4$ yields hybrids similar to ormosils. A precursor solution of titanium methacryloxytriisopropylate (TMT), a derivative of titanium tetra2 propoxide, was developed on stainless steel substrates and gelled: the hybrid film showed good blood compatibility. The TMT film reduced fibrinogen adsorption [268].

5.5.3 Biodegradable Hybrids: Gelatin–GPTMS Hybrids

Gelatin is extremely useful in biomedical field, e.g., as a delivery carrier of proteins [269], but it is suitable to be dissolved in an aqueous solution. The control of the dissolution rate is one of the topics of gelatin study, using silanes [270] or poly(lactic acid) [271]. Ren et al. employed GPTMS for controlling degradation in TRIS buffer solution. In addition, they added calcium ions so as to provide the hybrids with the apatite-forming ability [272]. The calcium ions uncoil the helical structure of gelatin strands into and random coils [273, 274]. From the amino residue analysis, they concluded that the epoxy group of the GPTMS molecules was preferably grafted to the lysine and histidine residues. Figure 5.11 represents schematically the structure of the gelatin–GPTMS hybrids. The Si–OH groups, from the hydrolysis of the Si–OCH_3 groups, are condensed with those of other molecules to form Si–O–Si skeleton or are involved to form the bridge between two fibrils. Thus, the mixing fraction (f_G) of GPTMS (= (GPTMS/(GPTMS + gelatin unit)) controls the degradation rate of the hybrids. For example, when f_G exceeds 0.5, the hybrids sustain in TRIS up to 40 days or longer periods with the weight decrease of <25 %. The hybrid with $f_G = 0.33$ is completely dissolved away within 30 days. The Ca-containing hybrids can deposit apatite in SBF within a day: that is, it is as active as Cerabone A-W® or 45S5 glass. Since those hybrids retain much water in the structure, freeze and drying procedure can introduce porosity. Ren et al. indicated [272] that the Ca-free hybrids with $f_G = 0.5$ and presoaked in 1 M NH_4OH gave pores of 5–10 μm in size (porosity, ~50 %) when frozen at −196 °C, 30–50 μm pores (~63 %) at −80 °C, and 300–500 μm pores (~80 %) at −17 °C. Presoaking made the freeze-drying procedure easy to occur by partially hydrolyzing the Si–O–Si bridging bonds, which ^{29}Si MAS NMR measurements confirmed by the increase in the fraction of T^2 (RSi(−O-)$_2$(OH)) and T^1 (RSi(−O-)(OH)$_2$) units. Bimodal pore structure is achieved by the application of the freeze-drying process twice to the wet gel: first freezing the gel at −17 °C to introduce large pores and the second freezing at −196 °C to introduce smaller pores in the wall of the pore cells. Osteoblast-like cells MC3T3-E1 were well proliferated on the gels of bimodal pore structure. Many globules rich in Ca covered the whole surface within two weeks, and bundles of collagen fibers were formed in 3 weeks. When a piece of gel pellet was implanted in the muscle of hind legs, the sign of calcification was observed within 2 weeks. Yet, it was unfortunate that the hybrids could not induct hard tissue, that is, the gelatin–GPTMS hybrids had no ability of bone induction.

Deguchi et al. implanted a small piece of the porous hybrids into the brain of rat for nerve cell regeneration [275]. The porous hybrid remained at the same site for 60 days, kept integrity of the brain shape, and attached well to the surrounding brain tissues without any damage. Yet, as found before for the osteoinduction ability, the hybrid has no ability to stimulate the regeneration of the brain cells. It is necessary to use basic fibroblast growth factor (bFGF) and epidermal growth factor (EGF).

Mahony et al. gave a short review on the gelatin–silane hybrids [270]. Munoz-Pinto et al. fabricated methacrylate-derived poly(dimethylsiloxane)star, combined with PEG-based hydrogels, which may be applicable to osteochondral regeneration matrices [276]. Thibault et al. attempt to fabricate hybrids of collagen HAp and non-collagenous proteins, mimicking the bone tissue structure [277]. Jayasuriya and Bhat employed chitosan and calcium phosphate hybrid microparticles, onto which mesenchymal stem cell attachment is expected and the cells are delivered to bone repairing site [278]. Gómez-Romero et al. prepared a book chapter from which conveys a concept of hybridization of organic and inorganic components. Some parts are shared for incorporation of biomolecules within inorganic matrices [279].

Shirosaki et al summarized biomedical applications of silica-based hybrids [280]. In addition, Kickelbick and Hüsing took the topics on porous hybrid materials into a book [281].

5.5.4 *Biodegradable Hybrids: Chitosan–GPTMS Hybrids*

Chitosan, like gelatin, can be used in a number of biomedical applications, such as wound dressings, drug delivery systems, and tissue defect fillers. For most medical applications, the polysaccharide network of chitosan should be cross-linked or bridged in order to improve its mechanical properties and to control biodegradation. A few reagents were known to be suitable for cross-linking, such as epoxy compounds, formaldehyde, or glutaraldehyde, but they are more or less cytotoxic when released into plasma as a result of biodegradation. Glycidyl methacrylate has epoxy and vinyl groups at each end and is a good candidate as linker for chitosan. However, glycidyl methacrylate behaves as a monovalent coupling reagent in this case because the vinyl groups would not polymerize under aqueous conditions with many ions and substances, most of which are fatal to the polymerization of vinyl groups. Chitosan absorbs amino groups on the chain, which are positively charged –NH_3^+ under the physiological pH. The epoxy group on an end of GPTMS would be grafted to those amino groups, as found for the gelatin cross-linking. Shirosaki et al. took GPTMS as the counterpart of chitosan hybridization [282], on which hybrids with varied GPTMS contents were coded as ChGx (x: 0–20 mol%), and examined the proliferation of MG63 osteoblastic cell. Even a small addition of GPTMS was effective in cell proliferation: In Fig. 5.12, Ch (chitosan only) was only partly covered by the cells after the cell culture for 6 days, whereas sample ChG05, as well as ChG10 and ChG20, was fully covered by the cells.

The same precursor solutions were freeze-dried to fabricate porous hybrids, for which the pore size increased with the freezing temperature: 50 μm at -80 °C and $\sim$100 μm at -20 °C. The porosity remained $\sim$90 %, regardless of the freezing temperature. MG63 cells proliferated well on the porous hybrids [283]. They were seeded on the top surface and migrated through the porous membrane to the bottom region. Although showing good cell proliferation characteristic, the ChGx membrane samples with little porosity caused severe inflammation of the surrounding tissues. Needless to say, the porous hybrids caused no such inflammation [284]. No matter how porous the scaffolds were, it was observed every now and then that the nutritious substances might be often supplied insufficiently. Their porous ChGx hybrids were highly active for the cell culture of human osteoblast (HOB).

As tissue engineering scaffolds are concerned, the use of porous chitosan–GPTMS hybrids is promising. Amado et al. [285] and Simoes et al. [286] employed the porous hybrids to repair rat sciatic nerve defects as a model for recovering from peripheral nerve injury. Figure 5.13 plots the data of withdrawal reflex latency, given

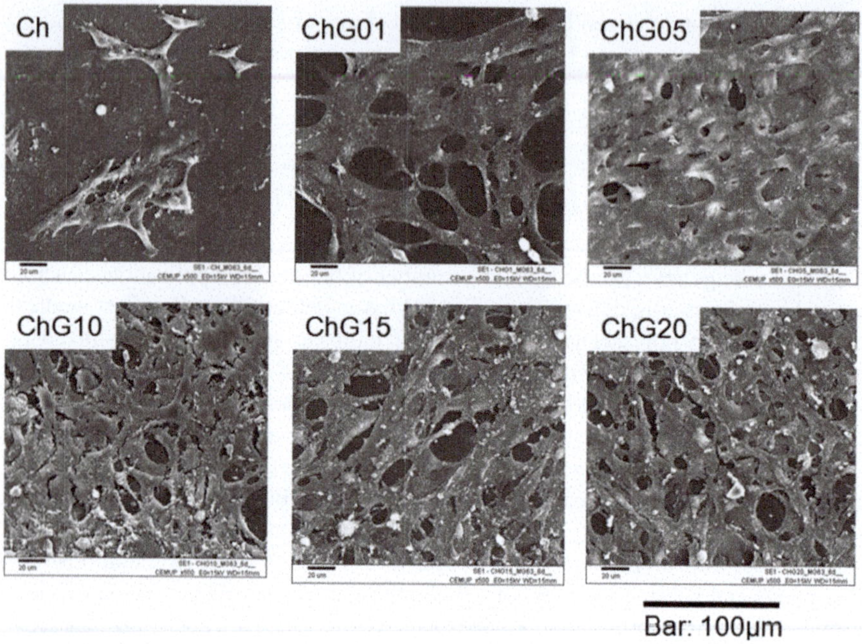

Fig. 5.12 MG63 cell culture for 6 days on chitosan–GPTMS hybrid sheets, coded as ChGx. Only a small addition of GPTMS drastically stimulates cell proliferation. Those with $x > 5$ are in a confluent stage (Reprinted from Ref. [282], copyright 2009, with permission from Elsevier)

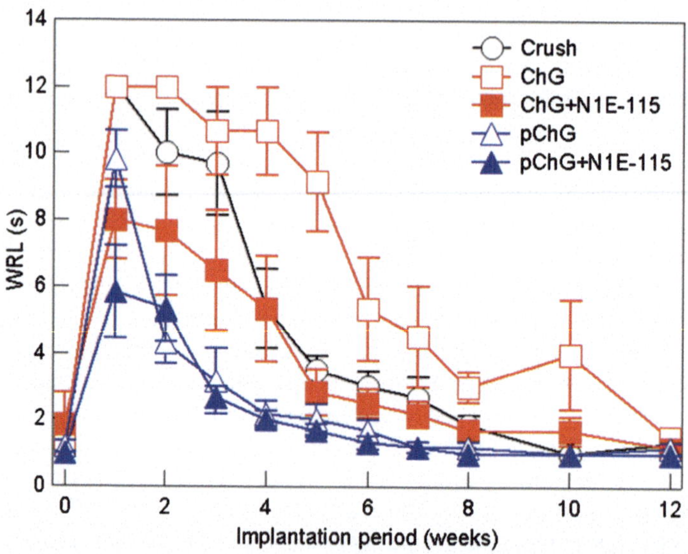

Fig. 5.13 Withdrawal reflex latency(s) is plotted as a function of the implantation period (weeks) for the membranes, porous (pChG: freeze-dried) and non-porous (ChG: xerogel), and with and without pre-impregnation of the nerve cells (+N1E-115). pChG was scarcely different from pChG +N1E-115. The non-porous membrane gave worse effects [286]

by Amado as a table. The shorter latency (time) means better recovery. Figure 5.13 compares four sets of experiments, different in pre-impregnation of the nerve cell, or porosity. The group without any treatment naturally showed the slowest recovery. Two porous membrane groups showed the fastest, but pre-impregnation of the cell in the pores gave very little effects on the recovery from the injury. That is, the porous microstructure was the key for the recovery.

The field of organic–inorganic hybrids is one of the busiest with countless numbers of publications, ideas, and materials popping up every day. It is therefore perfectly impossible to introduce each and every one.

5.6 Conclusive Remarks

We can now evaluate with ease the biomineralization behavior of biomedical ceramics through the use of Kokubo's SBF, but we should be reminded that SBF contains no physiological substances. One cannot avoid cell culture before in vivo experiment; however, different conditions exist between in vitro and in vivo environments. It is important to understand the correct usage of such in vitro techniques.

The ability of ceramic and metallic implants to form strong bonds to bone tissue or to soft tissues has been long discussed in terms of apatite-inducing ability. The concept behind many techniques is the same: how to stimulate apatite nucleation. We can always observe surface microstructures under a scanning electron microscope and locate or count the number of apatite agglomerates. When considering the real number of atoms on the surface, the nucleating sites are tremendously small. That may suggest that macroscopic thermochemistry would not be applicable, although we have no other alternatives.

In the long history of bioactive materials, four decades after the invention of Bioglass by Hench, some explanation or interpretation of specific phenomena might need modification to match newly discovered observations. A promising result evokes many researchers, attempting to think on the direction of the preceding explanation and establish their experiments on that basis. We have attempted to understand the mechanism of apatite orientation on the collagen, and we are close to the point, with a few promising models. Yet, every substance provides its own physicochemical potential to hydration and hydrolysis and polarizing any nearby substances. Inorganic chemists are much accustomed to ionic reactions that take so little time, but the apatite formation needs very long induction time in which invisible dissolution–deposition reactions surely take place. Chitosan hybrids, the last topic of this chapter, the xerogel of the hybrids, are sufficiently porous for the entrapment of water or other smaller molecules like glucose or sugars and oxygen molecules, yet the xerogel membrane caused inflammation when implanted. If the chemical species dissolved from Bioglass® stimulate several genes or factors, we can take the glass or related materials into use as delivery vehicles. What can the hybrids deliver to the regenerating tissue? What can titanium oxide layers do?

What are optimum ways for the atoms in the lattice to be arranged to induce the nucleation? The atoms in upward concave parts have higher chemical energy and tend to be dissolved, vice versa. Then, why many experiments suggest the importance of surface roughness? In atomic scales under which those ions and molecules are plying, cells are huge by several orders of magnitude. Detailed considerations and models are required.

Acknowledgment The author is very grateful of all the works introduced here and should apologize for not all work pertinent to this topic are described, as it is impossible.

References

1. Pourbaix M (1966) Atlas of electrochemical Equilibria in aqueous solutions. Pergamon Press, Oxford, p 504
2. Ohtsuki C, Aoki Y, Kokubo T, Bando Y, Neo M, Nakamura T (1995) Transmission electron microscopic observation of glass-ceramic A-W and apatite layer formed on its surface in a simulated body fluid. J Ceram Soc Japan 103:449–454
3. Chow LC (2009) Next generation calcium phosphate-based biomaterials. Dent Mater J 28:1–10
4. Ishikawa K (2010) Bone substitute fabrication based on dissolution-precipitation reactions. Materials 3:1138–1155
5. Hench LL (1991) Bioceramics: from concept to clinic. J Am Ceram Soc 74:1487–1510
6. Hench LL, Andersson ÖL (1993) Bioactive glasses. In: Hench LL, Wilson J (eds) Introduction to bioceramics. World Scientific, Singapore, pp 41–62
7. Hench LL, Day DE, Höland W, Rheinberger VM (2000) Glass and medicine. Intern J Appl Glass Sci 1:104–117
8. Cormack AN, Tilocca A (2012) Structure and biological activity of glasses and ceramics. Philos Trans R Soc A 370:1271–1280
9. Hoppe A, Güldal NS, Boccaccini AR (2011) A review of the biological response to ionic dissolution products from bioactive glasses and glass-ceramics. Biomaterials 32:2757–2774
10. Jones JR (2013) Review of bioactive glass: from Hench to hybrids. Acta Biomater 9:4457–4486
11. Clark AE, Pantano CG, Hench LL (1976) Auger spectroscopic analysis of bioglass corrosion films. J Am Ceram Soc 59:37–39; Hench LL (1975) Characterization of glass corrosion and durability. J Non-Crystal Solids 19:27–39
12. Hayakawa S, Tsuru K, Iida H, Ohtsuki C, Osaka A (1996) MAS NMR studies of apatite formation on 50CaO•50SiO2 glass in a simulated body fluid. Phys Chem Glasses 37:188–192
13. Hayakawa S, Tsuru K, Ohtsuki C, Osaka A (1999) Mechanism of apatite formation on a sodium silicate glass in a simulated body fluid. J Am Ceram Soc 82:2155–2160
14. Gross U, Stunz V (1985) The interface of various glasses and glass ceramics with a bony implantation bed. J Biomed Mat Res 19:251–271
15. Gross U, Müller-Mai C, Voigt C (1993) Ceravital® bioactive glass-ceramics. In: Hench LL, Wilson J (eds) Introduction to bioceramics. World Scientific, Singapore, pp 105–123
16. Vogel W, Höland W (1987) Development of bioglass ceramics for medical applications. Angew Chem Int Engl Ed 26:527–544
17. Vogt JC, Brandes G, Krüger I, Behrens P, Nolte I, Lenarz T, Stieve M (2008) A comparison of different nanostructured biomaterials in subcutaneous tissue. J Mater Sci Mater Med 19:2629–2636
18. Kokubo T (1991) Recent progress in glass-based materials for biomedical applications. J Ceram Soc 99:965–973

19. Neo M, Nakamura T, Yamamuro T, Ohtsuki C, Kokubo T (1993) Apatite formation on three kinds of bioactive mineral at an early stage in vivo: a comparative study by transmission electron microscopy. J Biomed Mater Res 27:999–1006
20. Kokubo T, Takadama H (2006) How useful is SBF in predicting in vivo bone bioactivity? Biomaterials 27:2907–2915
21. Cho SB, Nakanishi K, Kokubo T, Soga N, Ohtsuki C, Nakamura T, Kitsugi T, Yamamuro T (1995) Dependence of apatite formation on silica gel on its structure: effect of heat treatment. J Am Ceram Soc 78:1769–1774
22. Kokubo T, Kushitani H, Ohtsuki C, Sakka S, Yamamuro T (1992) Chemical reaction of bioactive glass and glass-ceramics with a simulated body fluid. J Mater Sci Mater Med 3:79–83
23. Round robin test: The 9th World Biomaterials Congress, Chengdu, China, 1–5 June 2012
24. Nakanishi K (1997) Pore structure control of silica gels based on phase separation. J Porous Mater 4:67–112
25. Cho SB, Nakanishi K, Kokubo T, Soga N, Ohtsuki C, Nakamura T (1996) Apatite formation on silica gel in simulated body fluid: its dependence on structures of silica gels prepared in different media. J Biomed Mater Res 33:145–151
26. Tsuru K, Kubo M, Hayakawa S, Ohtsuki C, Osaka A (2001) Kinetics of apatite deposition of silica gel dependent on the inorganic ion composition of simulated body fluids. Ceram Soc Jpn 109:412–418
27. Onuma K, Ito A (1998) Cluster growth model for hydroxyapatite. Chem Mater 10:3346–3351
28. Posner AS, Betts F (1975) Synthetic amorphous calcium phosphate and its relation to bone mineral structure. Acc Chem Res 8:273–281
29. Onuma K, Ito A, Tateishi T (1996) Investigation of a growth unit of hydroxyapatite crystal from the measurements of step kinetics. J Cryst Growth 167:773–776
30. Ducheyne P, Hench LL (1982) The processing and static mechanical properties of metal fibre reinforced bioglass. J Mater Sci 17:595–606
31. Hench LL, Andersson Ö (1993) Bioactive glass coatings. In: Hench LL, Wilson J (eds) Introduction to bioceramics. World Scientific, Singapore, pp 239–259
32. Ducheyene P, Martens M, Burssens A (1984) Materials, clinical and morphological evaluation of custom-made bioreactive-glass-coated canine. J Biomed Mater Res 18:1017–1030
33. Müller-Mai C, Schmitz HJ, Strunz V, Fuhrmann G, Fritz T, Gross UM (1989) Tissues at the surface of the new composite material titanium/glass-ceramic for replacement of bone and teeth. J Biomed Mater Res 23:1149–1168
34. Ferraris M, Rabajoli P, Paracchini L, Brossa F (1996) Vacuum plasma spray deposition of titanium particle/glass-ceramic matrix biocomposites. J Am Ceram Soc 79:1515–1520
35. Moritz N, Vedel E, Ylänen H, Jokinen M, Hupa M, Yli-Urpo A (2004) Characterisation of bioactive glass coatings on titanium substrates produced using a CO_2 laser. J Mater Sci Mater Med 15:787–794
36. Foppiano S, Marshall SJ, Saiz E, Tomsia AP, Marshall GW (2006) Functionally graded bioactive coatings: reproducibility and stability of the coating under cell culture conditions. Acta Biomater 2:133–142
37. Gomez-Vega JM, Saiz E, Tomsia AP (1999) Glass-based coatings for titanium implant alloys. J Biomed Mater Res 46:549–559
38. Gomez-Vega JM, Saiz E, Tomsia AP, Marshall GW, Marshall SJ (2000) Bioactive glass coatings with hydroxyapatite and Bioglass® particles on Ti-based implants. 1. Processing. Biomaterials 21:105–111
39. Vitale-Brovarone C, Verné E (2005) SiO_2-CaO-K_2O coatings on alumina and Ti6Al4V substrates for biomedical applications. J Mater Sci Mater Med 16:863–871
40. Osaka A (2012) Beyond current interpretation of bonding between silicate ceramics and bone. Phosphorus Res Bull 26:18–22
41. Nagayama H, Honda H, Kawahara H (1988) A new process for silica coating. J Electrochem Soc 135:2013–2016

42. Hishinuma A, Goda T, Kitaoka M, Hayashi S, Kawahara H (1991) Formation of silicon dioxide films in acidic solutions. Appl Surf Sci 48–49:405–408
43. Deki S, Aoi Y, Asaoka Y, Kajinami A, Mizuhata M (1997) Monitoring the growth of titanium oxide thin films by the liquid-phase deposition method with a quartz crystal microbalance. J Mater Chem 7:733–736
44. Yao T, Inui T, Ariyoshi A (1996) Novel method for Zirconium Oxide synthesis from aqueous solution. J Am Ceram Soc 79:3329–3330
45. Ozawa N, Ideta Y, Yao T, Kokubo T (2003) Apatite formation on polymers coated with Titania synthesized from an aqueous solution. In: Ben-Nissan B, Sher D, Walsh W (eds) Proceedings of the 15th international symposium on ceramics in medicine, Sydney, 4–8 Dec 2002. Key Eng Mater 240–242:71–74
46. Sato K, Onodera D, Hibino M, Yao T (2006) Development of bioactive organic polymer coated with ceramic thin films synthesized from aqueous solution. In: Nakamura T, Yamashita K, Neo M (eds) Proceedings of the 18th international symposium on ceramics in medicine, Kyoto, Japan, 5–8 Dec 2005. Key Eng Mater 309–311:771–774
47. Tanahashi M, Yao T, Kokubo Y, Minoda M, Miyamoto T, Nakamura T, Yamamuro T (1994) Apatite coating on organic polymers by a biomimetic process. J Am Ceram Soc 77:2805–2808
48. Balasa F, Kawashita M, Nakamura T, Kokubo T (2006) Formation of bone-like apatite on organic polymers treated with a silane-coupling agent and a titania solution. Biomaterials 27:1704–1710
49. Oyane A, Kawashita M, Kokubo T, Minoda M, Miyamoto T, Nakamura T (2002) Bone-like apatite formation on ethylene-vinyl alcohol copolymer modified with a silane coupling agent and titania solution. J Ceram Soc Jpn 110:248–254
50. Pino M, Stingelin N, Tanner KE (2008) Nucleation and growth of apatite on NaOH-treated PEEK, HDPE and UHMWPE for artificial cornea materials. Acta Biomater 4:1827–1836
51. Choi S-M, Yang W-K, Yoo Y-W, Lee W-K (2010) Effect of surface modification on the in vitro calcium phosphate growth on the surface of poly(methyl methacrylate) and bioactivity. Colloids Surf B Biointerfaces 76:326–333
52. Yokogawa Y, Reyes JP, Mucalo MR, Toriyama M, Kawamoto Y, Suzuki T, Nishizawa K, Nagata F, Kameyama T (1997) Growth of calcium phosphate on phosphorylated chitin fibres. J Mater Sci Mater Med 8:407–412
53. Yokogawa Y, Nishizawa K, Nagata F, Kameyama T (2001) Bioactive properties of chitin/chitosan-calcium phosphate composite materials. J Sol-Gel Sci Technol 21:105–113
54. Fu T, He L-P, Han Y, Xu K-W, Mai Y-W (2003) Induction of bonelike apatite on carbon–carbon composite by sodium silicate. Mater Lett 57:3500–3503
55. Furuzono T, Masuda M, Okada M, Yasuda S, Hi K, Tanaka R, Miyatake K (2006) Increase in cell adhesiveness on a poly(ethylene terephthalate) fabric by sintered hydroxyapatite nanocrystal coating in the development of an artificial blood vessel. ASAIO J 52:315–320
56. Furuzono T, Kishida A, Tanaka J (2004) Nano-scaled hydroxyapatite/polymer composite I. Coating of sintered hydroxyapatite particles on poly(γ-methacryloxypropyl trimethoxysilane)- grafted silk fibroin fibers through chemical bonding. J Mater Sci Mater Med 15:19–23
57. Korematsu A, Furuzono T, Yasuda S, Tanaka J, Kishida A (2005) Nano-scaled hydroxyapatite/polymer composite III. Coating of sintered hydroxyapatite particles on poly(4-methacryloyloxyethyl trimellitate anhydride)-grafted silk fibroin fibers. J Mater Sci Mater Med 16:67–71
58. Zhang X, Fan Z, Lu Q, Huang Y, Kaplan DL, Zhu H (2013) Hierarchical biomineralization of calcium carbonate regulated by silk microspheres. Acta Biomater 9:6974–6980
59. Nakamura A, Shishido A, Kishida I, Okada M, Furuzono T, Yokogawa Y (2004) TEM observation of hydroxyapatite nanocrystals ionically bonded onto the graft polymer-modified PET substrate. J Ceram Soc Jpn 116:100–104

60. Furuzono T, Wang P-L, Korematsu A, Miyazaki K, Oido-Mori M, Kowashi Y, Ohura K, Tanaka J, Kishida A (2003) Physical and biological evaluations of sintered hydroxyapatite/silicone composite with covalent bonding for a percutaneous implant material. J Biomed Mater Res Part B Appl Biomater 65B:217–226
61. Homeijer SJ, Barrett RA, Gower LB (2010) Polymer-Induced Liquid-Precursor (PILP) process in the non-calcium based systems of barium and strontium carbonate. Cryst Growth Des 10:1040–1052
62. Wolf SE, Leiterer J, Pipich V, Barrea R, Emmerling F, Tremel W (2011) Strong stabilization of amorphous calcium carbonate emulsion by Ovalbumin: gaining insight into the mechanism of 'Polymer-Induced Liquid Precursor' processes. J Am Chem Soc 133:12642–12649
63. Huang WH, Day DE, Kittiratanapiboon K, Rahaman MN (2006) Kinetics and mechanism of the conversion of silicate (45S5), borate and borosilicate glasses to hydroxyapatite in dilute phosphate solutions. J Mater Sci Mater Med 17:583–596
64. Han X, Day DE (2007) Reaction of sodium calcium borate glasses to form hydroxyapatite. J Mater Sci Mater Med 18:1837–1847
65. Li J, Shirosaki Y, Hayakawa S, Stamboulis A, Osaka A (2012) Sol-gel preparation of apatite-coated silica macrospheres from water glass and their adsorption of bovine serum albumin and lysozyme. J Ceram Soc Jpn 120:355–361
66. Li J, Shirosaki Y, Hayakawa S, Osaka A (2013) Revisiting structure of silica gels from water glass: an 1H and 29Si MAS and CP-MAS NMR study. J Sol-Gel Sci Technol 65:135–142
67. Chen S, Osaka A, Hayakawa S, Tsuru K, Fujii K (2008) Microstructure evolution in Stöber-type silica nanoparticles and their in vitro apatite deposition. J Sol-Gel Sci Technol 48:322–335
68. Liu C-H C, Maciel E (1996) The fumed silica surface: a study by NMR. J Am Chem Soc 118:5103–5119
69. Pham KN, Fullston D, Sagoe-Crentsil K (2007) Surface modification for stability of nano-sized silica colloids. J Colloid Interf Sci 315:123–127
70. Manzano M, Aina V, Aréan CO, Balas F, Cauda V, Colilla M, Delgado MR, Vallet-Regi M (2008) Studies on MCM-41 mesoporous silica for drug delivery: effect of particle morphology and amine functionalization. Chem Eng J 137:30–37
71. Chen S, Osaka A, Hayakawa S, Tsuru K, Fujii E, Kawabata K (2008) Novel one-pot sol-gel preparation of amino-functionalized silica nanoparticles. Chem Lett 37:1170–1171
72. Chen S, Hayakawa S, Shirosaki Y, Fujii E, Kawabata K, Tsuru K, Osaka A (2009) Sol–gel synthesis and microstructure analysis of amino-modified hybrid silica nanoparticles from aminopropyltriethoxysilane and tetraethoxysilane. J Am Ceram Soc 92:2074–2082
73. Pope EJA, Mackenzie JD (1986) Sol-gel processing of silica: II. The role of the catalyst. J Non-Cryst Solids 87:185–198
74. Anderson OH, Liu G-Z, Karlsson KH, Niemi L, Miettinen J, Juhanoja J (1990) In vivo behaviour of glasses in the SiO2–Na2O-CaO-P2O5–Al2O3–B2O3 system. J Mater Sci Mater Med 1:219–227
75. Brink M, Turunen T, Happonen R-P, Yli-Urpo A (1997) Compositional dependence of bioactivity of glasses in the system Na_2O-K_2O-MgO-CaO-B_2O_3-P_2O_5-SiO_2. J Biomed Mater Res 37:114–121
76. Di Z, Vedel E, Hupa L, Aro HT, Hupa M (2009) Predicting physical and chemical properties of bioactive glasses from chemical composition. Part 3: In vitro reactivity. Eur J Glass Sci Technol Part A 50:1–8
77. Moritz N, Vedel E, Ylänen H, Jokinen M, Hupa M, Yli-Urpo A (2004) Characterisation of bioactive glass coatings on titanium substrates produced using a CO2 laser. J Mater Sci Mater Med 15:787–802
78. Rajedran V, Begum AN, Azooz MA, El Batal FH (2002) Microstructural dependence on relevant physical–mechanical properties on SiO_2–Na_2O–CaO–P_2O_5 biological glasses. Biomaterials 23:4263–4275

79. Lossdörfer S, Schwartz Z, Lohmann CH, Greenspan DC, Ranly DM, Boyan BD (2004) Osteoblast response to bioactive glasses in vitro correlates with inorganic phosphate content. Biomaterials 25:2547–2555
80. Debdas R (2007) In vitro reactivity of Na_2O–MgO–SiO_2 glasses. J Phys Chem Solids 68:2321–2325
81. Daguano JK, Rogero SO, Crovace MC, Peitl O, Strecker K, dos Santos C (2013) Bioactivity and cytotoxicity of glass and glass-ceramics based on the 3CaO-P_2O_5–SiO_2–MgO system. J Mater Sci Mater Med. 24:2171–2180
82. Ebisawa Y, Sugimoto Y, Hayash T, Kokubo T, Ohura K, Yamamuro T (1991) Crystallization of (FeO, Fe_2O_3)-CaO-SiO_2 glasses and magnetic properties of their crystallized products. J Ceram Soc Jpn 99:7–13
83. Li G, Feng S, Zhou D (2011) Magnetic bioactive glass ceramic in the system CaO–P_2O_5–SiO_2–MgO–CaF_2–MnO_2–Fe_2O_3 for hyperthermia treatment of bone tumor. J Mater Sci Mater Med 22:2197–2206
84. Singh RK, Srinivasan A (2010) Apatite-forming ability and magnetic properties of glass-ceramics containing zinc ferrite and calcium sodium phosphate phases. Mater Sci Eng C 30:1100–1106
85. Zhang D, Leppäranta O, Munukka E, Ylänen H, Viljanen MK, Eerola E, Hupa M, Hupa L (2010) Antibacterial effects and dissolution behavior of six bioactive glasses. J Biomed Mater Res 93A:475–483
86. Hong Y-L, Chen X-S, Jing X-B, Fan H-S, Guo B, Gu Z-W, Zhang X-D (2010) Preparation, bioactivity, and drug release of hierarchical nanoporous bioactive glass ultrathin fibers. Adv Mater 22:754–758
87. Sepulveda P, Jones JR, Hench LL (2002) In vitro dissolution of melt-derived 45S5 and sol-gel derived 58S bioactive glasses. J Biomed Mater Res 61:301–311
88. Chrisodoulou I, Buttery LDK, Saravanapavan P, Tai G-P, Hench LL, Polak JM (2005) Dose- and time-dependent effect of bioactive gel-glass ionic-dissolution products on human fetal osteoblast-specific gene expression. J Biomed Mater Res B Appl Biomater 74B:529–537
89. Lei B, Chen X-F, Koh Y-H (2011) Effects of acidic catalysts on the microstructure and biological property of sol–gel bioactive glass microspheres. J Sol-Gel Sci Technol 58:656–663
90. Valeiro P, Pereira MM, Goes AM, Leite MF (2004) The effect of ionic products from bioactive glass dissolution on osteoblast proliferation and collagen production. Biomaterials 25:2941–2948
91. Zhang D, Jain H, Hupa M, Hupa L (2012) In-vitro degradation and bioactivity of tailored amorphous multi porous scaffold structure. J Am Ceram Soc 95:2687–2694
92. Arcos D, Vallet-Reggi M (2010) Sol-gel silica based biomaterials and bone tissue regeneration. Acta Biomater 6:2874–2888
93. Arcos D, Vila M, López-Noriega A, Rossignol F, Champion E, Oliveira FJ, Vallet-Reggí M (2011) Mesoporous bioactive glasses: mechanical reinforcement by means of a biomimetic process. Acta Biomat 7:2952–2959
94. Vaid C, Murugavel S (2013) Alkali oxide containing mesoporous bioactive glasses: synthesis, characterization and in vitro bioactivity. Mater Sci Eng C 33:959–968
95. Bellantone M, Coleman NJ, Hench LL (2000) Bacteriostatic action of a novel four-component bioactive glass. J Biomed Mater Res 51:484–490
96. Caturo M, Raucci M, De Gaetano F, Marrota A (2004) Antibacterial and bioactive silver-containing Na2O•CaO•2SiO2 glass prepared by sol-gel method. J Mater Sci Mater Med 15:831–837
97. Brown RF, Day DE, Day TE, Jung S, Rahaman MN, Fu Q (2008) Growth and differentiation of osteoblastic cells on 13–93 bioactive glass fibers and scaffolds. Acta Biomater 4:387–396
98. Fu Q, Rahaman MN, Bal SB, Brown RF (2010) Preparation and in vitro evaluation of bioactive glass (13–93) scaffolds with oriented microstructures for repair and regeneration of load-bearing bones. J Biomed Mater Res 93A:1380–1390

99. L-x B, Jung S, Day DE, Neidig K, Dusevich V, Eick D, Bonewald L (2012) Evaluation of bone regeneration, angiogenesis, and hydroxyapatite conversion in critical-sized rat calvarial defects implanted with bioactive glass scaffolds. J Biomed Mater Res Part A 100A:3267–3275
100. Liu X, Xie Z-P, Zhang C-Q, Pan H-B, Rahaman MN, Zhang X, Fu Q, Huang W-H (2010) Bioactive borate glass scaffolds: in vitro and in vivo evaluation for use as a drug delivery system in the treatment of bone infection. J Mater Sci Mater Med 21:575–582
101. Kasuga T, Hosoi Y, Nogami M, Niinomi M (2001) Apatite formation on calcium phosphate invert glasses in simulated body fluid. J Am Ceram Soc 84:450–452
102. Kasuga T (2005) Bioactive calcium pyrophosphate glasses and glass-ceramics. Acta Biomater 1:55–64
103. Fujii E, Kawabata K, Yohimatsu H, Hayakawa S, Tsuru K, Osaka A (2003) Structure and biomineralization of calcium silicate glasses containing fluoride ions. J Ceram Soc Jpn 111:762–766
104. Galliano PG, Lopes JMP (1995) Thermal behaviour of bioactive alkaline-earth silicophosphate glasses. J Mater Sci Mater Med 6:353–359
105. Brauer DS, Karpukhina N, O'Donnell MD, Law RV, Hill RG (2010) Fluoride-containing bioactive glasses: effect of glass design and structure on degradation, pH and apatite formation in simulated body fluid. Acta Biomater 6:3275–3282
106. Mneimne MG, Hill R, Bushby AJ, Brauer DS (2011) High phosphate content significantly increases apatite formation of fluoride-containing bioactive glasses. Acta Biomater 7:1827–1834
107. Lynch E, Brauer DS, Karpukhina N, Gillama DG, Hill RG (2012) Multi-component bioactive glasses of varying fluoride content for treating dentin hypersensitivity. Dent Mater 28:168–178
108. Cocchi M, Durante C, Lusvardi G, Malavasi G, Menabue L (2012) Evaluation of the behaviour of fluorine-containing bioactive glasses: reactivity in a simulated body fluid solution assisted by multivariate data analysis. J Mater Sci Mater Med 23:639–648
109. Wang Y-H, Osaka A, Miura Y (1989) Anionic conduction in lead oxyfluoride glasses. J Non-Cryst Solids 112:323–327
110. Brauer DS, Mneimne M, Hill G (2011) Fluoride-containing bioactive glasses: fluoride loss during melting and ion release in tris buffer solution. J Non-Cryst Solids 357:3328–3333
111. Massera J, Fagerlun S, Hupa L, Hupa M (2012) Crystallization mechanism of the bioactive glasses, 45S5 and S53P4. J Am Ceram Soc 95:607–613
112. Brink M (1997) The influence of alkali and alkaline earths on the working range for bioactive glasses. J Biomed Mater Res 36:109–117
113. Martín-Saavedra FM, Ruiz-Hernández E, Boré A, Arcos D, Vallet-Regí M, Vilaboa N (2010) Magnetic mesoporous silica spheres for hyperthermia therapy. Acta Biomater 6:4522–4531
114. Wang F, Tang Y-L, Zhang B-B, Chen B-D, Y-l W (2012) Preparation of novel magnetic hollow mesoporous silica microspheres and their efficient adsorption. J Colloid Interface Sci 386:129–134
115. Petchsang N, Pon-On W, Hodak JH, Tang IM (2009) Magnetic properties of Co-ferrite-doped hydroxyapatite nanoparticles having a core/shell structure. J Magn Magn Mater 321:1990–1995
116. Wu HC, Wang TW, Sun JS, Wang WH, Lin FH (2007) A novel biomagnetic nanoparticle based on hydroxyapatite. Nanotechnology 18:165601. doi:10.1088/0957-4484/18/16/165601
117. Maehara T, Konishi K, Kanmimori T, Aono J, Hirazawa H, Naohara T, Nomura S, Kikkawa H, Watanabe Y, Kawachi K (2005) Selection of ferrite powder for thermal coagulation therapy with alternating magnetic field. J Mater Sci Mater Med 40:135–138
118. Matsunaga T, Sakaguchi T (2000) Review: molecular mechanism of magnet formation in bacteria. J Biosci Bioeng 90:1–13
119. Matsunaga T, Okamura Y (2003) Genes and proteins involved in bacterial magnetic particle formation. TRENDS Microbiol 11:536–541
120. Tang YS, Wang D, Zhou C, Ma W, Zhang YQ, Liu B, Zhang S (2012) Bacterial magnetic particles as a novel and efficient gene vaccine delivery system. Gene Ther 19:1187–1195

121. Xynos ID, Edgar AJ, Buttery Lee DK, Hench LL, Polak JM (2001) Gene-expression profiling of human osteoblasts following treatment with the ionic products of Bioglass 45S5 dissolution. J Biomed Mater Res 55:151–157
122. Hench LL, Polak JM (2002) Third-generation biomedical materials. Science 295:1014–1017
123. Conzone SD, Day DE (2009) Preparation and properties of porous microspheres made from borate glass. J Biomed Mater Res Part A 88A:531–542
124. Pouxviel JC, Boilot JP, Smaihi M, Dauger A (1988) Structural study of aluminosilicate sols and gels by small angle X-ray and neutron scattering. J Non-Cryst Solids 106:147–152
125. Ramirez-del-Solar M, Esquvias L, Craievich AF, Zarzycki JJ (1992) Ultrastructural evolution during gelation of TiO2-SiO2 sols. Non-Cryst Solids 147&148:206–212
126. Ohtsuki C, Kokubo T, Takatsuka K, Yamamuro T (1991) Compositional dependence of bioactivity of glasses in the system CaO-SiO_2-P_2O_5 its in vitro evaluation. J Ceram Soc Jpn 99:1–6
127. Wang W, Huang D, Wang B, Darvell W, Day DE, Rahaman MN (2006) Preparation of hollow hydroxyapatite microspheres. J Mater Sci Mater Med 17:641–646
128. Huang W, Rahaman MN, Day DE, Miller BA (2009) Strength of hollow microspheres prepared by a glass conversion process. J Mater Sci Mater Med 20:123–129
129. Hayakawa S, Li Y, Tsuru K, Osaka A, Fujii E, Kawabata K (2009) Preparation of nanometer-scale rod array of hydroxyapatite crystal. Acta Biomater 5:2152–2160
130. Lotgering FK (1959) Topotactical reactions with ferrimagnetic oxides having hexagonal crystal structures. J Inorg Nucl Chem 9:113–123
131. Osaka A, Takahashi K (1983) Heats of solution of the glasses and crystals in the systems MO-P2O5 and bond energy relations in M(PO3)2 glasses. J Ceram Soc Jpn 91:395–398
132. Kasuga T, Abe Y (1999) Calcium phosphate invert glasses with soda and titania. J Non-Cryst Solids 243:70–74
133. Brow RK, Phifer CC, Turner GL, Kirkpatrick RJ (1991) Cation effects on ^{31}P MAS NMR chemical shifts of metaphosphate glasses. J Am Ceram Soc 74:1287–1290
134. Yang WH, Kirkpatrick RJ, Turner G (1986) ^{31}P and ^{29}Si magic-angle sample-spinning NMR investigation of the structural environment of phosphorus in alkaline-earth silicate glasses. J Am Ceram Soc 69:C222–C223
135. Hosono H, Abe Y (1995) Porous glass–ceramics composed of a titanium phosphate crystal skeleton. J Non-Cryst Solids 190:185–197
136. Kasuga T, Kimata T, Obata A (2009) Preparation of a calcium titanium phosphate glass–ceramic with improved chemical durability. J Am Ceram Soc 92:1709–1712
137. Parks GA (1965) The isoelectric points of solid oxides, solid hydroxides, and aqueous hydroxo complex systems. Chem Rev 65:177–198
138. Parks GA, de Bruyn PL (1962) The zero point of charge of oxides. J Phys Chem 66:969–973
139. Tengvall P, Lundström I (1992) Physico-chemical considerations of titanium as a biomaterial. Clin Mater 9:115–134
140. Uchida M, Kim HM, Kokubo T, Miyaji F, Nakamura T (2001) Bonelike apatite formation induced on zirconia gel in a simulated body fluid and its modified solutions. J Am Ceram Soc 84:2041–2044
141. Uchida M, Kim HM, Kokubo T, Tanaka K, Nakamura T (2002) Dependence of apatite formation on zirconia gels in a simulated body fluid. J Ceram Soc Jpn 110:710–715
142. Uchida M, Kim HM, Miyaji T, Kokubo F, Nakamura T (2002) Apatite formation on zirconium metal treated with aqueous NaOH. Biomaterials 23:313–317
143. Kokubo T, Matsushita T, Takadama H (2007) Titania-based bioactive materials. J Eur Ceram Soc 27:1553–1558
144. Kokubo T, Matsushita T, Takadama H, Kizuki T (2009) Development of bioactive materials based on surface chemistry. J Eur Ceram Soc 29:1267–1274
145. Uchida M, Kim HM, Kokubo T, Nawa M, Asano T, Tanaka K, Nakamura T (2002) Apatite-forming ability of a zirconia/alumina nano-composite induced by chemical treatment. J Biomed Mater Res 60:277–282

146. Miyazaki T, Kim HM, Kokubo T, Ohtsuki C, Kato H, Nakamura T (2001) Apatite-forming ability of niobium oxide gels in a simulated body fluid. J Ceram Soc Jpn 109:929–933
147. Miyazaki T, Kim HM, Kokubo T, Kato H, Nakamura T (2000) Bioactive tantalum metal prepared by NaOH treatment. J Biomed Mater Res 50:35–42
148. Miyazaki T, Kim HM, Kokubo T, Kato H, Nakamura T (2001) Induction and acceleration of bonelike apatite formation on tantalum oxide gel in simulated body fluid. J Sol-Gel Sci Technol 21:83–88
149. Kato H, Nakamura T, Nishiguchi S, Matsusue Y, Kobyashi M, Miyazaki T, Kim HM, Kokubo T (2000) Bonding of alkali- and heat-treated tantalum implants to bone. J Biomed Mater Res Appl Biomater 53:28–35
150. Li PJ, Ohtsuki C, Kokubo T, Nakanishi K, Soga N, de Groot K (1994) The role of hydrated silica, titania, and alumina in inducing apatite on implants. J Biomed Mater Res 28:7–15
151. Li P, Ohtsuki C, Kokubo T, Nakanishi K, Soga N, Nakamura T, Yamamuro T (1992) Apatite formation induced by silica gel in a simulated body fluid. J Am Ceram Soc 75:2094–2097
152. Abe Y, Kokubo T, Yamamuro T (1990) Apatite coating on ceramics, metals and polymers utilizing a biological process. J Mater Sci Mater Med 1:233–238
153. Taguchi T, Kishida A, Akashi M (1999) Apatite formation on/in hydrogel matrices using an alternate soaking process. III. Effect of physico-chemical factors on apatite formation on/in poly(vinyl alcohol) hydrogel matrices. J Biomater Sci Polym Ed 10:795–804
154. Takemoto M, Fujibayashi S, Neo M, Suzuki J, Kokubo T, Nakamura T (2006) Bone-bonding ability of a hydroxyapatite coated zirconia–alumina nanocomposite with a microporous surface. J Biomed Mater Res 78A:693–701
155. Kim HW, Kong YM, Bae CJ, Noh YJ, Kim HE (2004) Sol-gel derived fluor-hydroxyapatite biocoatings on zirconia substrate. Biomaterials 25:2919–1926
156. Nakamura S, Takeda H, Yamashita K (2001) Proton transport polarization and depolarization of hydroxyapatite ceramics. J Appl Phys 89:5386–5392
157. Itoh S, Nakamura S, Kobayashi T, Shinomiya K, Yamashita K (2006) Effect of electrical polarization of hydroxyapatite ceramics on new bone formation. Calcif Tissue Int 78:133–142
158. Okabayashi R, Nakamura M, Okabayashi T, Tanaka Y, Nagai A, Yamashita K (2009) Efficacy of polarized hydroxyapatite and silk fibroin composite dressing gel on epidermal recovery from full-thickness skin wounds. J Biomed Mater Res Appl Biomater B 90:641–646
159. Nakamura M, Nakamura S, Sekijima Y, Niwa K, Kobayashi T, Yamashita K (2006) Role of blood coagulation components as intermediators of high osteoconductivity of electrically polarized hydroxyapatite. J Biomed Mater Res A 79:627–634
160. Nakamura M, Inuzuka M, Hashimoto K, Nagai A, Yamashita K (2012) Polarized yttria-stabilized zirconia improves durability for degradation and apatite formation. Phosphorus Res Bull 26:77–80
161. Mariappan CR, Yunos DM, Boccaccini AR, Rolling B (2009) Bioactivity of electro-thermally poled bioactive silicate glass. Acta Biomater 5:1274–1283
162. Fujishima A, Honda K (1972) Electrochemical photolysis of water at a semiconductor electrode. Nature 238:37–38
163. Roy P, Berger S, Schmuki P (2011) Reviews: TiO_2 nanotubes: synthesis and applications. Angew Chem Int Ed 50:2904–2939
164. Yoko T, Kamiya K, Sakka S (1987) Photoelectrochemical properties of TiO_2 films prepared by the sol-gel method. J Ceram Soc Jpn 95:150–155
165. Dislich H, Hussman E (1981) Amorphous and crystalline dip coatings obtained from organometallic solutions: procedures, chemical processes and products. Thin Solid Films 77:129–139
166. Kasuga T, Hiramatsu M, Hoson A, Sekino T, Niihara K (1998) Formation of titanium oxide nanotube. Langmuir 14:3160–3163
167. Yun YJ, Chung JS, Kim SW, Hahn SH, Kim EJ (2004) Low-temperature coating of sol-gel anatase thin films. Mater Lett 58:3703–3706

168. Sheng YG, Liang LP, Xu Y, Wu D, Wu YH, Sun YH (2008) Low-temperature deposition of the high-performance anatase-titania optical films via a modified sol-gel route. Opt Mater 30:1310–1315
169. Daoud WA, Xin JH (2004) Low temperature sol-gel processed photocatalytic titania coating. J Sol-Gel Sci Technol 29:25–29
170. Uekawa N, Kajiwara J, Kakegawa K, Sasaki Y (2002) Low temperature synthesis and characterization of porous anatase TiO2 nanoparticles. J Colloid Interface Sci 250:285–290
171. Jensen MJ, Fuiere PA (2006) Low-temperature preparation of nanocrystalline anatase films through a sol-gel route. J Sol-Gel Sci Technol 39:229–233
172. Hu Y, Yuan CW (2005) Low-temperature preparation of photocatalytic TiO2 thin films from anatase sols. J Cryst Growth 274:563–568
173. Shirosaki Y (2009) Private communication: courtesy of Shirosaki, Y
174. Colby MW, Osaka A, Mackenzie JD (1988) Temperature dependence of the gelation of silicon alkoxides. J Non-Cryst Solids 99:129–139
175. Li PJ, de Groot K (1993) Calcium phosphate formation within sol-gel prepared titania in vitro and in vivo. J Biomed Mater Res 27:1495–1500
176. Li PJ, Kangasniemi I, de Groot K, Kokubo T (1994) Bonelike hydroxyapatite induction by a gel-derived titania on titanium substrate. J Am Ceram Soc 77:1307–1312
177. Kumar KN, Zaspals P, Keizer K, Burggraaf AJ (1992) Drying process in the formation of sol-gel-derived TiO2 ceramic membrane. J Non-Cryst Solids 147&148:375–381
178. Grosso D, Cagnol F, de AA Soler-Illia GJ, Crepaldi EL, Ameitsch H, Brunet-Bruneau A, Bourgeois A, Sanchez C (2004) Fundamentals of mesostructuring through evaporation-induced self-assembly. Adv Funct Mater 14:309–322
179. Pätsi ME, Jautaniemi JA, Rhiala JM, Peltola TO, Kangasniemi IMO (1998) Bonding strengths of titania sol-gel-derived coatings on titanium. J Sol-Gel Sci Technol 11:55–66
180. Areva S, Lindén M (2003) Calcium phosphate formation on chemically modified titanium. In: Ben-Nissan B, Sher D, Walsh W (eds) Proceedings of the 15th international symposium on ceramic in medicine, Sydney, 2002. Key Eng Mater 240–242:465–468
181. Areva S, Peltola T, Säliynoja E, Laajalehto K, Lindén M, Rosenholm JB (2002) Effect of albumin and fibrinogen on calcium phosphate formation on sol-gel derived titania coatings in vitro. Chem Mater 14:1614–1621
182. Klinger A, Steinberg D, Kohavi D, Sela MN (1997) Mechanism of adsorption of human albumin to titanium in vitro. J Biomed Mater Res 36:387–392
183. Chen Y-L, Zhang X-F, Gon Y-D, Zhao N-M, Zeng T-Y, Song X-Q (1999) Conformational changes of fibrinogen adsorption onto hydroxyapatite and titanium oxide nanoparticles. J Colloid Interface Sci 214:38–45
184. Peltola T, Pätsi M, Rahiala H, Kangasniemi I, Yli-Urpo A (1998) Effect of aging time of sol on structure and in vitro calcium phosphate formation of sol-gel-derived titania films. J Biomed Mater Res 41:504–510
185. Jokinen M, Pätsi M, Rahiala H, Peltola T, Ritala M, Rosenholm JB (1998) Influence of sol and surface properties on in vitro bioactivity of sol-gel-derived TiO2 and TiO2-SiO2 films deposed by dip-coating method. J Biomed Mater Res 42:295–302
186. Peltola T, Jokinen M, Rahiala H, Pätsi M, Heikkilä J, Kangasniemi I, Yli-Urpo A (2000) Calcium phosphate induction by sol-gel-derived titania coatings on titanium substrates in vitro. J Biomed Mater Res 51:200–208
187. Uchida M, Kim H-M, Kokubo T, Fujibayashi S, Nakamura T (2003) Structural dependence of apatite formation on titania gels in a simulated body fluid. J Biomed Mater Res 64A:164–170
188. Areva S, Paldan H, Peltola T, Närhi T, Jokinen M, Linden M (2004) Use of sol-gel derived titania coating for direct soft tissue attachment. J Biomed Mater Res 70A:169–178
189. Rossi S, Moritz N, Tirri T, Peltola T, Areva S, Jokinen M, Happonen RP, Närhi T (2007) Comparison between sol-gel-derived anatase- and rutile-structured TiO2 coatings in soft-tissue environment. J Biomed Mater Res 82A:965–974

190. Zhao JM, Liu JF, Wu JM, Tsuru K, Hayakawa S, Osaka A (2006) Apatite formation on rutile and anatase layers derived by hydrolysis of titanylsulfate in a simulated body fluid. J Ceram Soc Japan 114:253–258
191. Harmankaya N, Karlsson J, Palmquist A, Halvarsson M, Igawa K, Andersson M, Tengvall P (2013) Raloxifene and alendronate containing thin mesoporous titanium oxide films improve implant fixation to bone. Acta Biomater 9:7064–7073
192. Liu K, Lin XL, Zhao JS (2013) Toxic effects of the interaction of titanium dioxide nanoparticles with chemicals or physical factors. Int J Nanomed 8:2509–2520
193. Shimizu K, Imai H, Hirashima H, Tsukuma K (1999) Low-temperature synthesis of anatase thin films on glass and organic substrates by direct deposition from aqueous solutions. Thin Solid Films 35:220–224
194. Wu JM, Hayakawa S, Tsuru K, Osaka A (2002) In vitro bioactivity of anatase film obtained by direct deposition from aqueous titanium tetrafluoride solutions. Thin Solid Films 414:283–288
195. Wu JM, Xiao F, Hayakawa S, Tsuru K, Takemoto S, Osaka A (2003) Bioactivity of metallic biomaterials with anatase layers deposited in acidic titanium tetrafluoride solution. J Mater Sci Mater Med 14:1027–1032
196. Xiao F, Tsuru K, Hayakawa S, Osaka A (2003) In vitro apatite deposition on titania film derived from chemical treatment of Ti substrates with an oxysulfate solution containing hydrogen peroxide at low temperature. Thin Solid Films 441:271–276
197. Hayakawa S, Liu JF, Tsuru K, Osaka A (2006) Wet deposition of titania-apatite composite in cotton fibrils. J Sol-gel Sci Technol 40:253–258
198. Wu JM, Liu JF, Hayakawa S, Tsuru K, Osaka A (2007) Low-temperature deposition of rutile film on biomaterials substrates and its ability to induce apatite deposition in vitro. J Mater Sci Mater Med 18:1529–1536
199. Kokubo T, Miyaji F, Kim HM, Nakamura T (1996) Spontaneous formation of bonelike apatite layer on chemically treated titanium metals. J Am Ceram Soc 79:1127–1129
200. Kim HM, Miyaji F, Kokubo T, Kitsugi T, Nakamura T (1996) Preparation of bioactive Ti and its alloys via simple chemical surface treatment. J Biomed Mater Res 32:409–417
201. Kim HM, Miyaji F, Kokubo T, Nakamura T (1997) Apatite-forming ability of alkali-treated Ti metal in body environment. J Ceram Soc Jpn 105:111–116
202. Kim HM, Miyaji F, Kokubo T, Nakamura T (1997) Effect of heat treatment on apatite-forming ability induced by alkali treatment. J Mater Sci Mater Med 8:341–347
203. Takadama H, Kim HM, Kokubo T, Nakamura T (2001) An X-ray photoelectron spectroscopy study of the process of apatite formation on bioactive titanium metal. J Biomed Mater Res 55:185–193
204. Takadama H, Kim HM, Kokubo T, Nakamura T (2001) TEM-EDX study of mechanism of bonelike apatite formation on bioactive titanium metal in simulated body fluid. J Biomed Mater Res 57:441–448
205. Fujibayashi S, Nakamura T, Nishiguchi S, Tamura J, Uchida M, Kim H-M, Kokubo T (2001) Bioactive titanium: effect of sodium removal on the bone-bonding ability of bioactive titanium prepared by alkali and heat treatment. J Biomed Mater Res 56:562–570
206. Uchida M, Kim H-M, Kokubo T, Fujibayashi S, Nakamura T (2002) Effect of water treatment on the apatite-forming ability of NaOH-treated titanium metal. J Biomed Mater Res 63:522–530
207. Takemoto M, Fujibayashi S, Neo M, Suzuki J, Matsushita T, Kokubo T, Nakamura T (2006) Osteoinductive porous titanium implants: effect of sodium removal by dilute HCl treatment. Biomaterials 27:2682–2691
208. Kawai T, Kizuki T, Takadama H, Matsushita M, Unuma H, Nakamura T, Kokubo T (2010) Apatite formation on surface titanate layer with different Na content on Ti metal. J Ceram Soc Jpn 118:19–24

209. Pattanayak DK, Yamaguchi S, Matsushita M, Kokubo T (2011) Nanostructured positively charged bioactive TiO2 layer formed on Ti metal by NaOH, acid and heat treatments. J Mater Sci Mater Med 22:1803–1812
210. Kizuki T, Takadama H, Matsushita T, Nakamura T, Kokubo T (2010) Preparation of bioactive Ti metal surface enriched with calcium ions by chemical treatment. Acta Biomater 6:2836–2842
211. Yamaguchi S, Kizuki T, Takadama H, Matsushita T, Nakamura T, Kokubo T (2012) Formation of a bioactive calcium titanate layer on gum metal by chemical treatment. J Mater Sci Mater Med 23:873–883
212. Yamaguchi S, Takadama H, Matsushita T, Nakamura T, Kokubo T (2010) Apatite-forming ability of Ti–15Zr–4Nb–4Ta alloy induced by calcium solution treatment. J Mater Sci Mater Med 21:439–444
213. Fukuda A, Takemoto M, Saito T, Fujibayashi S, Neo M, Yamaguchi S, Kizuki T, Matsushita T, Niinomi M, Kokubo T, Nakamura T (2011) Bone bonding bioactivity of Ti metal and Ti–Zr–Nb–Ta alloys with Ca ions incorporated on their surfaces by simple chemical and heat treatments. Acta Biomater 7:1379–1386
214. Fawzy AS, Amer MA (2009) An in vitro and in vivo evaluation of bioactive titanium implants following sodium removal treatment. Dent Mater 25:48–57
215. Ravelingien M, Mullens S, Luyten J, Meynen V, Vinck E, Vervaet C, Remon JP (2009) Thermal decomposition of bioactive sodium titanate surface. Appl Surf Sci 255:9539–9542
216. Ravelingien M, Hervent AS, Mullens S, Luyten J, Vervaet C, Remon JP (2010) Influence of surface topography and pore architecture of alkali-treated titanium on in vitro apatite deposition. Appl Surf Sci 256:3693–3697
217. Aparicio S, Manero JM, Conde F, Pegueroles M, Planell JA, Vallet-Regi M, Gil FJ (2007) Acceleration of apatite nucleation on microrough bioactive titanium for bone- replacing implants. J Biomed Mater Res Part A 82:521–529
218. Kizuki T, Takadama H, Matsushita T, Nakamura T, Kokubo T (2013) Effect of Ca contamination on apatite formation in a Ti metal subjected to NaOH and heat treatments. J Mater Sci Mater Med 24:635–644
219. Kokubo T, Pattanayak DK, Yamaguchi S, Takadama H, Matsushita M, Kawai T, Takemoto M, Fujibayashi S, Nakamura T (2010) Positively charged bioactive Ti metal prepared by simple chemical and heat treatments. J R Soc Interf 7:S503–S513
220. Kawai T, Takemoto M, Fujibayashi S, Akiyama H, Yamaguchi S, Pattanayak DK, Doi K, Matsushita T, Nakamura T, Kokubo T, Matsuda S (2013) Osteoconduction of porous Ti metal enhanced by acid and heat treatments. J Mater Sci Mater Med 24:1707–1715
221. Spriano S, Brozoni M, Rosalbino F, Verné E (2005) New chemical treatment for bioactive titanium alloy with high corrosion resistance. J Mater Sci Mater Med 16:203–211
222. Wen HB, Liu Q, De Wijn JR, De Groot K, Cui FZ (1998) Preparation of bioactive microporous titanium surface by a new two-step chemical treatment. J Mater Sci Mater Med 9:121–128
223. Jonášová L, Müller FA, Helebrant A, Strnad J, Greil P (2004) Biomimetic apatite formation on chemically treated titanium. Biomaterials 25:1187–1194
224. Zhao CY, Zhu XD, Yuan T, Fan HS, Zhang XD (2010) Fabrication of biomimetic apatite coating on porous titanium and their osteointegration in femurs of dogs. Mater Sci Eng C 30:98–104
225. Eliaz N, Ritman-Hertz O, Aronov D, Weinberg E, Shenhar Y, Rosenman G, Weinreb M, Ron E (2011) The effect of surface treatments on the adhesion of electrochemically deposited hydroxyapatite coating to titanium and on its interaction with cells and bacteria. J Mater Sci Mater Med 22:1741–1752
226. Osaka A, Hayakawa S, Tsuru K, Takemoto S, Kawabe Y, Iwatani S (2001) In vitro biomimetic deposition of apatite on chemically and electrochemically treated titanium. J Aust Ceram Soc 37:1–8
227. Yang BC, Uchida M, Kim HM, Zhang XD, Kokubo T (2004) Preparation of bioactive titanium metal via anodic oxidation treatment. Biomaterials 25:1003–1010

228. Liang BJ, Fujibayashi S, Neo M, Tamura J, Kim HM, Uchida M, Kokubo T, Nakamura T (2003) Histological and mechanical investigation of the bone-bonding ability of anodically oxidized titanium in rabbits. Biomaterials 24:4959–4966
229. Zhao Y, Xiong TY, Huang WH (2010) Effect of heat treatment on bioactivity of anodic titania films. Appl Surf Sci 256:3073–3076
230. Yamamoto D, Iida T, Arii K, Kuroda K, Ichino R, Okido M, Seki A (2012) Surface hydrophilicity and osteoconductivity of anodized Ti in aqueous solutions with various solute ions. Mater Trans 53:1956–1961
231. Iwai-Yoshida M, Shibata Y, Wurihan, Suzuki D, Fujisawa N, Tanimoto Y, Kamijo R, Maki K, Miyazaki T (2012) Antioxidant and osteogenic properties of anodically oxidized titanium. J Mech Behav Biomed Mater 13:230–236
232. Hori N, Iwasa F, Tsukimura N, Sugita Y, Ueno T, Kojima N, Ogawa T (2011) Effects of UV photofunctionalization on the nanotopography enhanced initial bioactivity of titanium. Acta Biomater 7:3679–3691
233. Tsukimura N, Yamada M, Iwasa F, Minamikawa H, Att W, Ueno T, Saruwatari L, Aita H, Chious WA, Ogawa T (2011) Synergistic effects of UV photofunctionalization and micro-nano hybrid topography on the biological properties of titanium. Biomaterials 32:4358–4368
234. Shibata Y, Suzuki D, Omori S, Tanaka R, Murakami A, Kataoka Y, Baba K, Kamijo R, Miyazaki T (2010) The characteristics of in vitro biological activity of titanium surfaces anodically oxidized in chloride solutions. Biomaterials 31:8546–8555
235. Att W, Hori N, Takeuchi M, Ouyang JY, Yang Y, Anpo M, Ogawa T (2009) Biomaterials 30:5352–5363
236. Khang DW, Choi J, Im YM, Kim YJ, Jang JH, Kang SS, Nam TH, Song J, Park JW (2012) Role of subnano-, nano- and submicron-surface features on osteoblast differentiation of bone marrow mesenchymal stem cells. Biomaterials 33:5997–6007
237. Tengvall P, Elwing H, Sjöqvist L, Lundström I, Bjursten LM (1989) Interaction between hydrogen peroxide and titanium: a possible role in the biocompatibility of titanium. Biomaterials 10:118–120
238. Tengvall P, Lundström I, Sjöqvist L, Elwing H, Bjursten LM (1989) Titanium-hydrogen peroxide interaction: model studies of the influence of the inflammatory response on titanium implants. Biomaterials 10:166–175
239. Ohtsuki C, Iida H, Hayakawa S, Osaka A (1997) Bioactivity of titanium treated with hydrogen peroxide solutions containing metal chlorides. J Biomed Mater Res 35:39–47
240. Ohtsuki C, Unpublished data, private communication
241. Wang XX, Hayakawa S, Tsuru K, Osaka A (2000) Improvement of bioactivity of $H_2O_2/TaCl_5$-treated titanium after subsequent heat treatments. J Biomed Mater Res 52:171–176
242. Kaneko S, Tsuru K, Hayakawa S, Takemoto K, Ohtsuki C, Ozaki T, Inoue H, Osaka A (2001) In vivo evaluation of bone-bonding of titanium metal chemically treated with a hydrogen peroxide solution containing tantalum chloride. Biomaterials 22:875–881
243. Kim T, Suzuki M, Ohtsuki C, Masuda K, Tamai H, Watanabe E, Osaka A, Moriya H (2003) Enhancement of bone growth in titanium fiber mesh by surface modification with hydrogen peroxide solution containing tantalum chloride. J Biomed Mater Res Part B Appl Biomater 64B:19–26
244. Laleh M, Kargar F (2011) Formation of high bioactive nanoporous titania film by hybrid surface mechanical attrition treatment. Mater Let 65:2295–2298
245. Yoneyama Y, Matsuno T, Hashimoto Y, Satoh T (2013) In vitro evaluation of H2O2 hydrothermal treatment of aged titanium surface to enhance biofunctional activity. Dent Mater J 32:115–121
246. Wang XX, Hayakawa S, Tsuru K, Osaka A (2002) Bioactive titania gel layers formed by chemical treatment of Ti substrate with a H2O2/HCl solution. Biomaterials 23:1353–1357
247. Wu JM, Hayakawa S, Tsuru K, Osaka A (2002) Crystallization of anatase from amorphous titania in hot water and in vitro biomineralization. J Ceram Soc Jpn 110:78–80
248. Wu JM, Hayakawa S, Tsuru K, Osaka A (2003) Early apatite deposition on titanium treated by hydrogen peroxide. J Aust Ceram Soc 39:36–42

249. Wu JM, Tsuru K, Hayakawa S, Osaka A (2004) Low-temperature preparation of anatase and rutile layer on titanium substrate and their ability to induce in vitro apatite deposition. J Am Ceram Soc 87:1635–1642
250. Wang XX, Hayakawa S, Tsuru K, Osaka A (2001) A comparative study of in vitro apatite deposition on heat-, H_2O_2, and NaOH-treated titanium surfaces. J Biomed Mater Res 54:172–178
251. Wang XX, Yan W, Hayakawa S, Tsuru K, Osaka A (2003) Apatite deposition on thermally and anodically oxidized titanium surfaces in a simulated body fluid. Biomaterials 24:4631–4637
252. Sugino A, Uetsuki K, Tsuru K, Hayakawa S, Ohtsuki C, Osaka A (2008) Gap effect on the heterogeneous nucleation of apatite on thermally oxidized titanium substrate. Key Eng Mater 361–363:621–624
253. Sugino A, Uetsuki K, Tsuru K, Hayakawa S, Osaka A, Ohtsuki C (2008) Surface topography designed to provide osteoconductivity to titanium after thermal oxidation. Mater Trans 49:428–434
254. Sugino A, Tsuru K, Hayakawa S, Kikuta K, Kawachi G, Osaka A, Ohtsuki C (2009) Induced deposition of bone-like hydroxyapatite on thermally oxidized titanium substrates using a spatial gap in a solution that mimics a body fluid. J Ceram Soc Jpn 117:515–520
255. Shozui T, Tsuru K, Hayakawa S, Osaka A (2008) Enhancement of in vitro apatite-forming ability of thermally oxidized titanium surfaces by ultraviolet irradiation. J Ceram Soc Jpn 116:530–535
256. Uetsuki K, Akasaka K, Nakai S, Shirosaki Y, Hayakawa S, Osaka A (2011) Mechanism of stimulated apatite nucleation on Titania layer by UV-irradiation and autoclaving. Presented at the 11th Asian BioCeramics symposium in conjunction with the 22nd symposium on apatite, 30 Nov–2 Dec 2011, Tsukuba, Japan
257. Sato K (2007) Mechanism of hydroxyapatite mineralization in biological systems. J Ceram Soc Jpn 115:124–130
258. Sato K, Kogure T, Kumagai Y, Tanaka J (2001) Crystal orientation of hydroxyapatite induced by ordered carboxyl groups. J Colloid Interf Sci 240:133–138
259. Wang Y, Azais T, Robin M, Vallée A, Catania C, Legriel P, Pehau-Armaidet G, Babonneau F, Giraud-Guille MM, Nassif N (2012) The predominant role of collagen in the nucleation, growth, structure and orientation of bone apatite. Nat Mater 11:724–733
260. Nassif N, Gobeaux F, Seto J, Belamie E, Davidson P, Panine P, Mosser G, Fratzl P, Giraud Guille MM (2010) Self-assembled collagen-apatite matrix with bone-like hierarchy. Chem Mater 22:3307–3309
261. Landis WJ, Song MJ, Leith A, McEwen L, McEwen BF (1993) Mineral and organic matrix interaction in normally calcifying tendon visualized in three dimensions by high-voltage electron microscopic tomography and graphic image reconstruction. J Struct Biol 110:39–54
262. Landis W, Hodgens K, Song MJ, Arena J, Kiyonaga S, Marko M, Owen C, McEwen BF (1996) Mineralization of collagen may occur on fibril surfaces: evidence from conventional and high-voltage electron microscopy and three-dimensional imaging. J Struct Biol 117:24–35
263. Bewernitz MA, Gevayerm D, Long J, Cölfen H, Gower LB (2012) A metastable liquid precursor phase of calcium carbonate and its interactions with polyaspartate. Faraday Discuss 159:291–312
264. Hu Y, Mackenzie JD (1992) Rubber-like elasticity of organically modified silicates. J Mater Sci 27:4415–4420
265. Tsuru K, Ohtsuki C, Osaka A, Iwamoto T, Mackenzie JD (1997) Bioactivity of sol-gel derived organically modified silicates. J Mater Sci Mater Med 8:157–161
266. Yabuta T, Bescher EP, Mackenzie JD, Tsuru K, Hayakawa S, Osaka A (2003) Synthesis of PDMS-based porous materials for biomedical applications. J Sol-gel Sci Tech 26:1219–1222
267. Kataoka K, Nagao Y, Nukui T, Akiyama I, Tsuru K, Hayakawa S, Osaka A, Huh NH (2005) An organic-inorganic hybrid scaffold for the culture of HepG2 cells in a bioreactor. Biomaterials 26:2509–2516

268. Yoshioka T, Tsuru K, Hayakawa S, Osaka A (2004) Preparation of organotitanium molecular layers for biomedical applications. Mater Sci Eng C 24:901–905
269. Curcio M, Altimari I, Spizzirri UG, Cirillo G, Vittorio O, Puoci F, Picci N, Iemma F (2013) Biodegradable gelatin-based nanospheres as pH-responsive drug delivery systems. J Nanopart Res 15:1581–1592
270. Mahony O, Tsigkou O, Ionescu C, Minelli C, Ling L, Hanly R, Smith ME, Stevens MM, Jones JR (2010) Silica-gelatin hybrids with tailorable degradation and mechanical properties for tissue regeneration. Adv Funct Mater 20:3835–3845
271. Lu HX, Oh HH, Kawazoe N, Yamagishi K, Chen G (2012) PLLA–collagen and PLLA–gelatin hybrid scaffolds with funnel-like porous structure for skin tissue engineering. Sci Technol Adv Mater 13:064210. doi:10.1088/1468-6996/13/6/064210
272. Ren L, Tsuru K, Hayakawa S, Osaka A (2002) Novel approach to fabricate porous gelatin–siloxane hybrids for bone tissue engineering. Biomaterials 23:4765–4773
273. Ren L, Tsuru K, Hayakawa S, Osaka A (2001) Incorporation of Ca^{2+} ions in gelatin-siloxane hybrids through a sol-gel process. J Ceram Soc Jpn 109:406–411
274. Wüstneck R, Buder E, Wetzel R, Hermel H (1989) The modification of the triple helical structure of gelatin in aqueous solution, 3: the influence of cationic surfactants. Colloid Polym Sci 267:429–435
275. Deguchi K, Tsuru K, Hayashi T, Takaishi M, Nagahara M, Nagotani S, Sehara Y, Jin G, Zhang H, Hayakawa S, Shoji M, Miyazaki M, Osaka A, Huh NH, Abe K (2006) Implantation of a new porous gelatin–siloxane hybrid into a brain lesion as a potential scaffold for tissue regeneration. J Cereb Blood Flow Metab 26:1263–1273
276. Munoz-Pinto DJ, McMahon RE, Kanzelberger MA, Jimenez-Vergara AC, Grunlan MA, Hahn MS (2010) Inorganic–organic hybrid scaffolds for osteochondral regeneration. J Biomed Mater Res 94A:112–121
277. Thibault RA, Mikos AG, Kasper FK (2013) Scaffold/extracellular matrix hybrid constructs for bone-tissue engineering. Adv Healthcare Mater 2:13–24
278. Jayasuriya AC, Bhat A (2010) Fabrication and characterization of novel hybrid organic/inorganic microparticles to apply in bone regeneration. J Biomed Mater Res 93A:1280–1288
279. Gómez-Romero P, Sanches C, Hüsing N, Schubert U (2004) Porous inorganic-organic hybrid materials. In: Functional hybrid materials. Wiley, Weinheim
280. Shirosaki Y, Osaka A, Tsuru K, Hayakawa S (2012) Inorganic-organic sol-gel hybrids. In: Bio-glasses: an introduction. Wiley, Chichester
281. Kickelbick G, Hüsing N (2007) Hybrid materials: synthesis, characterization, and applications. Wiley-VCH, Weinheim
282. Shirosaki Y, Tsuru K, Hayakawa S, Osaka A, Lopes MA, Santos JD, Costa MA, Fernandes MH (2009) Physical, chemical and in vitro biological profile of chitosan hybrid membrane as a function of organosiloxane concentration. Acta Biomater 5:346–355
283. Shirosaki Y, Okayama T, Tsuru K, Hayakawa S, Osaka A (2008) Synthesis and cytocompatibility of porous chitosan-silicate hybrids for tissue engineering scaffold application. Chem Eng J 137:122–128
284. Mauricio AC (2009) Unpublished data, private communication
285. Amado S, Simoes MJ, Armada da Silva PAS, Luis AL, Shirosaki Y, Lopes MA, Santos JD et al (2008) Use of hybrid chitosan membranes and N1E-115 cells for promoting nerve regeneration in an axonotmesis rat model. Biomaterials 29:4409–4419
286. Simoes MJ, Amado S, Gärtner A, Armada da Silva PAS, Raimondo S, Vieira M, Luis AL, Shirosaki Y et al (2010) Italian. J Anat Embryol 115:175–195

Chapter 6
Signal Molecule-Calcium Phosphate Composites: Novel Approaches to Controlling Cellular and/or Biological Reactions and Functions

Xiupeng Wang, Ayako Oyane, and Atsuo Ito

Abstract Signal molecule-calcium phosphate (CaP) composites are formed in supersaturated CaP solutions containing signal molecules. The molecules coprecipitate with CaPs in the form of coating layers or particulates and are immobilized in the CaP matrix forming a nanocomposite of the molecule and CaP. Various substrates are used for the coprecipitation. The molecules thus immobilized include laminin, fibronectin, bone morphogenic protein-2 (BMP-2), fibroblast growth factor-2 (FGF-2), antibiotics, DNA, α-amylase, and immunogenic molecules. Solution chemistry, CaP phase, morphology, and molecule content affect biological activity of signal molecule-CaP composites. Depending on the choice of molecule, signal molecule-CaP composites have various applications including tissue regeneration, gene delivery, and cancer immunotherapy. For tissue regeneration, immobilization of signal molecules with CaP on a substrate can achieve a sustained regulation activity of the signal molecules and is applied to promote bone regeneration and soft tissue regeneration. DNA-CaP composite layers are surface-mediated gene delivery system that has gene delivery efficiency as high as that of a commercial lipid-based system. The efficiency has been improved further by the incorporation of cell adhesion molecules and lipids in the layers. Gene delivery systems using CaP composite layers are effective in enhancing cell differentiation and bone tissue regeneration in vitro and in vivo. Substituted tricalcium phosphate and mesoporous silica loaded with pathogen-associated molecular patterns using coprecipitation with CaP are used as an adjuvant for cancer immunotherapy. The composite adjuvants mixed with liquid-nitrogen-

X. Wang • A. Ito (✉)
Human Technology Research Institute, National Institute of Advanced Industrial Science and Technology (AIST), Central 6, 1-1-1 Higashi, Tsukuba, Ibaraki 305-8566, Japan
e-mail: atsuo-ito@aist.go.jp

A. Oyane
Nanosystem Research Institute, National Institute of Advanced Industrial Science and Technology (AIST), Central 4, 1-1-1 Higashi, Tsukuba, Ibaraki 305-8562, Japan

B. Ben-Nissan (ed.), *Advances in Calcium Phosphate Biomaterials*, Springer Series in Biomaterials Science and Engineering 2, DOI 10.1007/978-3-642-53980-0_6,

treated tumor tissue effectively triggered antitumor immune response and markedly inhibited the growth of rechallenged tumor cells (tumor recurrence model) in vivo.

Keywords Signal molecules • Calcium phosphate • Supersaturated calcium phosphate solution • Nanocomposite • Coatings • Tissue regeneration • Gene delivery • Cancer immunotherapy

6.1 Introduction

Biomaterials combined with signal molecules are designed to stimulate specific cellular and/or biological responses. Signal molecules are either physically mixed with, chemically bound with, embedded in, or adsorbed or immobilized on biomaterials. In particular, hydrophilic signal molecules are immobilized on the surface of metallic, polymeric, and ceramic biomaterials as coating layers of signal molecule-CaP composites. A signal molecule-CaP composite layer is fabricated by coprecipitation of a signal molecule and CaPs in a supersaturated CaP solution in the presence of the molecule. Once the signal molecule-CaP composite layer is implanted in the body, the signal molecule binds to cell-surface receptors or intracellular receptors of target cells, which generates a cascade of intracellular biochemical reactions that alter the behavior of the cells. Although CaPs, typically apatite (Ap) and tricalcium phosphate, elicit osteoconduction, signal molecule-CaP composites can elicit even specific non-osseous cellular reactions depending on the choice of signal molecule. Signal molecules include proteins, small peptides, steroids, polysaccharide, and foreign DNA. A foreign DNA molecule introduced into a cell (gene delivery) can also alter the behavior of the cell through expression of one or more genes in the introduced DNA. Although such DNA molecules usually are not termed "signal molecules," DNA-CaP composites for gene delivery are also described in this chapter.

6.2 Formation and Properties of Signal Molecule-CaP Composite Layers

6.2.1 Formation of Signal Molecule-CaP Composite Layers

A physiologically supersaturated CaP solution is supersaturated with respect to multiple CaP phases. The degree of supersaturation is defined using a geometrical mean as follows (Eq. 6.1):

$$S = \left(\frac{I}{Ks}\right)^{1/\nu} - 1 \tag{6.1}$$

where I is the ionic activity product of the solution with respect to a CaP, Ks is the solubility product of the CaP, and υ is number of ionic activity in the product (e.g., $\upsilon = 5$ and 9 for $(Ca^{2+})^3(PO_4{}^{3-})^2$ and $(Ca^{2+})^5(PO_4{}^{3-})^3(OH^-)$, respectively). Physiologically supersaturated CaP solutions such as body fluid, saliva, Kokubo's simulated body fluid (SBF), and Hank's solution are all supersaturated with respect to Ap and octacalcium phosphate (OCP) and nearly saturated with respect to amorphous calcium phosphate (ACP) in the pH range of 7.3–7.4 at 25 °C: for example, the S values of SBF are 12–19, 0.6–2.5, and −0.4 for Ap, OCP, and ACP, respectively, at pH 7.4 and 25 °C. Supersaturated CaP solutions contain prenucleation CaP clusters under physiological pH condition [1–5], which accounts for S being as high as 12–19 with respect to Ap. Owing to such a high value of S, Ap can be formed by both direct condensation of ions (classical route) and formation of precursors such as cluster aggregates or ACP followed by transformation into Ap (multistep route) [6].

Molecules present in a supersaturated CaP solution exhibit a variety of interactions with CaP crystals, precursors, and/or clusters in the solution depending on solution chemistry, pH, and temperature, which is yet to be fully understood. A protein molecule, a CaP crystal, precursors of the CaP crystal, and clusters can have a positive or a negative surface charge depending on solution chemistry and pH. It is when the molecule and CaP have opposite electrical charges that interaction can occur [7]. Thus, for example, the efficiency of coprecipitation of basic proteins largely differs between different supersaturated CaP solutions [8–10]. Temperature is another factor that influences the efficiency of coprecipitation owing to the temperature dependence of solubility and stability of CaPs [11]. Two different mechanisms have been proposed for the process of coprecipitation: one is molecular adsorption followed by crystal nucleation [12–14], and the other is molecular incorporation into ACP followed by amorphous-crystalline transformation [15]. The former is proposed by analogy with the fact that many noncollagenous acidic matrix proteins in bone promote Ap formation when they are immobilized on a substrate while they inhibit Ap formation when they are unimmobilized. Thus, once molecules are adsorbed on precipitated CaP, the adsorbed molecules act as the secondary nucleation sites of CaP crystals in a supersaturated CaP solution. In the latter mechanism, molecules, calcium ions, phosphate ions, and clusters are aggregated into an amorphous phase. As the molecule-containing ACP transforms to a polycrystalline phase, the molecules are captured on the surface or interstices of crystals. In both mechanisms, the final product is a nanocomposite of molecules and CaPs where the molecules are dispersed in the tens-to-hundred-nanometer-scale distances within the CaP matrix (Fig. 6.1) [12, 16].

Molecules thus immobilized so far include fibronectin [12], vitronectin [12], albumin [17, 18], collagen [19], amelogenin [20], laminin [21], BMP-2 [22], FGF-2 [10, 15], antibiotics [23, 24], L-ascorbic acid phosphate magnesium salt n-hydrate (AsMg) [25–27], DNA [28], α-amylase [29], and immunogenic molecules [30].

The molecule present in a supersaturated CaP solution controls the phase, size, and crystallinity of CaP precipitated. Albumin facilitated Ap crystallization in a

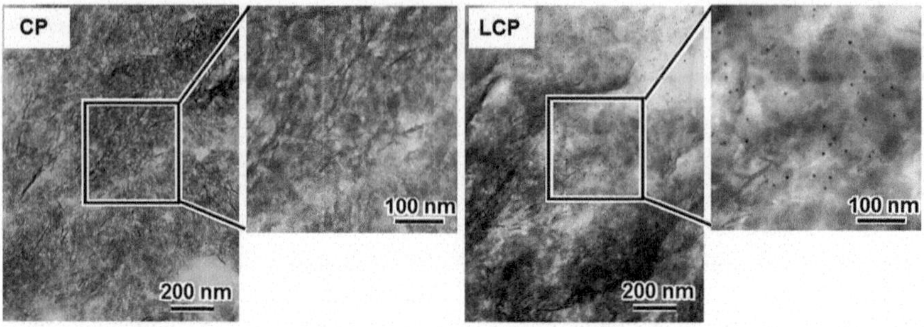

Fig. 6.1 Transmission immunoelectron microscopic photographs for an Ap layer (*CP*) and a laminin-Ap composite layer (*LCP*). *Black dots* in LCP correspond to laminin molecules (Reprinted from Oyane et al. [16], Copyright 2006, with permission from Elsevier)

supersaturated CaP solution where only OCP is formed in the absence of albumin [17]. Proteins that have particular peptide motifs present in dentin matrix protein 1 facilitated the transformation of ACP into Ap [31]. However, many molecules decrease the size and crystallinity of Ap or inhibit Ap crystallization [21, 24, 25, 32].

Supersaturated CaP solutions used for fabricating signal molecule-CaP composites are classified into (1) physiological saline, (2) SBF-based CaP solutions, (3) inhibitor-free CaP solutions, and (4) infusion fluid-based CaP solutions. Examples of physiological saline include Hanks' balanced salt solution, Dulbecco's phosphate-buffered saline, and phosphate-buffered saline (PBS) [14, 33–35]. SBF is a supersaturated CaP solution that has ion concentrations approximately equal to those of human blood plasma. 1.5 times concentrated SBF is prepared at pH 7.25. SBF with doubled Ca and P concentrations is prepared at pH 6.8 [36]. Bubbling carbon dioxide gas at a pressure of 0.1 MPa allows preparation of SBF concentrated as high as seven times [37]. Once supply of carbon dioxide gas is stopped, the gas is released out of the solution, leading to an increase in pH, thus increasing supersaturation and enhancing formation of CaP [37–39]. SBF and concentrated SBF are used for fabricating signal molecule-CaP composites or base coating of signal molecule-CaP composites [17, 40]. Physiological saline and SBF-based CaP solutions contain not only calcium and phosphate ions but also magnesium and carbonate ions that inhibit CaP formation. Removal of these inhibitor ions (inhibitor-free CaP solutions) accelerates formation of signal molecule-CaP composites [17, 21, 28, 41]. Physiological saline, and SBF-based and inhibitor-free CaP solutions contain organic buffering agents such as tris(hydroxymethyl)aminomethane (TRIS) and 4-(2-hydroxyethyl)-1-piperazineethanesulfonic acid (HEPES) except for those buffered with carbon dioxide gas. Besides buffering agents, these solutions do not necessarily guarantee biological safety for clinical use, owing to possible contamination by harmful impurities, microorganisms, viruses, and pyrogens. Infusion fluid-based CaP solutions have the advantage of biological safety over other classes of supersaturated CaP solutions. Infusion fluids are sterile, contain only trace amounts of pyrogens, and are approved officially for clinical use of injection. Aseptically mixing calcium-containing, phosphate-containing, and pH-adjusting infusion fluids allows the preparation of supersaturated CaP solutions that have a high level of biological safety [11, 19, 26, 42].

6.2.2 Material Properties of Signal Molecule-CaP Composite Layers

The CaP phase in signal molecule-CaP composite layers includes low-crystalline Ap [21, 24, 43], ACP [8], OCP, and/or an OCP-like phase [18, 20, 43, 44]. The thickness of the composite layer is from several hundred nanometer to some tens microns. The morphology and crystallinity of the matrix phase change with process parameters including solution chemistry and fabrication temperature. The Mg ion and molecule in the solution decrease the surface roughness of the layer through their inhibitory effect on the crystal growth of Ap, which results in a decrease in the crystal size of the formed Ap [45].

Information regarding the mechanical properties of signal molecule-CaP composite layers is available for some composite layers. The shear strength of the laminin-Ap composite layer depends on the moisture condition: the shear strength of the laminin-Ap composite layer is higher than that of the Ap layer under wet condition, while that of the former is lower than that of the latter under dry condition [46]. The adhesion strength values for 3- and 10-μm-thick laminin-Ap composite layers are 7 and 2 MPa, respectively, under dry condition, which are both lower than those for 3- and 10-μm-thick Ap layers, respectively [46]. Coatings with a Ca/P molar ratio of 1.30 and thicknesses of 15–23 μm prepared in supersaturated CaP solution in the presence of bovine serum albumin (BSA) had significantly higher critical loads in the scratch test than those with a Ca/P molar ratio of 1.33 and a thickness of 33 μm prepared in the absence of BSA [47]. However, the hardness of these coatings was not significantly influenced by the presence of BSA. A BMP-2-CaP composite layer had significantly higher critical loads (2.5 ± 0.37N) in the scratch test than the CaP layer (1.8 ± 0.08N) prepared in the absence of BMP-2 [44].

Immobilization enables the localization of signal molecules at specific body sites and their release in a sustained manner. On the contrary, free molecules cannot be retained at a local site for a long time because they rapidly diffuse from the site [48, 49]. Albumin [17], cytochrome *c* [8], and FGF-2 [50] immobilized in the signal molecule-CaP composite layers are released from the composite layers in physiological sodium chloride solution and cell-culture media (Fig. 6.2a). The release was sustained for 10–21 days, while these molecules adsorbed to the same substrate were released much faster and in some cases completely within 24 h. Collagen and fibronectin were immobilized firmly on an Ap ceramic and continued to be released into a physiological saline solution for at least 3 days [19, 51]. The DNA-CaP composite coating exhibited an initial burst of release during the first 8 h and a sustained release for a few days after exposure to a cell-culture medium

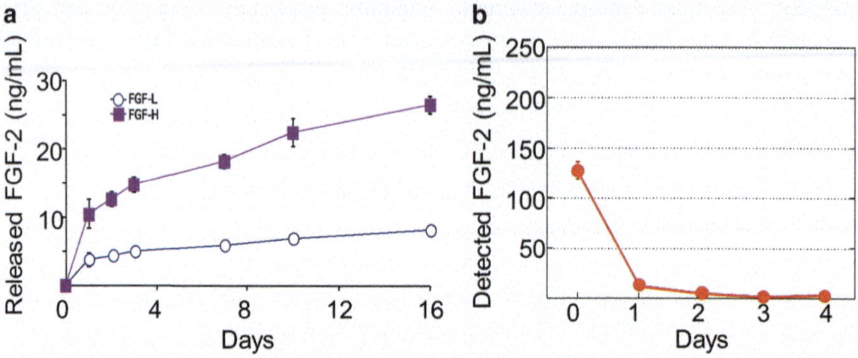

Fig. 6.2 (**a**) Cumulative release of FGF-2 from FGF-2-Ap composite layers containing FGF-2 at a low dose (FGF-L) and a high dose (FGF-H) in DMEM at 37 °C (Reprinted from Tsurushima et al. [50], Copyright 2010, with permission from Elsevier). (**b**) Decomposition of unimmobilized FGF-2 in DMEM at 37 °C

[28, 52]. An ascorbate-Ap composite coating resulted in slower ascorbate release in physiological saline solution than in the case of adsorbed ascorbate [53].

The biological activity of immobilized molecules is either decreased, preserved, or increased compared with that of unimmobilized ones. Biological activity may be decreased or lost when the molecular chemistry or configuration is changed by immobilization. This typically occurs when the chemical bonding of molecules to a substrate is too strong or the immobilizing reaction is degradative. Biological activity may be preserved when the molecular chemistry and configuration are unchanged by immobilization. The activity can be preserved even for a longer period than unimmobilized molecules since many biologically active and unimmobilized molecules have short lifetimes and lose their activity with time by natural denaturation or decomposition under physiological condition [54]. For example, in Dulbecco's Modified Eagle Medium (DMEM), the FGF-2-Ap composite layer preserved and released FGF-2 that is detectable with enzyme-linked immunosorbent assay (ELISA) even after 14 days [50, 55], while unimmobilized FGF-2 added directly to DMEM decomposes over 95 % within 48 h (Fig. 6.2b). The biological activity of immobilized molecules may be increased compared with unimmobilized molecules owing to increases in the molecular stability and local concentration, multivalency, and inhibition of cellular internalization of the molecules [54, 56].

The biological activity of signal molecule-CaP composites is characterized by bioassay. In particular, in vitro bioassay that reflects in vivo biological activity is useful and can be used for quality control of signal molecule-CaP composites. In vitro bioassay includes evaluation of the mitogenic activity of NIH3T3 and BHK-21 cells cultured with FGF-2-CaP composite layers [10, 27, 50], evaluation of the alkaline phosphatase (ALP) activity of rat bone marrow stromal cells cultured on BMP-2-CaP composite layers [22], and evaluation of cytokine secretion by THP-1 cells cultured with immunogenic molecules-CaP composites [30, 57].

6.3 Applications to Drug Delivery for Tissue Regeneration

Tissue loss or failure is one of the most frequent, devastating, and costly problems in human health care. Tissue engineering, which applies the principles of biology, engineering, and materials science, has emerged as potential means of growing new tissues and organs [58–60]. Signal molecules that regulate a variety of cellular processes, e.g., cell adhesion, proliferation, differentiation, and maturation, are crucial for tissue engineering or regenerative medicine to regulate cellular functions [58]. Immobilization of signal molecules with CaP on a substrate is a promising process to achieve a sustained regulation activity of the signal molecules [43]. To date, signal molecules have been integrated into CaP coatings for the purpose of promoting bone regeneration and soft tissue regeneration.

6.3.1 Bone Regeneration

Bone defects have been treated by surgery, using bone grafts such as autologous bone, allografts, or synthetic bone graft materials [61–63]. The major drawbacks of autologous bone are their limited supply and surgical side effects. Allografts have concerns related to host response and disease transmission and can be associated with infection and inflammation [64, 65]. Synthetic bone graft materials, typically CaPs, have no or clinically insufficient osteoinductive property. Tissue-engineered bone and biomaterials loaded with signal molecules are important alternatives. As one of the latter class, signal molecules such as BMP-2, FGF-2, ascorbate, collagen, fibronectin, amelogenin, and poly(L-lysine) are coprecipitated with CaPs to be immobilized on biomaterials to increase bone cell attachment, proliferation, and tissue regeneration.

BMP-2, a protein that induces the formation of bone and cartilage, is widely used for bone regeneration. BMP-2 in the BMP-2-CaP composite layers retains its bioactivity, e.g., it stimulated ALP activity of rat bone marrow stromal cells when the cells were seeded directly on these layers for 8 days [22, 44, 66, 67]. BMP-2-CaP composite layers are highly biocompatible, osteoconductive, and osteoinductive, and they promote ectopic bone formation [22, 44, 66, 67].

FGF-2 is one of several well-characterized growth factors; it is highly expressed in developing tissues, stimulates vascular endothelial cell proliferation and neovascularization, and regulates cell growth, differentiation, and migration [68–70]. FGF-2 at an appropriate dose can promote bone regeneration. FGF-2-CaP composite layers promoted the proliferation of osteoblastic MC3T3 and MG63 cells [34, 50]. These enhanced bone formation at an optimized FGF-2 dose compared with layers without FGF-2 in full-thickness skull defects in rats [50].

L-Ascorbic acid phosphate magnesium salt n-hydrate (AsMg)-Ap composite layers markedly enhanced osteoblastic MC3T3-E1 cell proliferation and differentiation in vitro [27]. Collagen-Ap composite layers obviously enhanced the attachment, proliferation, and differentiation of Saos-2 osteoblast-like cells [71–74]. Collagen-fibronectin-CaP composite layers promoted osteoblastic cell proliferation and differentiation and new bone formation in full-thickness skull defects in rabbits [19, 51]. Amelogenin-Ap composite layers increased type I collagen gene expression level, ALP activity, and osteocalcin content of human embryonic palatal mesenchymal preosteoblast cells [20, 75]. BSA-CaP composite layers showed high biocompatibility and osteoconductivity [76, 77]. Zinc/silicate-Ap composite layers enhanced the proliferation and differentiation of osteoblastic MC3T3-E1 cells [78, 79]. Poly(L-lysine)-, poly(L-glutamic acid)-Ap composite layers promoted initial osteoblast adhesion, spreading, and proliferation, and were critical to forming a stable tissue implant interface [80].

6.3.2 Soft Tissue Regeneration

Signal molecules are used as stimulators of soft tissue regeneration. Signal molecule-CaP composites are used for promoting soft tissue formation around percutaneous implants, accelerating vascularization in cerebral infarction lesions, promoting epithelial cell adhesion, and preventing epidermal downgrowth, among others.

Accelerated cell adhesion and tissue regeneration at the interface between the external fixation pin, a percutaneous implant, and soft tissues are required for decreasing infection around the percutaneous device. Several signal molecules were immobilized with Ap on titanium (Ti) external fixation pins to accelerate cell proliferation, differentiation, and tissue regeneration around the pin. Ti rods, which correspond to the stem part of the Ti external fixation pin, coated with AsMg-FGF-2-Ap composite layers markedly enhanced proliferation and procollagen type I gene expression of fibroblastic NIH3T3 cells [27]. Ti rods coated with zinc/silicate-Ap composite layers accelerated proliferation of fibroblastic NIH3T3 and osteoblastic MC3T3-E1 cells and differentiation of MC3T3-E1 cells in vitro [78, 79]. Ti screws coated with FGF-2-Ap composite layers exhibited a significantly higher bone-screw interface strength and a lower pin-tract infection rate than uncoated titanium screws after percutaneous implantation into the proximal tibial metaphyses in rabbits for 4 weeks (Fig. 6.3) [81].

Ti screws coated with the FGF-2-Ap composite layers showed a significantly higher wound healing rate than those coated with an Ap layer [82]. Ti screws coated with an AsMg-FGF-2-Ap composite layer significantly reduced the infection rate compared with those coated with an Ap layer after percutaneous implantation of the screws in both proximal tibial metaphyses in rabbits for 4 weeks [43]. It is suggested that the enhanced wound healing associated with the formation of Sharpey's fiberlike tissue triggered by FGF-2 leads to the reduction in pin-tract infection rate [82].

Besides Ti, stainless steel was coated with AsMg-Ap composite layers using an interfacial layer of mesoporous bioactive glass existing between the metal

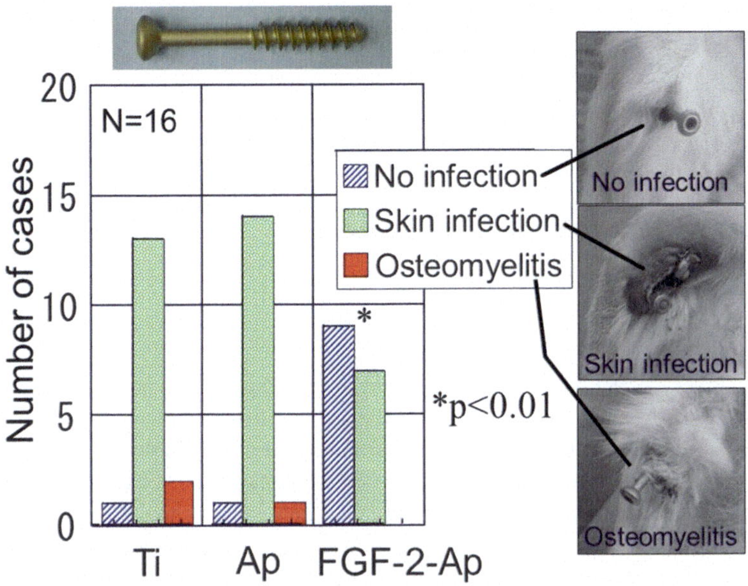

Fig. 6.3 Pin-tract infection around percutaneously implanted uncoated Ti screws (*upper left*, Ti) and those coated with Ap (Ap) and FGF-2-Ap composite layers (FGF-2-Ap). Infection rate for Ti screws coated with FGF-2-Ap composite layers was 44 % (7/16), while that for uncoated and Ap-coated Ti screws was 94 % (15/16), which is statistically significant ($p < 0.01$) [81]

and composite layers. The stainless steel coated with AsMg-Ap composite layers enhanced the proliferation of fibroblastic NIH3T3 cells in vitro [26]. Titanium or ethylene-vinyl alcohol copolymer (EVOH) coated with laminin-Ap composite layers showed greater epithelial cell adhesion than that uncoated and coated with Ap [21, 41]. The laminin-Ap composite layer is promising for preventing bacterial invasion through the interface around percutaneous implants such as dental implants, as adhesion of epithelial cells to surfaces of teeth or dental implants prevents bacterial invasion [83, 84]. EVOH coated with laminin-Ap composite layers had higher adhesion strength to the skin of rat than EVOH coated with Ap when they were percutaneously implanted [85]. However, there was no significant difference in epidermal downgrowth (which likely leads to bacterial infection through the interfacial space) between EVOH coated with laminin-Ap composite layers and EVOH coated with Ap.

Although FGF-2 is promising for treating brain infarction, intravenously administered FGF-2 has a short circulation half-life (0.5–3 min) and is sequestered rapidly in several organs [86]. An FGF-2-Ap composite layer was applied to prevent the progress of brain infarction in a rat cerebral ischemia model for progressive cerebrovascular disorder, called moyamoya disease [55]. The treatment of moyamoya disease includes the introduction of blood vessels to the brain from the soft tissue outside the skull through an opening or burr holes created in the skull. Burr hole plugs coated with FGF-2-Ap composite layers were implanted in the animal model. The plugs coated with an FGF-2-Ap composite layer showed an improved effectiveness of preventing the progress of brain infarction. The coated plugs yielded significantly smaller areas of brain ischemia and better capillary density than uncoated plugs and uncoated pugs plus direct FGF-2 administration [55].

6.4 Applications to Gene Delivery

6.4.1 *Gene Delivery: An Introduction*

Gene delivery is a fundamental technique in molecular biology for manipulating cellular characteristics, functions, and behavior by introducing foreign genes (DNA, RNA) into cells with the aid of viral or nonviral vectors. Table 6.1 shows major gene delivery systems. Physical gene delivery systems such as electroporation [87], microinjection [88], and gene gun [89] are excluded in this chapter.

Viral vectors such as adenoviruses, retroviruses, and lentiviruses are the most efficient. Viral vectors with a few exceptions (e.g., adenovirus) generally produce stable transgene expression almost permanently by introducing a foreign gene into the host cell's genome [90, 91]. A viral gene delivery system is a well-established method to manipulate cells and has long been studied for gene therapy applications. However, the viral systems have drawbacks such as toxicity (immunogenicity and oncogenicity), transgene overexpression, and difficulty in handling and large-scale production of recombinant viruses [90, 91].

Nonviral vectors (typically a plasmid including therapeutic genes) are safer and easier to use than viral vectors. Generally, nonviral vectors induce transgene expression only transiently (shorter than the cell lifespan) without affecting the host cell's genome. To enhance delivery efficiency, nonviral vectors are usually used in complex with transfection reagents such as lipids (of either liposomal or nonliposomal type), cationic polymers, and CaPs [92–94]. Nonviral gene delivery (also called transfection) systems have gained increased attention in tissue engineering applications as a tool to control cell behavior including multiplication and differentiation.

Table 6.1 Major gene delivery systems

System	Efficiency	Safety	Typical vectors/reagents used for delivery
Viral system	High	Low	Adenovirus, retrovirus, lentivirus
Lipid-based system	Medium	Medium	DOTAP[a], DOPE[b], DOSPA[c]
Polymer-based system	Medium	Medium	Polyethyleneimine Poly(L-lysine)
CaP-based system	Low	High	Ap, Carbonate Ap

[a]*N*-(1-(2,3-dioleoyloxy))-*N*,*N*,*N*-trimethylammonium propane methylsulfate
[b]1,2-dioleoyl-3-sn-phosphatidylethanolamine
[c]*N*-(2-((1,5,10,14-tetraazatetradecane-1-yl)carbonylamino]ethyl)-*N*,*N*-dimethyl-2,3-bis(oleoyloxy)-1-propanaminium

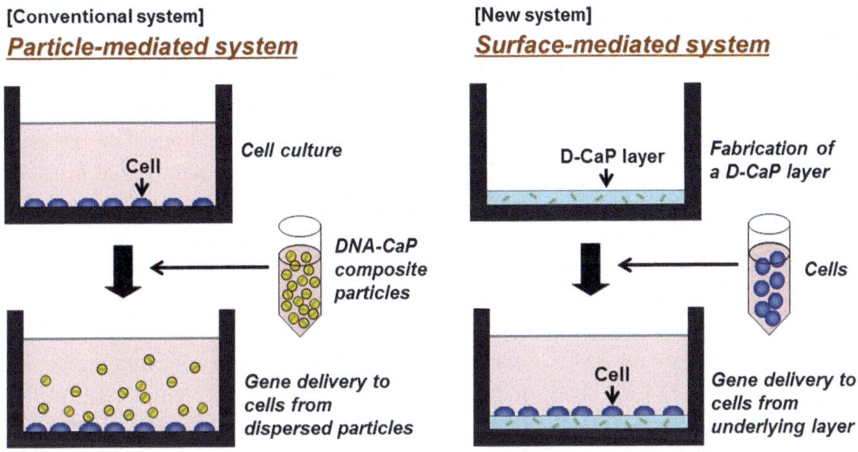

Fig. 6.4 Conventional (*left*, particle-mediated) and new (*right*, surface-mediated) CaP-based gene delivery systems (Reprinted from Oyane et al. [95], Copyright 2012, with permission from Elsevier)

Among various nonviral gene delivery systems developed hitherto, CaP-based systems have the advantages of safety, good biocompatibility, and a relatively simple and cost-effective production process. In the following sections, CaP-based gene delivery systems will be described with emphasis on a new system using DNA-CaP composite layers [95].

6.4.2 Gene Delivery Systems Using CaP Composite Layers

A conventional CaP-based gene delivery system [94] is generally mediated by nano-/microparticles of DNA-CaP composites. The DNA-CaP composite particles can be fabricated by mixing a phosphate ion solution and a calcium ion solution that is supplemented with DNA under neutral pH in a controlled manner. Thus precipitated DNA-CaP composite particles are either added to a culture medium bathing cells (Fig. 6.4 (left)) or injected into the body for the delivery of therapeutic genes into cells. The critical disadvantages of CaP-based gene delivery systems are their insufficient efficiency and poor reproducibility compared with other nonviral systems. Various approaches have been proposed to increase the efficiency of CaP-based gene delivery systems. For example, inhibitors of CaP crystal growth, i.e., block copolymers [96] or specific ions such as magnesium and carbonate [97, 98], were utilized to regulate the size and crystal structure of composite particles. Modification of composite particles with other transfection reagents [99] or cell adhesion molecules [100] was also proposed to enhance cell-particle interactions.

In 2004, Shen et al. proposed a new CaP-based gene delivery system [28]: a surface-mediated system using a DNA-CaP composite layer (D-CaP layer) that is composed of a matrix layer of CaP nanocrystals and DNA molecules immobilized within the layer. In this system, cells are seeded on the D-CaP layer that was previously fabricated on a substrate (Fig. 6.4 (right)). During the culture, the layer supports cell adhesion and growth on its surface with minimal toxicity. At the same time, the layer releases DNA molecules into the surrounding medium. The released DNA molecules or those in complex with calcium ions, CaP nano-sized clusters [1, 3], and/or CaP submicro- or microsized particles are taken up by the cells via endocytosis. In this way, the D-CaP layer mediates gene delivery to the cells adhering to the layer's surface. The gene delivery efficiency of the D-CaP layer was as high as that of a particle-mediated commercial lipid-based system.

Shen's gene delivery system has been refined and improved by modifying the D-CaP layer. In the late 2000s, Oyane et al. immobilized a cell adhesion molecule, laminin, within a D-CaP layer, thereby increasing gene delivery efficiency further [32, 101]. The gene delivery efficiency achieved with the laminin-immobilized D-CaP layer (DL-CaP layer) was 1–2 orders of magnitude higher than that achieved with the D-CaP layer for various cells [101]. Another cell adhesion molecule, fibronectin, also increased the gene delivery efficiency of the D-CaP layer when immobilized within the layer (resulting layer denoted as the DF-CaP layer) (Fig. 6.5), while a non-cell adhesion molecule, albumin, did not [32]. The role of cell adhesion molecules immobilized within the D-CaP layer has been proposed as follows [32]. Cell adhesion molecules immobilized within the layer enhance cell adhesion and spreading on the layer through ligand-receptor interactions (see the lower schematic in Fig. 6.5). As a result, a static microenvironment with low fluidity is formed at the interface between the cells and the layer. The DNA molecules released from the layer accumulate with time in this static microenvironment because the DNA release continues even after the cells have fully adhered and spread. As a consequence of the enlarged area of contact between the cell and the layer and the increased DNA concentration in this interfacial microenvironment, a more efficient gene delivery was accomplished on the DL-CaP and DF-CaP layers than on the D-CaP layer. Cell adhesion molecules released together with DNA from the layer might have also facilitated gene delivery by enhancing the cellular uptake of DNA.

In 2010, Sun et al. and Luong et al. showed that the immobilization of lipid transfection reagents within a D-CaP layer (resulting layer denoted as the DLp-CaP layer) is also effective in improving the gene delivery efficiency of the layer [40, 52]. Luong et al. demonstrated by fluorescent staining the colocalization of DNA and the lipid transfection reagent in the layer [40]. This colocalization occurs because lipid transfection reagents form stable complexes (lipoplexes) with DNA molecules through interactions between positively charged lipids and negatively charged DNA molecules. The DLp-CaP layer fabricated by a coprecipitation process (refer to Sect. 6.4.3) showed higher gene transfer efficiency than a CaP layer with superficially adsorbed lipoplexes [40, 103]. This result might derive from the presence of lipoplexes through the thickness of the DLp-CaP layer fabricated by the coprecipitation process, which causes a slow and sustained release of lipoplexes from the layer [103]. More recently, DLp-CaP layers have been prepared under different conditions using various types of lipid transfection reagent [104].

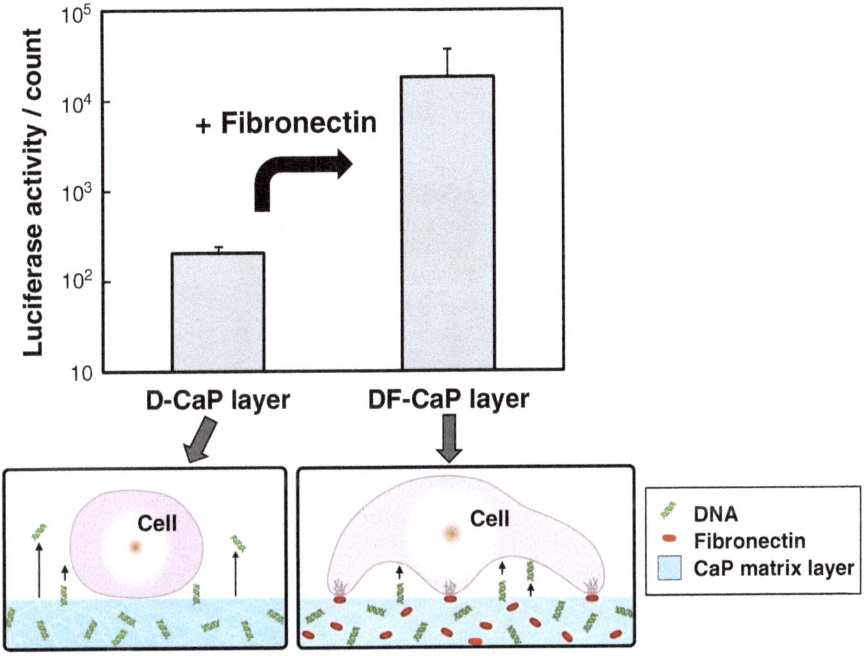

Fig. 6.5 Gene delivery efficiency of the D-CaP and DF-CaP layers for the CHO-K1 cells (*upper*) [102], and schematic of the cell-layer interface (*lower*) [32]

The gene delivery efficiency of the DLp-CaP layer is largely dependent on the molecular structure of lipids and the lipoplex content of the layer. The DLp-CaP layer fabricated under optimized conditions showed approximately 4 and 1 orders of magnitude higher gene delivery efficiency than the D-CaP and DF-CaP layers, respectively. Furthermore, the gene delivery efficiency achieved with the DLp-CaP layer was 2–3 orders of magnitude higher than that achieved with a conventional particle-mediated system using commercial lipid transfection reagents in the presence of serum. Given these results, the gene delivery system using the DLp-CaP layer is highly efficient as a nonviral system and has potential in tissue engineering applications.

6.4.3 Control of Gene Delivery

Surface modification of substrates for inducing CaP nucleation increases opportunity of application of the D-CaP layers to a wide range of substrates [95]. Such surface modification includes ACP precoating. Specifically, an ACP-assisted biomimetic process [95, 105] for fabrication of a D-CaP layer consists of a simple ACP precoating by dipping alternately in calcium and phosphate solutions followed

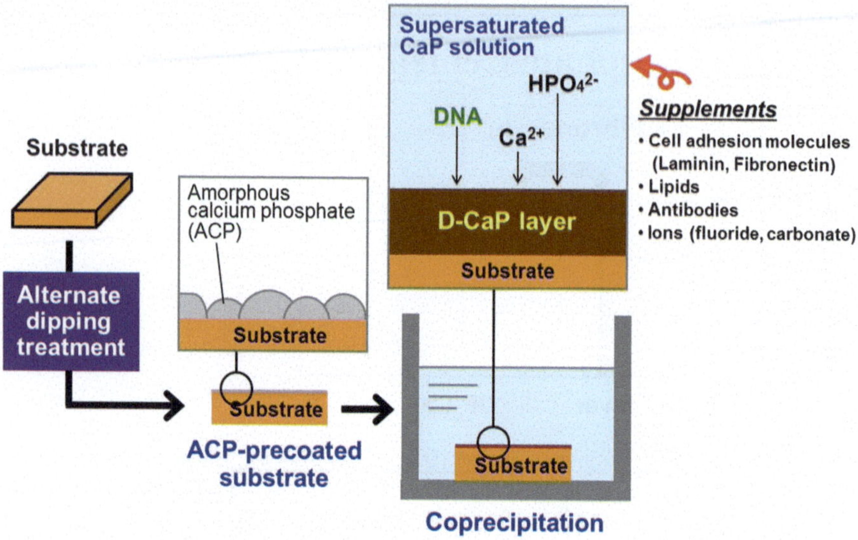

Fig. 6.6 Schematic of ACP-assisted biomimetic process

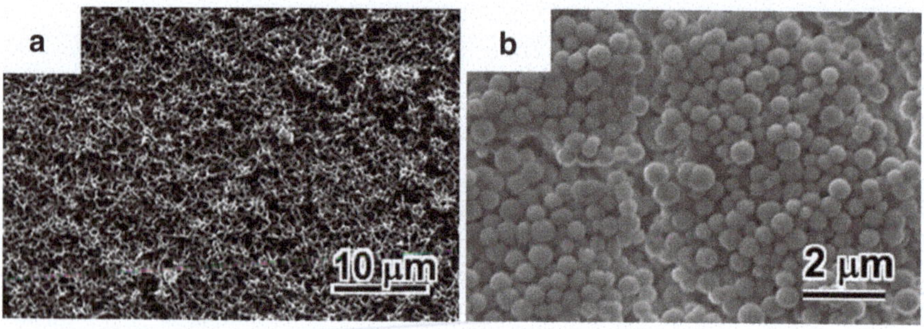

Fig. 6.7 SEM images of the surfaces of (**a**) a D-CaP layer of continuous film prepared in a metastable supersaturated CaP solution where the CaP is crystalline Ap and (**b**) a D-CaP layer of sphere assembly prepared in a labile supersaturated CaP solution where the CaP is ACP (Reproduced from Oyane et al. [107] by permission of The Royal Society of Chemistry)

by immersion in a supersaturated CaP solution supplemented with DNA (Fig. 6.6). The resulting D-CaP layer typically has a form of a continuous film with a submicron-sized cavernous structure (Fig. 6.7a) and is composed of low-crystalline Ap as the CaP crystalline phase [101, 102, 106]. Immobilization of macromolecules (e.g., fibronectin, lipids) within the D-CaP layer was achieved by supplementing these molecules to the supersaturated CaP solution in a certain concentration range.

The gene delivery efficiency of CaP composite layers can be controlled depending on the coprecipitation conditions such as the concentrations of inorganic ions, DNA, and supplemental macromolecules of the supersaturated CaP solution [28, 32,

40, 52, 101–103, 106]. These factors have an effect on gene delivery efficiency most likely by affecting the content of the DNA and supplemental macromolecules of the composite layer, macro- and crystal structures of the CaP phase, the profile of release of the DNA complexes, and/or physicochemical properties (e.g., particle size, surface charge, and dissolution kinetics) of the DNA complexes released from the layer [95]. For example, a higher laminin concentration of the supersaturated CaP solution leads to a higher laminin content of the DL-CaP layer, thereby increasing the layer's gene delivery efficiency [32, 101]. Similar correlations were also found between gene delivery efficiency and the contents of fibronectin [102], lipid [104], and DNA [32] of the composite layer. Immersion period in a supersaturated CaP solution (incubation time for coprecipitation) is another controlling factor affecting the gene delivery efficiency of the composite layer [40]. In fact, the gene delivery efficiency of the DLp-CaP layer decreased with increasing immersion period owing to the conformational change of DNA molecules: half of the supercoiled DNA changed into the nicked circular form within 48 h [40]. Macro- and crystal structures of the CaP phase is also a controlling factor affecting the gene delivery efficiency of the composite layer [107]. The D-CaP layer of sphere assembly (Fig. 6.7b) prepared in a labile supersaturated CaP solution showed higher gene transfer efficiency than D-CaP and DF-CaP layers of continuous films (Fig. 6.7a) fabricated via heterogeneous nucleation in a metastable supersaturated CaP solution [107].

The timing of gene delivery on the CaP composite layers can also be controlled depending on the coprecipitation conditions. The addition of sodium fluoride to a supersaturated CaP solution leads to the incorporation of fluoride ions into the DF-CaP layer via ionic substitution in the Ap crystal lattice [108]. Fluoride ions are present in trace amounts in Ap of bone tissue, and they decrease the solubility and dissolution rate of Ap. Therefore, the incorporated fluoride ions retard the dissolution of the DF-CaP layer and, consequently, delay the timing of gene expression in the cells cultured on the layer in a dose-dependent manner [108]. Such a timing-controlled gene delivery system using CaP composite layers would be useful for the effective induction of cell differentiation.

The CaP composite layers allow area-specific gene delivery on their surfaces, owing to gene delivery localized within the area of the layer. It was demonstrated that the gene expression level in the cells cultured on the DF-CaP layer was 45-fold higher than that in the cells cultured on a culture plate outside the layer, although the cells were cultured in the same medium in the same well, and the distance between them was only a few millimeters [102]. This result indicates that DNA was preferentially delivered to the cells adhering to the DF-CaP layer. Similar result was also obtained for a DLp-CaP layer [104]. Normally, it is difficult for conventional particulate vectors/transfection reagents to confine the area of gene delivery owing to their diffusion in the medium or in the body fluid. In contrast, the area of gene delivery can be confined to a specific location of a scaffold that is coated with a CaP composite layer as described above. Hence, a surface-mediated gene delivery system using CaP composite layers is advantageous over conventional particle-mediated systems in terms of the spatial control of gene delivery.

Cell-specific gene delivery is feasible with antibody-immobilized D-CaP layers with the aid of the specific antigen-antibody interaction. Immobilization of an anti-N-cadherin antibody within the D-CaP layer was effective in increasing the efficiency of gene delivery to the N-cadherin-positive P19CL6 cells but not to the N-cadherin-negative UV♀2 cells [106]. The increase in gene delivery efficiency was depleted by preblocking the P19CL6 cells with anti-N-cadherin antibody. Therefore, the antigen-antibody interaction occurring at the cell-layer interface should be responsible for the increased efficiency of gene delivery on the antibody-immobilized D-CaP layer. Antibodies have high specificities for particular antigens. Therefore, by selecting a suitable antibody for immobilization in a CaP composite layer, selective gene transfer to target cells in multiclonal cell systems, including in vivo systems, is feasible.

6.4.4 *Tissue Engineering Applications*

Gene delivery systems using CaP composite layers are effective in enhancing cell differentiation and tissue regeneration in vitro and in vivo. The DL-CaP layer with DNA carrying the gene of the nerve growth factor (NGF) induced neuronlike differentiation of neuronal PC12 cells in vitro [32]. The neuronlike differentiation was triggered by NGF secreted by the NGF-gene-transfected PC12 cells. DF-CaP and DLp-CaP layers with DNA carrying the BMP-2 gene were applied to bone tissue engineering [109–111]. In an in vitro study, the DF-CaP layer induced a twofold higher ALP activity and thus enhanced osteogenic differentiation of osteoblastic MC3T3-E1 cells than the CaP and D-CaP layers [109]. In a rat cranial bone defect model, the DF-CaP layer increased the BMP-2 content in the surrounding tissue to 107 pg/mg (the CaP layer, 58 pg/mg; the D-CaP layer, 46 pg/mg), thereby demonstrating the evidence of in vivo direct gene transfer. As a result, osteogenic differentiation and bone regeneration (at 8 weeks) were enhanced at the bone defect site (Figs. 6.8 and 6.9) [109]. Histological examination suggested good tissue compatibility with the CaP, D-CaP, and DF-CaP layers [109]. Moreover, even in an ectopic site (the dorsal subcutaneous tissue of rat), the DF-CaP layer induced a 49-fold increase in BMP-2 gene expression level and a fourfold increase in ALP gene expression level (at 4 weeks) compared with the CaP layer [111]. It is indicated that scaffolds coated with CaP composite layers loaded with DNA can be used for a variety of target cells and tissues by appropriately selecting genes according to the intended purpose.

The potential advantages of gene delivery over protein delivery in tissue regeneration include a higher stability of the DNA complexes and a longer sustainability of effectiveness associated with gene delivery. Many cytokines and growth factors are chemically unstable and have fragile molecular configurations, which lead to the decomposition or loss of full bioactivity in a short period in manufacturing processes and even in the body. Therefore, protein delivery systems often require high protein doses that range from micrograms to milligrams [112]. The delivery of the plasmid

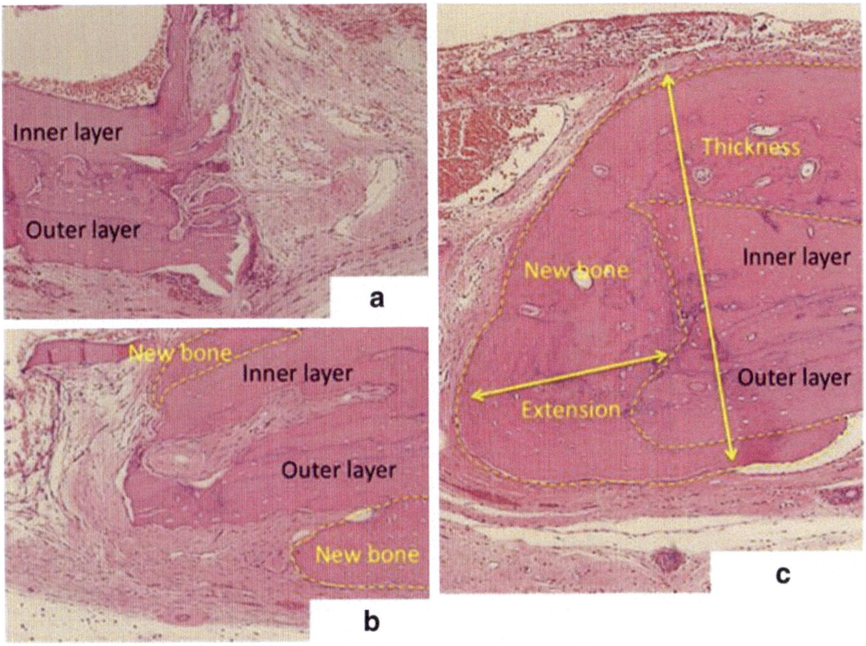

Fig. 6.8 Bone formation around burr hole plugs coated with the CaP (**a**), D-CaP (**b**), and DF-CaP (**c**) layers 8 weeks after the implantation in a rat cranial bone defect model (Reprinted from Zhang et al. [109], Copyright 2011 Zhang, W., Tsurushima, H., Oyane, A., Yazaki, Y., Sogo, Y., Ito, A., et al.; licensee BioMed Central Ltd.)

carrying the gene of a therapeutic protein rather than the protein itself might be an alternative and probably more effective approach. This is because plasmids are more economical than proteins to manufacture; moreover, they are more chemically stable when in complex with suitable transfection reagents compared with many therapeutic proteins. In nonviral gene delivery systems, the transfected cells serve as local bioreactors, express the exogenous genes, and continue to secrete the fresh recombinant proteins for a certain period in a paracrine/autocrine manner [113]. Such an in situ protein secretion by the autologous cells would prolong the therapeutic effect on the specific target. Note that proteins exhibit therapeutic activity immediately after they are delivered to the local site, whereas genes are not effective unless they are delivered into the cell nuclei and translated to their therapeutic protein products that are then finally secreted by the cell. In this respect, a safe and efficient system of delivery of genes to the intended cells at an intended location is of vital importance in medical applications. The gene delivery systems using CaP composite layers with the advantages of the safety of CaPs as well as controllable area, timing, affinity for cells, and delivery efficiency would be useful for achieving such gene delivery.

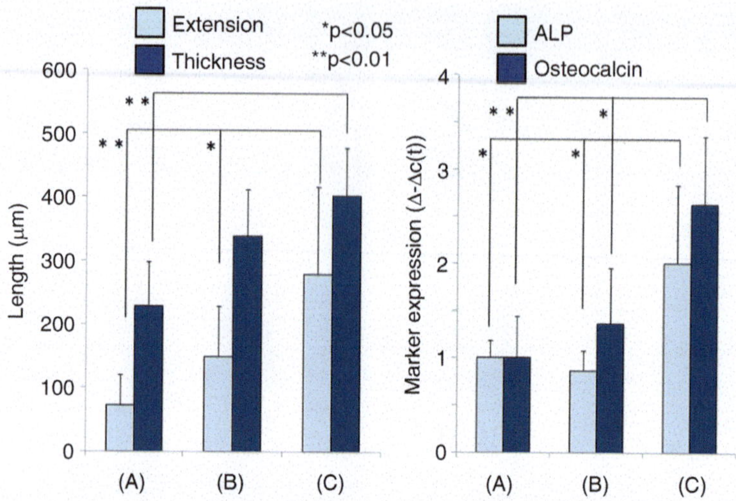

Fig. 6.9 Histomorphometric analysis for the bone and marker expression for the tissue around burr hole plugs coated with the CaP (*A*), D-CaP (*B*), and DF-CaP (*C*) layers 8 weeks after the implantation (Reprinted from Zhang et al. [109], Copyright 2011 Zhang, W., Tsurushima, H., Oyane, A., Yazaki, Y., Sogo, Y., Ito, A., et al.; licensee BioMed Central Ltd.)

6.5 Other Applications

6.5.1 Adjuvants for Cancer Immunotherapy

An adjuvant is a substance used in combination with a specific antigen that produces more immunity than the antigen used alone. Adjuvants serve to enhance the magnitude, breadth, quality, and longevity of specific immune responses to antigens and reduce the amount of antigen and/or number of immunizations required to achieve the desired immune responses [114, 115]. As conventional vaccine adjuvants, aluminum hydroxide, aluminum phosphate, and CaP (principally Ap) have been approved officially for human use. CaP is a safe material lacking immunopotentiating activity since it is a normal constituent of the body and is well tolerated and readily resorbed by the body [116]. The primary mode of action of the CaP adjuvant is targeting delivery of an immunogen to immune effector cells, generally via antigen-presenting cells [117]. In cancer immunotherapy, an immunopotentiating adjuvant combined with delivery function is crucial to triggering antitumor immune responses that include innate and adaptive immune responses [118, 119], because tumor cells show reduced antigen presentation and downregulate the immune responses of the body [119, 120]. Ceramic Ap particles combined with the patient's tumor antigens (immunogens) and heat shock proteins (immunopotentiating adjuvant) were safely administered as a therapeutic cancer vaccine and showed some encouraging clinical results in a human pilot study [121].

Pathogen-associated molecular patterns (PAMPs) are one of the most potent classes of immunopotentiating adjuvants lacking the function of targeting delivery. A promising strategy to enhance the immunopotentiating effect of PAMPs is to achieve a sustained release of PAMPs using a delivery system [122, 123], through which a synergistic effect between the two principal modes of action of adjuvants, i.e., the immunopotentiating and targeted delivery actions, is achieved.

Mesoporous silica (MS)-PAMP-CaP composite adjuvants were prepared using tuberculin purified protein derivative or hydrothermal extract of a human tubercle bacillus (*Mycobacterium tuberculosis*). The MS-PAMP-CaP composite adjuvants effectively induced activation of antigen-presenting cells, as evidenced by the enhanced GM-CSF secretion by THP-1 differentiated macrophages, probably owing to the efficient cellular uptake (delivery into the cells) of the MS-PAMP-CaP composites followed by the sustained release of PAMPs. The MS-PAMP-CaP composite adjuvants mixed with liquid-nitrogen-treated tumor tissue effectively triggered antitumor immune response and markedly inhibited the growth of rechallenged tumor cells in vivo (Fig. 6.10) [30, 57, 124].

6.5.2 Infection Control

An antibiotic-Ap composite may be a useful carrier for antibiotics. A common strategy to control infection is the use of a systemic antibiotic prophylaxis [125]. Attention has been focused on the localized use of therapeutic agents against infection. The advantages of local delivery may include a decrease in the side effects in systemic treatment and the possibility of higher dosages near the affected site, thereby improving efficacy and reducing the treatment duration [23, 24, 126, 127]. Chlorhexidine-Ap composite layers were formed on external fixation pins. An in vitro antimicrobial efficacy test of the chlorhexidine-Ap composite layers, evaluated using a *Staphylococcus aureus* culture, showed a larger "inhibition zone" formed around the composite layers than that of the chlorhexidine-free Ap layers. The chlorhexidine-Ap composite layers may greatly reduce the incidence of pin-tract infection associated with external fixation [126]. Tetracycline- and gatifloxacin-Ap composite layers were prepared on the surface of EVOH plates. The antibiotic-Ap composite layers showed antibacterial activity against *Escherichia coli* and *Staphylococcus aureus* and would be useful for infection control of percutaneous devices [24]. The cephalothin-, carbenicillin-, amoxicillin-, cefamandol-, tobramycin-, gentamicin-, and vancomycin-carbonated Ap composite layers were prepared on Ti alloy implants. The antibiotic-Ap composite layers showed inhibition of growth of *Staphylococcus aureus*, due to the release of antibiotics from the antibiotic-Ap composite layers [23, 127].

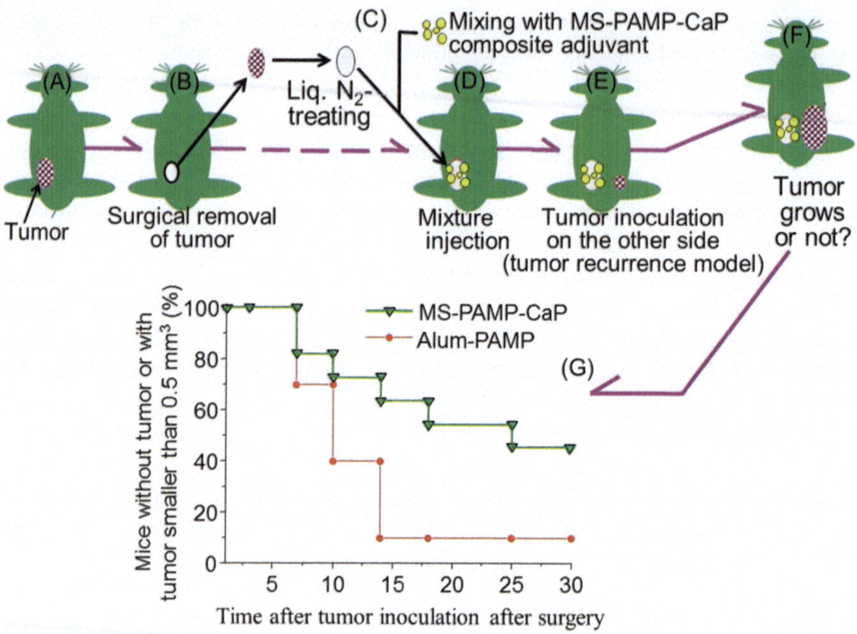

Fig. 6.10 Tumor (*A*) in the mouse is surgically removed (*B*). The tumor is killed in liquid nitrogen and mixed with the MS-PAMP-CaP adjuvant or commercial alum-PAMP adjuvant (*C*). Since killed tumor tissue contains plenty of autologous tumor antigens, the mixture now becomes individual-mouse-specific autologous cancer vaccine. Then, this mixture is injected to the mouse (*D*). The mouse without tumor recurrence at the original tumor site is subjected to inoculation of alive tumor cells (rechallenge) on the other side as a tumor recurrence model (*E*). If antitumor immunity is established owing to the tumor antigen and MS-PAMP-CaP adjuvant, no tumor grows or tumor growth is delayed (*F*). The mice in MS-PAMP-CaP adjuvant group showed significantly delayed tumor growth after rechallenge of the alive tumor cells ($p = 0.045$) compared with the commercial alum-PAMP adjuvant group (*G*) (Reprinted from Wang et al. [57], Copyright 2013, with permission from Elsevier)

6.5.3 Prevention of Thrombogenesis

Signal molecules are used to inhibit platelet adhesion, thus improving thromboresistance. Laminin-Ap composite layers coated on Ti plates exhibited significantly decreased platelet adhesion under blood flow condition compared with mirror polished uncoated Ti [18]. The laminin-Ap composite layers can be used to inhibit the thrombogenesis of blood-contacting medical devices. Laminin-Ap composite layers showed a lower surface roughness than Ap layers without laminin [45], which is favorable for inhibiting thrombogenesis. A decrease in the complexity of the surface microtexture decreases platelet adhesion [41, 128, 129].

A layer of vascular endothelial cells on the blood-contacting surface would provide an excellent antithrombogenic effect on the blood-contacting surface [130], as the endothelium is the physiological and most hemocompatible blood-contacting surface. The major limitation in forming a stable vascular endothelial cell layer has been a shortage of an extracellular matrix suitable for vascular endothelial adhesion, growth, and function [131, 132]. The laminin/FGF-2-Ap-composite-layer-based extracellular matrix can control vascular endothelial cell adhesion, growth, and retention and is thus expected to show an improved antithrombogenic effect [133, 134]. Laminin-Ap composite layers were prepared on Ti plate using a supersaturated CaP solution supplemented with laminin. The number of vascular endothelial cells adhering to the laminin-Ap composite layers was remarkably higher than that of cells adhering to the untreated Ti. Moreover, endothelial cells adhering to the laminin-Ap composite layers showed a significantly higher cell retention rate under physiological shear stress than those adhering to the untreated Ti [133]. FGF-2-AsMg-Ap-coated Ti plates were prepared by immersing Ti plates in supersaturated CaP solutions supplemented with FGF-2 and AsMg. The FGF-2-AsMg-Ap layer on the Ti plate accelerated the proliferation of endothelial cells compared with the as-prepared Ti. The vascular endothelial layer markedly inhibited in vitro platelet adhesion [134].

References

1. Onuma K, Ito A (1998) Cluster growth model for hydroxyapatite. Chem Mater 10:3346–3351
2. Kanzaki N, Treboux G, Onuma K, Tsutsumi S, Ito A (2001) Calcium phosphate clusters. Biomaterials 22:2921–2929
3. Oyane A, Onuma K, Kokubo T, Ito A (1999) Clustering of calcium phosphate in the system $CaCl_2$-H_3PO_4-KCl-H_2O. J Phys Chem B 103:8230–8235
4. Dey A, Bomans PHH, Muller FA, Will J, Frederik PM, de With G et al (2010) The role of prenucleation clusters in surface-induced calcium phosphate crystallization. Nat Mater 9:1010–1014
5. Habraken WJEM, Tao JH, Brylka LJ, Friedrich H, Bertinetti L, Schenk AS et al (2013) Ion-association complexes unite classical and non-classical theories for the biomimetic nucleation of calcium phosphate. Nat Commun 4:1507. doi:10.1038/ncomms2490
6. Erdemir D, Lee AY, Myerson AS (2009) Nucleation of crystals from solution: classical and two-step models. Acc Chem Res 42:621–629
7. Oyane A, Ootsuka T, Hayama K, Sogo Y, Ito A (2011) Enhanced immobilization of acidic proteins in the apatite layer via electrostatic interactions in a supersaturated calcium phosphate solution. Acta Biomater 7:2969–2976
8. Sogo Y, Ito A, Fukasawa K, Kondo N, Ishikawa Y, Ichinose N et al (2005) Coprecipitation of cytochrome C with calcium phosphate on hydroxyapatite ceramic. Curr Appl Phys 5:526–530
9. Sogo Y, Ito A, Onoguchi M, Li X, Oyane A, Ichinose N (2009) Formation of cytochrome C-apatite composite layer on NaOH- and heat-treated titanium. Mat Sci Eng C-Bio Sci 29:766–770
10. Sogo Y, Ito A, Onoguchi M, Oyane A, Tsurushima H, Ichinose N (2007) Formation of a FGF-2 and calcium phosphate composite layer on a hydroxyapatite ceramic for promoting bone formation. Biomed Mater 2:S175–S180
11. Li X, Wang XP, Ito A, Sogo Y, Cheng K, Oyane A (2009) Effect of coprecipitation temperature on the properties and activity of fibroblast growth factor-2 apatite composite layer. Mat Sci Eng C-Bio Sci 29:216–221

12. Rohanizadeh R, Padrines M, Bouler JM, Couchourel D, Fortun Y, Daculsi G (1998) Apatite precipitation after incubation of biphasic calcium-phosphate ceramic in various solutions: influence of seed species and proteins. J Biomed Mater Res 42:530–539
13. Couchourel D, Escoffier C, Rohanizadeh R, Bohic S, Daculsi G, Fortun Y et al (1999) Effects of fibronectin on hydroxyapatite formation. J Inorg Biochem 73:129–136
14. Daculsi G, Pilet P, Cottrel M, Guicheux G (1999) Role of fibronectin during biological apatite crystal nucleation: ultrastructural characterization. J Biomed Mater Res 47:228–233
15. Onuma K, Kanzaki N, Kobayashj N (2004) Association of calcium phosphate and fibroblast growth factor-2: a dynamic light scattering study. Macromol Biosci 4:39–46
16. Oyane A, Uchida M, Onuma K, Ito A (2006) Spontaneous growth of a laminin-apatite nano-composite in a metastable calcium phosphate solution. Biomaterials 27:167–175
17. Liu YL, Layrolle P, de Bruijn J, van Blitterswijk C, de Groot K (2001) Biomimetic coprecipitation of calcium phosphate and bovine serum albumin on titanium alloy. J Biomed Mater Res 57:327–335
18. Uchida M, Ito A, Furukawa KS, Nakamura K, Onimura Y, Oyane A et al (2005) Reduced platelet adhesion to titanium metal coated with apatite, albumin-apatite composite or laminin-apatite composite. Biomaterials 26:6924–6931
19. Sogo Y, Ito A, Matsuno T, Oyane A, Tamazawa G, Satoh T et al (2007) Fibronectin-calcium phosphate composite layer on hydroxyapatite to enhance adhesion, cell spread and osteogenic differentiation of human mesenchymal stem cells in vitro. Biomed Mater 2:116–123
20. Wen HB, Moradian-Oldak J (2003) Modification of calcium-phosphate coatings on titanium by recombinant amelogenin. J Biomed Mater Res A 64A:483–490
21. Uchida M, Oyane A, Kim HM, Kokubo T, Ito A (2004) Biomimetic coating of laminin-apatite composite on titanium metal and its excellent cell-adhesive properties. Adv Mater 16:1071–1074
22. Liu Y, Hunziker EB, Layrolle P, De Bruijn JD, De Groot K (2004) Bone morphogenetic protein 2 incorporated into biomimetic coatings retains its biological activity. Tissue Eng 10:101–108
23. Stigter M, de Groot K, Layrolle P (2002) Incorporation of tobramycin into biomimetic hydroxyapatite coating on titanium. Biomaterials 23:4143–4153
24. Oyane A, Yokoyama Y, Uchida M, Ito A (2006) The formation of an antibacterial agent-apatite composite coating on a polymer surface using a metastable calcium phosphate solution. Biomaterials 27:3295–3303
25. Ito A, Sogo Y, Ebihara Y, Onoguchi M, Oyane A, Ichinose N (2007) Formation of an ascorbate-apatite composite layer on titanium. Biomed Mater 2:S181–S185
26. Wang X, Li X, Onuma K, Ito A, Sogo Y, Kosuge K et al (2010) Mesoporous bioactive glass coatings on stainless steel for enhanced cell activity, cytoskeletal organization and AsMg immobilization. J Mater Chem 20:6437–6445
27. Wang X, Ito A, Sogo Y, Li X, Tsurushima H, Oyane A (2009) Ascorbate-apatite composite and ascorbate-FGF-2-apatite composite layers formed on external fixation rods and their effects on cell activity in vitro. Acta Biomater 5:2647–2656
28. Shen H, Tan J, Saltzman WM (2004) Surface-mediated gene transfer from nanocomposites of controlled texture. Nat Mater 3:569–574
29. Leonor IB, Alves CM, Azevedo HS, Reis RL (2009) Effects of protein incorporation on calcium phosphate coating. Mat Sci Eng C-Bio Sci 29:913–918
30. Li X, Wang X, Sogo Y, Ohno T, Onuma K, Ito A (2013) Mesoporous silica-calcium phosphate-tuberculin purified protein derivative composites as an effective adjuvant for cancer immunotherapy. Adv Health Mater 2:863–871
31. Tsuji T, Onuma K, Yamamoto A, Iijima M, Shiba K (2008) Direct transformation from amorphous to crystalline calcium phosphate facilitated by motif-programmed artificial proteins. Proc Natl Acad Sci USA 105:16866–16870
32. Oyane A, Tsurushima H, Ito A (2010) Highly efficient gene transfer system using a laminin-DNA-apatite composite layer. J Gene Med 12:194–206

33. do Serro APVA, Fernandes AC, Saramago BDV (2000) Calcium phosphate deposition on titanium surfaces in the presence of fibronectin. J Biomed Mater Res 49:345–352
34. Li Y, Lee IS, Cui FZ, Choi SH (2008) The biocompatibility of nanostructured calcium phosphate coated on micro-arc oxidized titanium. Biomaterials 29:2025–2032
35. Li Y, Lee IS, Cui FZ, Lin Z, Park JC, Chung SM (2008) Incorporation of cytochrome C with thin calcium phosphate film formed by electron-beam evaporation. Surf Coat Technol 202:5742–5745
36. Murphy WL, Mooney DJ (2002) Bioinspired growth of crystalline carbonate apatite on biodegradable polymer substrata. J Am Chem Soc 124:1910–1917
37. Togawa H, Kanzaki N, Tsutsumi S, Ito A (1996) Precipitation of apatite from high pressure simulated body fluid. In: Proceedings of 34th symposium on basic science of ceramics. Division of Basic Science, The Ceramic Society of Japan, Kyoto, pp 276–277
38. Ito A, Togawa H, Teraoka K, Tsutsumi S (1997) Chemical composition of apatite precipitated in a simulated body fluid concentrated using carbon dioxide gas and its application to a coating. In: Proceedings of 10th fall meetings of The Ceramic Society of Japan, p 76
39. Barrere F, Layrolle P, Van Blitterswijk C, de Groot K (2000) Fast formation of Ca-P coating on Ti6Al4V. Mater Res Soc Symp Proc 599:135–140
40. Luong LN, McFalls KM, Kohn DH (2009) Gene delivery via DNA incorporation within a biomimetic apatite coating. Biomaterials 30:6996–7004
41. Oyane A, Uchida M, Ito A (2005) Laminin-apatite composite coating to enhance cell adhesion to ethylene-vinyl alcohol copolymer. J Biomed Mater Res A 72A:168–174
42. Mutsuzaki H, Ito A, Sakane M, Sogo Y, Oyane A, Ebihara Y et al (2007) Calcium phosphate coating formed in infusion fluid mixture to enhance fixation strength of titanium screws. J Mater Sci-Mater Med 18:1799–1808
43. Wang XP, Ito A, Li X, Sogo Y, Oyane A (2011) Signal molecules-calcium phosphate coprecipitation and its biomedical application as a functional coating. Biofabrication 3:022001
44. Liu Y, de Groot K, Hunziker EB (2005) BMP-2 liberated from biomimetic implant coatings induces and sustains direct ossification in an ectopic rat model. Bone 36:745–757
45. Oyane A, Ishikawa Y, Yamazaki A, Sogo Y, Furukawa K, Ushida T et al (2008) Reduction of surface roughness of a laminin-apatite composite coating via inhibitory effect of magnesium ions on apatite crystal growth. Acta Biomater 4:1342–1348
46. Oyane A, Yokoyama Y, Kasahara M, Ichinose N, Saito M, Ito A (2009) Mechanical properties of a laminin-apatite composite layer formed on an ethylene-vinyl alcohol copolymer. Mat Sci Eng C-Bio Sci 29:1681–1686
47. Liu Y, Hunziker EB, Randall NX, de Groot K, Layrolle P (2003) Proteins incorporated into biomimetically prepared calcium phosphate coatings modulate their mechanical strength and dissolution rate. Biomaterials 24:65–70
48. Fu K, Klibanov AM, Langer R (2000) Protein stability in controlled-release systems. Nat Biotechnol 18:24–25
49. Langer R (1998) Drug delivery and targeting. Nature 392:5–10
50. Tsurushima H, Marushima A, Suzuki K, Oyane A, Sogo Y, Nakamura K et al (2010) Enhanced bone formation using hydroxyapatite ceramic coated with fibroblast growth factor-2. Acta Biomater 6:2751–2759
51. Sogo Y, Ishikawa Y, Kondo N, Uchimura E, Oyane A, Ohno T et al (2006) Coprecipitation of cell adhesion molecule with calcium phosphate on hydroxyapatite ceramic. Key Eng Mater 309–311:767–770
52. Sun BB, Tran KK, Shen H (2009) Enabling customization of non-viral gene delivery systems for individual cell types by surface-induced mineralization. Biomaterials 30:6386–6393
53. Ito A, Sogo Y, Ebihara Y, Wang X, Oyane A, Ichinose N (2009) Ascorbate-apatite composite layers formed on ceramic hydroxyapatite for promoting tissue regeneration. Arch BioCeram Res 9:155–158
54. Nur-E-Kamal A, Ahmed I, Kamal J, Babu AN, Schindler M, Meiners S (2008) Covalently attached FGF-2 to three-dimensional polyamide nanofibrillar surfaces demonstrates enhanced biological stability and activity. Mol Cell Biochem 309:157–166

55. Ito Y, Tsurushima H, Sato M, Ito A, Oyane A, Sogo Y et al (2013) Angiogenesis therapy for brain infarction using a slow-releasing drug delivery system for fibroblast growth factor 2. Biochem Biophys Res Commun 432:182–187
56. Ito Y (2008) Covalently immobilized biosignal molecule materials for tissue engineering. Soft Matter 4:46–56
57. Wang X, Li X, Ito A, Sogo Y, Ohno T (2013) Particle-size-dependent toxicity and immunogenic activity of mesoporous silica-based adjuvants for tumor immunotherapy. Acta Biomater 9:7480–7489
58. Langer R, Vacanti JP (1999) Tissue engineering. Science 260:920–926
59. Persidis A (1999) Tissue engineering. Nat Biotechnol 17:508–510
60. Nerem RM, Sambanis A (1995) Tissue engineering: from biology to biological substitutes. Tissue Eng 1:3–13
61. Vacanti CA, Upton J (1994) Tissue-engineered morphogenesis of cartilage and bone by means of cell transplantation using synthetic biodegradable polymer matrices. Clin Plast Surg 21:445–462
62. Petite H, Viateau V, Bensaid W, Meunier A, de Pollak C, Bourguignon M et al (2000) Tissue-engineered bone regeneration. Nat Biotechnol 18:959–963
63. Constantz BR, Ison IC, Fulmer MT, Poser RD, Smith ST, VanWagoner M et al (1995) Skeletal repair by in situ formation of the mineral phase of bone. Science 267:1796–1799
64. Lane JM, Tomin E, Bostrom MPG (1999) Biosynthetic bone grafting. Clin Orthop Relat Res 367 Suppl:S107–S117
65. Lane JM, Bostrom MP (1998) Bone grafting and new composite biosynthetic graft materials. Instr Course Lect 47:525–534
66. Liu Y, Hunziker EB, de Groot K, Layrolle P (2003) Introduction of ectopic bone formation by BMP-2 incorporated biomimetically into calcium phosphate coatings of titanium-alloy implants. Key Eng Mater 240–242:667–670
67. Liu Y, Hunziker EB, Van de Vaal C, de Groot K (2004) Biomimetic coatings vs. collagen sponges as a carrier for BMP-2: a comparison of the osteogenic responses triggered in vivo using an ectopic rat model. Key Eng Mater 254–256:619–622
68. Abraham JA, Mergia A, Whang JL, Tumolo A, Friedman J, Hjerrild KA et al (1996) Nucleotide-sequence of a bovine clone encoding the angiogenic protein, basic fibroblast growth-factor. Science 233:545–548
69. Mcgee GS, Davidson JM, Buckley A, Sommer A, Woodward SC, Aquino AM et al (1998) Recombinant basic fibroblast growth-factor accelerates wound-healing. J Surg Res 45:145–153
70. Okada-Ban M, Thiery JP, Jouanneau J (2000) Fibroblast growth factor-2. Int J Biochem Cell B 32:263–267
71. Chen Y, Mak AFT, Wang M, Li JS, Wong MS (2008) In vitro behavior of osteoblast-like cells on PLLA films with a biomimetic apatite or apatite/collagen composite coating. J Mater Sci-Mater Med 19:2261–2268
72. Chen Y, Mak AFT, Wang M, Li JS (2006) Composite coating of bonelike apatite particles and collagen fibers on poly L-lactic acid formed through an accelerated biomimetic coprecipitation process. J Biomed Mater Res B 77B:315–322
73. Chen Y, Mak AFT, Wang M, Li JS, Wong MS (2006) PLLA scaffolds with biomimetic apatite coating and biomimetic apatite/collagen composite coating to enhance osteoblast-like cells attachment and activity. Surf Coat Technol 201:575–580
74. Chen Y, Mak AFT, Wang M, Li JS (2005) Biomimetic coating of apatite/collagen composite on Poly L-lactic acid facilitates cell seeding. Proc Ann Int IEEE Eng Med Biol Soc 4:4087–4090
75. Du C, Schneider GB, Zaharias R, Abbott C, Seabold D, Stanford C et al (2005) Apatite/amelogenin coating on titanium promotes osteogenic gene expression. J Dent Res 84:1070–1074
76. Luong LN, Hong SI, Patel RJ, Outslay ME, Kohn DH (2006) Spatial control of protein within biomimetically nucleated mineral. Biomaterials 27:1175–1186

77. Lee WK, Im SM (2006) Effect of BSA substitution into calcium phosphate on the surface-mediated responses of bone-forming cells. J Ind Eng Chem 12:932–938
78. Wang X, Ito A, Sogo Y, Li X, Oyane A (2010) Zinc-containing apatite layers on external fixation rods promoting cell activity. Acta Biomater 6:962–968
79. Wang X, Ito A, Sogo Y, Li X, Oyane A (2010) Silicate-apatite composite layers on external fixation rods and in vitro evaluation using fibroblast and osteoblast. J Biomed Mater Res A 92:1181–1189
80. Spoerke ED, Stupp SI (2005) Synthesis of a poly (L-lysine)-calcium phosphate hybrid on titanium surfaces for enhanced bioactivity. Biomaterials 26:5120–5129
81. Mutsuzaki H, Ito A, Sakane M, Sogo Y, Oyane A, Ochiai N (2008) Fibroblast growth factor-2-apatite composite layers on titanium screws to reduce pin tract infection rate. J Biomed Mater Res B 86B:365–374
82. Mutsuzaki H, Ito A, Sogo Y, Sakane M, Oyane A, Ochiai N (2012) Enhanced wound healing associated with Sharpey's fiber-like tissue formation around FGF-2-apatite composite layers on percutaneous titanium screws in rabbits. Arch Orthop Trauma Surg 132:113–121
83. Ikeda H, Yamaza T, Yoshinari M, Ohsaki Y, Ayukawa Y, Kido MA et al (2000) Ultrastructural and immunoelectron microscopic studies of the peri-implant epithelium-implant (Ti-6Al-4V) interface of rat maxilla. J Periodontol 71:961–973
84. Ikeda H, Shiraiwa M, Yamaza T, Yoshinari M, Kido MA, Ayukawa Y et al (2002) Difference in penetration of horseradish peroxidase tracer as a foreign substance into the peri-implant or junctional epithelium of rat gingivae. Clin Oral Implan Res 13:243–251
85. Oyane A, Hyodo K, Uchida M, Sogo Y, Ito A (2011) Preliminary in vivo study of apatite and laminin-apatite composite layers on polymeric percutaneous implants. J Biomed Mater Res B 97B:96–104
86. Whalen GF, Shing Y, Folkman J (1989) The fate of intravenously administered bFGF and the effect of heparin. Growth Factors 1:157–164
87. Neumann E, Schaeferridder M, Wang Y, Hofschneider PH (1982) Gene-transfer into mouse lyoma cells by electroporation in high electric-fields. EMBO J 1:841–845
88. Capecchi MR (1980) High-efficiency transformation by direct micro-injection of DNA into cultured mammalian-cells. Cell 22:479–488
89. Yang N, Burkholder J, Roberts B, Martinell B, McCabe D (1990) In vivo and in vitro gene transfer to mammalian somatic cells by particle bombardment. Proc Natl Acad Sci USA 87:9568–9572
90. Schaffer DV, Koerber JT, Lim KI (2008) Molecular engineering of viral gene delivery vehicles. Annu Rev Biomed Eng 10:169–194
91. Flotte TR (2007) Gene therapy: the first two decades and the current state-of-the-art. J Cell Physiol 213:301–305
92. Fraley R, Subramani S, Berg P, Papahadjopoulos D (1980) Introduction of liposome-encapsulated Sv40 DNA into cells. J Biol Chem 255:431–435
93. Yamano S, Dai JS, Moursi AM (2010) Comparison of transfection efficiency of nonviral gene transfer reagents. Mol Biotechnol 46:287–300
94. Graham FL, van der Eb AJ (1973) A new technique for the assay of infectivity of human adenovirus 5 DNA. Virology 52:456–467
95. Oyane A, Wang XP, Sogo Y, Ito A, Tsurushima H (2012) Calcium phosphate composite layers for surface-mediated gene transfer. Acta Biomater 8:2034–2046
96. Kakizawa Y, Kataoka K (2002) Block copolymer self-assembly into monodispersive nanoparticles with hybrid core of antisense DNA and calcium phosphate. Langmuir 18:4539–4543
97. Chowdhury EH, Megumi K, Harada I, Kundu AK, Akaike T (2004) Dramatic effect of Mg^{2+} on transfecting mammalian cells by DNA/calcium phosphate precipitates. Anal Biochem 328:96–97
98. Chowdhury EH, Kunou M, Nagaoka M, Kundu AK, Hoshiba T, Akaike T (2004) High-efficiency gene delivery for expression in mammalian cells by nanoprecipitates of Ca-Mg phosphate. Gene 341:77–82

99. Sokolova V, Neumann S, Kovtun A, Chernousova S, Heumann R, Epple M (2010) An outer shell of positively charged poly(ethyleneimine) strongly increases the transfection efficiency of calcium phosphate/DNA nanoparticles. J Mater Sci 45:4952–4957
100. Kutsuzawa K, Chowdhury EH, Nagaoka M, Maruyama K, Akiyama Y, Akaike T (2006) Surface functionalization of inorganic nano-crystals with fibronectin and E-cadherin chimera synergistically accelerates trans-gene delivery into embryonic stem cells. Biochem Biophys Res Commun 350:514–520
101. Oyane A, Tsurushima H, Ito A (2007) Novel gene-transferring scaffolds having a cell adhesion molecule-DNA-apatite nanocomposite surface. Gene Ther 14:1750–1753
102. Oyane A, Murayama M, Yamazaki A, Sogo Y, Ito A, Tsurushima H (2010) Fibronectin-DNA-apatite composite layer for highly efficient and area-specific gene transfer. J Biomed Mater Res A 92A:1038–1047
103. Yazaki Y, Oyane A, Tsurushima H, Araki H, Sogo Y, Ito A et al (2014) Coprecipitation of DNA-lipid complexes with apatite and comparison with superficial adsorption for gene transfer applications. J Biomater Appl 28:937–945
104. Oyane A, Yazaki Y, Araki H, Sogo Y, Ito A, Yamazaki A et al (2012) Fabrication of a DNA-lipid-apatite composite layer for efficient and area-specific gene transfer. J Mater Sci-Mater Med 23:1011–1019
105. Oyane A (2010) Development of apatite-based composites by a biomimetic process for biomedical applications. J Ceram Soc Jpn 118:77–81
106. Yazaki Y, Oyane A, Araki H, Sogo Y, Ito A, Yamazaki A et al (2012) Fabrication of DNA-antibody-apatite composite layers for cell-targeted gene transfer. Sci Technol Adv Mater 13:064204
107. Oyane A, Araki H, Sogo Y, Ito A, Tsurushima H (2013) Spontaneous assembly of DNA-amorphous calcium phosphate nanocomposite spheres for surface-mediated gene transfer. Cryst Eng Commun 15:4994–4997
108. Yazaki Y, Oyane A, Sogo Y, Ito A, Yamazaki A, Tsurushima H (2011) Control of gene transfer on a DNA-fibronectin-apatite composite layer by the incorporation of carbonate and fluoride ions. Biomaterials 32:4896–4902
109. Zhang W, Tsurushima H, Oyane A, Yazaki Y, Sogo Y, Ito A et al (2011) BMP-2 gene-fibronectin-apatite composite layer enhances bone formation. J Biomed Sci 18:62
110. Wang XP, Ito A, Li X, Sogo Y, Hirose M, Oyane A et al (2013) DNA-lipid-apatite composite layers enhance gene expression of mesenchymal stem cells. Mater Sci Eng C-Mater 33:512–518
111. Wang X, Oyane A, Tsurushima H, Sogo Y, Li X, Ito A (2011) BMP-2 and ALP gene expression induced by a BMP-2 gene-fibronectin-apatite composite layer. Biomed Mater 6:045004
112. Bonadio J (2000) Tissue engineering via local gene delivery: update and future prospects for enhancing the technology. Adv Drug Deliv Rev 44:185–194
113. Fischer J, Kolk A, Wolfart S, Pautke C, Warnke PH, Plank C et al (2011) Future of local bone regeneration – protein versus gene therapy. J Cranio-Maxillo-Fac Surg 39:54–64
114. Wack A, Rappuoli R (2005) Vaccinology at the beginning of the 21st century. Curr Opin Immunol 17:411–418
115. Kenney RT, Edelman R (2003) Survey of human-use adjuvants. Expert Rev Vaccines 2:167–188
116. Gupta RK, Relyveld EH, Lindblad EB, Bizzini B, Benefraim S, Gupta CK (1993) Adjuvants – a balance between toxicity and adjuvanticity. Vaccine 11:293–306
117. Cox JC, Coulter AR (1997) Adjuvants – a classification and review of their modes of action. Vaccine 15:248–256
118. Pashine A, Valiante NM, Ulmer JB (2005) Targeting the innate immune response with improved vaccine adjuvant. Nat Med 11:s63–s68
119. Blattman JN, Greenberg PD (2004) Cancer immunotherapy: a treatment for the masses. Science 305:200–205

120. Schreiber RD, Old LJ, Smyth MJ (2011) Cancer immunoediting: integrating immunity's roles in cancer suppression and promotion. Science 331:1565–1570
121. Ciocca DR, Frayssinet P, Cuello-Carrion FD (2007) A pilot study with a therapeutic vaccine based on hydroxyapatite ceramic particles and self-antigens in cancer patients. Cell Stress Chaperon 12:33–43
122. Eisenbarth SC, Colegio OR, O'Connor W, Sutterwala FS, Flavell RA (2008) Crucial role for the Nalp3 inflammasome in the immunostimulatory properties of aluminium adjuvants. Nature 453:1122–U1113
123. Ali OA, Huebsch N, Cao L, Dranoff G, Mooney DJ (2009) Infection-mimicking materials to program dendritic cells in situ. Nat Mater 8:151–158
124. Wang X, Li X, Ito A, Sogo Y, Ohno T (2013) Pore-size dependent immunogenic activity of mesoporous silica-based adjuvants in cancer immunotherapy. J Biomed Mater Res A. doi:10.1002/jbm.a.34783
125. Green SA (1983) Complications of external skeletal fixation. Clin Orthop Relat Res 180:109–116
126. Campbell AA, Song L, Li XS, Nelson BJ, Bottoni C, Brooks DE et al (2000) Development, characterization, and anti-microbial efficacy of hydroxyapatite-chlorhexidine coatings produced by surface-induced mineralization. J Biomed Mater Res 53:400–407
127. Stigter M, Bezemer J, de Groot K, Layrolle P (2004) Incorporation of different antibiotics into carbonated hydroxyapatite coatings on titanium implants, release and antibiotic efficacy. J Control Release 99:127–137
128. Park JY, Gemmelll CH, Davies JE (2001) Platelet interactions with titanium: modulation of platelet activity by surface topography. Biomaterials 22:2671–2682
129. McCarthy PM, Smith WA (2002) Mechanical circulatory support – a long and winding road. Science 295:998–999
130. Lietz K, Miller LW (2008) Destination therapy: current results and future promise. Semin Thorac Cardiovasc Surg 20:225–233
131. Richardson TP, Peters MC, Ennett AB, Mooney DJ (2001) Polymeric system for dual growth factor delivery. Nat Biotechnol 19:1029–1034
132. Ge S, Chen J, Huang N (2009) The effect of immobilized laminin on titanium-oxide films to the behavior of human umbilical vein endothelial cells. Sheng Wu Yi Xue Gong Cheng Xue Za Zhi 26:97–100
133. He F, Wang X, Maruyama O, Kosaka R, Sogo Y, Ito A et al (2013) Improvement in endothelial cell adhesion and retention under physiological shear stress using a laminin-apatite composite layer on titanium. J R Soc Interface 10:20130014
134. Wang X, He F, Li X, Ito A, Sogo Y, Maruyama O et al (2013) Tissue-engineered endothelial cell layers on surface-modified Ti for inhibiting in vitro platelet adhesion. Sci Technol Adv Mater 14:035002

Chapter 7
Calcium Phosphate Cement

Kunio Ishikawa

Abstract Calcium phosphate cement (CPC) is a breakthrough of biomaterials aimed for the reconstruction of bone defect. Upon mixing its powder phase with its liquid phase, it sets to form apatite or dicalcium phosphate dihydrate. As a result of the setting reaction, CPC permits the application of minimum invasive surgery for the bone defect reconstruction. In this chapter, classification, setting reaction, and properties of CPCs are introduced along with the current trend of CPCs.

Keywords Calcium phosphate cement • Calcium phosphate bone cement • Bone substitutes • Apatite cement • Brushite cement • Apatite • Brushite • Setting reaction • Dissolution-precipitation

7.1 Introduction

Calcium phosphate cement (CPC) or calcium phosphate bone cement is defined as bone cement that forms calcium phosphate based on setting reaction of the cements. Based on the composition of final products, CPCs are classified into apatite cement (AC), apatite-forming cement and brushite cement (BC), brushite-forming cement. Initially, apatite cement was reported by Monma and Kanazawa in 1976 [1]. They found α-tricalcium phosphate set to form calcium-deficient hydroxyapatite (cd-HAp: $Ca_9(HPO_4)(PO_4)_5(OH)$) with Ca/P molar ratio of 1.5 when α-TCP was hydrated in water at 60–100 °C and pH between 8.1 and 11.4. In 1982, LeGerous proposed apatite cement as possible dental restoration materials [2]. Brown and Chow introduced combination of tetracalcium phosphate (TTCP: $Ca_4(PO_4)_2$) and dicalcium phosphate anhydrous (DCPA: $CaHPO_4$) or dicalcium phosphate dihy-

K. Ishikawa (✉)
Department of Biomaterials, Faculty of Dental Science, Kyushu University, 3-1-1, Maidashi, Higashi-ku, Fukuoka, Kyushu 812-8582, Japan
e-mail: ishikawa@dent.kyushu-u.ac.jp

B. Ben-Nissan (ed.), *Advances in Calcium Phosphate Biomaterials*, Springer Series in Biomaterials Science and Engineering 2, DOI 10.1007/978-3-642-53980-0_7,

drate (DCPD: $CaHPO_4{\cdot}2H_2O$) which sets in 30–60 min at physiological temperature when mixed with aqueous solution in 1986 [3–7]. On the other hand, brushite cement was invented by Lemaitre et al. in 1987 [8, 9].

Brushite cement is sometimes called DCPD cement. Brushite is the name of mineral, whereas DCPD is the abbreviation of chemical. Brushite cement is also sometimes referred to as β-tricalcium phosphate cement since the major component of the powder phase is β-tricalcium phosphate (β-TCP: β-$Ca_3(PO_4)_2$). In the following sections, the terms apatite cement (AC) and brushite cement (BC) will be used for the matter of simplicity.

7.2 Setting Reaction of CPC

Setting reaction of CPCs has a close relationship with the thermodynamical stability or the solubility of the calcium phosphate salts. Table 7.1 summarizes the properties of calcium orthophosphate in relation to the production of CPCs. The solubility of the calcium phosphate decreases as the Ca/PO_4 molar ratio or Ca/P molar ratio increases, with the exception of tetracalcium phosphate (TTCP: $Ca_4(PO_4)_2O$) which shows higher solubility than hydroxyapatite (HAp: $Ca_{10}(PO_4)_6(OH)_2$) even though Ca/P ratio is higher than HAp.

Figure 7.1 shows the phase diagram of calcium phosphates in relation to CPC. Hydroxyapatite (HAp) is the most stable phase thermodynamically when the pH is approximately 4.2 or higher. However, brushite or dicalcium phosphate dihydrate (DCPD) becomes the most stable phase thermodynamically when the pH is approximately lower than 4.2. When the pH level drops to approximately 2, monocalcium phosphate monohydrate (MCPM: $Ca(H_2PO_4)_2{\cdot}H_2O$) will become, in terms of thermodynamics, the most stable phase. It should be noted that apatite and brushite, final product of apatite cement and brushite cement, are the most stable

Table 7.1 Calcium orthophosphates and their solubility product constants (Ksp)

Compound	Abbreviation	Chemical formula	Ca/P	logKsp
Monocalcium phosphate monohydrate	MCPM	$Ca(H_2PO_4)_2{\cdot}H_2O$	0.5	Highly soluble
Monocalcium phosphate anhydrous	MCPA	$Ca(H_2PO_4)_2$	0.5	Highly soluble
Dicalcium phosphate dihydrate	DCPD	$CaHPO_4{\cdot}2H_2O$	1.0	6.59
Dicalcium phosphate anhydrous	DCPA	$CaHPO_4$	1.0	6.90
Octacalcium phosphate	OCP	$Ca_8H_2(PO_4)_6{\cdot}5H_2O$	1.33	96.6
α-Tricalcium phosphate	α-TCP	$Ca_3(PO_4)_2$	1.5	
β-Tricalcium phosphate	β-TCP	$Ca_3(PO_4)_2$	1.5	28.9
Hydroxyapatite	HAp	$Ca_{10}(PO_4)_6(OH)_2$	1.67	116.8
Tetracalcium phosphate	TTCP	$Ca_4(PO_4)_2O$	2.0	38–44

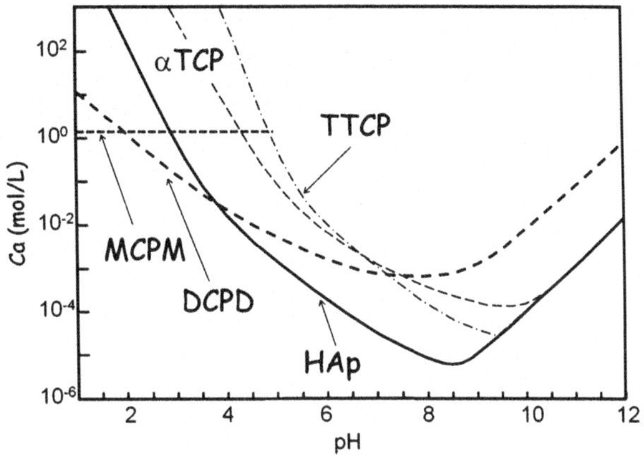

Fig. 7.1 Phase diagram of the solubility of several calcium phosphates as a function of pH. Solubility is expressed as the Ca concentration

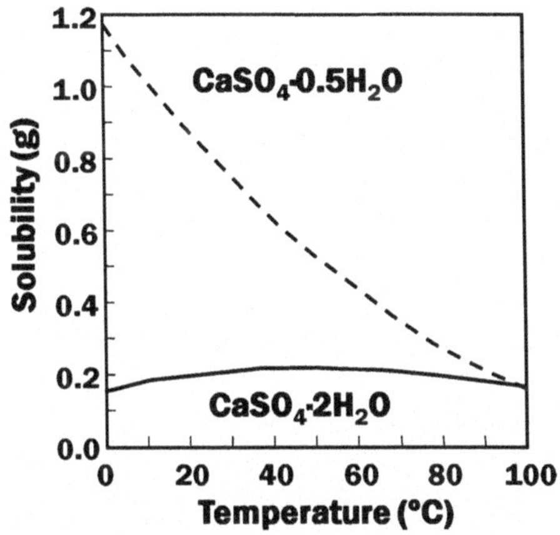

Fig. 7.2 Solubility of calcium sulfate hemihydrate and dihydrate as a function of temperature

phase thermodynamically at certain pH. Setting reaction of calcium phosphate cements is basically the same as the setting reaction of gypsum and is known as dissolution-precipitation reaction and entanglement of the precipitated crystals [10–16].

Gypsum, calcium sulfate dihydrate ($CaSO_4 \cdot 2H_2O$), and its dehydrated product calcium sulfate hemihydrate ($CaSO_4 \cdot 0.5H_2O$) are known as gypsum plaster or plaster of Paris (POP). Calcium sulfate hemihydrate is produced by heating gypsum to approximately 150 °C. Although they have the same chemical composition except for the hydrated water, their solubility is different as shown in Fig. 7.2.

For example, solubility of calcium sulfate hemihydrate is 0.9 g/100 mL at 20 °C. When calcium sulfate hemihydrate powder is mixed with water, it partially dissolves to supply calcium and sulfate ions which are equivalent to 0.9 g of calcium sulfate hemihydrate as shown in Eq. (7.1).

If calcium sulfate hemihydrate is the only chemical that could be in equilibrium with Ca^{2+} and $SO_4{}^{2-}$, the solution will reach equilibrium with respect to the calcium sulfate hemihydrate, and no further reaction will occur. However, the solution will also achieve equilibrium with calcium sulfate dihydrate, and its solubility is 0.2 g/100 mL, which is smaller than the solubility of calcium sulfate hemihydrate which is 0.9 g/100 mL. Therefore, the solution is supersaturated with respect to calcium sulfate dihydrate. This results in the precipitation of calcium sulfate dihydrate crystals as shown in Eq. (7.2). The precipitation of calcium sulfate dihydrate leads to undersaturation of the solution. Therefore, calcium sulfate hemihydrate will further be dissolved in the solution. These reactions continue successively, and the precipitated calcium sulfate dihydrates entangle each other to set [16]:

$$CaSO_4 \cdot 0.5H_2O \rightarrow Ca^{2+} + SO_4{}^{2-} + 0.5H_2O \tag{7.1}$$

$$Ca^{2+} + SO_4{}^{2-} + 2H_2O \rightarrow CaSO_4 \cdot 2H_2O \tag{7.2}$$

In the case of apatite cement also, setting reaction is the dissolution-precipitation reaction and entanglement of the precipitated apatite crystals [10–15]. For example, α-tricalcium phosphate (α-TCP) is known to form apatite upon setting [1]. α-Tricalcium phosphate is more soluble when compared with apatite as shown in Fig. 7.1. When α-tricalcium phosphate is mixed with water, it dissolves and supplies Ca^{2+} and $PO_4{}^{3-}$ into water as shown in Eq. (7.3). If α-tricalcium phosphate is the only chemical that could be in equilibrium with Ca^{2+} and $PO_4{}^{3-}$, the solution would just be in equilibrium with respect to the α-tricalcium phosphate, and no further reaction would take place. However, the solution is also in a state of equilibrium with calcium-deficient hydroxyapatite, and its solubility is smaller than the solubility of α-tricalcium phosphate. Therefore, the solution is said to be supersaturated with respect to calcium-deficient hydroxyapatite. This results in the precipitation of calcium-deficient hydroxyapatite crystals as shown in Eq. (7.4). The precipitation of calcium-deficient hydroxyapatite results in undersaturation of the solution. Therefore, α-tricalcium phosphate will be dissolved in the solution. These reactions continue successively, and the precipitated calcium-deficient hydroxyapatite crystals entangle each other to set. The overall reaction can be expressed as shown in Eq. (7.5):

$$3Ca_3(PO_4)_2 \rightarrow 9Ca^{2+} + 6PO_4{}^{3-} \tag{7.3}$$

$$9Ca^{2+} + 6PO_4{}^{3-} + H_2O \rightarrow Ca_9\,(HPO_4)\,(PO_4)_5\,(OH) \tag{7.4}$$

$$3Ca_3(PO_4)_2 + H_2O \rightarrow Ca_9\,(HPO_4)\,(PO_4)_5\,(OH) \tag{7.5}$$

Apatite cement can be made with various chemicals that contain calcium and phosphate. For example, an equimolar mixture of tetracalcium phosphate (TTCP: $Ca_4(PO_4)_2O$) and dicalcium phosphate anhydrous (DPCA: $CaHPO_4$) is known as

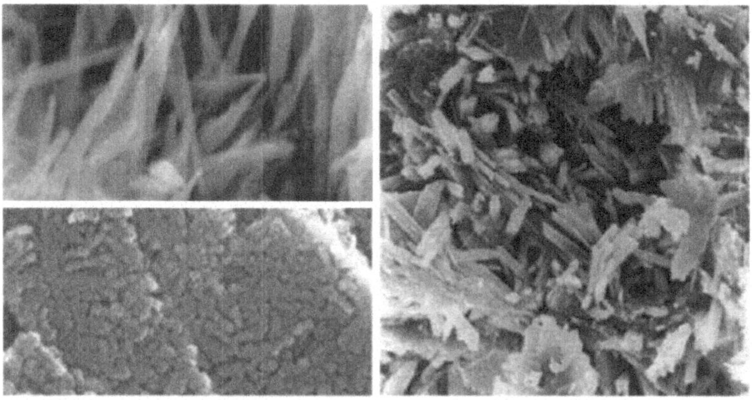

Fig. 7.3 SEM images of the set apatite cement made of TTCP and DCPA and set gypsum

typical apatite cement [3–7]. Apatite cement should contain calcium and phosphate in its composition so that apatite can be produced. The components should have suitable solubility in water since the setting reaction of the apatite cement is a dissolution-precipitation reaction. The cement paste should show moderate pH so that apatite is the most stable phase thermodynamically at that pH since setting reaction of the apatite cement is the dissolution-precipitation reaction.

Figure 7.3 summarizes the SEM images of (a) set gypsum and (b) set apatite cement made of an equimolar mixture of TTCP and DCPA. Basically, they showed the similar structure. In other words, precipitated needlelike crystals entangled each other to form set mass.

Brushite cement also sets in a similar setting reaction, dissolution-precipitation, and entanglement of precipitated crystal. The key difference of apatite cement and brushite cement is the final product. As stated earlier, brushite is the most stable phase when the pH is the approximately 2.0–4.2 (see Fig. 7.1). As a result, the components in brushite cement should contain calcium and phosphate that could form brushite, and the pH of the cement paste should be 2.0–4.2. One of the examples of the brushite cement is the mixture of β-tricalcium phosphate and monocalcium phosphate monohydrate. In this cement, monocalcium phosphate monohydrate shows relatively high solubility, and its dissolution results in acidic solution as shown in Eq. (7.6). Acidic solution results in the dissolution of β-tricalcium phosphate as shown in Eq. (7.7). The acidic solution in the cement paste containing Ca^{2+} and $HPO_4{}^{2-}$ will be supersaturated with respect to brushite. Therefore, brushite crystals are precipitated, and the precipitated brushite crystals entangle each other to set as shown in Eq. (7.8). The overall reaction can be expressed as shown in Eq. (7.9):

$$Ca(H_2PO_4)_2 \cdot H_2O \rightarrow Ca^{2+} + 2HPO_4{}^{2-} + 2H^+ + H_2O \qquad (7.6)$$

$$Ca_3(PO_4)_2 \rightarrow 3Ca^{2+} + 2PO_4{}^{3-} \quad (7.7)$$

$$4Ca^{2+} + 2PO_4{}^{3-} + 2HPO_4{}^{2-} + 2H^+ + H_2O + 7H_2O \rightarrow 4CaHPO_4 \cdot 2H_2O \quad (7.8)$$

$$Ca(H_2PO_4)_2 \cdot H_2O + Ca_3(PO_4)_2 + 7H_2O \rightarrow 4CaHPO_4 \cdot 2H_2O \quad (7.9)$$

Before the invention of CPCs, acrylic cement was the only bone cement in use. Acrylic bone cement also consists of a powder and liquid phase. Powder phase contains polymethyl methacrylate (PMMA), and liquid phase contains methyl methacrylate (MMA). When the powders and liquids are mixed, radical polymerization will occur based on the reaction of methyl methacrylate contained in the liquid phase and the polymerization initiator contained in the powder phase. MMA will also dissolve in PMMA and increases the viscosity of the paste during the setting or polymerization process. In the case of setting reaction of acrylic cement, significant heat is generated due to radical polymerization. Heat generation is natural since PMMA is more stable thermodynamically than MMA. However, heat generation should be avoided for biomaterials since it could damage surrounding tissue. Also, unreacted MMA is not ideal to human tissues.

Gypsum plaster also generates heat upon setting reaction as shown in Eq. (7.10):

$$CaSO_4 \cdot 0.5H_2O + 1.5H_2O \rightarrow CaSO_4 \cdot 2H_2O + 4,600 \text{ cal/mol} \quad (7.10)$$

Fortunately, heat generation is negligible in the case of CPCs at least for tissue response. Of course, heat is generated based on the setting reaction since apatite or brushite is the most stable phase thermodynamically. Thus, setting reaction of CPCs can be monitored by thermal analysis. However, heat generation due to setting reaction of CPC is limited, and consequently there is no need to pay attention to the heat generation in the case of CPC. It should be noted that this is a big advantage of CPCs for clinical use. Negligible heat generation due to the setting reaction of CPC can be explained by the relatively slow setting reaction when compared to the acrylic cement rather than the small difference in enthalpy. In other words, one of the factors that govern the temperature of the cement is the result of balance of generated heat and diffused heat. Diffusion of the generated heat is enough to prevent acute temperature increase if setting reaction takes relatively long time.

Another problem for the acrylic bone cement is the unreacted monomer, methyl methacrylate (MMA). Basically, MMA is toxic to human tissue. Fortunately, unreacted component of calcium phosphate cement does not cause toxic effect. In fact, TTCP usually remains unreacted in set TTCP-DCPA-type apatite cement. Unreacted TTCP acts as a filler of the cement and causes no adverse effect to tissue response.

On the other hand, it should be emphasized that CPCs show excellent tissue response only when set. In the other words, CPCs cause inflammatory response when they failed to set. All calcium phosphate powders including apatite powders are known to cause inflammatory response called crystalline inflammatory response. Therefore, an assurance in the setting reaction is one of the key advantages for the successful clinical results when using CPCs.

7.3 Regulations in Setting Reaction

Obviously, the key factor for the usefulness of calcium phosphate cement is its self-setting ability. Bone defect can be reconstructed using calcium phosphate cement without having a gap between the bone defect surface and set calcium phosphate cement. That is one of the key reasons why calcium phosphate bone cement shows better bone formation when compared to apatite block or apatite granular. When bone defect is reconstructed with apatite block, it is impossible to place apatite block into the bone defect without a gap being generated between the apatite block and bone defect. In the case of apatite granular, the gap between the granular and existing bone can be minimized. However, granular cannot be fixed at the bone defect and could be fluctuated. In contrast to the reconstruction using block or granular apatite, apatite cement can fill the bone defect without having a gap against the surface of bone defect, and the set apatite cement can supply concrete apatite surface.

Although apatite cement shows better bone-forming ability when compared to apatite block or apatite granular, apatite cement can cause inflammatory response when it fails to set as mentioned earlier. It should be emphasized that powder in micron size elicits inflammatory response even its composition is hydroxyapatite. Similar response is observed when apatite cement failed to set. For example, apatite cement powder would be released when apatite cement paste was rubbed by the covering skin before its setting reaction. Also, apatite cement powder would be released from apatite cement paste when apatite cement paste is exposed to body fluid before its setting reaction.

Figure 7.4 shows the appearance of apatite cement paste when implanted subcutaneously in rat. In this condition, cement paste is exposed to some pressure from the covering skin. Fast-setting apatite cement (left) which sets in 5 min sets even at this condition due to the rapid development of mechanical strength [14]. In contrast, conventional apatite cement (cAC) which sets in 30–60 min could not withstand this pressure since the development of mechanical strength takes time. Therefore, cAC disintegrated at this condition. When apatite cement failed to set, it causes inflammatory response.

Therefore, regulation of the setting reaction of apatite cement is important not only for its handling properties but also for its tissue response. Since setting reaction of calcium phosphate cement is based on dissolution-precipitation reaction and entanglement of the precipitated calcium phosphate crystals, particle size has an influence on the setting reaction. In other words, larger powder has smaller specific surface area, and rate of dissolution is slow. This results in calcium phosphate cement with longer setting time. Regulating particle size is especially important in the case of calcium phosphate cement that consists of multiple calcium phosphates

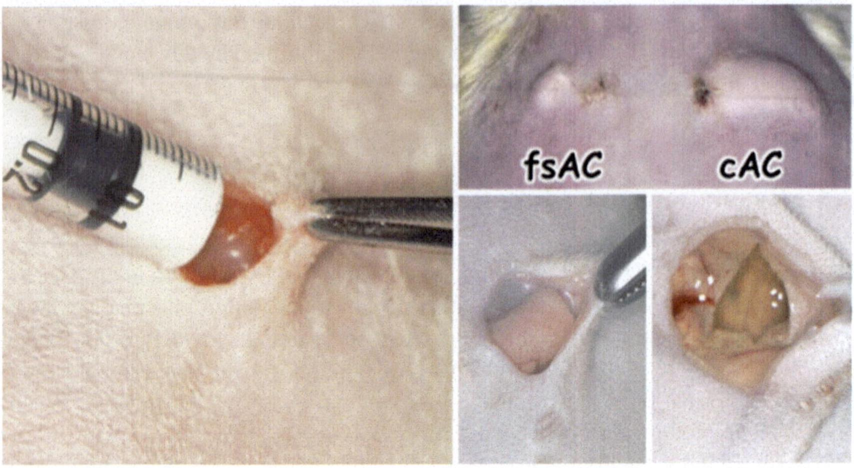

Fig. 7.4 Pictures of fast-setting apatite cement (*fsAC*) and conventional apatite cement (*cAC*) when the paste was implanted subcutaneously in rat

since the balanced supply of Ca^{2+} and $PO_4{}^{3-}$ based on the dissolution is important for the precipitation of the calcium phosphate.

In the case of apatite cement consisting of TTCP and DCPA, both TTCP and DCPA can supply Ca^{2+} and $PO_4{}^{3-}$ as shown in Eqs. (7.11) and (7.12). Then, Ca^{2+} and $PO_4{}^{3-}$ precipitated as hydroxyapatite crystals as shown in Eq. (7.13). The overall reaction can be expressed as shown in Eq. (7.14):

$$Ca_4(PO_4)_2O + H_2O \rightarrow 4Ca^{2+} + 2PO_4{}^{3-} + 2OH^- \tag{7.11}$$

$$CaHPO_4 \rightarrow Ca^{2+} + H^+ + PO_4{}^{3-} \tag{7.12}$$

$$4Ca^{2+} + 2PO_4{}^{3-} + 2OH^- + Ca^{2+} + H^+ + PO_4{}^{3-} \rightarrow 0.5Ca_{10}(PO_4)_6(OH)_2 \tag{7.13}$$

$$2Ca_4(PO_4)_2O + 2CaHPO_4 \rightarrow Ca_{10}(PO_4)_6(OH)_2 \tag{7.14}$$

However, Ca/PO_4 molar ratio supplied by TTCP and DCPA is different. TTCP which has Ca/PO_4 ratio of 2.0 supplies larger amount of Ca^{2+} for the formation of HAp which has Ca/PO_4 ratio of 1.67. In contrast, DCPA which has Ca/PO_4 ratio of 1.0 supplies less amount of Ca^{2+} for the formation of HAp which has Ca/PO_4 ratio of 1.67. Therefore, TTCP and DCPA should dissolve at the same rate for the formation of hydroxyapatite. Unfortunately, dissolution rate is different between TTCP and DCPA if the particle sizes are the same. TTCP dissolves much faster than DCPA as shown in Table 7.1.

Table 7.2 Effects of particle size on the compressive strength of calcium phosphate cement consisting of tetracalcium phosphate and dicalcium phosphate anhydrous

Average particle diameter (μm)		Ratio of the average particle diameter of TTCP/DCP	Compressive strength (MPa)
TTCP	DCPA		
1.6	11.9	0.13	0 (no setting)
12.4	11.9	1.04	7.1 ± 1.0
1.6	0.9	1.78	21.8 ± 4.4
12.4	0.9	13.78	51.0 ± 4.5

Table 7.2 summarizes the effect of particle size on mechanical strength of TTCP-DCPA-type apatite cement consisting of equimolar mixture of TTCP and DCPA when mixed with distilled water. In this experiment, TTCP and DCPA with different particle sizes were used. Particle sizes were 12.4 and 1.6 μm for TTCP and 11.9 and 0.9 μm for DCPA. Apatite cement consisting of a mixture of small TTCP (1.6 μm) with large DCPA (11.9 μm) did not reach setting. Compressive strength of set apatite cement increases with particle size ratio of TTCP-DCPA. Rate of DCPA dissolution is slower when the particle size or the surface areas are the same. Therefore, smaller DCPA with large surface area need to be used for the simultaneous dissolution or simultaneous supply of Ca^{2+} and $PO_4{}^{3-}$.

TTCP-DCPA-type apatite cement initially supplied for clinical use requires a setting time of 30–60 min. Based on the information from the cement supplier, they confirmed the setting reaction and advised to use new cement if the old cement failed to set. Obviously, 30–60 min was too long for clinical use.

Figure 7.5 shows the Ca^{2+} and $PO_4{}^{3-}$ concentrations in the cement powder suspension using equimolar mixture of 12.4 μm TTCP and 0.9 μm DCPA. As shown in the figure, $PO_4{}^{3-}$ concentration decreases until it was no longer detectable after 30 min, whereas Ca^{2+} remains in the solution. This result indicated that $PO_4{}^{3-}$ supply is the rate-determining step for the precipitation of hydroxyapatite even for mixtures of large TTCP and small DCPA. As stated already, DCPA supplies more $PO_4{}^{3-}$ for the precipitation of hydroxyapatite when compared to TTCP. Therefore, DCPA dissolution is the critical step for the setting reaction of apatite cement.

The results of chemical potential plot of cement powder suspension using equimolar mixture of 12.4 μm TTCP and 0.9 μm DCPA [12] are shown in Fig. 7.6. The figure reveals the solution is undersaturated with respect to HAp even though setting reaction of the apatite cement is a dissolution-precipitation reaction and entanglement of the precipitated apatite crystals. Therefore, precipitation reaction needs to be enhanced for quicker setting reaction.

We can enhance the precipitation reaction by using seed crystals. Doi et al. have prepared HAp at different temperatures from 40 to 100 °C. Setting time of TTCP-DCPA-type apatite cement became shorter by adding the HAp seed crystal. Furthermore, the setting time was shortened when seed crystal was added to HAp prepared at low temperature but resulted in poor crystallinity [17, 18].

Ruslin reported the effects of placement of HAp seed crystal in α-TCP-based apatite cement [19]. When α-TCP was partially hydrolyzed, HAp was formed on

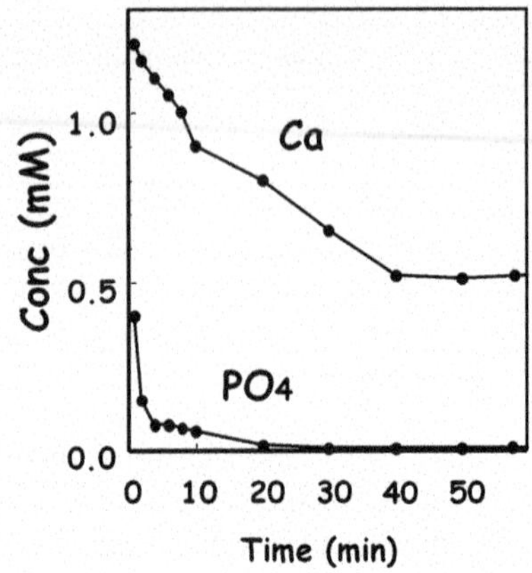

Fig. 7.5 Concentration of Ca^{2+} and PO_4^{3-} in TTCP-DCPA suspension in distilled water

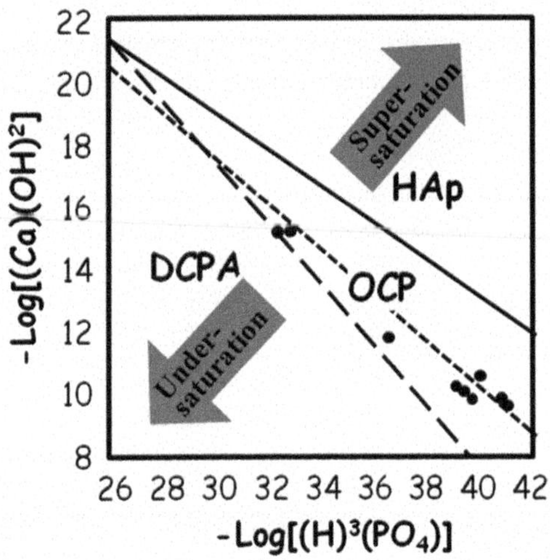

Fig. 7.6 Chemical potential plot of TTCP-DCPA in aqueous suspension

the surface of α-TCP powder, and this powder was used as the cement powder. The conversion to HAp was faster when the same amount of HAp was introduced externally as shown in Fig. 7.7.

What's more, when no HAp seed crystal or small amount of HAp seed crystal was introduced to apatite cement, conversion to HAp followed sigmoid curve which is typical for self-catalysis. Based on these observations, it was revealed that HAp shows seeding effect and its effect is more remarkable when HAp seed crystals were located on the surface of α-TCP powder. As shown in Eq. (7.3), α-TCP dissolves to supply Ca^{2+} and PO_4^{3-}. Then, Ca^{2+} and PO_4^{3-} will be supersaturated with respect to calcium-deficient apatite and precipitated as calcium-deficient apatite. When HAp seed crystal was located on the surface of α-TCP powder, dissolved Ca^{2+} and PO_4^{3-} from α-TCP is thought to be used immediately to grow HAp seed crystals.

Although the addition of HAp seed crystal was effective to shorten the setting time, unfortunately the mechanical strength of the set apatite cement was decreased.

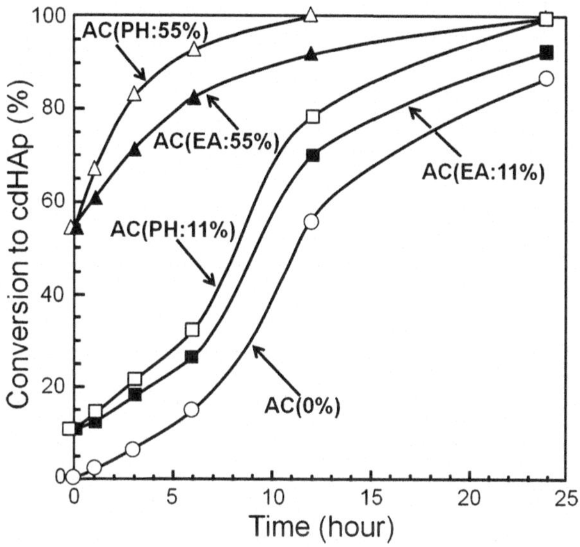

Fig. 7.7 Conversion of α-TCP-type apatite cement containing 0, 11, and 55 wt% seed HAp as a function of incubation time when kept at 37 °C and 100 % humidity

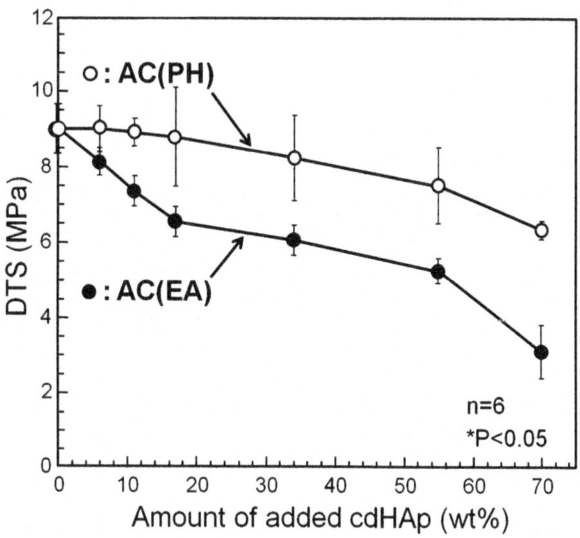

Fig. 7.8 Effects of placement of seed HAp on diametral tensile strength of α-TCP-type apatite cement. PH: HAp seed crystal was located on the surface of α-TCP by partial hydrolysis. EA: HAp seed crystal was externally added

The reduction in mechanical strength is thought to be the result of more frequent nuclei and limiting crystal growth. The decrease in mechanical strength of set apatite cement can be minimized by placing seed HAp on the surface of α-TCP powder by partial hydrolysis as shown in Fig. 7.8. Mechanical strength of the set apatite cement was closely related with the entanglement of precipitated HAp crystals. When HAp crystals were located on the surface of α-TCP, HAp crystals became longer, and interlocking reaction can be expected at higher density.

Table 7.3 Effects of liquid phase on the setting time of apatite cement consisting of TTCP and DCPA

Liquid	Concentration (mol/L)	Setting time (min)[a]
Distilled water	–	30–60
$Na_{1.8}H_{1.2}PO_4$	0.2	5
$Na_{1.8}H_{1.2}PO_4$	0.6	5
$Na_{1.8}H_{1.2}PO_4$	1.0	5
$K_{1.8}H_{1.2}PO_4$	0.2	5
$K_{1.8}H_{1.2}PO_4$	0.6	5

[a] Setting time was measured using Vicat needle method at 37 °C, and powder was mixed with liquid at powder-to-liquid ratio of 4.0

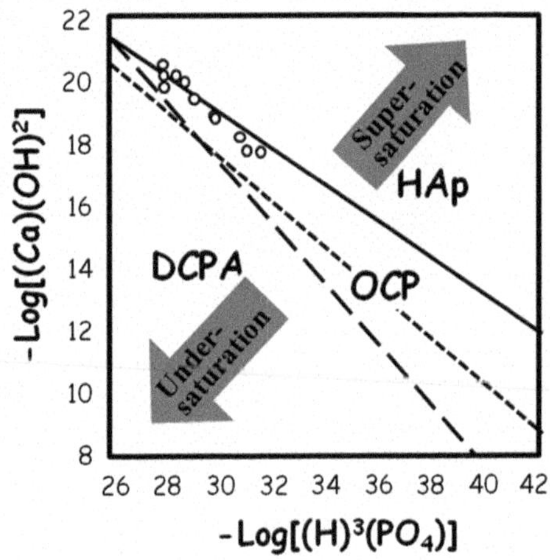

Fig. 7.9 Chemical potential plot of TTCP-DCPA in 0.5 mol/L $Na_{1.8}H_{1.2}PO_4$ (pH7.4) aqueous suspension

A more effective method to increase the setting reaction or the enhancement of apatite formation is the addition of PO_4^{3-} into the liquid phase of cement. As shown in Figs. 7.5 and 7.6, liquid portion of TTCP-DCPA paste is undersaturated with respect to HAp if TTCP-DCPA is mixed with water due to the limited supply of PO_4^{3-} based on the dissolution of DCPA.

Moreover, the addition of the PO_4^{3-} into the liquid phase could result in the immediate supersaturation of HAp and causes an immediate HAp formation upon dissolution of TTCP, which plays a more predominant role in the supply of Ca^{2+}. Consequently, the setting time of the apatite cement should be shortened.

Table 7.3 summarizes the effect of liquid phase on setting time of TTCP-DCPA-type apatite cement. Setting time of this apatite cement was 30 min when distilled water was used as the liquid phase. In contrast, setting time became 5 min when phosphate salts were used as the liquid phase [12, 14]. Basically, no effect was found on the type and concentration of phosphate salt employed in the experiment.

Figure 7.9 shows the chemical potential plot when TTCP-DCPA equimolar mixture was suspended in 0.5 mol/L $Na_{1.8}H_{1.2}PO_4$ aqueous solution with pH 7.4. As shown, the solution is equilibrium with HAp from the initial stage. Of course, this is caused by the PO_4^{3-} present in the solution.

In addition to seed crystals, the formation of apatite crystals can be essentially enhanced through the use of neutral phosphate salt solution or HAp. There are other approaches that we can use to shorten the setting time of apatite cement. These methods were employed more frequently in α-TCP-type apatite when compared to TTCP-DCPA-type apatite cement. This is due to the setting time of apatite cements free from setting accelerator. Setting time of TTCP-DCPA-type apatite cement was approximately 30–60 min even without setting accelerator. In fact, TTCP-DCPA-type apatite cement became clinically available without setting accelerator at the initial stage, and thus setting time was between 30 and 60 min. On the contrary, α-TCP-based apatite cement takes longer time to set (in the order of several hours) when compared to TTCP-DCPA-type apatite cement. Obviously, setting time, several hours, should be shortened for clinical use.

Chelating reaction was found to be an effective method to shorten the setting time and has been used in clinical applications [20, 21]. For example, succinic acid is added to the liquid phase in the case of Biopex®. Succinic acid ($HOOC(CH_2)_2COOH$) is dicarboxylic acid and forms chelate bonding with calcium phosphate powder. As a result of chelate formation with calcium phosphate powder, α-TCP powder sets in 5–10 min. It should be noted that succinic acid or the chelating agents are the inhibitor of apatite formation and dissolution of calcium phosphate [22–30]. In other words, apatite formation would be delayed when succinic acid is added to the liquid phase. Fortunately, there is no significant disadvantage to the tissue response even though HAp formation was delayed. Obviously, apatite will be formed gradually after steady dissolution of α-tricalcium phosphate since succinic acid has been used entirely for the initial setting reaction.

The situation is contrary in the case of brushite cement. Brushite cement sets immediately, and thus working time should be lengthened using a retarder [8, 9, 30]. Sulfate, pyrophosphate, and citrate are found as effective retarders [30]. Grover et al. discovered that adding 20 wt% calcium pyrophosphate ($Ca_2P_2O_7$) resulted in prolonged setting time by approximately 5 min. However, addition of calcium pyrophosphate resulted in a slight decrease in mechanical strength [23]. Calcium sulfate hemihydrate also prolongs the setting time to approximately 7 min when 20 % of calcium sulfate is added to brushite cement. Interestingly, the addition of calcium sulfate hemihydrate with 5 wt% calcium pyrophosphate results in a significant increase in mechanical strength. The recorded diametral tensile strength (DTS) of calcium sulfate hemihydrate with 5 wt% calcium pyrophosphate was 3 MPa, which was three times higher when compared to additive-free brushite cement. Bohner et al. found that effectiveness at increasing the setting time was in the order of pyrophosphate > citrate > sulfate. Basically, the mechanisms involved in extending the setting time using pyrophosphate and citrate ions were due to the inhibition of brushite crystallization. Hence, setting time was extended with increasing concentrations of the pyrophosphate and citrate ions. In the case of sulfate ion, the situation is more complex. Setting time increased from approximately 60 to 220 s when sulfuric acid concentration was increased from 0 to 0.1 mol/L and then shortened again with further increase in sulfuric acid concentration. Above 0.1 mol/L, $CaSO_4{\cdot}2H_2O$ is formed, and this salt is thought to act as a seed crystal of $CaHPO_4{\cdot}2H_2O$ due to the very close structure of $CaSO_4{\cdot}2H_2O$ and $CaHPO_4{\cdot}2H_2O$.

7.4 Regulations in Porosity

Obviously, intrinsic porous structure of the set calcium phosphate cements is due to the setting process of calcium phosphate cements, dissolution-precipitation reaction, and entanglement of the precipitated calcium phosphate crystals. Although apatite cement expands slightly due to the entanglement of precipitated apatite, volume of the set mass is almost the same with the volume of the paste. Therefore, bulk density and resulting porosity of the set cement can be regulated by the powder-to-liquid ratio of the paste and the molding pressure [31].

Figure 7.10 summarizes the effect of molding pressure and powder-to-liquid ratio (P/L ratio) on porosity of the set apatite cement. The figure shows smaller P/L ratio resulted in higher porosity of the set apatite cement. This is caused by the smaller P/L ratio that produces a larger amount of liquid in the paste, and this leads to a high degree of porosity in the final product. Similarly, higher molding pressure generates smaller porosity. This is caused by the exclusion of excess water from the paste when high pressure is used to pack the paste.

Figure 7.11 summarizes the relationship between the porosity and DTS of the set apatite cement. This relationship is in good agreement with the empirical equation presented by Duckworth for the relationship between mechanical strength and porosity as shown in Eq. (7.15) [32]:

$$S = S_0 \exp(-bP) \quad (7.15)$$

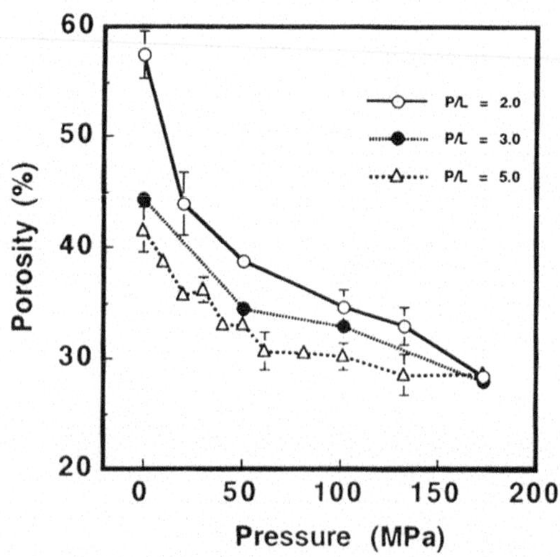

Fig. 7.10 Effects of the molding pressure and powder-to-liquid ratio on porosity of the set apatite cement

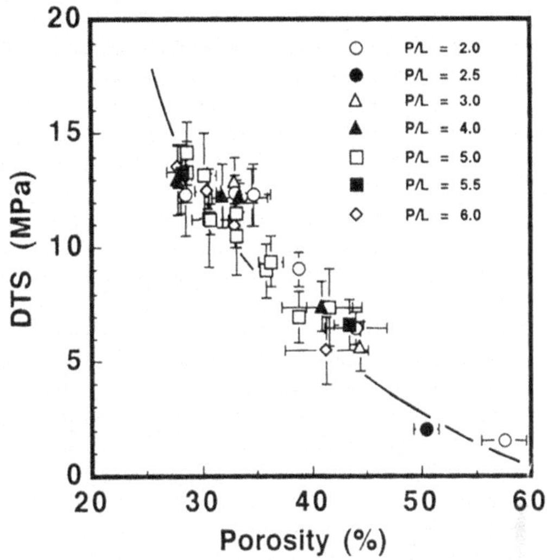

Fig. 7.11 Relationship between porosity of the apatite cement and diametral tensile strength (*DTS*) of set apatite cement

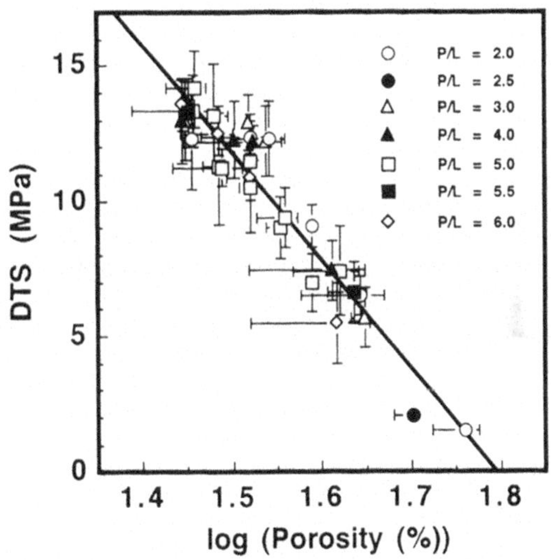

Fig. 7.12 Relationship between legalism of the porosity of the apatite cement and diametral tensile strength (*DTS*) of set apatite cement

where S is the observed mechanical strength of the porous material, S_0 is the ideal mechanical strength when there is no porosity, P is the porosity, and b is an empirical constant. By taking the natural logarithm of Eq. (7.15), Eq. (7.16) can be obtained:

$$\ln S = \mathrm{Ln} S_0 - bP \tag{7.16}$$

Figure 7.12 corresponds to Eq. (7.13):

$$\ln DTS = 4.637 - 0.067 \times P \tag{7.17}$$

Equation (7.17) is obtained in the case of apatite cement. S_0 or the ideal DTS when the porosity of the set apatite cement is zero can be estimated as 103 MPa which is similar to sintered hydroxyapatite.

Even though controlling the mechanical strength is possible by regulating the porosity of the set cement or powder-to-liquid ratio, a higher powder-to-liquid mixing ratio will lead to limited handling property or injectability. In other words, we have to find a balance between mechanical strength of the set apatite cement and handling property of the paste.

Pores stated in the Eqs. (7.15), (7.16), and (7.17) are micropore formed due to the entanglement of the precipitated apatitic crystals. Sometimes, macropores especially interconnected pores became important to allow penetration of the cells and tissues interior to the set calcium phosphate cement [33–44].

Several techniques have been proposed to produce macropores in calcium phosphate cements including porogen incorporation and bubble formation. Porogen addition is the simplest method to fabricate macroporous set calcium phosphates. Porogen should not dissolve, at least completely, during the mixing procedure. However, porogen needs to be dissolved when porogen is exposed to body fluid. As a result of dissolution of porogen, macrospore will be formed inside the set cement. Since porogen is dissolved in the body, porogen should not cause any toxic effect nor inflammatory response. Several porogens have been studied including mannitol, sucrose, sodium hydrogen carbonate, disodium hydrogen phosphate, polyglactin, poly(ε-caprolactone), poly(DL-lactic-co-glycolic acid), poly(L-lactic acid), and gelatin [40, 45–54]. In addition, there are many candidates to be used as porogen.

However, ideal porogen for calcium phosphate cements until now still remains unknown. This is due, at least in part, to the difficulty in finding ideal and harmless materials with proper solubility. In addition, it is not clear whether there is a proper solubility or not. Bone tissue is known to penetrate into the pores of calcium phosphate within 1 or 2 weeks. Therefore, porogen needs to be dissolved within 1 or 2 weeks at the bone defect. However, the body fluid circulation is limited at the bone defect, and most of the porogen is not exposed to body fluid but covered with the calcium phosphate. In fact, PLGA fiber-reinforced apatite cement showed limited resorption of PLGA.

The other method to create macropores into calcium phosphate cements is through the incorporation of gas in the cement paste. This can be further divided into two categories. One is the gas forming in the paste, and the other is the incorporation of air by air-entraining agents. The major advantage of using gas for the fabrication of porous calcium phosphate cement is the presence of pore when set. In other words, cell and tissue can penetrate interior to the cement immediately. In addition, there is no need to worry about the toxicity of the porogen. On the other hand, drawback of this method is the difficulty for pore regulation.

The formation of carbon dioxide bubbles by acid–base reaction of $NaHCO_3$/Na_2CO_3 and acidic reaction is a simple method for the production of macroporous cement [54–57]. For example, mixing of $NaHCO_3$ and NaH_2PO_4 in the cement paste results in the macroporous calcium phosphate cement since $NaHCO_3$ decomposes to form carbon dioxide when exposed to acidic solution such as NaH_2PO_4 as shown in Eq. (7.18). Na_2HPO_4 formed by this reaction will be used as an accelerator of the apatite formation:

$$NaHCO_3 + NaH_2PO_4 \rightarrow CO_2 + Na_2HPO_4 + H_2O \tag{7.18}$$

It should be noted that carbonate ion is used not only for the bubble formation but also for the formation of carbonate apatite (CO_3Ap) [58]. When carbonate apatite is formed, the mechanical strength of the set cement decreases more significantly with the porosity when compared to apatite cement free from carbonate. This indicated that carbonate apatite is weaker in mechanical strength when compared to hydroxyapatite. Based on the carbonate apatite formation and formation of interconnected porous structure which allows cell penetration interior to cement, resorption of the cement is much faster when compared to macroporosity-free apatite cement. For example, del Real et al. fabricated porous apatite cement using CO_2 formation method which was then used to reconstruct a bone defect (6.3 mm in diameter) in a goat model. After 2 weeks, bone formation had taken place inside the pores. At 10 weeks, 81 % of the initial cement was resorbed and new bone was deposited. On the other hand, 100 % of the initial cement will remain if there are no pores within the cement [56].

As air-entraining agents, various chemicals have been studied including sodium dodecyl sulfate, hexadecyltrimethylammonium chloride, polyethylene oxide, poly(ethylene oxide), albumin, and sugar surfactant [59–66]. Conversely to using carbon dioxide, air bubbles have to be introduced when using air-entraining agents. Also, relatively larger amount of air-entraining agent is needed to maintain the porous structure. Again, this is the important advantage for the penetration of cells into calcium phosphate cement.

For example, Mino-Farina et al. evaluated the usefulness of macrospore fabricated using air-entraining agent based on rabbit implant [59]. Macropore was introduced into α-TCP-type apatite cement using an air-entraining agent, dehydrated albumen. The porous paste was made by gentle mixing of cement paste and foamed albumen. Dense and porous α-TCP-type apatite cements were used for the reconstruction of a 6 mm diameter bone defect. Twelve weeks after the surgery, the ratio of tissue penetration into macroporous cement was 41 % compared to 22 % for dense cement. Furthermore, bone growth and revascularization were observed inside the central pores of the macroporous cement.

The importance of porous structure especially interconnected porous structure is clear for calcium phosphate cements when they are intended to replace bone. However, the ideal method for the fabrication of interconnected porous structure has not been established so far. At present, macropore fabrication and mechanical strength decrease should be balanced for the practical use of calcium phosphate cements.

7.5 Regulations in Anti-washout Property

Although calcium phosphate cements show excellent tissue response, they will cause inflammatory response when they fail to set due to powder release. Washout of the cement is one of the causes of the disintegration of cement paste. Cement paste should not be washed-out nor disintegrated. Although hemostasis is performed before the reconstruction of bone defect with calcium phosphate cement, complete hemostasis is sometimes not easily accomplished. Similarly, bleeding could sometimes occur after the bone defects have been filled with calcium phosphate cement. Moreover, hemostasis is impossible when bone defect is filled with the calcium phosphate cement using a syringe needle for minimum invasive surgery. Therefore, anti-washout properties are important for the calcium phosphate cement. Washout is caused by the penetration of body fluid into the calcium phosphate cements. Figure 7.13 illustrates the behavior of apatite cement in the bone defect. As illustrated in the figure, a struggle exists between the two reactions. One reaction is the setting and hardening reaction of the cement which is a dissolution-precipitation reaction and entanglement of the precipitated apatite crystals. The other reaction is the penetration of body fluid into cement paste, and this causes washout of the cement paste. The results of these two reactions will determine the overall behavior of the apatite cement. For that reason, both acceleration of setting reaction and inhibition of body fluid penetration should be carried out for the apatite cement to achieve anti-washout property.

Apatite formation or setting reaction is usually accelerated by the addition of neutral sodium phosphate or other additives [12, 14, 17–19]. Consequently, close attention should be paid to inhibit the penetration of body fluids. Gelling agent is one of the most effective additives that can be used for the prevention of body fluids penetrating into cement paste [15, 67–69]. Basically, cement powder or calcium phosphate powder has no strong interaction with the surrounding powder. Thus, body fluid can penetrate into the cement paste due to simple penetration or diffusion. This results in washout of the cement paste. On the contrary, when gelling agent is introduced to liquid phase, gelling agent prevents body fluid penetration into the cement paste. Furthermore, cement powder tends to have some bonding strength among each other through gelling agent even though the bonding strength is not high.

There are certain requirements for the gelling agent when used in the manufacture of anti-washout-type apatite cement. First, the gelling agent should not show any toxicity. Second, the gelling agent should have enough capability to prevent the

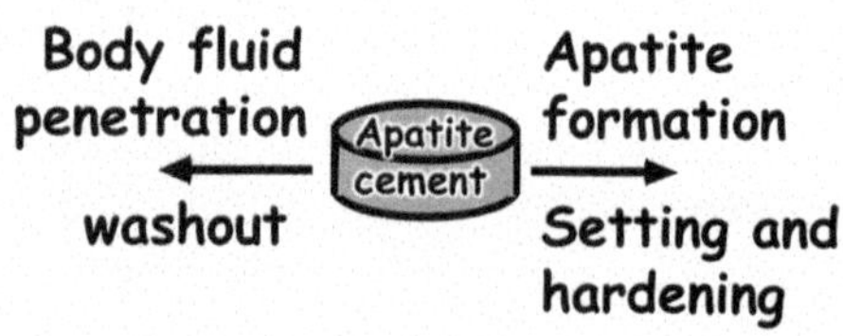

Fig. 7.13 Illustration of the reaction of apatite cement paste when exposed to body fluid

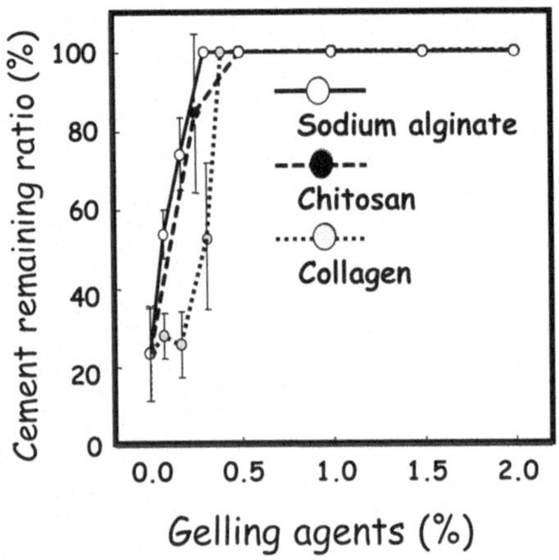

Fig. 7.14 The effects of gelling agents on the percentage of remaining cement paste after 24 h. The cement paste was immersed in serum at 37 °C immediately after mixing

body fluid penetrating into the cement paste. Fundamentally, all gelling agents prevent body fluid penetration into the cement. Therefore, concentration of the gelling agent is the factor. Third, the gelling agent should not inhibit the setting reaction of the cement. In other words, it should not inhibit dissolution-precipitation reaction. Unfortunately, gelling agent in general inhibits the dissolution-precipitation reaction. Hence, gelling agent should be chosen so that the degree of the inhibition will be minimal. Finally, the addition of gelling agent should not decrease the handling property or injectability. Fortunately, the addition of gelling agent seems to improve the handling property and injectability.

Figure 7.14 shows the effect of gelling agents on the percentage of remaining ratio of the cement paste. A percentage remaining ratio of zero indicates complete washed out, whereas 100 % indicates complete anti-washout. As shown in the figure, cement paste became anti-washout by adding gelling agent regardless of the type of gelling agent used. However, the amount of agent required to achieve complete anti-washout property varies for each gelling agent. This is normal since the properties such as viscosity are dependent on the gelling agent itself. Therefore, gelling agents should be chosen so that it will fulfill the requirement stated above.

7.6 Regulations in Injectability

Due to the setting reaction of calcium phosphate cement, bone defect can be reconstructed by calcium phosphate cement injected to the bone defect through syringe needle as shown in Fig. 7.15.

This allows minimum invasive surgery (Fig. 7.16). The key factor in determining the injectability of the cement paste is the viscosity of the cement paste, and the viscosity is governed by a number of factors including the viscosity of the liquid, liquid-to-powder mixing ratio (L/P mixing ratio), size of powder, shape of

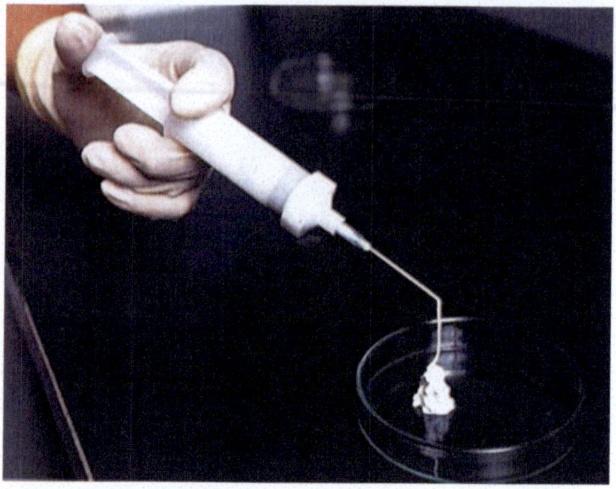

Fig. 7.15 Photograph of apatite cement injected from the syringe needle

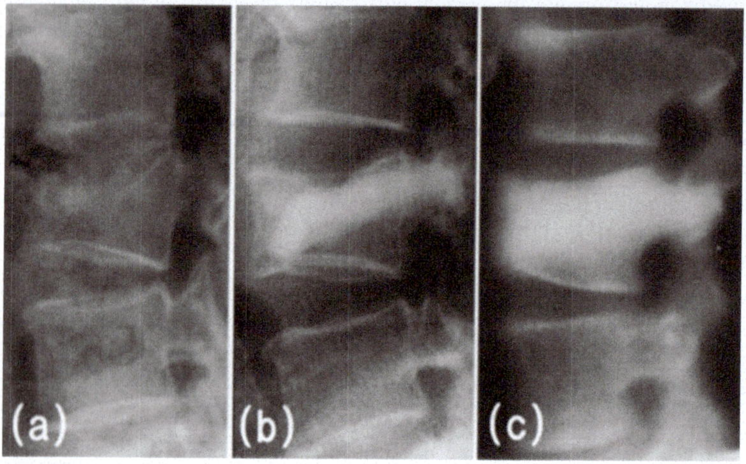

Fig. 7.16 Clinical case of fixation of repositioned compression fracture with apatite cement. Osteoporotic compression fracture of the 3rd lumbar vertebra shown in (**a**) was reconstructed with apatite cement paste as shown in (**b**) and (**c**) (Photos courtesy by Kochi Medical University)

powder, and time after mixing [70–82]. When viscosity of the paste is too low, the cement shows poor injectability. Only liquid phase or liquid phase containing limited powder is extracted from the syringe needle in such case. This phenomenon is explained as the filtration of paste using syringe needle. In other words, syringe needle acts as filter paper, and the cement powder and liquid are separated as a result of non-passing cement powder in the syringe needle.

Obviously, injectability is better when thicker syringe is employed due to less filtration effect. The thickness of the syringe needle is selected based on the type of surgery being carried out. For example, 10–13G syringe is commonly used for vertebroplasty [83]. It should be noted that liquid-to-powder mixing ratio changes when phase separation occurs between powder and liquid. Therefore, controlling of the injectability is important when it comes to clinical use. Although viscous liquid is important for the better injectability, the use of a liquid phase that is too viscous will cause an increase in force required to inject the cement paste from the syringe. In the case of manual injection, 100–300 N is used, and cement paste with 1,000 Pa·s viscosity can be injected manually from the syringe [84, 85]. Beyond that viscosity, machine injection should be employed.

Additives including sodium alginate, chitosan, polysaccharides, sodium glycerophosphate, lactic acid, glycerol, hydroxymethylcellulose, and polyvinyl alcohol (PVA) have been studied to improve injectability [70–82].

7.7 Difference Between Apatite Cements and Brushite Cements

Although both apatite cement and brushite cement are commercially available due to their usefulness for the reconstruction of bone defects, their behaviors in the bone defect are quite different especially with respect to resorption. Brushite cement resorbed much faster when compared to apatite cement. This difference is caused by the compositional difference in the final products. As the name represents, final product of apatite cement is apatite, whereas final product of brushite cement is brushite, and apatite is the most stable phase thermodynamically at physiological condition, and body fluid is supersaturated with respect to apatite. Therefore, no physicochemical dissolution occurs in the case of set apatite cement at physiological condition. Replacement of apatite cement with bone is caused by the resorption of apatite by osteoclasts. Osteoclasts produce Howship's lacuna and make inside the lacuna into weak acidic condition. As a result of acidic condition, apatite is dissolved similar to bone-remodeling process. Carbonate apatite is formed if carbonate ion is present during the setting reaction of apatite cement, and carbonate apatite shows higher solubility than hydroxyapatite at acidic condition. Therefore, apatite cement that forms carbonate apatite will be replaced to bone faster than apatite cement that forms carbonate-free apatite.

In contrast to apatite cement, final product of the brushite cements is brushite. Brushite is the most stable phase when pH is 2.0–4.2 and, thus, brushite is formed based on dissolution-precipitation reaction and entanglement of the brushite crystals results in the setting reaction. However, brushite is metastable phase at physiological pH and thus dissolves upon exposure to the body fluid. In other words, brushite cement is resorbed not only by the osteoclastic cell but also by physicochemical dissolution. It should be noted that dissolution of brushite not always means simple dissolution. Brushite or dicalcium phosphate dihydrate dissolves to supply Ca^{2+} and HPO_4^{2-} as shown in Eq. (7.19). Obviously, simple dissolution occurs when brushite cement is used where there is enough body fluid circulation:

$$CaHPO_4 \cdot 2H_2O \rightarrow Ca^{2+} + HPO_4^{2-} + 2H_2O \tag{7.19}$$

However, if body fluid circulation is limited, Ca^{2+} and HPO_4^{2-} dissolved from brushite are precipitated as apatite or carbonate apatite as shown in Eqs. (7.20) and (7.21). In each case, the overall reaction is shown in Eqs. (7.22) and (7.23). Note that the equations are simplified. For example, stoichiometric hydroxyapatite ($Ca_{10}(PO_4)_6(OH)_2$) is not formed, but Ca-deficient hydroxyapatite ($Ca_{10-x}(HPO_4)_x(PO_4)_{6-x}(OH)_{2-x}$) is produced at body temperature. Likewise, carbonate content of carbonate apatite is different and thus should be expressed as $Ca_{10-a}(CO_3)_b(PO_4)_{6-c}(OH)_{2-d}$. Eqs. (7.20), (7.21), (7.22), and (7.23) are assumed for us to understand the general idea of the transformation of brushite to hydroxyapatite or carbonate apatite:

$$10Ca^{2+} + 6HPO_4^{2-} + 2H_2O \rightarrow Ca_{10}(PO_4)_6(OH)_2 + 8H^+ \tag{7.20}$$

$$10Ca^{2+} + 4HPO_4^{2-} + 3CO_3^{2-} + 2H_2O \rightarrow Ca_{10}(PO_4)_4(CO_3)_3(OH)_2 + 6H^+ \tag{7.21}$$

$$10CaHPO_4 \cdot 2H_2O \rightarrow Ca_{10}(PO_4)_6(OH)_2 + 4HPO_4^{2-} + 8H^+ + 18H_2O \tag{7.22}$$

$$\begin{aligned} &10CaHPO_4 \cdot 2H_2O + 3CO_3^{2-} \\ &\rightarrow Ca_{10}(PO_4)_4(CO_3)_3(OH)_2 + 6HPO_4^{2-} + 6H^+ + 18H_2O \end{aligned} \tag{7.23}$$

Precipitated hydroxyapatite or carbonate apatite shows osteoconductivity and excellent tissue response. Similarly, precipitated hydroxyapatite or carbonate apatite regulates the dissolution of the metastable brushite at physiological condition.

Nonetheless, brushite cement dissolves much faster than apatite cement. If body fluid circulation is proper, brushite cement is replaced to bone. For example, Apelt et al. reported that brushite cement was used for the reconstruction of bone defects in sheep, and it almost completely resorbed after 6 months, whereas apatite cement did not show any remarkable change for the same period of time [86].

7.8 Application for Local Drug Delivery Devices

Non-exothermic setting reaction of calcium phosphate cement is a major advantage when used as a carrier of drug delivery systems since temperature-sensitive drug such as biological molecule can be loaded in the set cement [87]. In general, drugs are incorporated into the cement by blending drug powder with the cement powder.

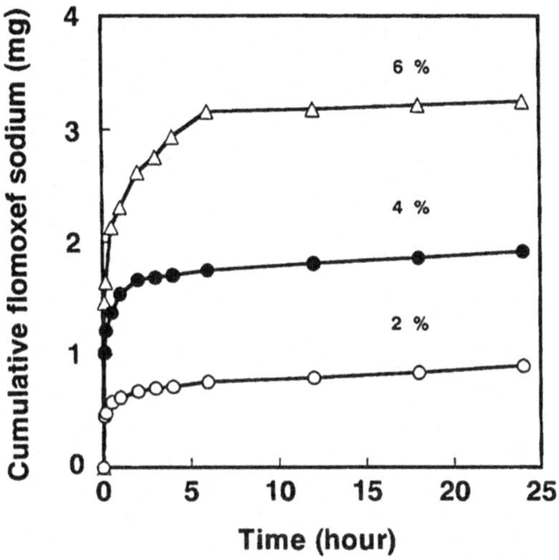

Fig. 7.17 Drug release characteristic of set apatite cement containing various amounts of drug (flomoxef sodium)

Obviously, drugs can be introduced to the liquid phase if its amount is limited. Drug incorporated in the powder and/or liquid phase would be homogenously distributed inside the cement based on mixing the cement powder with liquid. Upon mixing, cement will set based on dissolution-precipitation reaction and entanglement of the precipitated crystals. Basically, drug will not be incorporated in the apatite or brushite crystal lattice but located between the entangled crystals. Therefore, drug loaded into the cement showed simple drug release character for skeletal system as shown in Fig. 7.17 [88]. Initial burst release is caused mainly by diffusion of the drug from pores [89–94]. Initial burst is more popular in the case of brushite cement rather than apatite cement. One of the reasons of this difference is thought to be the difference in absorption properties with drug.

Drug release profile from the calcium phosphate cements can be modified by employing another drug delivery system in the cement. For example, drug-loaded polymer can be introduced in the calcium phosphate cement. By employing other systems, drug release profile can be regulated. For example, burst release of the drug can be avoided. Also, dissolved polymer creates pores, and thus cells and tissue can be penetrated into the pores [95].

7.9 Currently Available Calcium Phosphate Cement

Calcium phosphate cement became commercially available in the 1990s. At present, many apatite cements and brushite cements became commercially available. Tables 7.4 and 7.5 summarize the examples of current apatite cement and brushite cement.

Table 7.4 Example of the commercially available apatite cement and its composition

Registered name (Manufacturer)	Composition
Biopex®-R (Mitsubishi Materials)	Powder: α-TCP + TTCP + DCPD + HAp + $Mg_3(PO_4)_2$ Liquid: succinic acid, chondroitin sulfate, and sodium hydrogen sulfite
Primafix® (NGK Spark Plug Co)	Powder: TTCP + DCPD Liquid: sodium dextran sulfate sulfur 5
Cerapaste® (NGK Spark Plug Co)	Powder: TTCP + DCPA Liquid: sodium dextran sulfate sulfur 5
BoneSource® (Stryker)	Powder: TTCP(73 %) + DCPA(27 %) Liquid: sodium phosphate solution
Norian SRS® (Synthes)	Powder: α-TCP(85 %) + $CaCO_3$(12 %) + MCPM(3 %) Liquid: disodium phosphate solution
Norian CRS® (Synthes)	Powder: α-TCP(85 %) + $CaCO_3$(12 %) + MCPM(3 %) Liquid: disodium phosphate solution
Norian SRS® Fast Set Putty (Synthes)	Not documented
Norian CRS® Fast Set Putty (Synthes)	Not documented
Calcibon® (Biomet)	Powder: α-TCP(61 %) + DCPA(26 %) + $CaCO_3$(10 %) + HAp(3 %) Liquid: disodium phosphate solution
Mimix™ (Biomet)	Powder: TTCP + α-TCP + $C_6H_5O_7Na_3 \cdot 2H_2O$ Liquid: citric acid
QuickSet Mimix™ (Biomet)	Not documented
Cementek® (Teknimed)	Powder: TTCP + α-TCP + $Ca(OH)_2$ + sodium glycerophosphate Liquid: acidic calcium phosphate
Cementek® LV (Teknimed)	Powder: TTCP + α-TCP + $Ca(OH)_2$ + sodium glycerophosphate + dimethylsiloxane Liquid: acidic calcium phosphate
α-BSM® (ETEX)	Powder: ACP(50 %) + DCPD(50 %) Liquid: saline
Biobon®[a] (ETEX)	Powder: ACP(50 %) + DCPD(50 %) Liquid: saline
Embarc® (ETEX)	Powder: ACP(50 %) + DCPD(50 %) Liquid: saline
KyphOs™ (Kyphon)	Powder: α-TCP(77 %) + $Mg_3(PO_4)_2$(14 %) + $MgHPO_4$ (4.8 %) + $ScCO_3$(3.6 %) Liquid: 3.5 mol/L diammonium hydrogen phosphate
Callos™ (Skeletal Kinetics)	Not documented
Rebone (Shanghai Rebone Biomaterials Co Ltd.)	Powder: TTCP + DCPA Liquid: water

[a]Biobon® is the trade name of α-BSM in Europe

Table 7.5 Example of the commercially available brushite cement and its composition

Registered name (Manufacture)	Composition
ChronOS™ Inject	Powder: β-TCP(73 %) + MCPM(21 %) + $MgHPO_4 \cdot 3H_2O$(5 %) + $MgSO_4$(<1 %) + $Na_2H_2P_2O_7$(<1 %)
(Norian)	Liquid: 0.5 % sodium hyaluronate
Eurobone®	Powder: β-TCP(98 %) + $Na_4P_2O_7$(2 %)
(Kasios)	Liquid: 3 mol/L H_3PO_4 + 0.1 mol/L H_2SO_4
VitalOs	Component 1: β-TCP(1.34 g) + $Na_2H_2P_2O_7$(0.025 g) 0.05 mol/L pH7.4 PBS
(CalciOs)	Component 2: MCPM (0.78 g) + $CaSO_4 \cdot 2H_2O$ + 0.05 mol/LH_3PO_4

References

1. Monma H, Kanazawa T (1976) The hydration of α-tricalcium phosphate. Yogyo-Kyokai-Shi 84:209–213
2. LeGeros RZ, Chahayeb A, Shulman A (1982) Apatite calcium phosphates: possible dental restorative materials. J Dent Res 61:343–347
3. Brown WE, Chow LC (1985) Dental restorative cement paste, US Patent No. 4,518,403
4. Brown WE, Chow LC (1986) A new calcium phosphate, water-setting cement. In: Brown PW (ed) Cement research progress. American Ceramic Society, Westerville, pp 351–379
5. Brown WE, Chow LC (1986) Combination of sparingly soluble calcium phosphate cements in slurries and paste as mineralizers and cements. US Patent No. 4,612,059
6. Chow LC, Takagi S (2001) A natural bone cement. A laboratory novelty led to the development of revolutionary new biomaterials. J Res Natl Inst Stand Technol 106:1029–1033
7. Chow LC, Takagi S, Constantino PD, Friedman CD (1991) Self-setting calcium phosphate cement. In: Material research society symposium proceedings. Materials Research Society, vol 179, pp 3–24
8. Lemaitre J, Mirtchi A, Mortier A (1987) Calcium phosphate cements for medical uses: state of the art and perspectives of development. Silic Ind Ceram Sci Technol 52:141–146
9. Mirtchi AA, Lemaitre J, Terao N (1989) Calcium phosphate cements: study of the b-tricalcium phosphate – monocalcium phosphate system. Biomaterials 10:475–480
10. Mirtchi AA, Lemaitre J, Munting E (1989) Calcium phosphate cements: action of setting regulators on the properties of the β-tricalcium phosphate monocalcium phosphate cements. Biomaterials 10:634–638
11. Kuntze RA (1984) The chemistry and technology of gypsum. American Society for Testing and Materials, Philadelphia, STP 861
12. Ishikawa K, Takagi S, Chow LC, Ishikawa Y (1995) Properties and mechanisms of fast-setting calcium phosphate cements. J Mater Sci Mater Med 6:528–533
13. Ishikawa K (2010) Bone substitute fabrication based on dissolution-precipitation reaction. Materials 3:1138–1155
14. Miyamoto Y, Ishikawa K, Fukao H, Sawada M, Nagayama M, Kon M, Asaoka K (1995) In vivo setting behaviour of fast-setting calcium phosphate cement. Biomaterials 16:855–860
15. Ishikawa K, Miyamoto Y, Takechi M, Toh T, Kon M, Nagayama M, Asaoka K (1997) Non-decay type fast-setting calcium phosphate cement: hydroxyapatite putty containing an increased amount of sodium alginate. J Biomed Mater Res 36(3):393–399
16. Sekiya M (1964) Gypsum. Kasai Press, Osaka
17. Doi Y, Takezawa Y, Shibata S, Moriwaki Y, Wakamatsu N, Horiguchi H, Uno K, Yamamoto K (1989) Self-setting apatite. New materials as canal filling and bone substitute. MRS Int'l Mtg Adv Mats 1:415–420

18. Doi Y (1993) Self-setting apatite cement. New Ceram 5:47–54
19. Ruslin (2011) Effects of partial hydrolysis on basic properties of alpha-tricalcium phosphate based apatite cement. Ph.D. thesis
20. Unezaki Y, Eto T, Inoue H, Minamigawa K, Sugihara F (1993) A study of hardening material consisted of tetracalcium phosphate dicalcium phosphate dehydrate and citric acid. J Jpn Prosthodont Soc 37:61–66
21. Unezaki Y, Ryumon H, Inoue H, Okuda H, Onishi H, Minamigawa K (1996) Histocompatibility of a bone graft cement consisting of tetracalcium phosphate dicalcium phosphate dehydrate and citric acid. Bioceramics 9:251–253
22. Fleish H, Neuman WF (1961) Mechanisms of calcification: role of collagen, polyphosphates, and phosphatase. Am J Physiol 200:1296–1300
23. Grover LM, Gbureck U, Young AM, Wright AJ, Barralet JE (1995) Temperature dependent setting kinetics and mechanical properties of beta-TCP-pyrophosphoric acid bone cement. J Mater Chem 15:4955–4962
24. Eidelman N, Meyer JL, Brown WE (1990) Effect of pyrophosphate on growth of OCP and OHAp crystals. J Dent Res 69:119
25. Meyer JL (1984) Can biological calcification occur in the presence of pyrophosphate? Arch Biochem Biophys 231:1–8
26. Sharma VK, Johnsson M, Sallis JD, Nancollas GH (1992) Influence of citrate and phosphocitrate on the crystallization of octacalcium phosphate. Langmuir 8:676–679
27. Marshall RW, Nancollas GH (1969) The kinetics of crystal growth of dicalcium phosphate dihydrate. J Phys Chem 73:3838–3845
28. Fleisch H, Maerki J, Russell RGG (1966) Effect of pyrophosphate on dissolution of hydroxyapatite and its possible importance in calcium homeostasis. Proc Soc Exp Biol Med 122:317–320
29. Christoffersen J, Christoffersen MR (1981) Kinetics of dissolution of calcium hydroxyapatite IV. The effect of some biologically important inhibitors. J Cryst Growth 53:42–54
30. Bohner M, Lemaitre J, Ring TA (1996) Effects of sulfate, pyrophosphate and citrate ions on the physicochemical properties of cements made of beta tricalcium phosphate-phosphoric acid-water mixtures. J Am Ceram Soc 79:1427–1434
31. Ishikawa K, Asaoka K (1995) Estimation of ideal mechanical strength and critical porosity of calcium phosphate cement. J Biomed Mater Res 29(12):1537–1543
32. Yamane M (1980) The role and characteristic of gypsum products in dentistry. J Soc Mater Sci Jpn 29:421–427
33. Kroese-Deutman HC, Wolke JG, Spauwen PH, Jansen JA (2006) Closing capacity of cranial bone defects using porous calcium phosphate cement implants in a rabbit animal model. J Biomed Mater Res Part A 79:503–511
34. Hulbert SF, Morrison SJ, Klawitter JJ (1972) Tissue reaction to three ceramics of porous and non-porous structures. J Biomed Mater Res 6:347–374
35. Holmes RE (1979) Bone regeneration within a coralline hydroxyapatite implant. Plast Reconstr Surg 63:626–633
36. Holmes RE, Bucholz RW, Monney V (1986) Porous hydroxyapatite as a bone-graft substitute in metaphyseal defects. J Bone Joint Surg 68:904–911
37. Eggli PS, Muller W, Schenk RK (1988) Porous hydroxyapatite and tricalcium phosphate cylinders with two different pore size ranges implanted in the cancellous bone of rabbits. Clin Orthop 232:127–138
38. Schliephake H, Neukam FW, Klosa D (1991) Influence of pore dimensions on bone ingrowth into porous hydroxylapatite blocks used as bone graft substitutes. A histometric study. Int J Oral Maxillofac Surg 20:53–58
39. Cook SD, Thongpreda N, Anderson RC, Thomas KA, Haddad RJ Jr, Griffin CD (1987) Optimum pore size for bone cement fixation. Clin Orthop 223:296–302
40. Takagi S, Chow LC (2001) Formation of macropores in calcium phosphate cement implants. J Mater Sci Mater Med 12:135–139
41. Xu HHK, Quinn JB, Takagi S, Chow LC, Eichmiller FC (2001) Strong and macroporous calcium phosphate cement: effects of porosity and fiber reinforcement on mechanical properties. J Biomed Mater Res 57:457–466

42. Xu HHK, Quinn JB, Takagi S, Chow LC (2004) Fast-setting calcium phosphate scaffolds with tailored macropore formation rates for bone regeneration. J Biomed Mater Res 68A:725–734
43. Xu HHK, Simon CG (2004) Self-hardening calcium phosphate cement-mesh composite: reinforcement, macropores, and cell response. J Biomed Mater Res 69:267–278
44. Zhang Y, Xu HHK, Takagi S, Chow LC (2006) In-situ hardening hydroxyapatite-based scaffold for bone repair. J Mater Sci Mater Med 17:437–445
45. Xu HHK, Eichmiller FC, Giuseppetti AA (2000) Reinforcement of a self-setting calcium phosphate cement with different fibers. J Biomed Mater Res 52:107–114
46. Xu HHK, Eichmiller FC, Barndt PR (2001) Effects of fiber length and volume fraction on the reinforcement of calcium phosphate cement. J Mater Sci Mater Med 12:57–65
47. Ruhe PQ, Boerman OC, Russel FGM, Spauwen PH, Mikos AG, Jansen JA (2005) Controlled release of rhBMP-2 loaded poly(DL-lactic-co-glycolic acid)/calcium phosphate cement in vivo. J Control Release 106:162–171
48. Ruhe PQ, Hadberg EL, Padron NT, Spauwen PHM, Jansen JA, Mikos AG (2005) Biocompatibility and degradation of poly(DL-lactic-co-glycolic acid)/calcium phosphate cement composites. J Biomed Mater Res A74:533–544
49. Link DP, van den Dolder J, Jurgens WJFM, Wolke JGC, Jansen JA (2006) Mechanical evaluation of implanted calcium phosphate cement incorporated with PLGA microparticles. Biomaterials 27:4941–4947
50. Tajima S, Kishi Y, Oda M, Maruta M, Matsuya S, Ishikawa K (2006) Fabrication of biporous low-crystalline apatite based on mannitol dissolution from apatite cement. Dent Mater J 25(3):616–620
51. Habraken WJEM, Wolke JGC, Mikos AG, Jansen JA (2006) Injectable PLGA microsphere/calcium phosphate cements: physical properties and degradation characteristics. J Biomater Sci Polym Ed 17:1057–1074
52. Plachokova A, Link D, van den Dolder J, van den Beucken J, Jansen JA (2007) Bone regenerative properties of injectable PGLA-CaP composite with TGF-b1 in a rat augmentation model. J Tissue Eng Regen Med 1:457–464
53. Shimogoryo R, Eguro T, Kimura E, Maruta M, Matsuya S, Ishikawa K (2009) Effects of added mannitol on the setting reaction and mechanical strength of apatite cement. Dent Mater J 28(5):627633
54. Bodde EWH, Habraken WJEM, Mikos AG, Spauwen PHM, Jansen JA (2009) Effect of polymer molecular weight on the bone biological activity of biodegradable polymer/calcium phosphate cement composites. Tissue Eng Part A 15(31):3184–3191
55. del Real RP, Wolke JG, Vallet-Regi M, Jansen JA (2002) A new method to produce macropores in calcium phosphate cements. Biomaterials 23:3673
56. del Real RP, Ooms E, Wolke JG, Vallet-Regi M, Jansen JA (2003) In vivo response to porous calcium phosphate cement. J Biomed Mater Res A 65:30–36
57. Klijn RJ, van den Beucken JJJP, Lanao RPF, Veldhuis G, Leeuwenburgh SC, Wolke JGC, Meijer GJ, Jansen JA (2012) Three different strategies to obtain porous calcium phosphate cements: comparison of performance in a rat skull bone augmentation model. Tissue Eng Part A 18:1171–1182
58. Miyamoto Y, Toh T, Ishikawa K, Yuasa T, Nagayama M, Suzuki K (2001) Effect of added $NaHCO_3$ on the basic properties of apatite cement. J Biomed Mater Res 54(3):311–319
59. Ginebra MP, Boltong MG, Fernandez E, Planell JA, Driessens FCM (1995) Effect of various additives and temperature on some properties of an apatitic calcium phosphate cement. J Mater Sci Mater Med 6:612–616
60. Sarda S, Fernandez E, Nilsson M, Planell JA (2002) Influence of air-entraining agent on bone cement macroporosity. Key Eng Mater 218–220:335–338
61. Sarda S, Nilsson M, Balcells M, Fernandez E (2003) Influence of surfactant molecules as air-entraining agent for bone cement macroporosity. J Biomed Mater Res Part A 65:215–221
62. Ginebra-Molins MP, Planell-Estany JA, Gil-Mur FX (2006) Injectable, self-setting calcium phosphate foam. Patent WO2006/030054

63. Ginebra MP, Delgado JA, Harr I, Almirall A, Del Valle S, Planell JA (2007) Factors affecting the structure and properties of an injectable self-setting calcium phosphate foam. J Biomed Mater Res Part A 80:351–361
64. Delgado JA, Harr I, Almirall A, del Valle S, Planell JA, Ginebra MP (2005) Injectability of a macroporous calcium phosphate cement. Key Eng Mater 284–286:157–160
65. Hesaraki S, Nemati R (2009) Cephalexin-loaded injectable macroporous calcium phosphate bone cement. J Biomed Mater Res Part B 89:342–352
66. Miño-Fariñaa N, Muñoz-Guzóna F, López-Peñaa M, Ginebrab MP, Valle-Fresnob S, Ayalac D, González-Cantalapiedra A (2009) Quantitative analysis of the resorption and osteoconduction of a macroporous calcium phosphate bone cement for the repair of a critical size defect in the femoral condyle. Vet J 179:264–272
67. Ishikawa K, Miyamoto Y, Kon M, Nagayama M, Asaoka K (1995) Non-decay type fast-setting calcium phosphate cement: composite with sodium alginate. Biomaterials 16(7):527–532
68. Miyamoto Y, Ishikawa K, Takechi M, Yuasa M, Kon M, Nagayama M, Asaoka K (1996) Non-decay type fast-setting calcium phosphate cement: setting behaviour in calf serum and its tissue response. Biomaterials 17(14):1429–1435
69. Takechi M, Miyamoto Y, Ishikawa K, Yuasa M, Nagayama M, Kon M, Asaoka K (1996) Non-decay type fast-setting calcium phosphate cement using chitosan. J Mater Sci Mater Med 7(6):317–322
70. Ishikawa K, Matsuya S, Nakagawa M, Udoh K, Suzuki S (2004) Basic properties of apatite cement containing spherical tetracalcium phosphate made with plasma melting method. J Mater Sci Mater Med 15(1):13–17
71. Ishikawa K, Takeuchi A, Suzuki Y, Koyano K (2008) Effects of thermal treatment on injectability and basic properties of apatite cement containing spherical tetracalcium phosphate made with plasma melting method. J Ceram Soc Jpn 116:63–67
72. Khairoun I, Boltong MG, Driessens FCM, Planell JA (1998) Some factors controlling the injectability of calcium phosphate bone cements. J Mater Sci Mater Med 9:425–428
73. Khairoun I, Driessens FC, Boltong MG, Planell JA, Wenz R (1999) Addition of cohesion promotors to calcium phosphate cements. Biomaterials 20(4):393–398
74. Santini MT, Cametti C, Formisano G, Flamma F, Perilli R (2002) Effects of hyaluronan viscous materials on cell membrane electrical properties. J Biomed Mater Res 41(2):211–220
75. Ginebra MP, Rilliard A, Fernandez E, Elvira C, San Roman J, Planell JA (2001) Mechanical and rheological improvement of a calcium phosphate cement by the addition of a polymeric drug. J Biomed Mater Res 57(10):113–118
76. Andrianjatovo H, Lemaıtre J (1995) Effects of polysaccharides on the cement properties in the monocalcium phosphate/α-tricalcium phosphate system. Innov Tech Biol Med 16S(1):140–147
77. Leroux L, Hatim Z, Freche M, Lacout JL (1999) Effects of various adjuvants (lactic acid, glycerol, and chitosan) on the injectability of a calcium phosphate cement. Bone 25(2):S31–S34
78. Belkoff SM, Mathis JM, Jasper LE, Deramond H (2001) An ex vivo biomechanical evaluation of a hydroxyapatite cement for use with vertebroplasty. Spine 26(14):1542–1546
79. Borzacchiello A, Sanginario V, Ambrosio L, Ginebra MP, Planell JA (2003) Characterization of an injectable hydrogel composite for orthopedic applications. In: Proceedings of the second international conference on new biomedical materials. Cardiff, UK, 6–8 Apr 2003
80. Sarda S, Fernandez E, Nilsson M, Balcells M, Planell JA (2002) Kinetic study of citric acid influence on calcium phosphate bone cements as water-reducing agent. J Biomed Mater Res 61(4):653–659
81. Gbureck U, Barralet JE, Spatz K, Grover LM, Thull R (2004) Ionic modification of calcium phosphate cement viscosity. Part I: Hypodermic injection and strength improvement of apatite cement. Biomaterials 25(11):2187–2195
82. Barralet JE, Grover LM, Gbureck U (2004) Ionic modification of calcium phosphate cement viscosity. Part II: Hypodermic injection and strength improvement of brushite cement. Biomaterials 25(11):2197–2203

83. Dang L, Wardlaw D, Hukins DW (2007) Removal of nucleus pulposus from the intervertebral disc – the use of chymopapain enhances mechanical removal with rongeurs: a laboratory study. BMC Musculoskelet Disord 8:122
84. Carrodeguas RG, Lasa BV, Del Barrio JS (2005) Injectable acrylic bone cements for vertebroplasty with improved properties. J Biomed Mater Res B Appl Biomater 68(1):94–104
85. Gbureck U, Spatz K, Thull R, Barralet JE (2005) Rheological enhancement of mechanically activated alpha-tricalcium phosphate cements. J Biomed Mater Res B Appl Biomater 73(1):1–6
86. Apelt D, Theiss F, El-Warrak AO, Zlinszky K, Bettschart-Wolfisberger R, Bohner M, Matter S, Auer JA, von Rechenberg B (2004) In vivo behavior of three different injectable hydraulic calcium phosphate cements. Biomaterials 25:1439–1451
87. Ginebra MP, Traykova T, Planell JA (2006) Calcium phosphate cements: competitive drug carriers for the musculoskeletal system? Biomaterials 27:2171–2177
88. Takechi M, Miyamoto Y, Ishikawa K, Nagayama M, Kon M, Asaoka K, Suzuki K (1998) Effects of added antibiotics on the basic properties of anti-washout-type fast-setting calcium phosphate cement. J Biomed Mater Res 39(2):308–316
89. Tamimi F, Torres J, Bettini R, Ruggera F, Rueda C, López-Ponce M (2008) Doxycycline sustained release from brushite cements for the treatment of periodontal diseases. J Biomed Mater Res A85:707–714
90. Bohner M, Lemaître J, VanLanduyt P, Zambelli PY, Merkle HP, Gander B (1997) Gentamicin-loaded hydraulic calcium phosphate bone cement as antibiotic delivery system. J Pharm Sci 86:565–572
91. Bohner M, Lemaître J, Merkle HP, Gander B (2000) Control of gentamicin release from a calcium phosphate cement by admixed poly(acrylic acid). J Pharm Sci 89:1262–1270
92. Hofmann MP, Mohammed AR, Perrie Y, Gbureck U, Barralet JE (2009) High-strength resorbable brushite bone cement with controlled drug-releasing capabilities. Acta Biomater 5:43–49
93. Liu W, Chang J (2009) In vitro evaluation of gentamicin release from a bioactive tricalcium silicate bone cement. Mater Sci Eng C29:2486–2492
94. Stallmann HP, Faber C, Slotema ET, Lyaruu DM, Bronckers ALJJ, Amerongen AVN et al (2003) Continuous-release or burst-release of the antimicrobial peptide human lactoferrin1-11(hLF1-11) from calcium phosphate bone substitutes. J Antimicrob Chemother 52:853–855
95. Ginebra MP, Canal C, Espanol M, Pastorino D, Montufar EB (2012) Calcium phosphate cements as drug delivery materials. Adv Drug Deliv Rev 64:1090–1110

Chapter 8
Characterization of Calcium Phosphates Using Vibrational Spectroscopies

Christian Rey, Olivier Marsan, Christèle Combes, Christophe Drouet, David Grossin, and Stéphanie Sarda

Abstract Vibrational spectroscopies are extensively used for the characterization of calcium phosphates either as natural biological minerals (bone, teeth, ectopic calcifications) or as biomaterials (bioceramics, coatings, composites). The present review begins with a theoretical description of expected spectra for the main calcium phosphate phases (i.e., brushite, monetite, octacalcium phosphate, tricalcium phosphates, apatites, amorphous calcium phosphate) followed by the analysis of real spectra, line positions and assignments, and observed anomalies. In the second part, the spectra of complex well-crystallized ion-substituted apatites and other calcium phosphates, as well as solid solutions, are investigated, and the information gained regarding the substitution types and ion distributions are derived. Finally, we will examine and interpret the spectra of nanocrystalline apatites considering the ion substitution effects and the existence of a surface hydrated layer. Quantification processes and spectra treatments are briefly presented and discussed. Examples of the use of vibrational spectroscopies for biomaterials and biominerals characterization will be detailed for coating evaluations, including spectroscopic imaging, following up on mineral cement setting reactions, adsorption studies, near infrared investigations of surface water, residual strains determinations in bone, orientation of apatite crystals in biological tissues, and crystallinity and maturity of bone mineral.

Keywords FTIR and Raman spectra • Phosphate • Carbonate • Apatite • Coating • Cements • Adsorption • Mechanical strains • Crystal orientation • Bone crystallinity and maturity

---

C. Rey (✉) • O. Marsan • C. Combes • C. Drouet • D. Grossin • S. Sarda
CIRIMAT-Carnot Institute, University of Toulouse, UMR CNRS-UPS-INPT 5085, ENSIACET, Toulouse, France
e-mail: christian.rey@ensiacet.fr

B. Ben-Nissan (ed.), *Advances in Calcium Phosphate Biomaterials*, Springer Series in Biomaterials Science and Engineering 2, DOI 10.1007/978-3-642-53980-0_8,

8.1 Introduction

Calcium phosphate (Ca–P) biominerals, especially apatites, are complex structures affording many ion substitutions and vacancies, which may be poorly crystallized. Their study by diffraction techniques does not always give information on fine structural details such as the presence and location of CO_3^{2-}, HPO_4^{2-}, or OH^- groups. Vibrational spectroscopies bring, in addition to structural identification, this valuable information and may be used for a quantitative determination on a very limited amount of material. They may also yield, in favorable cases, information on the orientation of molecular species and crystals; in addition, microscopic techniques can also be used for local investigations on biological tissues or materials, and they allow a rather accurate mapping of specific mineral characteristics.

Several techniques involve transitions between vibrational levels. This review is mainly focused on FTIR and Raman spectroscopies, which are used extensively. Vibrational spectra of different Ca–P of biological interest will first be described with an emphasis on apatites. The effect of ion substitutions and vacancies will be illustrated, showing how local environments disturb the vibrational spectra. This phenomenon can be used for the characterization of surface species in nanocrystalline compounds. Many other uses of vibrational spectroscopies have been published, for example, in adsorption studies, follow-up of calcium phosphate cement setting, analyses of coatings, near infrared (NIR) investigations of surface water, or biological mineralizations. These will be briefly discussed in the last section of this chapter.

8.2 Basic Spectra and Line Assignments

8.2.1 *Theoretical Considerations*

A vibration is defined by a periodic variation of the interatomic distance in a compound. In the simple case of a diatomic molecule, A-B, the vibration frequency can be modeled using the simple Hook's law in the approximation of a harmonic oscillator. The frequency of vibration, ν, is given by

$$\nu = \frac{1}{2\pi c}\sqrt{\frac{k}{\mu}}$$

where κ is the force constant associated with the chemical bond and μ is the reduced mass: $\mu = m_A * m_B/(m_A + m_B)$ with m_A and m_B the mass of atoms A and B. For more complex molecular species, different types of vibrations are possible, which can be determined theoretically [1]. Two types of vibrations with different energy domains are recognized for molecular species other than diatomic

Table 8.1 Vibrational characteristics of molecular ions involved in calcium phosphates

Molecular ion (symmetry)	Vibrational domains, symmetry, and activity of the free ions (R: Raman activity and IR: infrared activity)					
	ν_1	ν_2	ν_3		ν_4	
PO_4^{3-} (T_d)	A_1 (R)	E (R)	T_2 (IR, R)		T_2 (IR, R)	
Position (cm^{-1})	938	420	1,017		567	
HPO_4^{2-} (C_{3v})	A	E	A +	E	A +	E
	(IR, R)	(IR, R)	(IR, R)	(IR, R)	(IR, R)	(IR, R)
Positions (cm^{-1})	988	394	862	1,076	537	537
CO_3^{2-} (D_{3h})	A'_1	A''_2	E'		E'	
	(R)	(IR)	(IR, R)		(IR, R)	
Positions (cm^{-1})	1,064	879	1,415		680	

ones: stretching vibrations, corresponding to an elongation of chemical bonds, and bending vibrations, corresponding to angular variation between two chemical bonds. Stretching vibrations exhibit a higher energy than the bending ones.

In crystalline solids several types of vibration may occur. In addition to acoustic modes, two main types are identified, "internal vibrations" associated with molecules and molecular ions with covalent bonds that are present in the solid and "external vibrations" corresponding to the vibrations of species and ions in their crystallographic site [2–4]. Internal vibrations are generally close to the vibration energy of the free molecule/ions and allow the identification of molecular species in the solid. However, variations will appear in the energies of internal vibrations and in their relative intensities which depend on the environments of these molecular species in the solid. Such variations allow a precise identification of mineral structures in most cases. Although external vibration modes also depend on the crystal structure, their energy is lower than that of internal vibrations, and they are more easily accessed using Raman spectroscopy. Among these external vibrations, two types of movements may be recognized: translation modes and libration modes, which can be viewed as partial rotation of molecular groups in the crystal. Libration movements of OH^- ions and H_2O molecules occur at a relatively high energy compared to non-protonated molecules, and the corresponding lines are frequently found among the internal vibrations of other species like phosphate or carbonate. To complete the description of vibrational spectra, overtone and combination lines, which involve multi-quanta excitations, can be observed, although with much weaker intensities than fundamental lines.

The main molecules and molecular ions found in calcium phosphates are orthophosphate groups: PO_4^{3-}, HPO_4^{2-}, $H_2PO_4^-$ and also H_2O, OH^-, CO_3^{2-}. The vibrational characteristics of the "free" CO_3^{2-} and PO_4^{3-} ions are shown in Table 8.1 [5, 6], with the symmetry group and vibrational domains. We will use the denominations of the spectroscopic domains of the free molecules/ions to describe and discuss the different spectra in this paper. Although specific domains can be used for protonated phosphate species [5, 7], the P–O vibrational regions remain close to those of the PO_4^{3-} group and they will be discussed by reference to this ion. In protonated species additional lines are expected due to the O–H bond. The stretching of the O–H bonds in HPO_4^{2-} and $H_2PO_4^{-}$ groups are generally broad and appear with a low to medium intensity. However, the P-(OH) bonds in HPO_4^{2-} and $H_2PO_4^{-}$ are longer and weaker than the P–O bond in the PO_4^{3-} ion, and the corresponding stretching bands are shifted towards lower wavenumbers. These bands are very sensitive to hydrogen bonding [5, 8, 9]. In contrast the weakening of the P–OH bond is associated with a strengthening of the remaining P–O bonds, whose stretching vibrations are shifted towards higher wavenumbers, whereas bending vibrations are shifted towards lower wavenumbers. The symmetry alterations induced by protonation occurring in HPO_4^{2-} can conveniently be described using distorted PO_4 edifices belonging to C_{3v} symmetry (although the symmetry of the real free ions is lower). These species have been included in Table 8.1.

The vibrational modes of "free" molecular ions and molecules are conveniently determined using molecular group theory [1], which is used to name and distinguish the vibrational modes. Group theory also allows determination of the infrared (IR) and Raman (R) observance of the vibrational modes, their "activity," which is related to the physical interactions between electromagnetic radiations and vibrational energy levels involved in these spectroscopic methods [2–4].

In crystalline solids two main alterations have been identified: the site symmetry effect and the factor group symmetry [2–4]. The site symmetry effect corresponds to an alteration in vibrational energy levels due to the symmetry lowering of the "free" molecule or polyatomic ion related to its position in a well-defined crystallographic site; these effects are shown in Tables 8.2, 8.3, and 8.4 for different crystalline calcium phosphates in different structures [5, 9–14]. Considering PO_4^{3-} ions in apatites with a hexagonal unit cell (space group $P6_3/m$; Table 8.3), for example, the site symmetry is C_s, as only a symmetry plane is preserved from the original tetrahedral symmetry. In consequence, the degeneracy of vibrational modes E (degeneracy: 2) and T_2 (degeneracy: 3) of the "free" PO_4^{3-} species is raised, and instead of one vibrational level, several non-degenerated modes occur. All these vibrational modes are active in IR and R and a "splitting" of the ν_2, ν_3, and ν_4 lines is predicted. In addition, ν_1 and ν_2 modes are now active in IR, although they were not observed for the free ion.

The factor group treatment provides a complete prediction of the vibrational levels of a crystal for both internal and external vibration modes. This approach takes into consideration the whole content of the unit cell, including the correlations between the vibrations of similar groups in a crystal that may interfere with each other in a confined environment. These considerations result in additional vibrational levels of molecules and molecular ions as shown in Tables 8.2, 8.3, and 8.4. The number of predicted lines may vary considerably according to the structure. For compounds containing HPO_4^{2-}, OH^- ions, and water molecules, line broadenings are observed related to hydrogen bonding. In addition, libration transitions, which have not been considered here, appear in addition to bending and stretching lines.

The factor group may lead to weak shifts so, when numerous lines are expected, individual components are hindered by line broadening and cannot be distinguished.

Table 8.2 Internal vibrations of phosphate groups in non-apatitic calcium phosphates of interest (PO_4^{3-}-containing compounds)

Tetracalcium phosphate (TTCP); $Ca_4(PO_4)_2O$; monoclinic $P2_1$ [10]			
	ν_1 PO_4	ν_2 PO_4	ν_3, ν_4 PO_4
Site symmetry: C_1	A(IR-R)	2A(IR-R)	3A(IR-R)
Factor group: C_2	2A(IR-R)	4A(IR-R)	6A(IR-R)
	2B(IR-R)	4B(IR-R)	6B(IR-R)
Number of lines IR	4	8	12
Number of lines R	4	8	12
α-Tricalcium phosphate (α-TCP); $Ca_3(PO_4)_2$; monoclinic $P2_1/a$ [12]			
	ν_1 PO_4	ν_2 PO_4	ν_3, ν_4 PO_4
Site symmetry: C_1	A(IR,R)	2A(IR-R)	3A(IR-R)
Factor group: C_{2h}	$12A_g$(R)	$24A_g$ (R)	$36A_g$(R)
	$12A_u$(IR)	$24A_u$ (IR)	$36A_u$(IR)
	$12B_g$(R)	$24B_g$ (R)	$36B_g$(R)
	$12B_u$(IR)	$24B_u$ (IR)	$36B_u$(IR)
Number of lines IR	24	48	72
Number of lines R	24	48	72
β-Tricalcium phosphate (β-TCP); $Ca_3(PO_4)_2$; trigonal R3c [12]			
	ν_1 PO_4	ν_2 PO_4	ν_3, ν_4 PO_4
Site symmetry C_3	A(IR-R)	E(IR-R)	A(IR-R)
			E(IR-R)
Site symmetry C_1	A(IR-R)	2A(IR-R)	3A(IR-R)
Factor group C_{3v}	$3A_1$(IR-R)	$2A_1$(IR-R)	$5A_1$(IR-R)
	E(IR-R)	4E(IR-R)	5E(IR-R)
Number of lines IR	4	6	10
Number of lines R	4	6	10

Molecular group theory, site symmetry, and factor group treatments do not allow the prediction of spectra with their line positions and intensities.

This information can be provided by quantum chemistry calculations [15]. For mineral structures with disordered or partially occupied sites and for solid solutions, factor group theory is more difficult to apply. For amorphous structures like amorphous calcium phosphates, the spectra prediction may rely on the symmetry of basic structural units, Posner's clusters (Table 8.5) [16], although the S_6 symmetry of these clusters has been discussed and lower symmetry, C_1 or C_3, has been proposed depending on the environment [17].

8.2.2 *Spectra of Well-Defined Stoichiometric Calcium Phosphates*

The FTIR and Raman spectra of the most important calcium phosphates are shown in Figs. 8.1 and 8.2. Line positions are reported in Tables 8.6 and 8.7.

Table 8.3 Internal vibrations of phosphate groups in apatites for different structures and symmetries

Apatite; hexagonal $P6_3/m$ [11]			
	ν_1 PO_4	ν_2 PO_4	ν_3, ν_4 PO_4
Site symmetry: C_s	A′(IR-R)	A′(IR-R), A″(IR-R)	2A′(IR-R), A″(IR-R)
Factor group: C_{6h}	A_g (R), E_{2g} (R), B_u E_{1u}(IR),	A_g(R), E_{2g}(R), B_u, E_{1u}(IR), B_g, E_{1g}(R), A_u (IR), E_{2u}	$2A_g$(R), $2E_{2g}$(R), $2B_u$, $2E_{1u}$(IR), B_g, E_{1g}(R), A_u (IR), E_{2u}
Number of lines IR	1	2	3
Number of lines R	2	3	5
Apatite; hexagonal $P6_3$ [12]			
	ν_1 PO_4	ν_2 PO_4	ν_3, ν_4 PO_4
Site symmetry: C_1	A (IR,R)	2A (IR-R)	3A (IR-R)
Factor group: C_6	A(IR-R), B, E_1(IR-R), E_2(R)	2A(IR-R), 2B, $2E_1$(IR-R), $2E_2$(R)	3A(IR-R), 3B, $3E_1$(IR-R), $3E_2$(R)
Number of lines IR	2	4	6
Number of lines R	3	6	9
Apatite; monoclinic $P2_1/b$			
	ν_1 PO_4	ν_2 PO_4	ν_3, ν_4 PO_4
Site symmetry C_1	A(IR,R)	2A(IR-R)	3A(IR-R)
Factor group C_{2h}	$3A_g$(R), $3B_g$(R), $3A_u$(IR), $3B_u$(IR)	$6A_g$(R), $6B_g$(R), $6A_u$(IR), $6B_u$(IR)	$9A_g$(R), $9B_g$(R), $9A_u$(IR), $9B_u$(IR)
Number of lines IR	6	12	18
Number of lines R	6	12	18

Very often for complex structures, the assignments are difficult to obtain due to the superimposition of elementary fundamental vibrations. Theoretical calculated spectra can, in principle, be obtained if the crystal structure is known, and a few reports have been published on this subject [15].

Generally speaking, the spectra observed for well-crystallized stoichiometric calcium phosphates like apatite correspond to the theoretical prediction, although some anomalies can be noted like the observation of superimposed E_{2g} and A_g modes for the apatite spectra in the ν_1 PO_4^{3-} domain in Raman or other anomalies [11]. Detailed investigations have discussed the occurrence of faint lines revealed by second derivatives of the spectra and the adequacy of the $P6_3/m$ model for hexagonal hydroxyapatite [11, 20, 21] (factor group C_{6h}), compared to the real local symmetry (factor group C_6). The structure of stoichiometric hydroxyapatite, corresponding to a monoclinic unit cell, space group $P2_1/b$, should theoretically lead to spectra with additional lines which are not all observed. The ordering of OH^- anions in the structure, related to the monoclinic superstructure, seems to have little effect on the vibration movements of the PO_4^{3-} ions, which is very analogous in hydroxyapatite to that of a truly $P6_3/m$ symmetry like that of fluorapatite [11, 22].

The spectra of tricalcium phosphates (TCP) and tetracalcium phosphates (TTCP) are particularly complex, and all predicted lines cannot be distinguished and identified due to superimposition, except for the ν_1 lines of TTCP which are

Table 8.4 Internal vibrations of phosphate groups in calcium phosphates of interest (HPO_4^{2-}-containing compounds)

Octacalcium phosphate (OCP); $Ca_8(PO_4)_4(HPO_4)_2$, $5H_2O$; triclinic P−1 * HPO_4^{2-} [14]			
	ν_1 PO_4	ν_2 PO_4	ν_3, ν_4 PO_4
Site symmetry: C_1	A(IR,R)	2A(IR, R)	3A(IR, R)
Factor group: C_i	4+2*A_g(IR)	8+4*A_g(IR)	12+6*A_g(IR)
	4+2*B_u (R)	8+4*B_u(R)	12+6*B_u(R)
Number of lines IR	4+2*	8+4*	12+6*
Number of lines R	4+2*	8+4*	12+6*
Anhydrous dicalcium phosphate (DCPA) or monetite; $CaHPO_4$; triclinic P−1			
Site symmetry: C_1	A(IR, R)	2A(IR, R)	3A(IR, R)
Group factor: C_i	2A_g(R)	4A_g(R)	6A_g(R)
	2A_u(IR)	4A_u(IR)	6A_u(IR)
Number of lines IR	2	4	6
Number of lines R	2	4	6
Dicalcium phosphate dihydrate (DCPD) or brushite; $CaHPO_4$; monoclinic Ia [5]			
Site symmetry: C_1	A(IR-R)	2A(IR-R)	3A(IR-R)
Site symmetry: C_s	A′(IR-R)	A′(IR-R)	2A′(IR-R)
		A″(IR-R)	A″(IR-R)
Factor group: C_s	A′(IR-R)	2A′(IR-R)	3A′(IR-R)
	A″(IR-R)	2A″(IR-R)	3A″(IR-R)
Number of lines IR	2	4	6
Number of lines R	2	4	6

Table 8.5 Vibrations of phosphate groups in amorphous calcium phosphate (ACP) assuming a S_6 symmetry of the Posner's clusters [16]

	ν_1 PO_4	ν_2 PO_4	ν_3, ν_4 PO_4
Symmetry S_6	A_u(IR), E_u(IR)	2A_u(IR), 2E_u(IR)	3A_u(IR), 3E_u(IR)
	A_g(R), E_g(R)	2A_g(R), 2E_g(R)	3A_g(R), 3E_g(R)
Number of lines IR	2	4	6
Number of lines R	2	4	6

relatively thin and well resolved. The case of α-TCP is special due to a very large unit cell with numerous phosphate groups, giving numerous lines with a poor resolution. Strong lines are observed in the FTIR ν_2 PO_4 domain of TTCP, like in oxyapatite [23], possibly related to the presence of oxide ions in these structures.

Other types of lines can be observed corresponding to the libration movements of protonated species like OH^- ions for hydroxyapatite or H_2O- and HPO_4^{2-}-related lines for brushite and octacalcium phosphates. On Raman spectra several external vibrations can be detected at low wavenumbers. Several differences between the spectra of different calcium phosphate phases allow their identification and, to some extent, their quantification. Overtone and combination bands can be seen

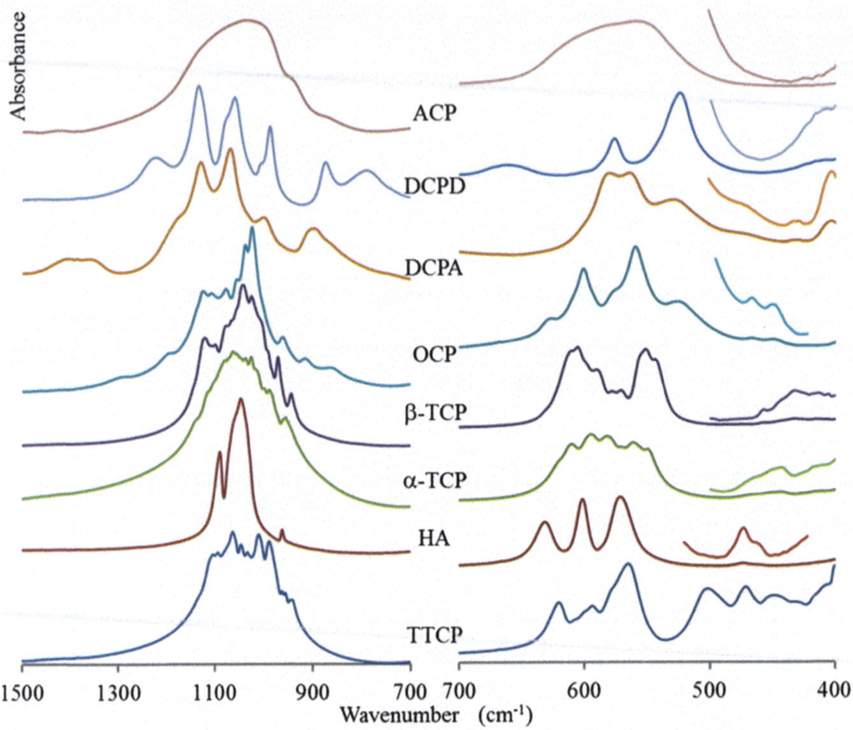

Fig. 8.1 FTIR spectra of calcium phosphates in the domains of internal vibrations of phosphate ions

on some spectra. For hydroxyapatite and related compounds, the most frequently observed overtone/combination is a group of lines at 2,200–1,950 cm^{-1} [11].

These weak intensity lines do not seem to have received much attention and they are sometimes misinterpreted. Overtone and combination bands of protonated molecules are also used in near infrared (NIR) characterization of calcium phosphates. Lines assignments have been proposed in the case of the simplest spectra like apatite [11, 12, 20, 22, 24, 25]. For the amorphous calcium phosphate, the lines appear very broad and dissymmetric, suggesting the existence of several components. It seems however difficult, using FTIR and Raman data, to contribute to the discussion concerning the symmetry of real Posner's clusters.

8.3 Methods and Techniques

The vibrational spectra of solids are relatively complex, and several techniques have been used to improve band resolution and assignment. Spectra obtained at low temperatures, for example, may show narrower lines, improving the band

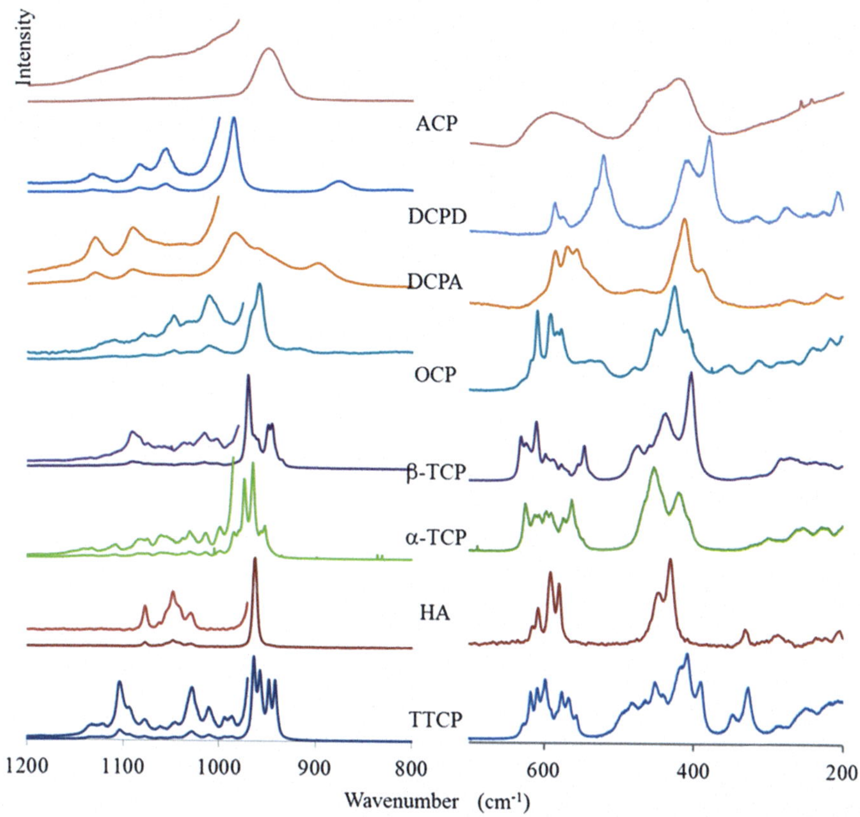

Fig. 8.2 Raman spectra of calcium phosphates in the domains of internal vibrations of phosphate ions (for comparison purposes the wavenumber axis is in reverse order, like for the FTIR spectra)

resolution in certain cases [9, 18]. Among specific techniques applied to vibrational spectroscopies are isotopic substitutions and the use of dichroic properties. Data computing is also largely used, as in other domains of spectroscopy.

8.3.1 Isotopic Substitutions

One of the strengths of vibrational spectroscopies is the possible use of stable isotopic substituted molecules or molecular ions that can be incorporated into a material as molecular probes [18, 24]. Isotopic substitutions allow the identification of vibrating groups when some doubt or suspicion is raised, follow-up of chemical reactions or transformations of calcium phosphates, or simply shifts of weak hidden lines superimposed on other absorption bands.

Table 8.6 FTIR line positions of calcium phosphates (cm^{-1}; *m* medium, *s* strong, *sh* shoulder, *v* very, *w* weak)

	TTCP	HA	α-TCP	β-TCP	OCP	DCPA	DCPD	ACP
ν_3 PO_4						1,400 w		
						1,350 w		
					1,295 w		1,215 m	
					1,193 w	1,175 m,sh		
					1,137 vvw	1,128 s	1,132 s	
				1,119 s	1,121 s			
	1,105 w				1,103 s			
	1,093 w	1,092 s		1,094 w,sh				
	1,073 w			1,080 w,sh	1,077 s		1,070 s	
	1,062 s		1,055 s		1,055 s	1,064 s	1,060 s	
	1,046 s	1,040 vs	1,039 s	1,041 vs				1,040 s
	1,033 m		1,025 s		1,037 s			
			1,013 s		1,023 s			
	1,010 s		997 s	1,010 w,sh	1,000 vvw		1,000 w,sh	
	989 s		984 s					
ν_1 PO_4				972 s		992 m	984 s	
	962 w	962 w			962 w			
	956 w		954 m					
	946 w			945 m				949 w,sh
	941 w							
P-OH of					917 w			
HPO_4^{2-}					861 w	892 m	872 m	
ν_4 PO_4	620 w		613 m		627 vw			
	594 w	601 m	597 m	602 m	601 m			
			585 m	589 w				
	571 s	575 m,sh	563 m		575 w	576 s	577 m	
		561 m	551 m	550 m	560 m	563 s		560 m
	501 w			541 m	524 w	525 m	526 s	
ν_2 PO_4	471 m	472 vw	471 w			480		
		462 sh	463 w		466 vw			
			454 w					
	450 w		430 w	432 vw	449 vw	428 vw	418 sh	
	429 w		415 w			405 m	400 m	
	399 m					398 sh		
References	[10]	[12]	[13]	[12]	[14]	[12]	[18]	

The isotopic shift (position ratio between identical vibration modes of the unsubstituted and isotopic substituted molecules) can vary according to the atom substituted in the molecule and the vibrational mode considered. For diatomic vibrators like the OH^- ion, the shift between OH^- and its deuterated equivalent OD^- is given using Hook's derived formula. The position ratio between the protonated and deuterated ion stretching line is theoretically close to 0.7276, the square root of the reduced mass ratios, which in fact is observed experimentally.

Table 8.7 Raman line positions of calcium phosphates (cm^{-1}; *m* medium, *s* strong, *sh* shoulder, *v* very, *w* weak)

	TTCP	HA	α-TCP	β-TCP	OCP	DCPA	DCPD	ACP
ν_3 PO_4						1,131 m	1,132 vw	
	1,119 vw						1,119 vw	1,118 w
	1,101 w				1,112 w			
	1,091 sh	1,077 w	1,077 w	1,090 w	1,079 vw	1,094 m	1,079 w	
	1,076 vw	1,064 w					1,061 m	
		1,057 w	1,058 w		1,052 w			
	1,045 vw	1,048 w			1,048 w			1,050 w
		1,041 w						
		1,034 w			1,036 vw			
	1,026 w	1,029 w	1,027 w		1,027 vw			
	1,008 w		1,012 w	1,015 w	1,011 m			
			998 w		1,005 w,sh			
ν_1 PO_4	983 vw		976 s					
	961 vs	964 vs	964 s	970 s	966 s	988 s	986 s	
	956 vs		954 sh	948 s	959 vs			
	946 s							951 s
	940 s							
P-OH st. of					916 w	900 m		
HPO_4^{2-}					874 w		878 m	
ν_4 PO_4	615 vw	614 w	620 w		619 vw			
	608 vw	607 w	610 w	612 w	609 mw			
	597 w	591 w	593 w		591 m	588 m	588 w	594 m
	576 vw	580 w	577 w		577 m	563 m		
	566 sh		563 w					
	556 vw			549 w				
	495 sh				523 w, b		525 w	
ν_2 PO_4	481 sh			480 w				
	463 sh	448 w	451 w		451 m			451 m
	449 w	433 w		439 w				
	414 sh		421 w		427 m	420 w		419 m
	407 w			408 w	409 m		411 w	
	389 w				353 w	394 w	381 w	
References	[10]	[19]	[13]	[19]	[14]	[20]	[19]	

For more complex molecules, the isotopic shift depends only on the mass ratios of the atoms and can be determined according to the Teller–Redlich product rule [26]. The replacement of ^{12}C by ^{13}C in the carbonate ion, for example, gives different shifts depending on the vibration domain. The line position ratios are, respectively, 1,000, 0.9686, 0.9723, and 0.9963 for the ν_1, ν_2, ν_3, and ν_4 domains. The replacement of ^{16}O by ^{18}O in PO_4 groups has been used in early studies [24]. However, as a total substitution of ^{16}O by ^{18}O could not be achieved, the spectra were rendered more complex by virtue of the different possible substitutions.

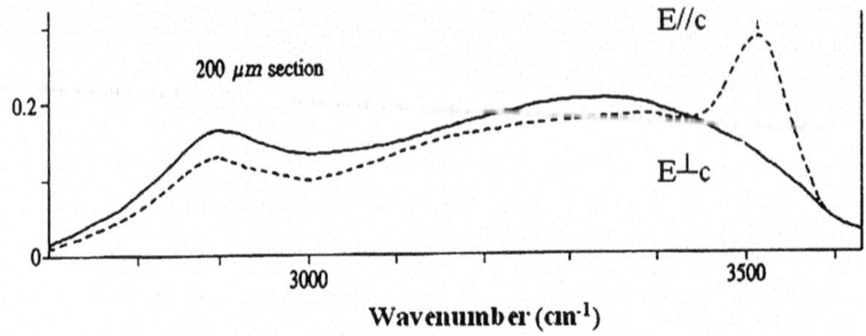

Fig. 8.3 Example of dichroism on dahlite monocrystals (IR spectra). *Dotted line*: OH stretching vibration, when the electric vector of the IR beam is parallel to the c-axis of the hexagonal structure; the OH line shows a maximum height. This line is not observed when the electric vector is perpendicular to the c-axis. These data indicate that the OH^- ion is parallel to the c-axis (Reprinted from Ref. [7]. Copyright 1994. With permission from Elsevier)

8.3.2 Dichroism

Dichroism corresponds to the change in line intensities related to the polarization of the IR or Raman beams with respect to the crystallographic axis. It can be used when monocrystals are available with shapes and morphologies compatible with the techniques in use for spectra recording. The activities of the different vibrational modes in polarized IR and Raman can be determined using factor group theory. Conversely, dichroism can be used to determine the orientation of crystals in a material or a biological tissue. One of the most interesting examples is that of the orientation of OH^- groups in hydroxyapatites [7]. Early works on natural monocrystals of dahlite (a carbonated hydroxyapatite) have shown that OH^- groups are parallel to the c-axis of the hexagonal structure (Fig. 8.3). Conversely, this orientation can be used to determine the orientation of hydroxyapatite crystals in materials or biological tissues like dental enamel [26].

8.3.3 Data Computing

The actual techniques of vibrational spectra acquisition in general permit the recording of spectra of high quality with excellent resolution and signal/noise ratio. However, very frequently an intrinsic broadening persists, related to the substance itself. Many computing techniques have been proposed to improve spectral resolution and line identifications. The easiest ones are second derivative and FTIR self-deconvolution [11, 21, 27]. A drawback is an enhancement of sharp slope changes in the spectra, whereas broad lines remain mostly unchanged and a lowering of the signal on noise ratio. Second derivative changes considerably the aspect of the spectra. With self-deconvolution, the aspect of the spectra is preserved, but spurious bands may appear in case of overdeconvolution [28]. These resolution enhancement techniques are often associated with curve-fitting procedures, extensively used nowadays for quantitative evaluations. However, these techniques are difficult to validate, and, very often, several solutions may appear for the same spectrum, which leads to some heterogeneity in the published reports [29, 30] with variable numbers of lines and assignments. The line shape is an important parameter in curve-fitting; however, no definitive rule can be provided, and the best fitting parameters might not always correspond to the most relevant ones from a physical-chemical point of view. Whenever possible, the peak fitting procedure and line assignments should be supported by other data involving, for example, isotopic substitution, chemical analyses, or correlation with other techniques such as solid-state NMR. Curve-fitting techniques lead to a peak area or integrated intensity allowing quantitative determinations. It is very difficult, in the case of solids, to use the absolute line intensities, and generally the results are given as intensity ratios in a given domain. These integrated intensity ratios are often considered to represent the molecular composition of a phase or the composition of a mixture of phases. However, line intensity ratios should not be confused with molecular or phase ratios. The molecular extinction coefficients between molecules in different environments or in different phases can be very different, and appropriate standardization curves are needed to determine a chemical composition.

Other elaborate techniques such as principal component analysis can be applied to collections of spectra to determine the individual components involved in the series [31]. However, this technique presupposes, implicitly, that discrete individual compounds with invariable line positions are involved and thus excludes the existence of apparent continuous band shifts often observed in solid solutions. Many other techniques are available, including specialized data treatment software combining chemometrics and spectroscopy.

8.4 Substituted Well-Crystallized Calcium Phosphates

Very often biological apatites and other calcium phosphates can incorporate substitution ions, and the corresponding spectra can be strongly altered. Thus, in addition to phase identification, vibrational spectroscopies also allow the identification of site occupancies in crystalline solids and interactions between species in close proximity.

8.4.1 Substituted Apatites and Their Solid Solutions

Several types of substituted apatites may be found, from simple solid solutions involving different cations in stoichiometric apatites to complex substitutions involving coupled replacements and vacancies. The spectra interpretation, including line assignments, for substituted compounds is considered to derive from those for pure, non-substituted compounds. However, at the molecular level, the differences in mineral ion environments due to solid solutions may be perceived as disruptions in the crystal periodicity and as alterations in the vibrator environments and symmetry. Thus, there is some ambivalence in interpreting spectra of substituted apatites considering either the global crystallographic structure or the local environments of the vibrating species.

8.4.1.1 Cation-Substituted Stoichiometric Apatites

The spectra of cationic solid solutions can often be related to those of pure compounds. An illustrative example is given by strontium–calcium hydroxyapatites. In the series Ca_{10-x} Sr_x $(PO_4)_6$ $(OH)_2$, the phosphate and OH lines are shifted between those of the end terms; pure calcium and strontium hydroxyapatites. The infrared lines are globally shifted towards lower wavenumbers when a large, heavy cation replaces a smaller, lighter one. This phenomenon is often related to the unit cell volume and, indirectly, to the substitution ratio. The number of lines, however, remains consistent for all spectra of the series with that for a stoichiometric calcium or strontium hydroxyapatite. The shift of simple lines like the Raman ν_1 PO_4 (Fig. 8.4) can be linearly correlated to the substitution ratio, even if the distribution of cations between the two cationic sites of the structure is not homogeneous in this kind of substitution. Similar observations have been reported by Bigi et al. [32]. This behavior is not, however, always observed, and discrepancies have been reported for lead–calcium apatites, for example [33].

Line broadening is generally observed for substituted apatites, which increases progressively with the substitution rate, reaching a maximum at about half substitution and decreasing when approaching the end point. Line broadening is generally related to the irregularity of the atomic array, often referred to as lattice strain, although several causes may be involved [34]. As the substitution ratio increases, the disorder increases and is attested to by line broadening. At a low level of substitutions, a dissymmetry of the Raman ν_1 PO_4 line is clearly observed, suggesting a slight unresolved band shift.

The position and shape of the FTIR or Raman stretching OH vibration follows the same rules (not shown). When we look at the FTIR OH libration line, however, a large gap exists between the extremes of the solid solution (from 633 cm^{-1} for calcium hydroxyapatite to 535 cm^{-1} for strontium hydroxyapatite), and the shift is no longer progressive and linear but seems to correspond to new line formations which could be tentatively assigned to a change in the cationic environments of the OH species, as shown for the Ca_9 Sr_1 $(PO_4)_6$ $(OH)_2$ sample (Fig. 8.5), where two OH libration lines can be distinguished.

Interestingly, for other types of hydroxyapatites, for example, calcium arsenate hydroxyapatites, the position of the OH stretching and libration lines is close to those of calcium phosphate, suggesting that it is the cationic environment of the

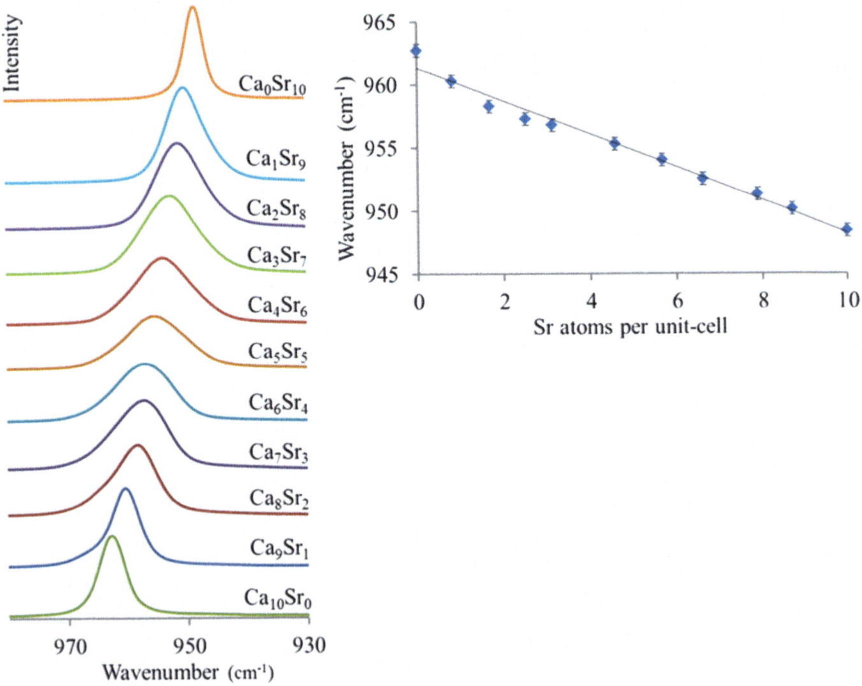

Fig. 8.4 Raman spectra of Sr–Ca hydroxyapatite solid solution in the ν_1 PO_4 domain and quasi-linear variation in the position of the Raman ν_1 PO_4 line as a function of the cationic composition

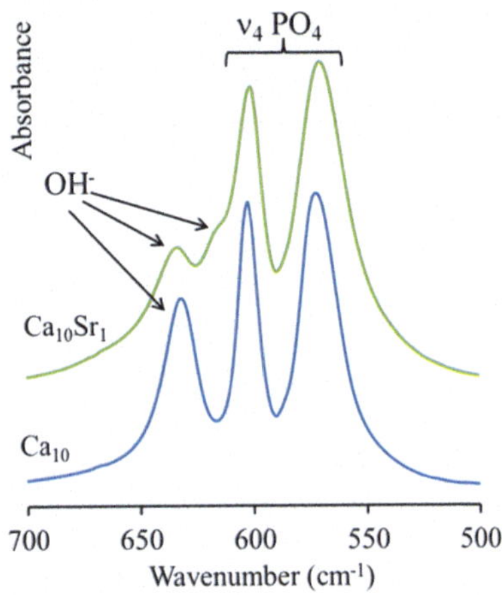

Fig. 8.5 FTIR spectra of OH^- libration line showing the formation of a second shifted OH^- line in Ca_9Sr_1 hydroxyapatite (2), in addition to the OH^- line of Ca_{10} hydroxyapatite (the assignment to the OH^- ion has been confirmed by deuteration, not shown)

OH^- ions that determines their vibrational and libration frequencies. The observation of several lines could then possibly be related to the local cationic environments of the OH vibrators and could potentially give information on clustering of cations in the apatite structure.

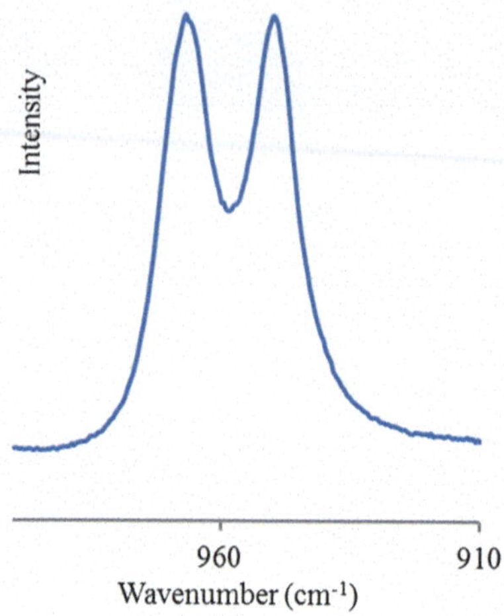

Fig. 8.6 Raman spectra in the ν_1 PO_4 domain of oxyapatite (with undetected OH^- line by Raman). The two lines at 966 and 951 cm^{-1} correspond to phosphate ions close to a O^{2-} ion or a vacancy

8.4.1.2 Substituted Anions and Nonstoichiometric Apatites

The replacement of phosphate ions in stoichiometric apatite by other ions like $AsO_4{}^{3-}$ or $VO_4{}^{3-}$, for example, in lead fluorapatite, $Pb_{10}(PO_4)_{6-x}(VO_4)_xF_2$, induces an alteration in both molecular anion spectra, with a quasi-linear shift of lines relative to each anion, proportional to the substitution ratio, like in cation-substituted apatites [35]. This lines shift with the substitution ratio could probably be used to support the formation of a homogeneous solid solution.

The observation of the oxyapatite, Ca_{10} $(PO_4)_6$ O, spectra is interesting as it involves strong alterations in the infrared and Raman lines compared to its parent phase hydroxyapatite. The Raman ν_1 PO_4 line, for example (Fig. 8.6), is split into two components at 951 and 966 cm^{-1} which has been related to the formation of a vacancy in the monovalent anionic sites (OH^- sites) due to water release and the formation of O^{2-} ions [23]:

$$Ca_{10}(PO_4)_6(OH)_2 \rightarrow H_2O + Ca_{10}(PO_4)_6O \qquad (8.1)$$

In oxyapatite, one half unit cell contains either a vacancy or an oxide ion corresponding to two kinds of local phosphate environments.

For a similar apatite, type A carbonate apatite, Ca_{10} $(PO_4)_6$ CO_3, also containing one bivalent anion and a vacancy per unit cell, the ν_1 Raman phosphate line is also split into two lines at 947 and 957 cm^{-1} [20].

Additionally, a general feature of this kind of apatite with a vacant anionic monovalent site is a rather specific phosphate line in the ν_3 PO_4 domain of the FTIR spectra at around 1,140 cm^{-1}. Such a line is observed, for example, in oxyapatite, type A carbonated apatite, sulfoapatite Ca_{10} $(PO_4)_6$ S, and peroxyapatite Ca_{10} $(PO_4)_6$ O_2 and has been related to the presence of bivalent ions and vacancies

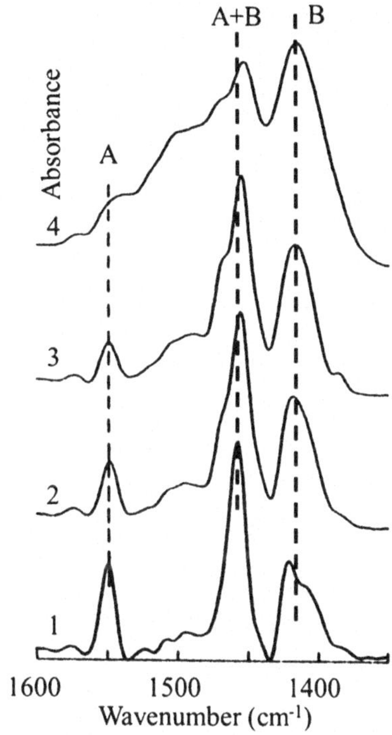

Fig. 8.7 Self-deconvoluted FTIR spectra in the ν_3 CO_3 domain of carbonate ions in mixed type AB carbonated apatites with increasing carbonate concentration (in weight %). 1–1.3 %; 2–2.8 %; 3–3.5 %; 4–10 %. At low concentrations, relatively thin lines can be seen for type A and B carbonate. As the concentration increases, new lines appear corresponding to interactions between carbonate species, and a line broadening associated with a loss of resolution is observed (Reproduced with permission from [37])

[36]. Interestingly, a line near this position is also observed in HPO_4^{2-}-containing apatites, which has been assigned in this case to a P–O stretching of HPO_4^{2-} ions in the apatite structure. It should be observed, however, that these apatites, like type B carbonated apatites (carbonate ions substituting phosphate ions), are considered to contain OH^- vacancies [7]. However, the 1,140 cm^{-1} line is not detected in type B carbonated apatites.

Another alteration observed in the spectrum of oxyapatite is an enhancement of the ν_2 PO_4 line compared with other apatites, which has not yet received a definitive explanation.

Among illustrative examples of substituted apatites are type AB carbonate apatites containing carbonate species replacing both the phosphate ions (type B) and hydroxide ions (type A) of hydroxyapatite: Ca_{10} $(PO_4)_{6-x}$ $(CO_3)_x$ $(OH)_{2-x-2y}$ $(CO_3)_y$ [37]. At very low carbonate content, the carbonate species are dispersed in the crystals, and relatively thin and well-resolved carbonate bands can be observed (Fig. 8.7). This is generally the case when low amounts of substituents are used. When the carbonate concentration increases, the lines become broader, as expected in solid solutions, and, interestingly, new lines appear that have been attributed to interactions between carbonate species [37, 38] and also to the effect of coupled substitution like Na–CO_3 for Ca–PO_4, for example [39].

8.4.2 Other Substituted Calcium Phosphates

A few other examples of FTIR or Raman investigations of other substituted calcium phosphates have been proposed. Quillard et al., for example, have shown that the spectra of sodium- and potassium-containing β-TCP could be interpreted in a quantitative manner by evaluating the line intensities related to the alteration in the phosphate environments produced by this substitution [40].

8.5 Nanocrystalline Biomimetic Apatites

Nanocrystals are characterized by a very high surface area, and vibrational spectroscopies can be used to get information on the surface species. Several reports have been published revealing specific features considering nanocrystalline apatites of biological origin as well as synthetic biomimetic apatites [41, 42].

8.5.1 Surface Characteristics of Biomimetic Nanocrystalline Apatites

An interesting set of data is the comparison of FTIR spectra obtained on freshly precipitated nanocrystalline apatites in either the wet or dry state (Fig. 8.8) [43]. As water strongly absorbs IR radiation, such spectra are obtained either by using the attenuated total reflectance (ATR) technique or more simply by transmission through a thin layer of a suspension deposited on a polyethylene membrane. The data show that the spectra in the ν_1, ν_3 phosphate domain differ strongly.

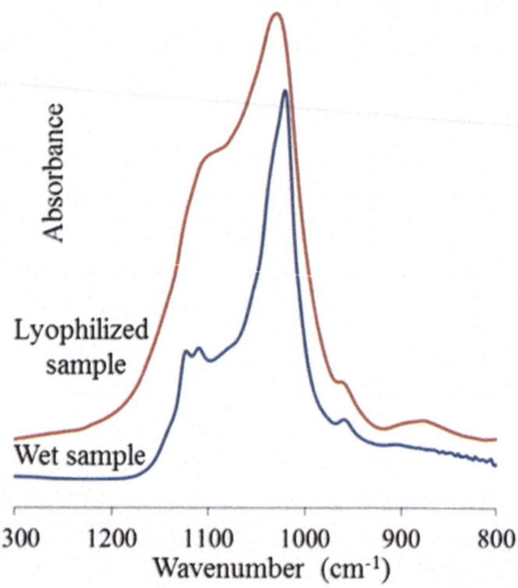

Fig. 8.8 FTIR spectra of biomimetic nanocrystalline apatites in the ν_1, ν_3 PO_4 domain: in a wet state (transmission through a thin layer on polyethylene); after freeze-drying (in a KBr pellet)

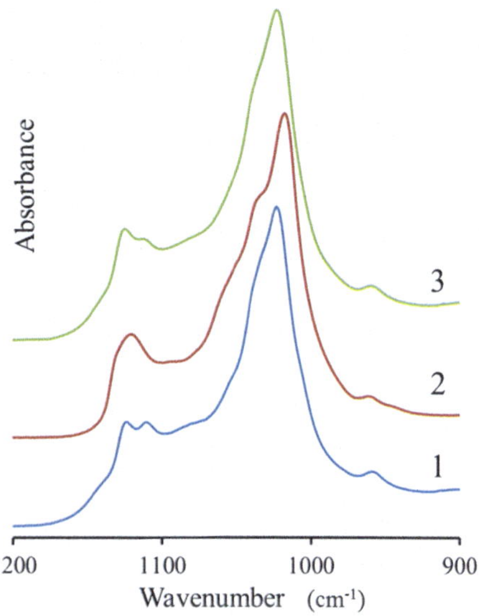

Fig. 8.9 FTIR spectra of biomimetic apatites in a wet state: *1* original sample; *2* sample 1 exchanged in a NH_4HCO_3 solution (1 M) for 5 min; *3* sample 2 exchanged back for 5 min with a 1 M $(NH_4)_2HPO_4$ solution. Illustration of the alteration related to carbonate ion uptake and the reversibility of the surface ion exchange (Reproduced with permission from [43])

In the wet state, relatively narrow lines are obtained, whereas in the dry state, a loss of resolution and band broadening are observed. The transition appears progressively on drying, and it has been assigned to the existence of a structured hydrated layer on the surface of these nanocrystals, which is destroyed upon drying leaving amorphous-like domains. When carbonate is present, such a hydrated layer with relatively thin spectral lines can also be observed, although with less clarity. Interestingly, ion exchanges, which can be easily realized, alter the structure of the hydrated layer, but these changes are reversible and the original features can be reestablished by reverse exchange reactions (Fig. 8.9).

At this point it should be recalled that vibrational spectroscopies are sensitive to local environments and surface environments can be very easily modified. Thus, the observation of an amorphous-like structure using vibrational spectroscopies does not necessarily mean that there is an amorphous phase precursor to the apatite formation. The example above shows that amorphous domains may form on the surface of existing nanocrystals but these do not constitute an isolated phase with defined boundaries, as would be the case with a precursor phase.

Considering the structure of the hydrated layer, FTIR shows that carbonate-free layers are close although not identical to OCP environments as predicted by Brown [44]. For the carbonated hydrated layer, we did not find three-dimensional model structures with comparable spectroscopic characteristics.

From ion exchange experiments, the characteristics of surface carbonate species can be determined (Fig. 8.10), either in the wet state or after drying and amorphization [43]. If the dried sample shows line positions and shapes analogous to those of amorphous calcium carbonate, distinct bands positions can be seen on wet samples, demonstrating again the role of water in the spectroscopic characteristics of surface species.

Fig. 8.10 FTIR spectra of biomimetic nanocrystalline apatites with surface carbonate ions in the ν_3 CO_3 domain: *1* after freeze-drying (in a KBr pellet); *2* in the wet state (transmission through a thin layer on polyethylene) (Reproduced with permission from [43])

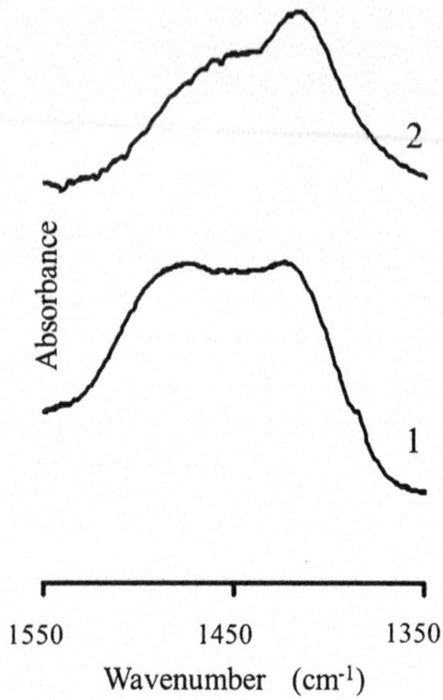

8.5.2 *Characterization of Nanocrystalline Apatites Using Isotopic Substitution*

Isotopic substituted molecular ions can be incorporated as molecular probes into a material to follow alterations in their environments or chemical reactions. These can be used, for example, in apatite nanocrystals to identify sites of carbonate incorporation and alterations in the nanocrystals upon aging.

8.5.2.1 Surface Carbonate in Biomimetic Nanocrystalline Apatites

^{13}C carbonate is easily available and can be used to follow the carbonate species in exchange reactions involving the hydrated layer. When a ^{13}C carbonate-containing solution is put in contact with a ^{12}C carbonated nanocrystalline apatite, a surface equilibration occurs. The FTIR spectra were analyzed in the ν_2 CO_3 domain (Fig. 8.11). The isotopic shift is large enough in this domain to completely separate the ^{12}C and ^{13}C carbonate bands. The data show that the ^{12}C carbonate spectrum is mainly composed of thin lines at 879 and 871 cm^{-1}, respectively, assigned to type A and B carbonate. After contact with the ^{13}C carbonate-containing solution, the ^{13}C domain shows a broad line, characteristic of surface "amorphous" carbonate, without signs of ^{13}C carbonate incorporation in the apatite sites. The ^{12}C species present in the apatite domains are not modified by the ^{13}C carbonate solution treatment. The ^{13}C carbonate uptake is associated with a decrease in surface HPO_4^{2-} ions detectable by FTIR [45], consistent with a surface ion exchange.

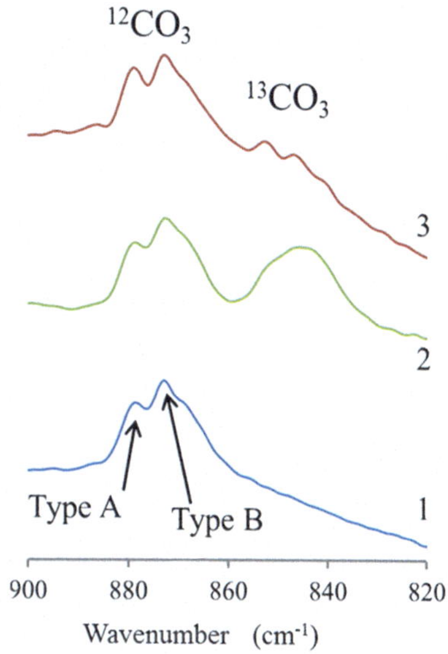

Fig. 8.11 Self-deconvolved FTIR spectra in the ν_2 CO_3 domain: *1* original precipitated ^{12}C carbonate apatite matured for 1 day; *2* original apatite 1 treated in 1 M ^{13}C carbonate solution for 20 min; *3* apatite 2 exchanged in 1 M HPO_4^{2-} solution for 20 min. All samples were freeze-dried after washing

It is possible to exchange back the surface ^{13}C carbonate in a second reaction, with HPO_4^{2-} ions (Fig. 8.11; spectrum 3); the data show that only the ^{13}C surface species have been removed and that once again the apatite's ^{12}C type A and B carbonate remains unchanged. Very faint lines corresponding to apatite carbonate type A and type B are seen in the ^{13}C domain, corresponding to a very small uptake of surface carbonate into the growing apatite domains, due to the brief maturation process taking place during the time of the exchange reaction.

These experiments clearly show the existence of two domains for the carbonate ions inside the nanocrystalline apatite domains (type A and B carbonates) that are stable and nonreactive and on the surface of these domains, comprising a hydrated layer in which carbonate ions can be easily trapped.

8.5.2.2 Maturation Process

Solution exchanges can also be used to pursue the incorporation of carbonate species during aging into nanocrystalline apatites, which is also referred to as maturation.

In these sets of experiments, the nanocrystalline apatites were first precipitated into a ^{12}C or a ^{13}C carbonate-containing solution. After different periods of aging, the solutions were exchanged and the ^{12}C carbonated samples were separated and put in ^{13}C carbonate solutions and vice versa. The spectra obtained after recovering and freeze-drying the samples were analyzed in the ν_2 CO_3 domain. The data are shown only for the ^{13}C-precipitated and then ^{12}C-treated samples (Fig. 8.12).

The samples corresponding to solution substitution at time 0, immediately after precipitation, contain essentially all ^{12}C carbonate. When the solution exchanges

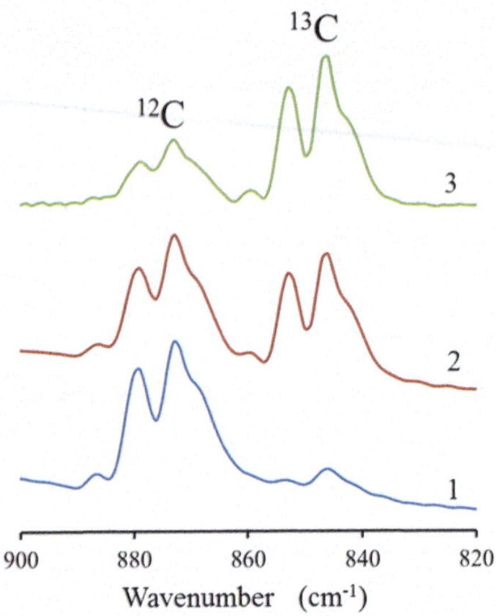

Fig. 8.12 Self-deconvoluted FTIR spectra in the ν_2 CO_3 domain of apatites prepared in a ^{13}C carbonate-containing solution (1 M) matured for different times and put in ^{12}C carbonate solution for 3 additional weeks. *1* initial maturation time 0 in the ^{13}C precipitation solution, most carbonate species are incorporated as ^{12}C during the 3 weeks after the solution exchanges; *2* 3 days maturation in the ^{13}C solution before the exchange; *3* 9 days maturation in the ^{13}C solution before the exchange. The ^{13}C carbonate line intensity increases progressively as the initial maturation time increases, whereas the ^{12}C carbonate line intensity decreases (Reprinted from Ref. [45]. Copyright 2007. With permission from Elsevier)

occur later after precipitation, however, the proportion of ^{13}C carbonate increases and that of ^{12}C carbonate decreases. The first noteworthy observation is that the carbonate ions are incorporated in these nanocrystalline apatites during aging and that they are not trapped in the apatite domains during the fast precipitation. The carbonate taken up during precipitation exists essentially as easily exchangeable surface carbonate. The second observation is that the ratios between type A and type B locations do not vary significantly with time of uptake during aging and that species already in the apatite domain are not altered. The third phenomenon revealed by these experiments is that the ability to incorporate carbonate ions slows down considerably with time reflecting a loss of reactivity of the nanocrystals on aging related to the decrease of proportion of the unstable surface hydrated layer which nourishes the growth of the apatite domains.

The comparison of apatites precipitated in $^{13}CO_3$ solutions, aged for 3 days, then treated in $^{12}CO_3$ solutions with symmetrical samples precipitated in $^{12}CO_3$ solutions and aged for 3 days, and then treated in $^{13}CO_3$ solutions (Fig. 8.13) indicates, in addition, that the line resolution is always better for the first carbonate species to enter ($^{13}CO_3$ and $^{12}CO_3$, respectively), which can be interpreted as an improvement in the local organization possibly related to the growth of the apatite domains at the expense of the unstable hydrated surface layer.

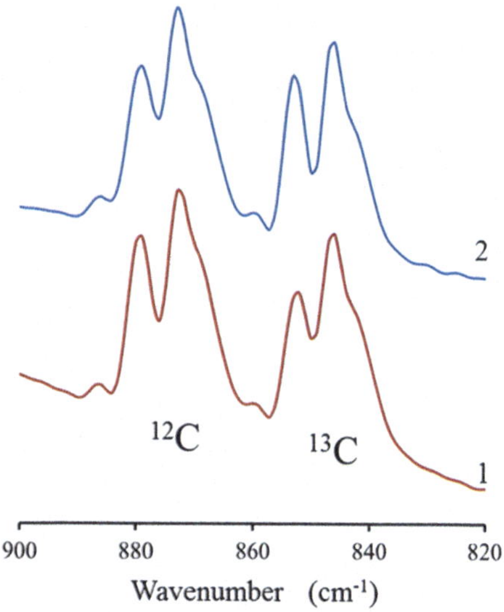

Fig. 8.13 Deconvoluted spectra in the ν_2 CO_3 domain of: *1* apatites precipitated in the ^{12}C carbonate-containing solution matured for 3 days and put in ^{13}C carbonate solution for 3 additional weeks and *2* apatites precipitated in the ^{13}C carbonate-containing solution matured for 3 days and put in ^{12}C carbonate solution for 3 additional weeks. The first trapped carbonate species are more resolved and correspond to their environments with better crystallinity (Reprinted from Ref. [45]. Copyright 2007. With permission from Elsevier)

8.6 Examples of the Use of Vibrational Spectroscopies in Biominerals and Biomaterials Involving Calcium Phosphates

8.6.1 Plasma Sprayed Coating

Plasma spraying of hydroxyapatite (HA) is largely used to improve the biological activity and biointegration of orthopedic metal implants [46–48]. However, it is well established that HA decomposes during plasma spraying, leading to the formation of different phases [48–50]. This reported decomposition has several advantages and drawbacks for the behavior of the coatings after implantation. Plasma sprayed coatings are mainly composed of crystalline HA and oxyapatite (OA) embedded into a relatively soluble amorphous phase (ACP). Sometimes CaO, TTCP, and α- or β-TCP are also present, generally in small proportions. In order to determine the material's quality, several standards have been published regarding the coating's chemical composition (Ca/P ratio), phase composition, and crystallinity (ISO 13779-3:2008). Most of these characterizations are based essentially on X-ray diffraction (XRD) analyses. However, several additional parameters that are more difficult to determine, such as the main phase proportions and their distribution within the coating and more specifically the amount of amorphous phase, are not considered in the standards, although they could be related to the coating behavior in vitro and in vivo. All the phases detected in a plasma sprayed coating can theoretically be distinguished by Raman spectroscopy, especially the most important, in some instances with better sensitivity than by XRD. In addition, Raman scattering allows local investigations of the coating's heterogeneity [50–53].

Fig. 8.14 Raman spectra of plasma sprayed coating in the ν_1 PO_4 domain showing the main phases: amorphous calcium phosphate (ACP), oxyapatite (OA), and hydroxyapatite (HA) (Reprinted from Ref. [54]. Copyright 2012. With permission from Elsevier)

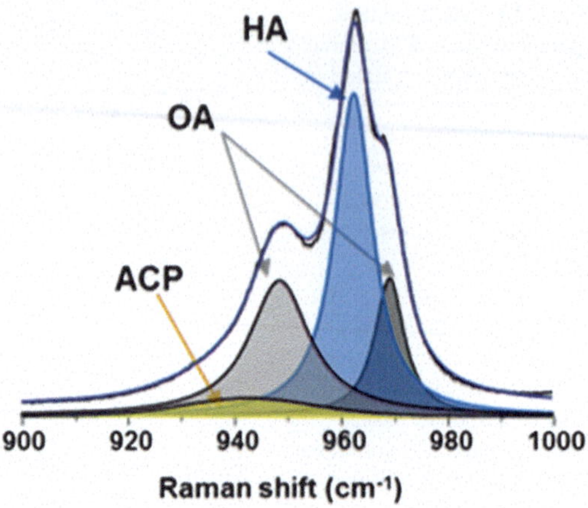

Micro-Raman imaging based on different representations from the same data set may provide a powerful means to study structural alterations and visualize the distribution of phases within heterogeneous plasma sprayed HA coatings. The $\nu_1 PO_4$ domain, with strong thin lines, seems well adapted for imaging (Fig. 8.14) [54]. The ACP especially is characterized by a broad Raman line around 950 cm^{-1}, and all crystalline phases show lines distinct from that of apatite at 961 cm^{-1}. The OA, so difficult to distinguish by other methods, exhibits very specific Raman scattering lines at about 951 and 966 cm^{-1}, as mentioned earlier [23]. CaO is the only phase that cannot be detected in this domain.

An accurate mapping of the different phases in HA coatings can be obtained by micro-Raman imaging involving curve-fitting in the ν_1 PO_4 domain, extraction of the characteristic line(s) associated with specific phases, and of their relative intensities. It should be noticed that at this stage, without accurate standardization, the data represent only the relative integrated intensities of lines associated with a specific phase and their relative variation, but not their real content in the coating. In the example shown in Fig. 8.15, we can see the distribution of the HA, OA, and ACP in a cross section of a coating obtained using a low-energy plasma spray device [54].

The domains rich in oxyapatite appear relatively narrow and dispersed. Two types of OA-rich domains can be distinguished, those found within the amorphous phase, which may correspond in part to a recrystallization process, and those contiguous to HA domains, possibly formed by dehydration during the particles' flight. HA-rich domains might correspond to solid particle cores. It clearly appears that HA-rich domains exist in zones with low amorphous content.

In addition to a heterogeneous distribution of phases through the thickness of the deposit, there is also a heterogeneous distribution on its surface, and very different Raman spectra are collected depending on the location [55]. Therefore, Raman microspectroscopy can be used as a routine nondestructive tool to obtain rapid analysis of the composition of apatite coatings and even of different domains

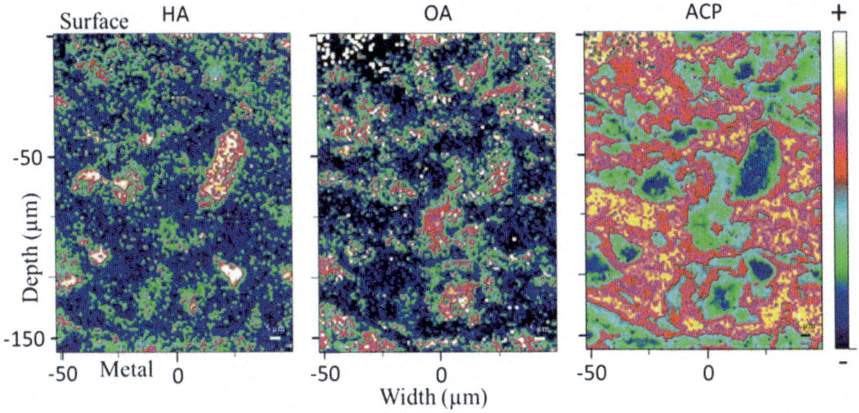

Fig. 8.15 Raman mapping of the main calcium phosphate constituents in a cross section of a plasma sprayed coating obtained using a low-energy mini-torch [55]. Relative areas of specific lines: HA, hydroxyapatite ($962 \pm 1\ cm^{-1}$); OA, oxyapatite ($957 \pm 1\ cm^{-1}$); and ACP, amorphous calcium phosphate ($948 \pm 2\ cm^{-1}$). The amorphous phase appears as a binder. Islands of HA are surrounded and superimposed to OA. HA is never totally absent suggesting a recrystallization from the amorphous phase

of a splat. This technique could be adapted for the chemical characterization of the coating directly on biomedical implants. Image analyses could then be used to describe the coating characteristics with accuracy.

8.6.2 Setting Reactions of Calcium Phosphate Cements

Calcium phosphate cements have been widely used as bone substitute materials since the 1980s, and generally FTIR and Raman spectroscopy are involved in the characterization of the set cements. Interestingly, this technique can also be implemented to study the cement paste composition during setting and hardening and thus provides kinetics data on the chemical reaction(s) involved during these processes. Generally it is only the physical setting that is examined according to standards.

Two methods can be used for such a study: (1) lyophilization of cement paste after different maturation periods (water removal stops the chemical reaction) and then preparation of a KBr pellet of the sample for transmission mode FTIR analysis and (2) direct real-time FTIR analysis of cement paste using a horizontal attenuated total reflectance device equipped with a standard ZnSe monocrystal [56]. This technique allows direct follow-up of the cement setting reactions and kinetics. We present herewith an example of this kind of FTIR analysis on vaterite $CaCO_3$–dicalcium phosphate dihydrate (DCPD) mixed cement to study the influence of a solid phase co-grinding treatment on the cement setting reaction [57].

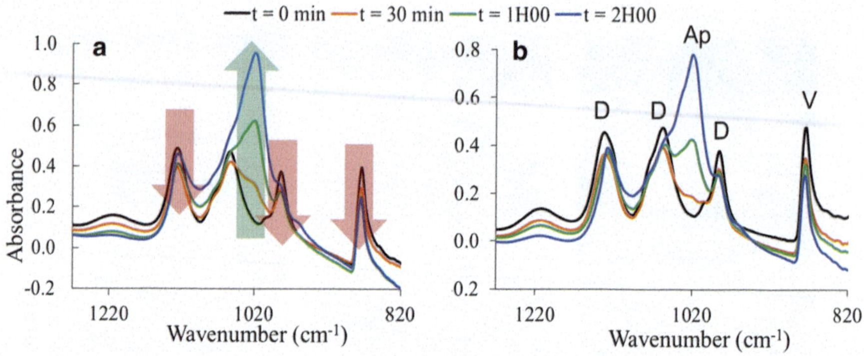

Fig. 8.16 Real-time evolution of the FTIR spectra of a cement paste at 37 °C: (**a**) the cement paste prepared with unground solid phase; (**b**) the cement paste prepared with co-ground solid phase (*D* DCPD, *V* vaterite, *Ap* apatite) (Reproduced with adaptation from Ref. [56]. Copyright 2011. With permission from Elsevier)

It has previously been shown that the setting reaction of the reference cement is based on the chemical reaction of DCPD on vaterite, leading to a solid form composed of nanocrystalline carbonated apatite analogous to bone mineral associated with untransformed vaterite $CaCO_3$.

Hydrogen phosphate groups in brushite (at 985, 1,058, 1,132, and 1,222 cm^{-1}), phosphate groups in apatite (at 1,020 cm^{-1}), and carbonate groups in vaterite (at 876 cm^{-1}) can be identified by FTIR spectroscopy. We focused on examination of modifications in the phosphate and carbonate domains of the spectrum.

Figure 8.16a illustrates the setting reaction of a reference cement paste: a decrease in the brushite and vaterite lines is associated with an increase in the apatite lines. Figure 8.16b shows the evolution of the FTIR spectrum (in the range 1,270–820 cm^{-1}) of a cement paste made of previously co-ground brushite and vaterite powders. Significant differences can be seen regarding the progression of the setting reaction, especially during the first hour of paste evolution [56]. Interestingly, 30 min after paste preparation, the intensity of the band (shoulder) at 1,020 cm^{-1} characteristic of apatite is lower in the case of the co-ground cement than in the case of the reference cement. This marked difference in 1,020 cm^{-1} band intensity is also visible if we compare spectra obtained after 1 h (Fig. 8.16a, b), thus indicating a significant effect of co-grinding on cement setting reaction kinetics. This effect is also marked when comparing the decrease in intensity of the weak phosphate band of DCPD at 1,222 cm^{-1} for both cements: a delay in the decrease in intensity of this band is noted for the cement paste prepared with a co-ground solid phase, especially if we compare spectra corresponding to 1 h of cement paste evolution (Fig. 8.16a b).

This kind of study can easily be transposed to other systems and allow a convenient and precise evaluation of the effect of additives, pretreatments, or impurities on cement setting and hardening reactions.

8.6.3 Adsorption of Biomolecules and Drugs

Bioactive molecules often exhibit a high binding affinity for calcium phosphate surfaces through ionic end groups. Adsorption properties of apatites are involved in biological molecule chromatography and in the regulation of biological processes like biomineralization [58–60]. In the biomaterials field, adsorption of drugs on apatitic surfaces can be used to confer a therapeutic activity to substitutive biomaterials based on calcium phosphate [61]. FTIR and Raman spectroscopies appear to be powerful tools in understanding the interactions of bioactive molecules with apatitic surfaces; they have been widely utilized, for example, to study bisphosphonate adsorption on apatite in vitro [62, 63] or, potentially, in vivo, using surface-enhanced Raman spectroscopy (SERS) [64]. Bisphosphonate molecules (BPs) are used as successful antiresorptive agents for the prevention and treatment of bone diseases such as osteoporosis. They present a high affinity for apatitic surfaces and prevent mineral dissolution and bone resorption, inhibiting osteoclast activity [65]. The adsorption equilibrium of such drugs with apatitic surfaces can be described by a Langmuir isotherm, and follow-up of the variation in the mineral ion content of the solution after adsorption indicates that the adsorption reaction can be described as an ion exchange process between phosphonate groups of BPs molecules in solution and phosphate groups on the apatitic surface [66].

Raman microspectroscopy provides a powerful way to acquire information about chemical composition at a molecular level, even in aqueous environments. Moreover most BP molecules contain aromatic or conjugated domains and are therefore strong Raman scatterers. For example, considering the Raman spectra of biomimetic apatitic nanocrystals after adsorption of a bisphosphonate, tiludronate (Fig. 8.17), several vibration bands attributable to tiludronate are observed.

Some of them, especially those of phosphonate groups, are hidden by those from phosphate ions of the substrate. However, additional lines appear at 745 and 1,575 cm^{-1} corresponding to C–S and aromatic ring chain vibrations, assigned to tiludronate. Thus, the spectroscopic data from adsorbed molecules permits to confirm the presence of BPs on apatitic supports, and the irreversibility of such adsorption processes on solution diluting or sample washing [67]. Quantitative determinations can be performed directly on such systems, and a linear variation is obtained for the line area ratio of 746 or 1,575 cm^{-1} lines of tiludronate on the 961 cm^{-1} phosphate line of apatite (Fig. 8.17). These determinations could be improved using statistical analysis and chemometric methods.

8.6.4 Near Infrared Spectroscopy

Near infrared spectroscopy (NIR) may also be considered as an interesting complementary tool for physicochemical characterizations, for example, where the analysis of adsorbed water molecules is concerned. Indeed, water absorption bands in the NIR region (composed of combination transitions and overtones, [68]) are

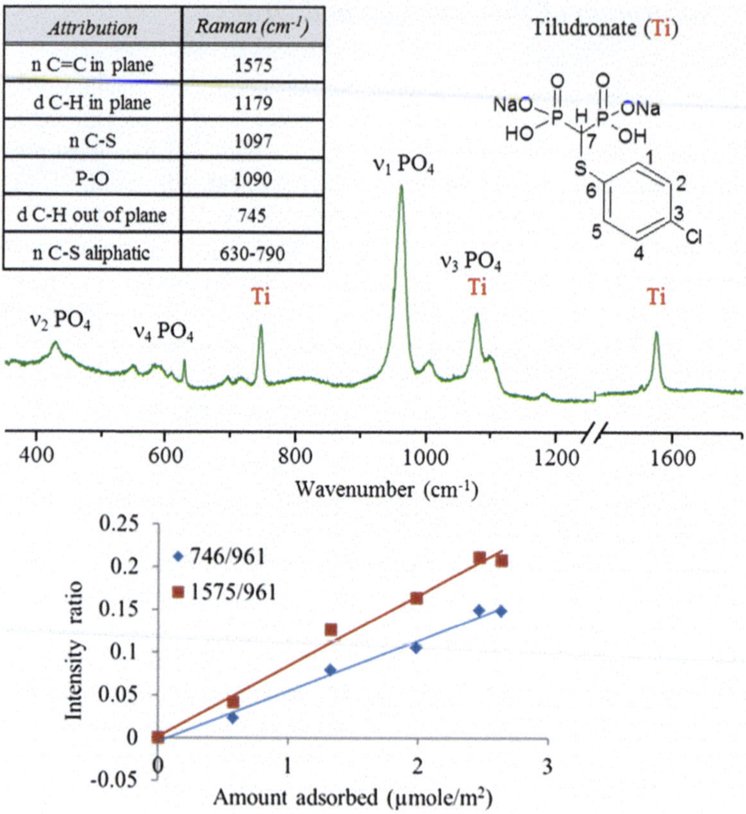

Attribution	Raman (cm-1)
n C=C in plane	1575
d C-H in plane	1179
n C-S	1097
P-O	1090
d C-H out of plane	745
n C-S aliphatic	630-790

Fig. 8.17 Raman spectrum of a biomimetic nanocrystalline apatite after adsorption of tiludronate and variation of the intensity ratio of tiludronate lines at 746 and 1,575 cm^{-1} on the ν_1 PO_4 apatite line at 961 cm^{-1} [67]

characterized by weaker extinction coefficients than in the mid-IR region where the absorption due to water molecules can approach saturation, especially for samples exhibiting a high surface area. NIR analyses have, for instance, been exploited to explore surface hydration phenomena on nanocrystalline apatite samples, including surfaces with cationic substituent such as Mg^{2+} ions [69]. In this type of experiment, some biomimetic samples (preliminarily outgassed at room temperature) were equilibrated with water vapor and analyzed by NIR in situ, to follow interaction phenomena with surface water molecules.

NIR absorption bands due to water molecules in the 6,800–7,200 cm^{-1} range may be overlapped by harmonic vibrations of apatitic OH^- ions; therefore, attention can be focused on the more specific $\delta + \nu_{asym}$ combination mode of water molecules located at lower frequencies, in the 5,500–4,500 cm^{-1} region: this mode was indeed shown to be rather sensitive to hydrogen bonds involving water molecules, leading to a variety of NIR contributions due to molecules experiencing different types of interactions with the surface [68, 70].

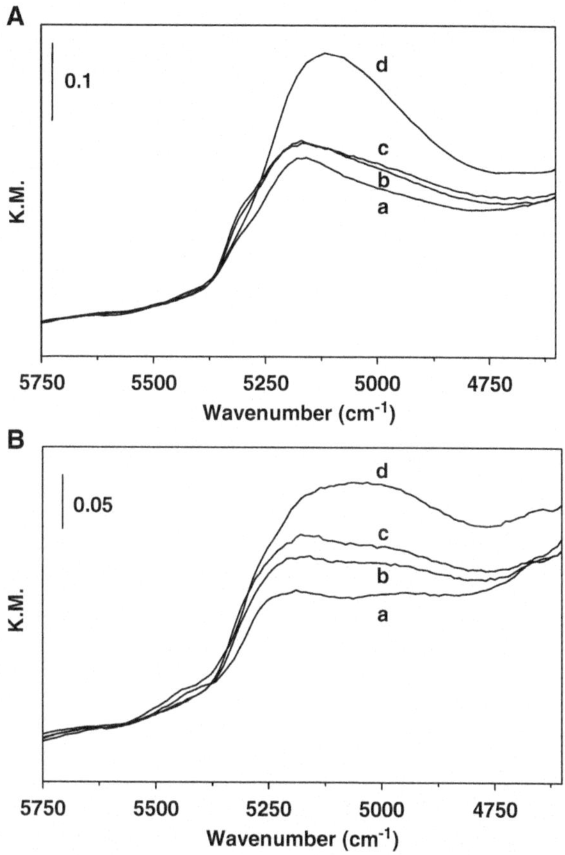

Fig. 8.18 NIR spectra in the 5,750–4,720 cm^{-1} range of nanocrystalline apatite (nap). Panel **A**: samples in contact with water vapor: line a- nap at 1 day maturation; line b- nap-1d with 0.9 % Mg on the surface obtained by ionic exchange; line c- nap-1d with 1.3 % Mg; line d- nap-1d with 3.0 % Mg (d). Panel **B**: samples after outgassing at room temperature for 1 h (Reprinted from Ref. [69]. Copyright 2009. American Chemical Society)

The $\delta + \nu_{asym}$ H_2O band for water adsorbed on nanocrystalline apatite [69] (Fig. 8.18A, line a) was found to be multicomponent in nature, with a main absorption around 5,170 cm^{-1}, attributed to H_2O molecules acting as donors of two equivalent H bonds, and two shoulders at about 5,300 (narrow) and 5,000 (broad) cm^{-1} attributed to the OH moieties (non H-bonded and H-bonded, respectively) of water molecules acting as donors of a single H bond [68, 69, 71]. The presence of water molecules in direct contact with the crystal's surface, as well as water overlayers, was assumed. The introduction of Mg^{2+} ions by way of Ca^{2+}/Mg^{2+} surface exchanges in solution was found to result in an increased overall intensity in the $\delta + \nu_{asym}$ H_2O band (Fig. 8.18A, lines b and c), unveiling additional water adsorption capabilities for Mg-enriched samples. NIR spectroscopy thus suggested that apatite samples enriched with Mg^{2+} retained more water at their surface than Mg-free counterparts. Although the increase in the amount of adsorbed water did not appear to be strictly proportional to the Mg^{2+} content, the ion distribution on the surface of the nanocrystals is bound to vary upon Mg enrichment, and these findings may be linkable to the greater interaction of Mg^{2+} ions with H_2O molecules as compared to Ca^{2+}.

The residual $\delta + \nu_{asym}$ pattern found after contact with water vapor and subsequent outgassing at room temperature (thus solely representative of "irreversibly" adsorbed water molecules) was also investigated [69]. The related NIR absorption profile then mostly exhibited two partially overlapped components at ca. 5,190 cm^{-1} and ca. 4,950 cm^{-1} (Fig. 8.18B, line a). In the case of samples enriched with Mg^{2+}, a broad component appeared in the range 5,150–5,000 cm^{-1}. In all these cases, the absence of high-frequency components suggested that both O–H groups from "irreversibly" adsorbed H_2O molecules were probably involved in hydrogen bonds.

Such NIR findings thus illustrate the coexistence of various types of adsorbed water on nanocrystalline apatites (as witnessed by changes in relative intensities and positions), and the nature of surface cations (e.g., Ca^{2+}, Mg^{2+}) was shown to have a direct effect on water adsorption capabilities. These modifications are, however, probably not limited to water molecules in direct contact with the surface (Fig. 8.18B) but could also involve water overlayers (Fig. 8.18A).

8.6.5 Pressure Effects and Residual Strains

Vibrational energy levels are sensitive to pressure exerted on crystals, and they offer an interesting ability to detect residual strains. Generally when a sufficiently high pressure (on the order of several GPa) is applied to a crystal, the FTIR or Raman lines are shifted to higher wavenumbers as shown in the case of fluorapatite $Ca_{10}(PO_4)_6F_2$ (Fig. 8.19) [71].

Shifts towards lower wavenumbers are also possible and have been reported for water molecules and for ions involved in strong hydrogen bondings [73]. The increase in pressure is also associated with line broadening and a loss of resolution. In several cases phase transitions under pressure have been reported. The observed shifts ($d\nu$) are proportional to the applied stress (dP), and the slopes ($d\nu/dP$) have been reported for some calcium phosphates (Table 8.8) [72–74]. The $d\nu/dP$ values depend on the vibrational mode and may vary considerably, as for monetite, for example, where the negative value reported for the 1,070 cm^{-1} line is attributed to strong hydrogen bonding involving the $HPO_4{}^{2-}$ ions. Very similar values are observed for the ν_1 lines of apatite samples. When pressure initiates a phase transition, $d\nu/dP$ variations generally show a discontinuity.

There are only a few studies involving solid solutions such as carbonated apatites [75, 76]. In their study of type B carbonate apatite and bone mineral, de Carmejane et al. [75] showed that $d\nu/dP$ was much higher for the ν_1 phosphate line than for the ν_1 carbonate line. They attributed this difference to the greater rigidity of carbonate ions compared to phosphate. In all cases the alterations of the spectra under isostatic pressure were found to be reversible and disappeared when the pressure was released.

Several authors have claimed that it was possible to determine residual strains in several cases, in coatings and in bone mineral, for example. In both cases, however,

Fig. 8.19 FTIR spectra of fluorapatite submitted to different pressures, showing the line shifts towards higher wavenumbers (Reprinted from Ref. [72]. Copyright 1996. With permission from Elsevier)

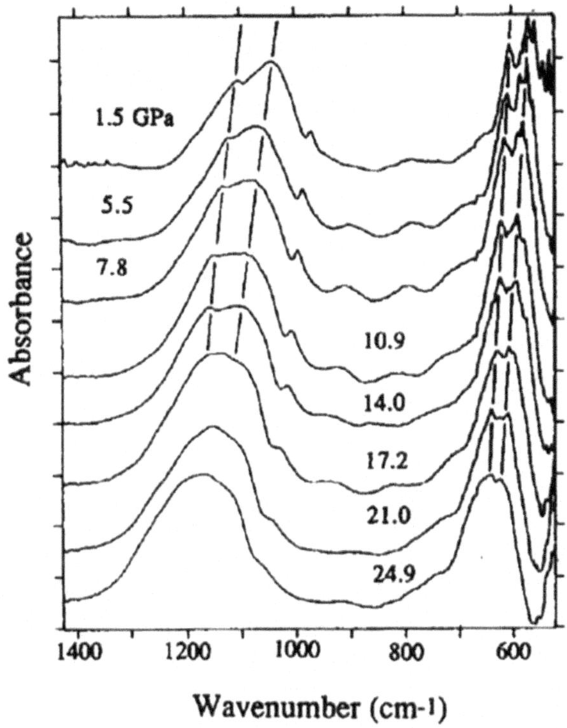

Table 8.8 Infrared line shifts as a function of the applied pressure: dν/dP (cm^{-1}.kbar^{-1}) for different representative lines of calcium phosphates in the ν_1, ν_3 domain, at room temperature

Compound	Line position without pressure (cm^{-1})	dν/dP Low-pressure phase	dν/dP High-pressure phase
$Ca_{10}(PO_4)_6F_2$	1,095 (ν_3)	0.56	–
fluorapatite (FA)	964 (ν_1)	0.42	–
$Ca_{10}(PO_4)_6(OH)_2$	1,089 (ν_3)	0.58	0.06
hydroxyapatite (HA)	1,033 (ν_3)	0.46	0.06
	963 (ν_1)	0.41	0.08
$CaHPO_4$ monetite	1,132 (ν_3)	0.26	
(DCPA)	1,070 (ν_3)	−0.11	
	996 (ν_1)	0.29	
$CaHPO_4$, $2H_2O$ brushite	1,141 (ν_3)	0.64	0.50
(DCPD)	1,066 (ν_3)	0.31	0.27
	998 (ν_1)	0.48	0.34

the line displacements observed could be due to the existence of solid solutions with different compositions. In the case of bone [77], the Raman spectra at a zone indented with a cylindrical indenter were analyzed using multivariate factor analysis. The data revealed that additional mineral factors appeared in the floor of the indent. These new factors were attributed to pressure alterations in the mineral phase. It should be noted that these alterations appeared at relatively low pressures (0.4–1.2 GPa) compatible with physiological loadings. The possibility of obtaining permanent alterations, though the effect of pressure was found to be reversible, has been related to the difference between an isostatic pressure, preventing ion and water displacement, and axial loading. The organic matrix was found to be affected near the indent edge. The new factor appearing there was assigned to a loss of the collagen triple helical structure resulting in a disordered state of the protein related to a rupture of cross-links. Similar observations have been published related to fatigue microdamage in bone [78].

8.6.6 Orientation of Crystals

The orientation of apatite crystals in biological tissues has often been studied by electron micro-diffraction. Although Raman and FTIR spectroscopies can also be used to determine crystal orientation, the spatial resolution of FTIR is too broad to analyze crystals with small sizes and can only give information on collections of crystals in textured domains. Micro-Raman spectroscopy offers a unique tool for assessing the orientation of crystals within rather small domains of a few μm^3, with some constrains due to the use of common optics on a single axis for both the excitation and the scattered beam [79]. Micro-Raman spectroscopy has been used for the determination of crystal orientations in tooth enamel and in bone. In enamel, comprised of well-crystallized apatites and exhibiting a well-resolved Raman spectrum, clear data can be obtained on specifically identified lines, and the apatite crystals have been found to be oriented with the c-axis of the hexagonal structure perpendicular to the tooth surface [25]. In bone the spectral resolution is lower and lines are superimposed. In addition, the orientation of crystals has to be compared to that of collagen fibers, which vary within an osteon and even a lamella. The data are presented mainly as variations in intensity ratios of chosen lines of the collagen matrix and the mineral [80]. An angular dependence of the spectra of the collagen matrix and bone mineral can be detected, indicating orientation correlations (Fig. 8.20). Using these correlations, variations in the orientation of crystals could be detected within an osteon lamellae using polarized Raman microscopy.

8.6.7 Maturity and Crystallinity of Bone Mineral

Bone mineral is a nanocrystalline apatite, and it evolves with age in a similar manner to synthetic biomimetic nanocrystalline apatites: the nanocrystals exhibit, just after their formation in early embryonic bone, a well developed hydrated

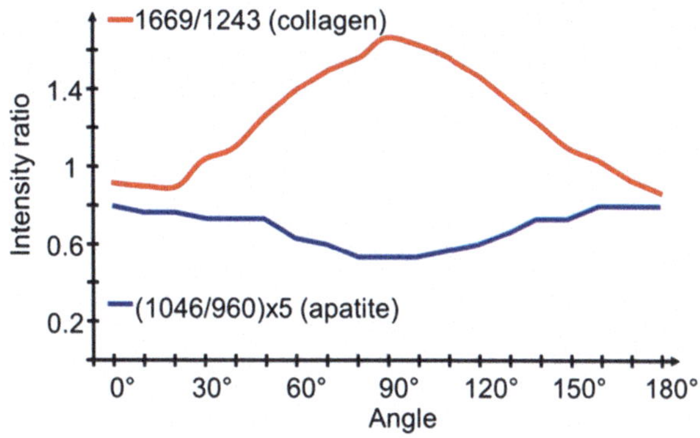

Fig. 8.20 Angular variations in the lines intensity ratios of bone Raman microspectra of an osteon lamella as a function of sample orientation with respect to the polarization of the incident beam. Collagen fibres: 1,669/1,243 cm^{-1}; apatite crystals: 1,046/960 cm^{-1} (Redraw from [80])

layer rich in HPO_4^{2-} and non-apatitic carbonate species [81]. Upon aging, this layer, which is thermodynamically less stable than apatite, is progressively replaced by stable apatite domains, and carbonate ions are progressively incorporated in the apatite domains. The precise characterization of bone mineral would then necessitate the determination of both the extension and the content of the hydrated layer and the apatite domain.

Maturation of bone mineral is related to its changes with age and is often associated with an improvement in the crystallinity of the apatite phase, first determined by X-ray diffraction [82]. Later spectroscopic methods using a specific ratio of phosphate bands were correlated to XRD determinations of apatite crystallinity [29, 31], and a certain confusion exists about the maturation and crystallinity of bone mineral. Maturity can be defined as the ratio between non-apatitic surface environments present in the hydrated layer of the bone crystals and apatite environments. Crystallinity is related to the size and strains of crystallized apatite domains and ignores the surface hydrated layer. Although in many cases these two parameters evolve concomitantly, this might not always be the case, as shown by the example of fluorotic bone [80], and a careful characterization of bone mineral should separate these two parameters. The crystallinity of the apatite domains can be determined by XRD; however, such determinations at a microscopic scale are difficult, and a crystallinity index can be obtained using the FTIR line broadening of the ν_4 apatite line at 600 cm^{-1}. A proposed maturity index is obtained by determining the ratio of the integrated intensity of a line at 1,030 cm^{-1} assigned to phosphate ions in the apatite domain, with that of a line at 1,110 cm^{-1} assigned to phosphate groups in non-apatitic domains [83]. The results on human bone compared to synthetic samples show a greater amount of non-apatitic environments in bone mineral and a poor correlation with the crystallinity index specifically related to the apatite domain as it is defined in this study. Although we are still far from complete knowledge of the content and proportion of apatitic and non-apatitic domains, this first approach confirms the importance of non-apatitic domains in bone mineral characteristics and their possible stabilization or renewal.

8.7 Conclusion

The use of vibrational spectroscopies for the characterization of calcium phosphates will continue to develop because of their several major advantages, including the possibility of reaching micrometric domains and the related imaging ability, the ease and rapidity of information recording, and their relatively low cost. One of the major advantages of these techniques is their ability to give very reproducible and accurate information on nanocrystalline calcium phosphates. Future developments will include analyses of line shapes and improvements in curve-fitting techniques in the case of solid solutions and ion interactions with the possibility, thanks to theoretical spectra predictions, of reaching inhomogeneities of ion distributions in the crystals. Other developments will include analyses of images and association with chemometric techniques. These techniques, which can easily be automated, will also permit unitary control of medical devices, each device being analyzed and provided with its own characteristics. The standards in use will have to take these developments into account and adaptations should follow. The techniques related to vibrational spectroscopies have evolved rapidly with ultrafast vibrational spectroscopy or multidimensional spectroscopy, opening new possibilities in material science and chemistry.

Acknowledgments We are grateful to Gérard Leroy for discussions regarding the content of this chapter, and we thank Imane Demnati, Solene Tadier, and Patricia Pascaud for allowing us to use the results of their Ph.D. thesis in Figs. 8.15, 8.16, and 8.17.

References

1. Bishop DM (1993) Group theory and chemistry. Dover Publications, New York
2. Ross SD (1972) Inorganic infrared and Raman spectra. McGraw-Hill, Maidenhead
3. Farmer VC (ed) (1974) The infrared spectra of minerals. Mineralogical Society, London
4. Santhyanarayana DN (2011) Vibrational spectroscopy. New Age International Publisher, New Delhi
5. Casciani F, Condrate RA Sr (1979) The vibrational spectra of brushite. $CaHPO_4$·$2H_2O$. Spectrosc Lett 12:699–713
6. White WB (1974) The carbonate minerals. In: Farmer VC (ed) The infrared spectra of minerals Mineralogical society monograph, 4th edn. Mineralogical Society, London
7. Elliott JC (1994) Structure and chemistry of the apatites and other calcium orthophosphates. Elsevier, Amsterdam
8. Bertoluzza A, Battaglia MA, Bonora S, Monyi P (1985) Hydrogen bonds in calcium acidic phosphates by infrared and Raman spectra. J Mol Struct 127:35–45
9. Trpkovska M, Soptrajanov B, Malkov P (1999) FTIR re-investigation of the spectra of synthetic brushite and its partially deuterated analogues. J Mol Struct 480–481:661–666
10. Posset U, Löcklin E, Thull R, Kiefer W (1998) Vibrational spectroscopic study of tetracalcium phosphate in pure polycrystalline form and as a constituent of a self-setting bone cement. Biomed Mater Res 40:640–645
11. Markovic M, Fowler BO, Tung MS (2004) Preparation and characterization of a comprehensive hydroxyapatite reference standard. J Res Natl Inst Stand Technol 109:553–568

12. Fowler BO, Moreno EC, Brown WE (1996) Infrared spectra of hydroxyapatite octacalcium phosphate and pyrolysed octacalcium phosphate. Arch Oral Biol 11:477–492
13. Jillavenkatesa A, Condrate RA Sr (1998) The infrared and Raman spectra of α- and β-tricalcium phosphate ($Ca_3(PO_4)_2$). Spectrosc Lett 31:1619–1634
14. Fowler BO, Markovic M, Brown WE (1993) Octacalcium phosphate. 3. Infrared and Raman vibrational spectra. Chem Mater 5:1417–1423
15. Ulian G, Valdre G, Corno M, Ugliengo P (2013) The vibrational features of hydroxylapatite and type A carbonated apatite: a first principle contribution. Am Miner 98:752–759
16. Treboux G, Layrolle P, Kanzaki N, Onuma K, Ito A (2000) Symmetry of Posner's cluster. J Am Chem Soc 122:8323–8324
17. Yin X, Stott J (2003) Biological calcium phosphates and Posner's cluster. J Chem Phys 118:3717–3723
18. Petrov I, Soptrajanov B, Fuson N, Lawson JR (1967) Infrared investigation of dicalcium phosphates. Spectrochim Acta 23A:2636–2646
19. Penel G, Leroy G, van Landuyt P, Flautre B, Hardouin P, Lemaitre J, Leroy G (1999) Raman microspectrometry studies of brushite cement: in vivo evolution in a sheep model. Bone 25(suppl 2):81S–84S
20. Penel G, Leroy G, Rey C, Bres E (1998) Micro-Raman spectral study of the PO_4 and CO_3 vibrational modes in synthetic and biological apatites. Calcif Tissue Int 63:475–481
21. Walters MA, Leung YC, Blumenthal NC, LeGeros RZ, Konsker KA (1990) A Raman and infrared spectroscopic investigation of biological hydroxyapatite. J Inorg Biochem 39:193–200
22. Penel G, Leroy G, Rey C, Sombret B, Huvenne JP, Bres E (1997) Infrared and Raman microspectrometry study of fluor- fluor-hydroxy- and hydroxy-apatites powders. J Mater Sci Mater Med 8:271–276
23. Trombe JC (1973) Decomposition et réactivité d'apatites hydroxylées et carbonatée. Ann Chim Paris 8:251–269
24. Fowler BO (1973) Infrared studies of apatites. I. Vibrational assignments for calcium, strontium and barium hydroxyapatites utilizing isotopic substitution. Inorg Chem 13:94–207
25. Tsuda H, Arends J (1994) Orientation micro-Raman spectroscopy on hydroxyapatite single crystals and human enamel crystallites. J Dent Res 73:1703–1710
26. Herzberg G (1968) Molecular spectra and molecular structure. II Infrared and Raman spectra of polyatomic molecules. D. Van Nostrand Company, London
27. Rey C, Collins B, Goehl T, Glimcher MJ (1989) The carbonate environment in bone mineral. A resolution enhanced Fourier transform infrared spectroscopy study. Calcif Tissue Int 45:157–164
28. Kaupinnen JK, Moffatt DJ, Mantsch HH, Cameron DG (1981) Fourier self-deconvolution: a method for resolving intrinsically overlapped bands. Appl Spectrosc 35:271–276
29. Pleshko N, Boskey A, Mendelsohn R (1991) Novel infrared spectroscopic method for the determination of crystallinity of hydroxyapatite minerals. Biophys J 60:786–793
30. Galadeta SJ, Paschalis EP, Betts F, Mendelsohn R, Boskey AL (1996) Fourier transform infrared spectroscopy of the solution mediated conversion of amorphous calcium phosphate to hydroxyapatite: new correlations between X-ray diffraction and infrared data. Calcif Tissue Int 58:9–16
31. Morris MD, Drumm CA (1995) Microscopic Raman line–imaging with principal component analysis. Appl Spectrosc 49:1331–1337
32. Bigi A, Boanini E, Capuccini C, Gazzano M (2007) Strontium-substituted hydroxyapatite nanocrystals. Inorg Chim Acta 360:1009–1016
33. Hadrich A, Lautié A, Mhiri T (2001) Vibrational study and fluorescence bands in the FT-Raman spectra of $Ca_{10-x}Pb_x(PO_4)_6(OH)_2$ compounds. Spectrochim Acta Part A 57:1673–1681
34. de Mul FFM, Otto C, Greve J, Arends J, ten Bosch JJ (1998) Calculation of the Raman line broadening on carbonation in synthetic hydroxyapatite. J Raman Spectrosc 19:13–21
35. He Q, Liu X, Hu X, Li S, Wang H (2011) Solid solution between lead fluorapatite and lead fluorvanadate apatite: mixing behavior, Raman feature and thermal expansivity. Phys Chem Miner 38:741–752

36. Trombe JC, Montel G (1973) Sur le spectre d'absorption infrarouge des apatites dont les tunnels contiennent des ions bivalents et des lacunes. CR Acad Sci Paris 276:1271–1274
37. Barroug A, Rey C, Trombe JC (1994) Precipitation and formation mechanism of type AB carbonate apatite analogous to dental enamel. Adv Mater Res 1–2:147–153
38. Fleet ME, Liu X (2007) Coupled substitution of type A and B carbonate in sodium bearing apatites. Biomaterials 28:916–926
39. Legeros RZ, LeGeros JP (1996) Carbonate apatite: formation and properties. Bioceramics 9:161–164
40. Quillard S, Paris M, Deniard P, Gildenhaar R, Berger G, Obadia L, Bouler JM (2011) Structural and spectroscopic characterization of a series of potassium and/or sodium-substituted β-tricalcium phosphate. Acta Biomater 7:1844–1852
41. Eichert D, Drouet C, Sfihi H, Rey C, Combes C (2007) Nanocrystalline apatite-based biomaterials: synthesis, processing and characterization. In: Kendal JB (ed) Biomaterials research advances. Nova Science, New York, pp 93–143
42. Jäger C, Welzel T, Meyer-Zaika W, Epple M (2006) A solid-state NMR investigation of the structure of nanocrystalline hydroxyapatite. Magn Reson Chem 44:573–580
43. Eichert D, Combes C, Drouet C, Rey C (2005) Formation and evolution of hydrated surface layers of apatites. Key Eng Mater 284–286:3–6
44. Brown WE, Mathew M, Chow LC (1984) Roles of octacalcium phosphate in surface chemistry of apatites. In: Misra DN (ed) Adsorption and surface chemistry of hydroxyapatite. Plenum Press, New York, pp 13–28
45. Rey C, Combes C, Drouet C, Sfihi H, Barroug A (2007) Physico-chemical properties of nanocrystalline apatites: implications for biomaterials and biominerals. Mater Sci Eng C 27:198–205
46. Leeuwenburgh SCG, Wolke JGC, de Jansen JA, Groot K (2008) Calcium phosphate coatings. In: Kokubo T (ed) Bioceramics and their clinical applications. Woodhead Publishing Limited, Cambridge, pp 464–484
47. Sun L, Berndt CC, Gross KA, Kucuk A (2001) Material fundamentals and clinical performance of plasma sprayed hydroxyapatite coatings: a review. J Biomed Mater Res 58:570–592
48. Gross KA, Berndt C, Herman H (1998) Amorphous phase formation in plasma-sprayed hydroxyapatite coatings. J Biomed Mater Res Part A 39:407–414
49. Carayon M, Lacout J-L (2003) Study of the Ca/P atomic ratio of the amorphous phase in plasma-sprayed hydroxyapatite coatings. J Solid State Chem 172:339–350
50. Demnati I, Grossin D, Combes C, Rey C (2013) Plasma sprayed apatite coatings: review of physical-chemical aspects and their biological consequences. J Med Biol Eng 34:1–7. doi:10.5405/jmbe.1459
51. Yan L, Leng Y, Weng L-T (2003) Characterization of chemical inhomogeneity in plasma-sprayed hydroxyapatite coatings. Biomaterials 24:2585–2592
52. Podlesak H, Pawlowski L, d'Haese R, Laureyns J, Lampke T, Bellayer S (2010) Advanced microstructural study of suspension plasma sprayed hydroxyapatite coatings. J Therm Spray Technol 19:657–664
53. Weinlaender M, Beumer J, Kenney EB, Moy PK (1992) Raman microprobe investigation of the calcium phosphate phases of three commercially available plasma-flame-sprayed hydroxyapatite-coated dental implants. J Mater Sci Mater Med 3:397–401
54. Demnati I, Parco M, Grossin D, Fagoaga I, Drouet C, Barykin G, Combes C, Braceras I, Goncalves S, Rey C (2012) Hydroxyapatite coating on titanium by a low energy plasma spraying mini-gun. Surf Coat Technol 206:2342–2353
55. Demnati I (2011) Développement et caractérisation de revêtements bioactifs d'apatite obtenus par projection plasma à basse énergie: application aux implants biomédicaux. PhD thesis, Institut National Polytechnique de Toulouse
56. Tadier S (2009) Etude des propriétés physico-chimiques et biologiques de ciments biomédicaux à base de carbonate de calcium: apport du procédé de co-broyage. PhD thesis, Institut National Polytechnique de Toulouse

57. Tadier S, Le Bolay N, Rey C, Combes C (2011) Co-grinding significance for calcium carbonate-calcium phosphate mixed cement. Part I: effect of particle size and mixing on solid phase reactivity. Acta Biomater 7:1817–1826
58. Cummings LJ, Snyder MA, Brisack K (2009) Protein chromatography on hydroxyapatite columns. Methods Enzymol 463:387–404
59. Tamerler C, Sarikaya M (2009) Molecular biomimetics: nanotechnology and bionanotechnology using genetically engineered peptides. Philos Trans A Math Phys Eng Sci 367:1705–1726
60. Goldberg HA, Warner KJ, Hunter GK (2001) Binding of bone sialo-protein osteopontin and synthetic polypeptides to hydroxyapatite. Connect. Tissue Res 42:25–37
61. Al-Kattan A, Errassifi F, Sautereau AM, Sarda S, Dufour P, Barroug A, Dos Santos I, Combes C, Grossin D, Rey C, Drouet C (2010) Medical potentialities of biomimetic apatites through adsorption, ionic substitution, and mineral/organic associations: three illustrative examples. Adv Eng Mater 12:B224–B233
62. Juillard A, Falgayrac G, Cortet B, Vieillard MH, Azaroual N, Hornez JC, Penel G (2010) Molecular interactions between zoledronic acid and bone: an in vitro Raman microspectroscopic study. Bone 47:895–904
63. Cukrowski I, Popovic L, Barnard W, Paul SO, van Roovyen PH, Liles DC (2007) Modeling and spectroscopic studies of bisphosphonates-bone interactions. The Raman, NMR and crystallographic investigations of Ca-HEDP complexes. Bone 41:668–678
64. Xie HN, Stevenson R, Stone N, Hernandez-Santana A, Faulds K, Graham D (2012) Tracking bisphosphonates through a 20 mm thick porcine tissue by using surface-enhanced spatially offset Raman spectroscopy. Angew Chem Int Ed Engl 51:8509–8511
65. Rodan GA, Fleisch HA (1996) Bisphosphonates: mechanisms of action. J Clin Invest 97:2692–2696
66. Pascaud P, Gras P, Coppel Y, Rey C, Sarda S (2013) Interaction between a bisphosphonate, tiludronate, and biomimetic nanocrystalline apatites. Langmuir 29:2224–2232
67. Pascaud P (2012) Apatite nanocrystallines biomimétiques comme modèles de la réactivité osseuse: étude des propriétés d'adsorption et de l'activité cellulaire d'un bisphosphonate, le tiludronate. Thesis INPT, University of Toulouse
68. Burneau A, Barres O, Gallas JP, Lavalley JC (1990) Comparative study of the surface hydroxyl groups of fumed and precipitated silicas. 2 Characterization by infrared spectroscopy of the interactions with water. Langmuir 6:1364–1372
69. Bertinetti L, Drouet C, Combes C, Rey C, Tampieri A, Coluccia S, Martra G (2009) Surface characteristics of nanocrystalline apatites: effect of Mg surface enrichment on morphology, surface hydration species, and cationic environments. Langmuir 25:5647–5654
70. Takeuchi M, Bertinetti L, Martra G, Coluccia S, Anpo M (2009) States of H_2O adsorbed on oxides: an investigation by near and mid infrared spectroscopy. Appl Catal A Gen 307:13–20
71. Ishikawa T, Wakamura M, Kondo S (1989) Surface characterization of calcium hydroxylapatite by Fourier transform infrared spectroscopy. Langmuir 5:140–144
72. Williams Q, Kettle E (1996) Infrared and Raman spectra of $Ca_5(PO_4)_6F_2$-fluorapatite at high pressures: compression-induced changes in phosphate site and Davydov splitting. J Phys Chem Solids 57:417–422
73. Xu J, Butler IS, Gilson DFR (1999) FT-Raman and high-pressure infrared spectroscopic studies of dicalcium phosphate dihydrate ($CaHPO_4$:$2H_2O$) and anhydrous dicalcium phosphate (CaHPO4). Spectrochem Acta Part A 55:2801–2809
74. Xu J, Gilson DFR, Butler IS, Stangel I (1996) Effect of high external pressures on the vibrational spectra of biomedical material: calcium hydroxyapatite and calcium fluorapatite. J Biomed Mater Res 30:239–244
75. de Carmejane O, Morris MD, Davis MK, Stixrude L, Tecklenburg M, Rajachar RM, Kohn DH (2005) Bone chemical structure response to mechanical stress studied by high pressure Raman spectroscopy. Calcif Tissue Int 76:207–213
76. Fleet ME, Liu X, Liu X (2011) Orientation of channel carbonate ions in apatite: effect of pressure and composition. Am Miner 96:1148–1157

77. Carden A, Rajachar RM, Morris MD, Kohn DH (2003) Ultrastructural changes accompanying the mechanical deformation of bone tissue: a Raman imaging study. Calcif Tissue Int 72:166–175
78. Timlin JA, Carden A, Morris MD (2000) Raman spectroscopic imaging markers for fatigue-related microdamage in bovine bone. Anal Chem 72:2229–2236
79. Tsuda H, Arends J (1997) Raman spectroscopy in dental Research: a short review of recent studies. Adv Dent Res 11:539–547
80. Falgayrac G, Facq S, Leroy G, Cortet B, Penel G (2010) New method for Raman investigation of the orientation of collagen fibrils and crystallites in the Haversian system of bone. Appl Spectrosc 64:775–780
81. Rey C, Combes C, Drouet C, Glimcher MJ (2009) Bone mineral: update on chemical composition and structure. Osteoporos Int 20:1013–1021
82. Bonar LC, Roufosse AH, Sabine WK, Grynpas MD, Glimcher MJ (1983) X-ray diffraction studies of the crystallinity of bone mineral in newly synthesized and density fractionated bone. Calcif Tissue Int 35:202–209
83. Farlay D, Panczer G, Rey C, Delmas PD, Boivin G (2010) Mineral maturity and crystallinity index are distinct characteristics of bone mineral. J Bone Miner Metab 28:433–445

Chapter 9
A Review of Hydroxyapatite Coatings Manufactured by Thermal Spray

C.C. Berndt, Md. Fahad Hasan, U. Tietz, and K.-P. Schmitz

Abstract Modification of orthopaedic prostheses by the incorporation of a biocompatible coating is attractive due to the attributes that arise from the biomaterial design of the interface. Hydroxyapatite (HA) is a favoured ceramic that has served functionalities such as enhancing fixation and stabilisation of the implant. The HA can be termed as "intelligent" because it responses to the physiochemical environment and adapts itself accordingly. There has been a great deal of clinical case histories and scientific discovery that have elucidated the mechanisms that enable HA coatings to perform successfully. However, there is a major link missing in this fundamental research, i.e. establishing a relationship between the processing parameters by which a coating is manufactured and the corresponding performance. Thus, the current work addresses this major issue by looking at the design criteria for HA biomaterial coatings. The prime issues that are addressed include (1) the relationship of the thermal spray devices and the manufacturing parameters to the so-formed phase structure, (2) limitations of thermal spray methods in achieving an appropriate HA coating that may exhibit specific functionalities, (3) the creation of specific phases via thermal spray methods and the importance of positioning these

C.C. Berndt (✉)
Industrial Research Institute Swinburne (IRIS), Swinburne University of Technology, Internal Main H66, PO Box 218, Hawthorn, VIC 3122, Australia

Department of Materials Science and Engineering, Stony Brook University, Stony Brook 11794, NY, USA
e-mail: cberndt@swin.edu.au

Md.F. Hasan • U. Tietz
Industrial Research Institute Swinburne (IRIS), Swinburne University of Technology, Internal Main H66, PO Box 218, Hawthorn, VIC 3122, Australia
e-mail: mdfahadhasan@swin.edu.au; ulrike.tietz@stryker.com

K.-P. Schmitz
Institute for Biomedical Engineering, University of Medicine, University of Rostock, Friedrich-Barnewitz-Str.4, D-18119 Rostock, Germany
e-mail: Klaus-Peter.Schmitz@uni-rostock.de

B. Ben-Nissan (ed.), *Advances in Calcium Phosphate Biomaterials*, Springer Series in Biomaterials Science and Engineering 2, DOI 10.1007/978-3-642-53980-0_9,

phases at specified locations within the coating, and (4) the nature of porosity that is created by a thermal spray method and how manufacturing parameters influence this microstructural characteristic.

Keywords Thermal spray coating • Hydroxyapatite • Materials considerations • Microstructural design • Manufacturing parameters • Review

9.1 Introduction

9.1.1 *Biomaterials*

Biomaterials are critical components to replace a part or a function of the body in a safe, reliable, economic, and physiologically acceptable manner. The goal of using biomaterials is to improve human health by restoring the function of natural living tissues and organs in the body. Therefore, it is necessary to understand the properties, functions, and structures of biological materials. The success of a biomaterial used in an implant depends on the properties and biocompatibility of the implant, the health condition of the recipient and the competency of the surgeon who monitors its progress.

Biomaterials are a worldwide multi-billion-dollar industry that is increasing every day. Biomaterials have helped to improve, support, and sustain the lives of over 20 million patients over the last decade, and this number increases by 10 % per year. The market for organ replacement and prostheses exceeds $300 billion US dollars per year and represents between 7 and 8 % of total worldwide healthcare spending. In the USA, the cost of therapies enabled by organ replacement technology exceeds 1 % of the gross national product [1]. These large expenses highlight the importance of biomaterial development. As a consequence, research in this area is essential to improve materials and reduce costs.

This area of materials science is shaped by medical needs, materials characterisation and design; basic research; advanced technological development; patient expectation; ethical considerations; industrial involvement, and federal regulation [2]. Such multidisciplinary research requires expertise and techniques used in a wide variety of subjects such as materials science, chemistry, molecular and cell biology, mathematics, engineering, biomechanics, computer modelling, manufacturing, medicine, and genetics.

9.1.2 *Hydroxyapatite*

The applications of biomaterials are expanded daily. Metallic devices for orthopaedic applications have been successful with many thousands implanted annually to stabilise fractures. Metallic biomaterials have an increasing demand for joint replacements since they possess the mechanical strength required to withstand the high loads imposed in uniaxial directions on load-bearing joints. Many metals and alloys have been used, which differ slightly in properties and biological response. Disadvantages in selecting metals include harmful ion release [3] and a lower quality of biological response compared with other materials. Thus, to provide protection and enhance the healing process, biocompatible coatings have been applied onto metals. Hydroxyapatite is well accepted as a bioactive and biocompatible coating closely resembling the mineral phase in bone and able to form a strong implant–bone interfacial bond to improve prosthesis fixation [4, 5].

A prime goal in modern orthopaedics and bioengineering is to improve the fixation time and longevity of implant anchorage in the human body. The introduction of hydroxyapatite is a scientific milestone in achieving these favourable outcomes because it enhances the on-growth of natural bone due to an identical chemical structure. Used as coatings, cement, and scaffolds; hydroxyapatite has proved its bioactivity in many studies. A faster on-growth of bone matrix onto the implant enables an accelerated load transmission between both components and, therefore, an earlier mobilisation of the patient. Furthermore, good integration of the implant with natural bone benefits the long-term performance, including less pain and greater time intervals between revision operations.

Nevertheless, some aspects of hydroxyapatite as a coating material are not fully understood. Especially the in vivo long-term behaviour of the material, including the time-dependent dissolution accompanied by changes of mechanical properties, needs further investigation. Many studies have examined the influence of several hydroxyapatite parameters on its structural and mechanical properties as well as on its bioactivity.

This chapter summarises the state of the art with regard to the thermal spray processing of hydroxyapatite materials to enable a foundation for focused studies. Developments in this area have correlated in vitro studies to in vivo performance, and this work is summarised from the perspective of investigating the influences on hydroxyapatite coating behaviour. The specific objective of this extended work is to design microstructures of hydroxyapatite coatings with better long-term stability for coated orthopaedic and dental implants.

Several methods and techniques have been introduced to coat hydroxyapatite on metal. The list includes immersion coating, dip coating followed by sintering, ion-beam sputter coating, flame spraying, plasma spraying, high-velocity oxy-fuel spraying, electrophoretic deposition, solution deposition, sol-gel, and laser surface engineering [6–8]. Among all of these methods, plasma spray is the most commonly used method for the application of hydroxyapatite coatings that has also received approval from the US FDA (Food and Drug Administration).

9.2 Literature Review

9.2.1 *Hydroxyapatite*

Hydroxyapatite (HA)[1] is a hydrated calcium phosphate mineral. In 1788, Proust and Klaprota recognised the similarity between calcium phosphate bioceramics and the mineral component of the bone [9]. The development of many commercial and non-commercial calcium phosphate materials, including ceramic HA, β-TCP, coralline HA, and biphasic calcium phosphates, was based on this similarity. In 1920, Albee successfully repaired a bony defect with a calcium phosphate reagent, depicted as a triple calcium phosphate compound [10].

The production of ceramic materials for use in dental and medical applications was developed by Levitt and Monroe in the late 1960s and early 1970s [11]. The research continued in the mid-1970s by researchers in the USA, Europe, and Japan where they worked simultaneously but independently on the development and commercialisation of hydroxyapatite [11].

Calcium phosphate ceramics have been used for dental implants, orthopaedics, maxillofacial surgery, periodontal treatment, alveolar ridge augmentation, and otolaryngology for about 30 years [12]. They are employed as a coating material that must be applied onto a tougher substrate due to their inherent brittleness under load-bearing applications. HA coatings are used commercially for hip and knee replacements [13].

9.2.1.1 Structure and Phase Diagram

Werner [9] was the first scientist who named hydroxyapatite as a mineral in 1786. The name was derived from the Greek word "to deceive" [9]. The chemical formula of HA is $Ca_{10}(PO_4)_6(OH)_2$, and it has a Ca/P ratio of 1.67. It is important to keep the ratio of 1.67 in mind since this is a clear marker for the presence of HA.

HA is the most abundant naturally occurring phosphate on earth. Sometimes it can also be referred to as hydroxylapatite [14, 15], calcium hydroxyapatite, or apatite. HA has a composition and chemical formula that is identical to that of bone. It is a brittle ceramic with a calculated density of 3.22 g/cm^3. Synthetic HA is considered to be a stoichiometric material, whereas biological apatites are generally considered as non-stoichiometric due to vacancies or substitutions that may occur within the structural lattice.

HA is monoclinic with lattice parameters of $a = 9.4214$ A, $b = 2a$, $c = 6.8814$ A, $\gamma = 120°$ and a lattice volume of 528.8 A^3. Figure 9.1 represents the crystal structure that is commonly attributed to HA. The unit cell contains Ca, PO_4, and OH ions

[1] The accepted convention for the abbreviation is either "HA", "HAp" or occasionally "Hap".

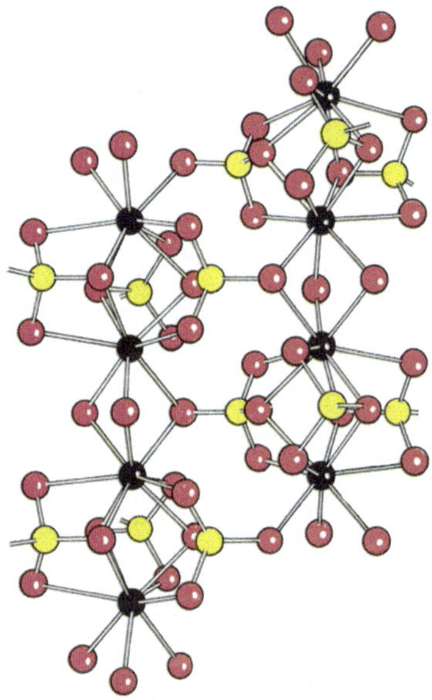

Fig. 9.1 Fluorapatite crystal structure [16]. Note that the only difference between the fluorapatite and HA cells is that the HA unit cell is slightly larger. *Black* = calcium, *Yellow* = phosphorous, *Pink* = oxygen

Table 9.1 Chemical composition of hydroxyapatite (Ravaglioli and Krajewik [20]; Lacout [21]

Symbol	Chemical formula	Chemical definition	Ca/P
MCP	$Ca(H_2PO_4)_2$	Monocalcium phosphate hydrate	0.5
DCPA	$CaHPO_4$	Dicalcium phosphate anhydrous	1.00
DCPD	$CaHPO.2H_2O$	Dicalcium phosphate dihydrate	1.00
OCP	$Ca_8H_2(PO4)_6.5H_2O$	Octacalcium phosphate	1.33
α-TCP	α-$Ca_3(PO_4)_2$	α-Tricalcium phosphate	1.5
β-TCP	β-$Ca_3(PO_4)_2$	β-Tricalcium phosphate	1.50
TTCP	$Ca_4(PO_4)_2O$	Tetracalcium phosphate	2.00
OHA	$Ca_{10}(PO_4)_6(OH)_{2-2x}O_x$	Oxyhydroxyapatite	1.67
OA	$Ca_{10}(PO_4)_6O$	Oxyapatite	1.67
HA	$Ca_{10}(PO_4)_6(OH)_2$	Hydroxyapatite	1.67

closely packed to represent the apatite structure. The *c*-axis is perpendicular to three equivalent *a*-axes at an angle of 120°.

HA, like all apatites, has a hexagonal system with space group $P6_3/m$ [11, 17]. The acceptance of a hexagonal $P6_3$ structure provides a poor least squares fit to XRD data. Therefore, two monoclinic models have been suggested: P21/b [18] and P21 [19]. Their chemical composition and Ca/P ratios are summarised in Table 9.1.

Figure 9.2a shows the phase diagram of HA with no water present and (b) at a partial water pressure of 500 mmHg. Figure 9.2a indicates that HA can decompose into other calcium phosphates such as tetracalcium phosphate (TTCP), tricalcium phosphate (TCP), monetite (C_2P), and mixtures of calcium oxide (CaO) and C_4P. Figure 9.2b shows that HA is stable up to 1,550 °C. The two renditions of the phase

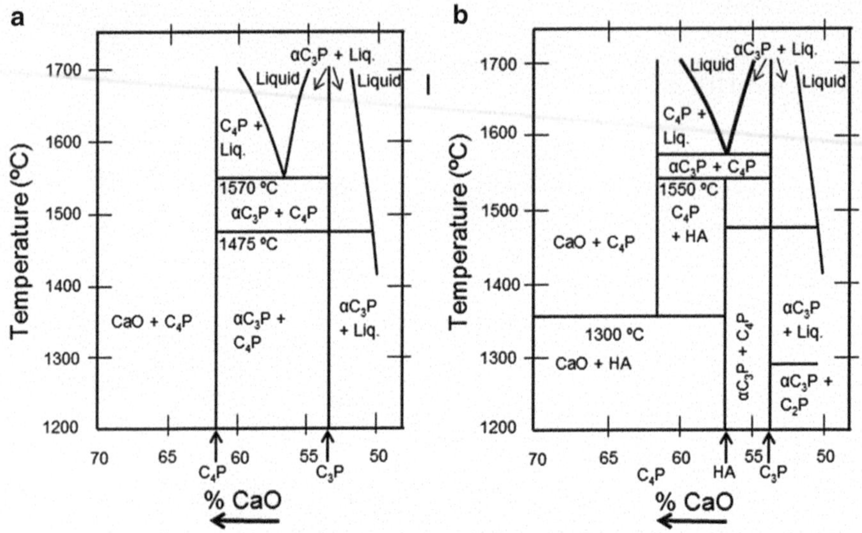

Fig. 9.2 (**a**) Phase diagram of the system CaO–P_2O_5 at high temperature. No water present. (**b**) Phase diagram of the system of Cao-P_2O_5 at high temperature and at a partial water pressure of 500 mmHg. (Note: There are many references to the hydroxyapatite phase diagram. The following references are examples where information can be accessed (White et al. [22]; Gross et al. [23]))

diagram indicate that the phase equilibrium of HA is influenced greatly by the partial pressure of water in the surrounding atmosphere. Fang et al. [24] reported the effect of stoichiometry on the thermal stability of HA from experiments where HA powder samples with Ca/P ratios remained within 1.52–1.68 when heated to 1,100 °C.

These potential changes in phase structure are of direct relevance since the DC plasma operates under high pressures at atmospheric conditions that comprise water vapour.

9.2.1.2 Comparison of Hydroxyapatite and Bone

HA, due to its apatite structure, contains structural sites that allow substitution of other ions. For example, if there is a deficiency in either calcium or carbonate species, then sodium (Na^+), magnesium (Mg^{2+}), acid phosphate (HPO_4), potassium (K^+), carbonate (CO_3^{2-}), fluoride (F^-), and chloride (Cl^-) ions may be substituted as minor elements. The trace elements of strontium (Sr^{2+}), barium (Ba^{2+}), and lead (Pb^{2+}) may also be observed. Synthetic HA and the main constituents of the bone are compared in Table 9.2.

There are different methods available to deposit calcium phosphate, and their mechanical properties vary accordingly. Likewise, HA powder differs in grain size and in composition because of different preparation methods for the HA scaffold materials. Small grain size provides greater fracture toughness. Table 9.3 shows a

Table 9.2 Comparison of bone and hydroxyapatite ceramics (Nicholson [25])

Constituents (wt.%)	Bone	HA[a]
Ca	24.5	39.6
P	11.5	18.5
Ca/P ratio	1.65	1.67
Na	0.7	Trace
K	0.03	Trace
Mg	0.55	Trace
CO_3^{2-}	5.8	–

[a]HA hydroxyapatite

Table 9.3 Mechanical properties of HA and bone (Lee [26]; Herschler et al. [27])

	Cortical bone	Cancellous bone	HA scaffolds
Compressive strength (MPa)	130–180	4–12	350–450
Tensile strength (MPa)	50–151	1–5	38–48
Young's modulus (GPa)	12–18	0.1–0.5	7–110

comparison of mechanical properties of cortical bone, cancellous bone, and HA scaffolds where large variations can be observed.

9.2.1.3 Dissolution Behaviour

Hydroxyapatite is very stable in physiological media. However, the dissolution rates of other phases formed due to the high temperature of the plasma spray process are more pronounced. The phases that appear in the HA coating are tricalcium phosphate ($Ca_3(PO_4)_2$, TCP, i.e. α-TCP and/or β-TCP), tetracalcium phosphate ($Ca_4P_2O_9$, i.e. TTCP), calcium oxide (CaO), oxyhydroxyapatite (OHA), and oxyapatite (OA). Hydroxyapatite may also exist as an amorphous phase, ACP. The dissolution order is as follows [11, 28]:

$$\mathrm{CaO > TCP > ACP > TTCP > OHA/OA > HA}$$

Among these phases, CaO is known to be biocompatible when incorporated into a silicate glass. However, it dissolves significantly faster than the other phases in the $CaO–P_2O_5$ phase diagram, and therefore, CaO is considered as a detrimental phase for orthopaedic applications. The dissolution of a HA coating increases with an increase in porosity and surface area and a decrease in particle size and crystallinity. Coatings sprayed at lower power (27.5 kW) demonstrated crystalline HA, whereas coatings sprayed at higher power (42 kW) exhibited amorphous phases [29].

The dissolution of unstable phases in the coating leads to an undesirable reduction of the mechanical strength in a coating. It should be kept in mind though that these dissolved phases have been shown to enhance bone tissue growth [30, 31] so that there is a compromise between dissolution rate and growth rate. Ducheyne et al. [30] compared the performance of three calcium phosphate coatings (polylactic acid/calcium-deficient HA, calcium-deficient HA, and oxyhydroxyapatite/α-TCP/β-TCP) with an uncoated implant in vivo. The calcium phosphate-coated implants were observed to permit a greater degree of bone growth than the uncoated implant.

9.2.1.4 Thermal Behaviour

Plasma-sprayed HA coatings are formed with a significantly different crystal structure, phase composition, and morphology than the original starting powder. This outcome arises because the plasma spray process involves melting of particles that causes thermal decomposition and changes the phase balance of the individual particles [32]. The changes occurring within the plasma flame need to be understood to ensure that the coating produced has the required composition.

The heating of HA leads to three processes. They are (1) evaporation of water, (2) dehydroxylation, and (3) decomposition. Hydroxyapatite has the property to absorb water that may be present on the surface of the powder and trapped within pores [33]. The absorbed water begins to evaporate when heated and is followed by water within the lattice structure [34]. The dehydroxylation reaction reported by several authors [34, 35] is as follows, where V represents a vacancy and $x < 1$:

$$\begin{aligned}&\mathrm{Ca_{10}(PO_4)_6(OH)_2 \rightarrow Ca_{10}(PO_4)_6(OH)_{2-2\mathit{x}}O_\mathit{x}V_\mathit{x} + \mathit{x}H_2O}\\&\text{Hydroxyapatite} \rightarrow \text{Oxyhydroxyapatite}\end{aligned} \tag{9.1}$$

$$\begin{aligned}&\mathrm{Ca_{10}(PO_4)_6(OH)_{2-2\mathit{x}}O_\mathit{x}V_\mathit{x} \rightarrow Ca_{10}(PO_4)_6O_\mathit{x}V_\mathit{x} + (1-\mathit{x})\,H_2O}\\&\text{Oxyhydroxyapatite} \rightarrow \text{Oxyapatite}\end{aligned} \tag{9.2}$$

The first step involves the formation of a hydroxyl ion-deficient product, known as oxyhydroxyapatite (OHA). OHA consists of a bivalent oxygen ion and a vacancy substitute for two monovalent OH^- ions of HA [34]. In the second step, dehydroxylation leads to the formation of oxyapatite. In the presence of water, oxyhydroxyapatite and oxyapatite can transform back to hydroxyapatite [28].

Hydroxyapatite decomposes into other phases at high temperature. HA retains its crystal structure up to a critical point, beyond which complete and irreversible decomposition occurs. During decomposition, HA converts into other calcium phosphate phases such as β-tricalcium phosphate (β-TCP) and tetracalcium phosphate (TTCP). Firstly, oxyapatite transforms into tricalcium phosphate and tetracalcium phosphate. In the next step, tricalcium phosphate and tetracalcium phosphate convert into calcium oxide [34, 36, 37]. The chemical equilibria can be described by means of the three following equations:

Table 9.4 Thermal effects of hydroxyapatite (Levingstone [38])

Temperature (°C)	Reaction(s)
25–200	Evaporation of absorbed water
200–600	Evaporation of lattice water
600–800	Decarbonation
800–900	Dehydroxylation of HA forming partially or completely dehydroxylated oxyhydroxyapatite
1,050–1,400	HA decomposes to form β-TCP and TTCP
<1,120	β-TCP is stable
1,120–1,470	β-TCP is converted to α-TCP
1,550	Melting temperature of HA
1,630	Melting temperature of TTCP, leaving behind CaO
1,730	Melting of TCP

$$\begin{aligned} &Ca_{10}(PO_4)_6O_xV_x \rightarrow 2Ca_3(PO_4)_2\,(\beta) + Ca_4(PO_4)_2O \\ &\text{Oxyapatite} \rightarrow \text{Tricalcium phosphate} + \text{Tetracalcium phosphate} \end{aligned} \tag{9.3}$$

$$\begin{aligned} &Ca_3(PO_4)_2 \rightarrow 3CaO + P_2O_5 \\ &\text{Tricalcium phosphate} \rightarrow \text{Calcium oxide} + \text{Phosphorus pentoxide} \end{aligned} \tag{9.4}$$

$$\begin{aligned} &Ca_4(PO_4)_2O \rightarrow 4CaO + P_2O_5 \\ &\text{Tetracalcium phosphate} \rightarrow \text{Calcium oxide} + \text{Phosphorus pentoxide} \end{aligned} \tag{9.5}$$

It is difficult to predict the exact temperatures for these reactions because they occur over a wide temperature range that depends on factors related to the environment and the HA composition. Table 9.4 lists the reactions that occur as HA is heated from room temperature to 1,730 °C, keeping in mind that these have not been validated under the extreme environments of a DC plasma process.

9.2.2 *Hydroxyapatite Powder*

HA feedstock is the foundation for each thermal spray process. The ASTM standard F 1609 [39], which is comparable with other standards from FDA or ISO, provides limitations for feedstock concerning crystallinity, particle form, and in vivo and in vitro behaviour. Therefore, several common parameters for the feedstock have become accepted. Usually, a fully crystalline pure HA powder is the basis, which is generally manufactured by using phosphate-containing and calcium ion-containing ingredients. After mixing both components, calcination leads to the HA feedstock [40].

The ASTM Standard Specification (ASTM designation: F1185-88 [41]) states that surgical implants require a minimum of 95 % of HA content, established by a quantitative X-ray diffraction (XRD) analysis, while the concentration of trace elements should be limited, e.g. arsenic 3 ppm, cadmium 5 ppm, mercury 5 ppm, and lead 30 ppm. The HA phase is required by the International Standards Institute (ISO 13778-1: 2000, Implants for surgery, Hydroxyapatite – Part 1: Ceramic hydroxyapatite) [42] to exhibit a crystallinity of at least 45 %. The maximum allowable total limit of all heavy metals is 50 ppm. The Ca/P ratio for HA used for surgical implants must be between 1.65 and 1.82 [41].

The quality of coatings depends on the shape of HA powders for plasma spray deposition. The particles are melted or partly melted in the plasma flame; thus, the morphology of the powder particles relates directly to the heating rate. Irregularly shaped particles exhibit a higher degree of particle heating within the plasma flame due to their greater surface area to volume ratio than spherical particles [43]. Spherical particles have better flow properties than angular particles and can be more reliably transported to the plasma flame.

Powder with a narrow range of particle sizes will result in a more consistent coating. The particles must also be capable of withstanding the spray environment. For example, Cheang and Khor [44] observed that weakly agglomerated HA powders fragment within the plasma stream giving a new distribution of smaller particles that influences the coating microstructure.

9.3 Human Bone

Since the main intention of HA implant coatings is to support the growth of human bone tissue on the implant surface, it is necessary to understand the structure of this tissue and its modelling and remodelling behaviour. In this way, the intention is to design an artificial microstructure that mimics the performance criteria of natural bone.

In general, there are two types of bone tissue, the high and the low porous ones, called the compact and the trabecular bone [45]. With 75–95 % porosity [45], the trabecular bone (also called cancellous or spongy bone) is mostly found in the epiphysis, the ends of long bones [46]. There the matrix is formed of 200 μm thick [45] trabeculae. The trabeculae matrix formation directions follow the principal stress axes [47] within the bone that allows the transfer of high loads along these axes. Overall, the trabeculae of the cancellous bone form 80 % of the bone surface [48].

The high-density bone is found in the middle parts of long bones, the diaphysis, and in the outer parts of bones, where it forms the bone shell that is termed cortical bone. With 80–85 % of the skeletal bone mass, it provides protection and strength for the whole bone [48]. This compact matrix shows a porosity from 5 to 10 % [45, 49]. Within the pores of the matrix, there are tissue types that display different morphologies and character [47], the detail of which is considered out of scope for this current chapter.

Primary bone is located on the bone surface. A new bone structure will be arranged parallel to this shell structure and is termed as "lamellae". The bone matrix itself is continuously changing. Therefore, the primary structure will be replaced by the secondary bone. It is interesting to note that the substructure of the bone has a morphology of 200 μm in diameter and consists of approximately 16 layers [45] that are surrounded by a cement line. This dimensional feature is similar to the dimensions of a single HA splat that is formed via thermal spray processing.

9.3.1 The Composite Structure of Bone

Bone is composed of collagen, HA mineral, water, and particles of noncollagenous proteins and proteoglycans [45, 50]. In general, 30 % of the bone matrix is organic substance (collagen), and 70 % is inorganic (with water being ~25 % and HA ~45 %) [45, 51]. Collagen is a protein that exists in many organs and tissues in the human body. Due to its solubility and a constant blood flow in the bone matrix, other components such as fluoride and carbonate can add impurities to the HA bone substructure [45].

As seen in the investigation of Robinson and Elliott (1957) [52] on dog bones, which are comparable to human bones, most of the organic matrix is composed of collagen. Furthermore, it is interesting that over 50 % of the HA apatite minerals are found within the collagen fibres, which may be proof that collagen structures are fundamental for the mineralisation of the bone.

Modelling and remodelling – forming and resorbing of bone material – are permanent processes in bone tissue. Four different bone cells are responsible for this behaviour: osteoclasts, osteoblasts, osteocytes, and bone lining cells [49].

Osteoclasts are multinuclear, amoebic cells [45, 53], covering nearly one per cent of the bone surface [49]. These cells are in charge for the resorption of the bone matrix. The cells produce acids to demineralise the bone surface and, afterwards, dissolve the bone collagen with enzymes [45]. Using this process, osteoclasts can resorb bone to a depth of tens of micrometres per day [45].

Osteoblasts (Fig. 9.3) exist on the surface of bone-forming areas [53]. They are mononuclear, cuboidal cells [45] with an approximate diameter of 20 μm [53]. The main task of these cells is to produce collagen and other components of the organic bone matrix [45, 53]. This process takes place to an amount of ~1 μm per day, which is termed the bone apposition rate [45]. Studies have shown that osteoblasts are, as well, connected with the bone resorption process; that is, it has been suggested that osteoblasts control the activities of osteoclasts [53].

Some osteoblasts enclose themselves into the matrix during the bone modelling process. Approximately 10 % of them will transform into *osteocytes*, which are responsible for the long-term functionality of the bone matrix [49]. These cells are connected with each other and the bone surface via a wide-ranging net of channels, the canaliculi [45, 53]. These tunnels enable communication and the transport of minerals into the bone matrix [45], which enables the matrix internal mineralisation process.

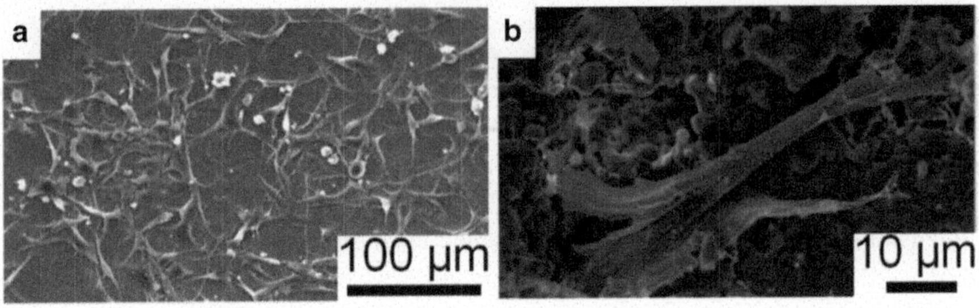

Fig. 9.3 Osteoblasts on implant surface (**a**) by Ball et al. [54] and (**b**) by Ng et al. [55] (Reprinted with permission. The copyright is held by the referenced sources)

9.3.2 *Bone Modelling and Remodelling*

There are two bone formation processes, i.e. the endochondral and the intramembranous modelling processes [56]. The specialised cells need an unmineralised tissue to mineralise bone matrix as a foundation. But when a bone grows, this interim, softer matrix needs to withstand loads that affect the bone. Therefore, cartilage, which is able to resist high compressive pressures, provides a base for the bone-mineralising cells [45]. Long bones grow along their length axis. Thus, two bone-growing zones are located near the ends of the bone [45]. Later, osteoclasts and osteoblasts will remodel the bone, and secondary bone matrix will be mineralised [56]. These processes are called the primary and the secondary ossification.

After modelling the primary bone matrix, permanent remodelling processes take place in the whole skeleton. The main purpose is to react to changes in stress [57] caused by different loads on the bone, e.g. generated by changes in daily activities or age- and disease-related alterations. Thereby, Wolff's law proclaims that less strain causes degradation of bone, whereas overstraining causes increased production of bone matrix in this area. Furthermore, remodelling enables the body to repair small damage of the bone matrix [57]. Therefore, at any time, approximately 20 % of the trabecular bone is situated within a remodelling process, and every bone surface region will be remodelled nearly every second year [45, 57].

The remodelling process takes place in separate regions at the bone surface matrix, depending on where it is necessary. Osteoclasts and osteoblasts work together in so-called basic multicellular units, BMUs, resorbing old and creating new tissue [45, 57]. Activation and movement of BMUs is a not a sufficiently investigated field. It is assumed that osteocytes can sense stresses in the bone matrix and, therefore, these cells transfer signals to the BMUs to activate remodelling of this part of the bone in accordance to the changed needs [57].

9.3.3 Mechanical Properties of Bone

Bone is a non-orthotropic material. Therefore, cortical and trabecular bone can be differentiated in terms of mechanical properties. The porosity of trabecular bone is much higher than that of compact bone, and thus, the density and Young's modulus are lesser in this tissue. Additionally, it is important to note the load direction during measurement of the mechanical properties of the bone. Since the bone matrix grows along the main stress axes, the bone properties change longitudinal or transverse to this direction as seen in Table 9.5.

As reflected in Table 9.5, the property differences between HA and collagen are significant due to the material properties. Bone is a composite of both materials, and thus, the bulk values of the bone lie between those of collagen and HA, depending on the degree of mineralisation. Finite element studies of Jäger and Fratzl [63] have indicated that the mineral concentration and the mineral arrangement influence the whole bone properties significantly.

9.4 Hydroxyapatite Coatings

9.4.1 Historical Development of the Natural Material

In 1979, the American Society of Testing and Materials (ASTM) enacted the ASTM standard C633-79 (now updated to C633-01), a standard test method for adhesion or cohesive strength of flame-sprayed coatings [64]. Although the thermal spray manufacturing process has been in use for over 90 years, their application to clinical implants began in the 1980s [40], for example, with the material and clinical research by Osborn (in 1985 and 1987) [65, 66]. Further studies, especially concerning sprayed HA coatings, such as by Mornachon (in 1985) [67] and De Groot (in 1987) [15], presented evidence of promising clinical implementation.

Naturally grown HA is located in many countries, e.g. Switzerland, Germany, Italy, and the USA [68]. The HA feedstock material is now produced synthetically for clinical applications to guarantee quality.

9.4.2 Manufacturing Processes

The manufacturing process of the coating greatly influences the coating properties since the microstructure will reflect the process. Therefore, good knowledge and understanding of this method is essential for analysing, developing, and upgrading HA coatings. Various methods, as mentioned in Sect. 9.1.2, have been developed

Table 9.5 Typical mechanical properties for human bone (Non-marked values after R.B. Martin et al. [45])[a]

ID	Property	Cortical bone	Cancellous bone	Average bone	Bone material HA	Bone material collagen
1	Young's modulus [GPa]	8–24 [50]	0.07–0.49	20 [58][b]	130 [50]	0.05 [58]
	Longitudinal	17.4 22.5 [59][c] 25.8 [59][d]				
	Transverse	9.6	13.4 [59]			
	Bending	14.8				
2	Shear modulus [GPa]	3.51				
3	Poisson's ratio	0.39		0.3 [60]		
4	Tensile yield stress [MPa]			100 [58][e]		20 [58][e]
	Longitudinal	115				
5	Tensile ultimate stress [MPa]					
	Longitudinal	133				
	Transverse	51				
6	Compressive yield stress					
	Longitudinal [MPa]	182				
	Transverse [MPa]	121				
7	Compressive ultimate stress					
	Longitudinal [MPa]	195				
	Transverse [MPa]	133				
8	Shear yield stress [MPa]	54				
9	Shear ultimate stress [MPa]	69				
10	Bending ultimate stress [MPa]	208.6				
11	Tensile ultimate strain [%]			0.03 [58][f]		35 [58][f]
	Longitudinal	0.0293				
	Transverse	0.0324				
12	Compressive ultimate strain					
	Longitudinal [%]	0.0220				
	Transverse [%]	0.0462				
13	Shear ultimate strain [%]	0.33				
	Hardness [MPa]	–				
	Longitudinal	611 [59][g] 736 [59][h]				
	Transverse		468 [59]			
14	Density [g/cm^3]	1.8–2.0 1.8 [62]	1.0–1.4	2.11 [61][i]	2.0 [45, 50]	1.0 [45, 50]

[a]Yield stress and strain mark the point of change between elastic and plastic forming. Ultimate stress and strain mark the point of maximum load
[b]0.45° of mineralisation
[c]Tibial osteons
[d]Tibia interstitial lamellae
[e]No note on kind of load on the bone. 0.45° of mineralisation
[f]No note on kind of load on the bone. 0.45° of mineralisation
[g]Tibial osteons
[h]Tibia interstitial lamellae
[i]Ca/P ratio: 1.67

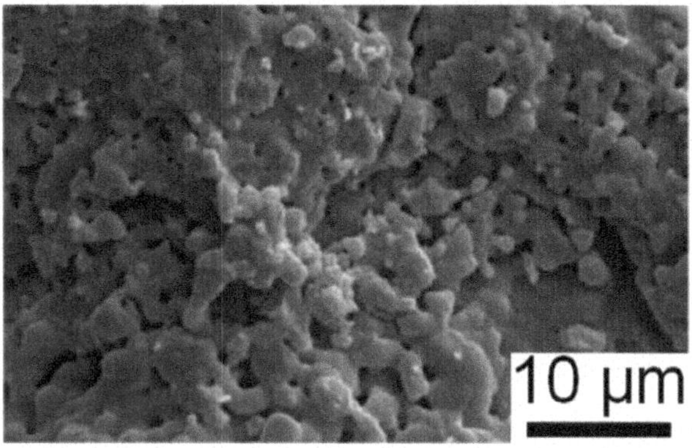

Fig. 9.4 Typical structure of a sprayed hydroxyapatite coating (Ng et al. [55]. Reprinted with permission. The copyright is held by the referenced source)

to deposit HA onto an implant surface, such as biomimetry [69, 70], dip coating [71], sol-gel methods [72–74], immersion coatings [6, 75], plasma sintering [76], ion beam-assisted deposition (IBAD) [77], electrophoretic deposition [8, 78–80], pulsed laser deposition [81], electrohydrodynamic spraying [82] and thermal spray techniques [83, 84] such as plasma [85], flame [86], and high-velocity oxygen fuel (HVOF) [87].

Many of these processes have disadvantages, which make the manufacturing inefficient or which do not fulfil mechanical and clinical expectations. Reasons for failure [40] include (1) the impurity of the HA coating, (2) poor bonding strength between the coating and implant, and (3) changes in structure and properties of the implant metal or the HA coating due to the processing heat.

Among these techniques, thermal spray, in particular plasma spray, has been approved by the FDA for the deposition of HA coatings [88]. The plasma spray method can prepare large-scale coatings that exhibit good adhesion to substrates of complex shape [40, 89]. Plasma spraying has the ability to produce specialised coatings with functional properties such as biocompatibility, fixation, corrosion, and wear resistance that is beneficial to the field of biomedical engineering [90–92]. The plasma spray method (1) offers good chemical and microstructural control, (2) can be used on difficult surfaces and implant shapes, (3) has demonstrated an ability to form coatings of variable thickness, and (4) exhibits good biocorrosion and substrate fatigue resistance [40]. Figure 9.4 depicts the typical surface of a HA coating deposited by a plasma spray method.

9.5 Thermal Spraying

Thermal spray employs high temperature and velocity to melt the powder or wire as a feedstock and deposit one material onto the surface of another. Thermal spray methods can be divided into two major classes: (1) chemical energy of the combustion gases that power the flame spray torch and (2) electric currents providing energy for plasma generators.

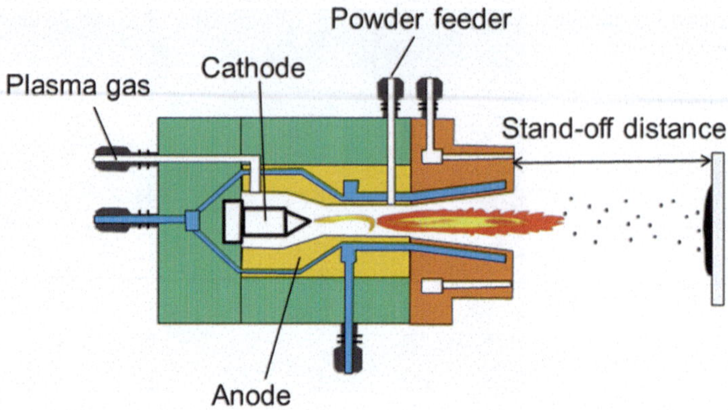

Fig. 9.5 Plasma spray system (CACT [94]. Reprinted with permission. The copyright is held by the referenced source)

9.5.1 Plasma Spray Operation

Plasma spray is regarded as the most versatile of all the thermal spray processes. The plasma spray process uses the latent heat of two ionised inert gases to create the heat source. The most common gases used to create the plasma are argon as the primary and hydrogen or helium as the secondary gases. However, the gas use depends on the type of material to be sprayed and intended application.

The plasma spray process is able to melt a large array of ceramic materials. The plasma spray system consists of an electronically controlled power supply, a PLC-based operator control station, a gas mass flow system, a closed-loop water chilling system, a powder feeder, and a plasma torch [93]. The plasma spray torch (Fig. 9.5) consists of a copper anode and a tungsten cathode, which are both cooled by water. Plasma gas (argon, nitrogen, hydrogen, helium) surrounds the cathode and exits the torch by passing through the anode nozzle. A high-voltage discharge between the cathode and anode ionises the plasma-forming gas so that a high heat source is created.

The plasma temperature may be nearly 10,000 °C, into which the feedstock of HA powder is injected. Any powders injected into the plasma flame will melt and subsequently be deposited onto the substrate to form a coating [95]. The particle velocities of plasma spraying are higher than flame and wire arc spraying, therefore producing more dense coatings and surfaces that demonstrate a more fine topography. Figure 9.5 shows a typical torch and plasma spray coating process.

The advantages of plasma spray have been widely recognised in many industries. The unique features that characterise plasma spray processing are that (1) it is simple and flexible, (2) coating parameters can be controlled by appropriate setting of parameters, (3) a uniform coating is produced, (4) an ability to melt many metals, ceramics, or composites, and (5) high deposition rates.

The feedstock powder particles are accelerated to a high velocity, heated up and, depending on their size, are totally or partly molten (Fig. 9.6). The spherical droplets

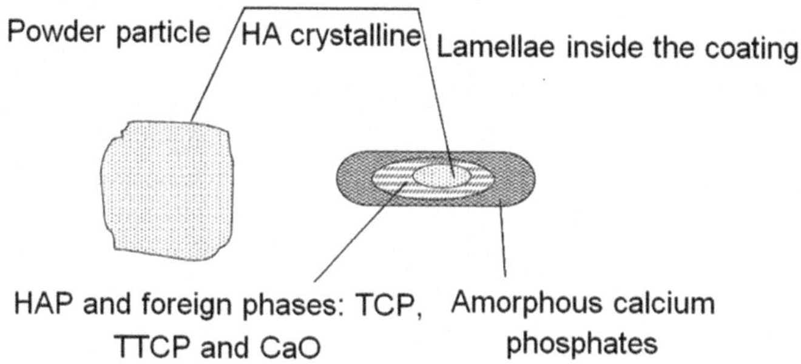

Fig. 9.6 Possible phase development in half melted hydroxyapatite powder particle (Deram et al. [96]. Reprinted with permission. The copyright is held by the referenced source)

Fig. 9.7 Typical hydroxyapatite splat on a metal surface with one large and several smaller pores (Li et al. [98]. Reprinted with permission. The copyright is held by the referenced source)

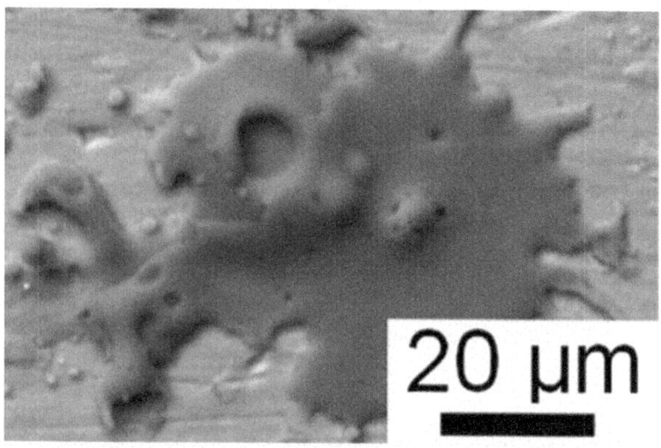

Fig. 9.8 Plasma spray coating of hydroxyapatite on TiAl6V4 (Narayanan et al. [99]. Reprinted with permission. The copyright is held by the referenced source)

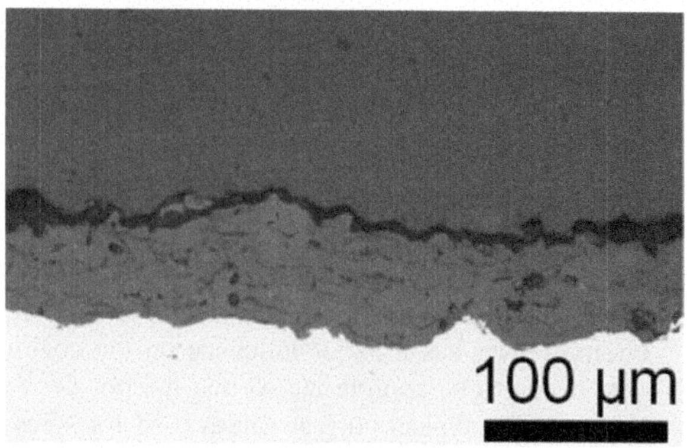

form disc-shaped splats [97] on impact against the implant surface (Fig. 9.7). The transit time, or residence time, between gun and implant surface is of the order of 2–6 ms, during which time the HA particles heat up and cool down to form HA phases within the coating (Fig. 9.8). Thermal spray parameters such as the feedstock characteristics and thermal spray parameters control the character and amount of the HA phases.

Table 9.6 Primary and secondary parameters for thermal spray processes [38]

Primary parameters	Secondary parameters
Powder particle morphology	Plasma flame temperature
Powder particle composition	Plasma flame velocity
Powder injection angle	Dwell time in plasma flame
Plasma-forming gas	Particle velocity
Plasma-forming gas flow rate	Particle melting
Current	Substrate temperature
Power	Particle quench rate
Carrier gas	Residual stress development
Carrier gas flow rate	Coating thickness
Standoff distance	
Substrate material	
Substrate surface properties	
Substrate preheating	
Traverse velocity	

Since the implant material is not heated during the process, plasma spraying is called a cold method, which has the advantage of avoiding metallurgical change or damage to the implant metal [100]. Furthermore, plasma spraying produces coatings with good density and strength and minimised contamination by other elements during the manufacturing process [100].

9.5.2 Plasma Spray Process Parameters

The properties of plasma spray coatings are affected by as many as 50 process parameters [101]. Some parameters can be controlled directly and are called primary parameters, whereas the secondary parameters are determined by the primary parameters (Table 9.6).

The desired, preferred coatings may be manufactured when the parameters that influence the coatings are fully understood. The main parameters of the plasma spray process are power, plasma-forming gas, carrier gas, powder feed rate, standoff distance, and torch traverse velocity.

Plasma power has a major influence on the coating. The power of the spray process needs to be appropriate so that the powder can melt adequately to form the coating. The typical current values used for spraying HA coatings are in the range of 350–1,000 A and are equivalent to 15–60 kW.

Cizek et al. [102] and Guessasma et al. [103] studied the effect of power on the temperature of the plasma flame velocity of the particle. They reported that a high current or power level caused an increase in particle temperature and velocity. Cizek et al. [102] found that high power levels result in an increased flame temperature that gives rise to a greater degree of particle melting. Increasing the power level also increased the velocity of the plasma flame.

A net power increase of 10 kW was observed to cause an increase of 80 °C in particle temperature and an increase of 60 ms^{-1} in particle velocity. Increased power lead to a decrease in the purity and crystallinity of HA coatings as demonstrated by Tsui et al. [104] and Sun et al. [105]. The findings of Yang et al. [106] contradicted these findings [104, 105] with crystallinity increasing with increasing current. Tsui et al. [104] reported that the porosity level and extent of microcracking decreased with an increase in power. Quek et al. [107] demonstrated that dense, less porous coatings evolved when high currents were employed.

The plasma-forming gas has a major role on the coating properties. There are four main gases used in the plasma spray process: argon, helium, hydrogen, and nitrogen. The choice of the plasma gas depends on many factors, such as the design features of the torch, in particular the electrode materials [108]. However, argon is used as the primary gas because it is relatively inexpensive, is easily ionised, and exhibits inert properties [43]. Argon demonstrates a velocity from 600 to 2,200 ms^{-1} as reported by Fauchais et al. [109]. Helium, an expensive gas, is used in special cases because it produces a high-temperature plasma flame of high enthalpy. Nitrogen and hydrogen are diatomic gases that give rise to a plasma jet with higher thermal conductivity than monatomic argon, and this helps heat transfer to the feedstock particles. Leung et al. [110] reported that the size and shape of the jet and the momentum that the carrier gas imparts on the powder particles vary with regard to the gases used.

Plasma gas flow rate and power to the plasma torch must be properly balanced or optimised to achieve a stable plasma flame. Gas flow rate has a direct effect on particle velocity, since increasing the gas flow rate during spraying leads to an increase in particle velocity [103]. Guessasma et al. [103] also demonstrated that increasing the gas flow rate from 30 to 50 standard litres per minute (SLPM) resulted in an increase in the average particle velocity from 186 to 269 ms^{-1} and also a slight increase in particle temperature from $2{,}516 \pm 131$ °C to $2{,}526 \pm 203$ °C.

The carrier gas transports the powder to the plasma torch and directs it through the central region of the plasma. The velocity of the powder carrier gas is critical, particularly when the powder injector is radial to the plasma flame. A low flow rate would fail to convey the powder effectively to the plasma jet, and a high flow rate may cause the feedstock to overshoot the hottest region of the jet. In a radial injected plasma torch, the powder particles are forced into the plasma flame perpendicular to the direction of the flame. In such a fashion, most particles attain their maximum velocity by passing through the hottest region of the plasma along its central jet axis. The ideal carrier gas flow rate would inject particles into the plasma jet at a momentum similar to that of the plasma jet.

Different carrier gases influence different particle flows into the plasma jet. Argon is most commonly used as the carrier gas [111]. Leung et al. [110] demonstrated that nitrogen exhibited a gas momentum that was 37 % greater than that of argon, and for helium it was 10 % less compared to argon. The nitrogen carrier gas achieved the highest radial distance between the particle trajectory centre and the torch axis due to conferring the greatest momentum. Mawdsley et al. [112]

demonstrated that carrier gas flow rate had an effect on the thickness of plasma-sprayed coatings with a high carrier gas flow rate leading to an increase in coating thickness.

The powder, also termed as the feedstock, is transported to the plasma flame by means of a powder delivery tube that may be up to 10 m in length. The delivery rate of the feedstock has two consequences with regard to the coating build-up. Firstly, the powder feed rate influences the coating thickness since an increased flow rate increases the quantity of particles and, therefore, the coating thickness for a set transverse speed. Whereas this is an attribute from the perspective of the manufacturing economics, it should be kept in mind that a very high flow rate may give rise to incomplete melting that results in highly porous coatings. Incomplete melting increases the proportion of the unmelted powders that may bounce off the substrate surface and give rise to a low deposition efficiency. Secondly, it has been reported that the feed rate affects the temperature of the plasma flame. High feed rates infer high carrier gas flows that, with an associated increase in number of particles, may reduce the flame temperature [38].

The distance between the torch and the substrate is termed as the spray distance or standoff distance (SOD). SOD influences the velocity of the particle and the length of time that the particles are exposed to the plasma flame, thus influencing the degree of particle melting. A longer SOD may cause a reduction in the velocity of the droplets during spraying due to the frictional forces from the ambient environment. A shorter SOD would indicate that the substrate experiences more of the heating effects from the plasma flame. Thus, SOD affects the substrate temperature [38]. Kweh et al. [113], for example, demonstrated that coating properties deteriorated with increasing spray distance.

Sun et al. [105] studied the effects of varying SOD from 80 to 160 mm and reported that longer spray distances cause increased particle melting, lower porosity, and a greater number of microcracks. Lu et al. [114] investigated spray distances of 80–200 mm and suggested that at longer spray distances, the particles began to cool and resolidify, thereby allowing formation of a coating with increased crystallinity. Cizek et al. [102] measured the change in temperature and velocity as the spray distance increased from 50 to 150 mm. A decrease in particle temperature of 220 °C and a velocity decrease of 90 ms^{-1} were observed over this SOD range.

The velocity at which the plasma torch travels is called the torch traverse velocity. Traverse velocity has an effect on cooling, thickness, recrystallisation, and residual stress development. Traverse speeds used for spraying vary greatly, with values ranging from 75 [115] to 750 mms^{-1} [107] being reported.

9.5.3 *High-Velocity Oxygen-Fuel Spraying*

The high-velocity oxygen-fuel spray (HVOF) process has been investigated [87, 116] for HA processing. In this process, the feedstock powder is injected in a water-cooled high-pressure combustion chamber that has a long barrel [117]. Oxygen and

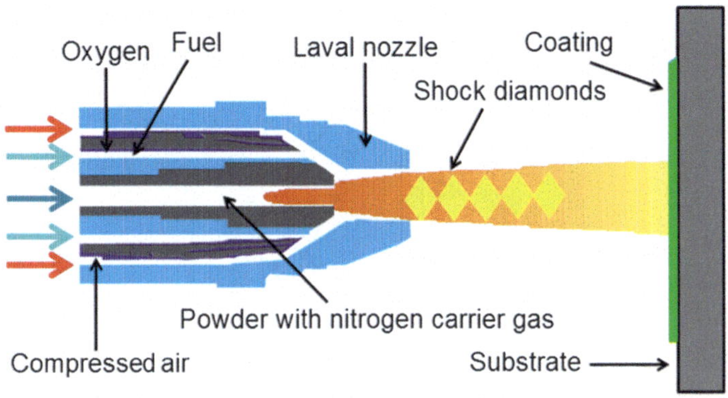

Fig. 9.9 High-velocity oxy-fuel apparatus (Anonymous [118]. Reprinted with permission. The copyright is held by the referenced source)

Table 9.7 Calcium-containing compounds in the calcium phosphate system (After Gross and Berndt [119][a])

Calcium phosphate	Chemical formula	Short ID	Ca/P ratio
Hydroxyapatite	$Ca_{10}(PO_4)_6(OH)_2$	HA, Hap, HAp	1.67
Tricalcium phosphate	$Ca_3(PO_4)_2$ (as α- or β-phases)	C_3P, TCP	1.5
Tetracalcium phosphate	$Ca_4P_2O_9 4CaO$	C_4P, TTCP	2
Calcium oxide	CaO	CaO	–
Calcium pyrophosphate	$Ca_2P_2O_7$	CPP	1
Oxyapatite	$Ca_{10}(PO_4)_6O$	OA	1.67

[a]Note: Some of this data appears in Table 9.1. Only those phases appearing in thermal-sprayed HA are presented in the current table

a fuel gas such as hydrogen [116, 118] combust and establish a high-pressure flame that is able to melt or partly melt the HA feedstock (Fig. 9.9). Coatings produced by means of the HVOF process exhibit good density and strength with low residual tensile stresses. A main advantage is that the feedstock particles do not need to be fully melted to create a high-quality coating [117].

9.5.4 *Coating Phases*

There are six possible calcium-containing compounds known in the calcium phosphate system: hydroxyapatite, tricalcium phosphate, tetracalcium phosphate, calcium oxide, calcium pyrophosphate, and oxyapatite (Table 9.7).

Not every compound appears in HA coatings since these are controlled by the spray process and parameters. The amorphous and the crystalline phases of HA are dominant. Alpha and/or beta phases of tricalcium phosphate and tetracalcium

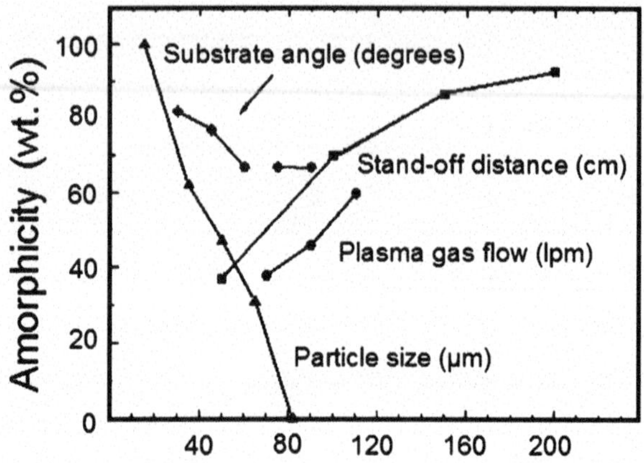

Fig. 9.10 Causes for an increase or decrease of the amorphous phase in a plasma-sprayed hydroxyapatite coating (Gross et al. [121]. Reprinted with permission. The copyright is held by the referenced source)

phosphate are often also present. The amorphous HA phase may develop instead of a crystalline phase due to the rapid solidification conditions during the splat quenching process where cooling rates of 1×10^6 degrees per second may exist. Thus, the HA does not have adequate time to crystallise [120, 121].

It has been mentioned previously that the spray parameters gave rise to coating layers that may exhibit variable thickness. A decrease of the layer depth, for example, by employing a low feedstock delivery rate, leads to higher cooling rates since heat can be transferred more rapidly away from the splat, thus leading to HA with an amorphous character (Fig. 9.10). This same effect may be achieved by altering the spray angle so that the impacting particle is more likely to smear across the substrate surface. Increasing the droplet heat has the same effect since the particle viscosity is decreased so that there is more fluid upon flattening against the implant surface. Alternatively, the thermal spray process may be performed at a higher velocity, e.g. affected by a higher primary gas flow that increases the cooling rate by flattening the coating layers.

It is possible to form an oxide layer on the implant metal surface due to heating effects caused by the initial particle layers. These layers, together with the thermal flux from the plasma, may exhibit increased cooling rates due to enhanced heat transfer and thereby increase the proportion of the amorphous phase.

An increase of the surface roughness of the implant material will reduce the flattening response of splats and, therefore, reduce the cooling rate. It is more likely that crystalline phases will evolve under such conditions.

The tendency for the amorphous phase to appear near the metal surface has been reported [40, 120, 121] for the above reasons but also arises due to the high thermal diffusivity of titanium (8×10^{-2} cm^2s^{-1}) [121]. The coating roughness increases during the evolution of the coating, and this leads to less heat conduction that presents conditions for enhanced crystallisation. Thus, the presence of crystalline HA is expected to be revealed on the coating surface.

The evolution of amorphous phase depends on the dehydroxylation rate [104, 119, 121], i.e. the reduction of OH^- groups, during the residence time of the

HA droplets in the plasma flame. Dehydroxylation can commence at 900 °C and increases at higher temperatures [23]. An increase of dehydroxylation enhances the amount of amorphous phase [121] and is influenced by the thermal spray parameters. For example, a longer SOD should decrease the amount of amorphous phase since larger droplets have time to form and so the cooling rate would be less. However, due to a longer flight time in the hot plasma, more dehydroxylation takes place, and consequently the crystalline phase is less, as shown in the study of Gross et al. (1998) [121].

There will also be particle size effects such that smaller particles will be heated more rapidly and more completely, hence exhibiting a greater degree of dehydroxylation [121]. If the feedstock contains less OH^- groups and there is further dehydroxylation during the spray process, then the amount of amorphous phase increases [122]. Studies have demonstrated that the amorphous phase dissolves much more rapidly in vitro and in vivo than the crystalline phase. It will be absorbed by the bone-growing cells and enhance bone growth. However, this beneficial effect is offset by the fact that defects form in the HA coating that may cause mechanical weakness in the coating [40].

The crystalline phase consists of unmelted or partially molten HA feedstock and recrystallised molten particles [121], which underwent less rapid cooling and, therefore, did not transform to the amorphous phase. The crystalline phase dissolves in vitro and in vivo less rapidly than the amorphous phase [40]. Hence, crystalline HA provides the coating with enhanced long-term mechanical properties, which is of special importance at the interface between the coating and implant to guarantee a durable bond strength. Even though the amorphous phase seems to enhance bone growth more than the crystalline phase, it is important to have an appropriate amount of crystalline splats within the coating, especially towards the implant surface, to support good mechanical properties.

Heat treatment of the implant after the coating process can increase the proportion of the crystalline phase by transforming regions of the amorphous phase [119, 121]. The splats, formed by partly molten droplets, can consist of a crystalline core in a shell of amorphous phase. Upon reheating, hydroxylation may occur and support transformations into the crystalline phase, which is then able to spread and crystallise within the amorphous regions of the coating. The downside of such heat treatment is the propensity for cracking within the coating [119]. Cracks may result from stress evolution and influence structural integrity in the coated implant.

The advantages and disadvantages of different ratios of amorphous and crystalline HA phases in a coating have been demonstrated in many studies. Overgaard et al. [123] studied 16 dogs in 1999 where they implanted HA-coated implants in the knee, with crystallinities of 50 and 75 %. After 16 and 32 weeks, each group was tested with regard to mechanical properties and bone growth rates. Within the first 16 weeks, the 50 % crystalline implants exhibited more bone growth on the coating surface. This phase structure accounted for the higher shear strength measured since there was a better connection to bone tissue. After 32 weeks, the bone growth and the mechanical properties of the 50 % crystalline implants did not increase substantially.

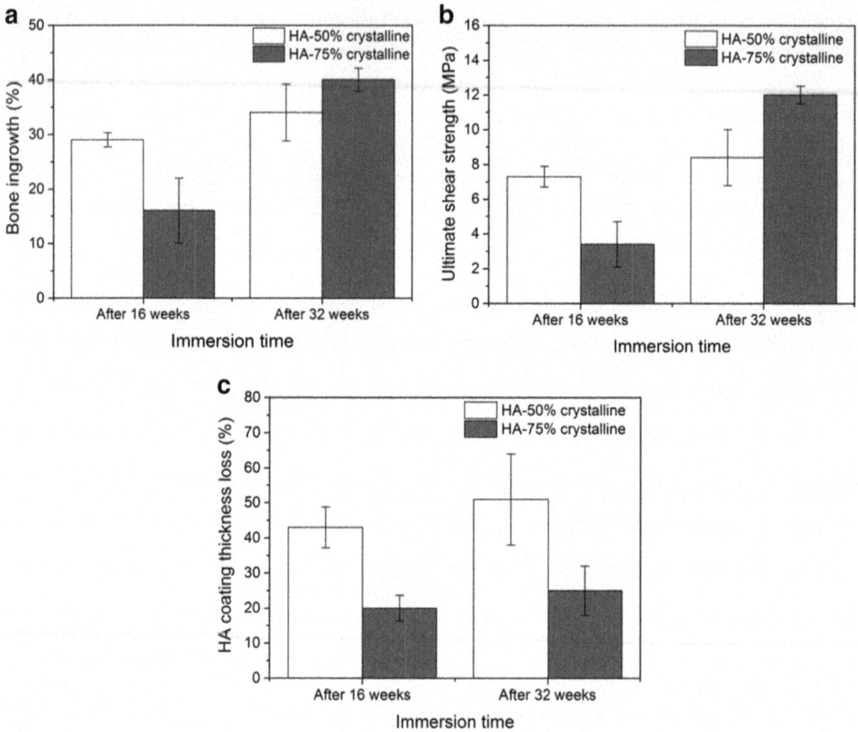

Fig. 9.11 Properties of HA-coated implants with 50 and 75 % crystallinity (After Overgaard et al. [123])

However, the 75 % crystalline implants exhibited more bone growth than the other implants, as well as enhanced mechanical properties (Fig. 9.11).

A conclusion of the above study is that higher crystallinity rates may not support fast bone growth initially. However, the crystalline HA offers a stable platform and adequate mechanical properties that presents an environment for slow bone growth. The slow growth leads to better mechanical properties and a stable, long-term coating. The stability of the HA coating is evidenced by means of the development of the coating thickness. That is, within the study period, the coating thicknesses of the 50 % crystalline implants were reduced by one half, whereas the thicknesses of the 75 % crystalline implants were reduced by 25 %, on average.

Tricalcium phosphate phases are relatively stable over a large temperature range [119]; therefore, they are often detected in thermal-sprayed HA coatings. Only the structure of the phase varies. For example, at high temperatures, a polymorph α-phase exists, which transforms under slow cooling into a β-phase or under fast cooling into a metastable tricalcium phosphate [119]. Gross and Berndt (1998) [119] indicated that tricalcium phosphate can be observed predominantly when the spray process encourages heat transfer to the feedstock particles. Under such low heat excursions, for example, on the surface of a coating as it builds up where amorphous and crystalline hydroxyapatite phases have solidified, the tricalcium phosphate can be located in greater amounts. Since tricalcium phosphate requires long periods at high temperature to form, it will solidify mostly in a higher dehydroxylated area [119].

In vivo, the degeneration rate of the alpha phase is higher than the beta tricalcium phosphate [124]. This characteristic of phase transformation is similar to that of the amorphous HA phase, i.e. it can enhance early bone growth but also weaken the mechanical properties of the coating.

Tetracalcium phosphate has similar thermo-physical characteristics as tricalcium phosphate and, therefore, can be found under the same conditions and in the same areas as this phase. Furthermore, it dissolves in vivo nearly as quickly as the tricalcium phosphate phases [125] with equal consequences for the HA coating.

Oxyapatite crystallises when the dehydroxylated melt of the feedstock particles cools slowly. If the cooling rate is higher, the amorphous phase of HA evolves as described earlier [23]. Preferably, oxyapatite crystallises on the structures of tri- and tetracalcium phosphate and, hence, can be localised in areas of this phase [119].

One of the properties of oxyapatite is to transform into crystalline HA under hydroxylation [23]. Thus, when oxyapatite comes into contact with water, e.g. in the body fluid, it absorbs OH- groups and converts into crystalline HA. Therefore, oxyapatite will under in vitro and in vivo conditions be mostly located in lamellae within the central regions of the HA coating [23] where fluid is less likely to have penetrated.

Calcium oxide reacts rapidly in an aqueous environment [119] and shows no biocompatible properties [40] and should, therefore, be avoided in HA implant coatings.

9.5.5 Design of Experiment (DOE) Methods

Much of the experimental work in the deposition of HA by thermal spray methods has been executed in an unstructured fashion. The precise thermal spray parameters, for instance, may not be documented, and the reproducibility of the experimental outcomes can be questioned since there is no strong evidence of statistical outcomes. Thus, in the current work, it is appropriate to explore methods of investigation that will lead to results that present scientific rigour.

The statistical experimental approach is usually termed as "design of experiment" (DOE) methods. Fisher in the early 1920s [126] developed a method to carry out agricultural experiments in which the effects of properties such as fertiliser, sunshine, and rain on a crop were determined. Further improvements in the DOE technique were brought about by Dr. Taguchi in the 1940s [126]. A number of special orthogonal arrays were introduced that made the implementation of DOE easier. The DOE method has been applied across a wide range of disciplines.

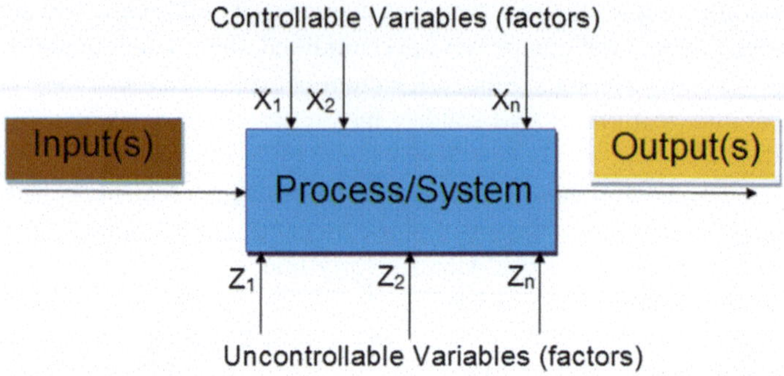

Fig. 9.12 The general model of a process/system (Antony et al. [128]. Reprinted with permission. The copyright is held by the referenced source)

In the DOE technique, the parameters to be changed in the experiment are termed as "factors" or "variables" [127]. The different possibilities for a factor are called the levels. Levels can be either qualitative or quantitative. The measured output from the experiment is termed as the response. Once the experiment has been run, the effect of each factor can be evaluated by comparing the average response change with the factor changed. Responses can then be represented as a polynomial regression equation of the following form:

$$y = b_0 + \sum b_j X_j + \sum b_{ij} X_i X_j + \sum b_{ijk} X_i X_j X_k \tag{9.6}$$

where i, j, and k vary from 1 to the number of variables; the coefficient b_0 is the mean of the responses for the whole experiment; the b_j coefficient represents the effect of the variable X_j; and b_{ij} and b_{ijk} are the coefficients of regression that represent the effects of interactions of the variables X_iX_j and $X_iX_jX_k$, respectively [38].

In performing a DOE, there is a need to input process or machine variables to observe corresponding changes in the output process. The information gained from properly planned experiments can be used to improve the performance of products. Figure 9.12 shows the general model of a process/system.

In every process, there are some variables or factors that can be controlled easily, and some are hard to control during normal production or standard conditions. In Fig. 9.12, the outputs are performance characteristics that are measured to assess process and/or product performance. The controllable variables can be measured during an experiment and such variables have a key role to play in the process characterisation. Uncontrollable variables, which may influence the process characterisation, are difficult to control during an experiment. It is important to determine optimal settings of controllable variables to minimise the effect of the uncontrollable variables [128].

Three aspects of design that pertain to thermal spray methods are analysed under DOE methods by processes such as factors, levels, and responses (Fig. 9.13). Factors, such as power, powder feed rate, and standoff distance, can be either

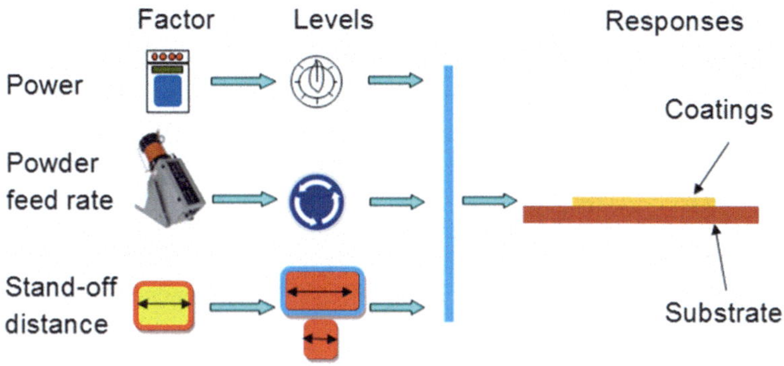

Fig. 9.13 Coating build-up (Moresteam et al. [129]. Reprinted with permission. The copyright is held by the referenced source)

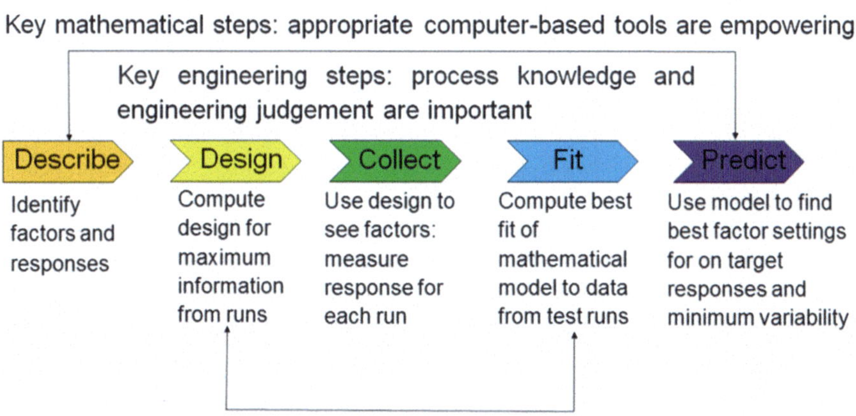

Fig. 9.14 Steps of design of experiment (SAS et al. [130]. Reprinted with permission. The copyright is held by the referenced source)

controllable or uncontrollable variables. Levels include the settings of these parameters. In this case, coatings are potentially influenced by the factors and their respective levels. Experimenters often design a series of tests to avoid optimising the process for one response at the expense of another. Based on this, the DOE technique can be flowcharted as shown in Fig. 9.14.

Different DOE methods have been developed, including factorial experiments and fractional factorial experiments and response surface methodology techniques, such as the central composite design, the Box–Behnken design, and Taguchi orthogonal arrays. The potential application of DOE in manufacturing processes includes [128] (1) improved process yield, stability, and capability; (2) reduced process variability and improved product performance; and (3) development of a relationship between key process inputs and output(s). DOE methods provide quality information from a smaller number of experiments.

9.6 Coating Properties

Of fundamental importance for developing and upgrading implant coatings is knowledge of the microstructural and mechanical properties and their parameters and influences. Therefore, the aspects of microstructure, porosity, coating thickness, and mechanical properties are investigated in this section. Within the examination of coating properties, it must be considered that, firstly, the coating consists of different phases with diverse properties and, secondly, the microstructures that form within a coating are composed mostly of nonunique phases that are assembled as a mixture of phases.

9.6.1 Optimisation of Hydroxyapatite Coatings

DOE is a suitable technique that provides maximum information on the basis of a minimum number of experiments. The benefits of DOE have been demonstrated in studies of plasma-sprayed coatings for materials, such as zirconia [131], titanium nitride [132], alumina [112] and alumina-titania [133]. DOE has been applied to plasma-sprayed HA coatings by Dyshlovenko et al. [134, 135], Cizek et al. [102] and Levingstone [38].

The HA coating consists of several layers of overlapping splats, formed of fully or partially molten feedstock. The flat, round-shaped splats are approximately 50–60 μm in diameter and 5 μm thick [98]. The microstructure depends on the spray parameters, which explains the coexistence of flat and layered splats with spheroidised particles [40]. The splats consist of grains, which are smaller at the fringe and larger in the centre (up to 5 μm) [98]. Figure 9.15 demonstrates the nano-grained structure of a HA splat.

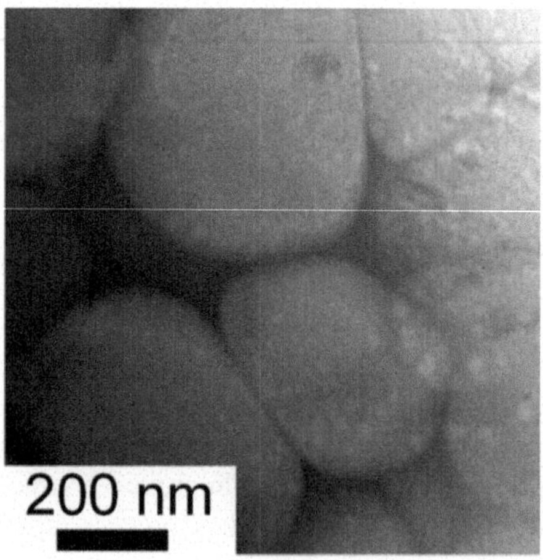

Fig. 9.15 Grains within a HA coating splat (Li et al. [98]. Reprinted with permission. The copyright is held by the referenced source)

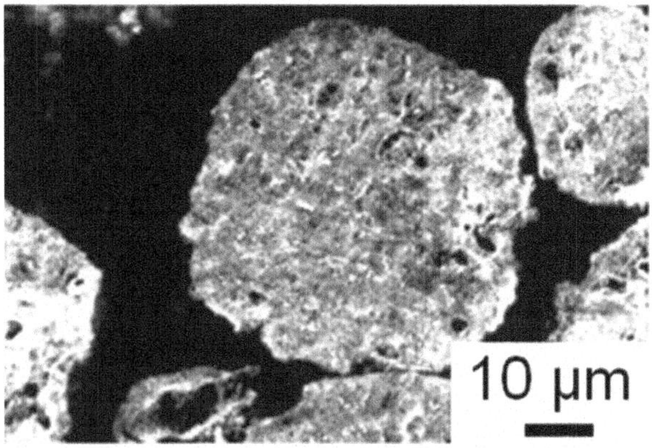

Fig. 9.16 Typical HA coating cross section that shows porosity within the splat microstructure (Li et al. [98]. Reprinted with permission. The copyright is held by the referenced source)

The coating shrinks during cooling, and the relieve of stresses leads to microcracks, which are a major stress relaxation mechanism in ceramics [136]. The presence of pores is responsible for the open microstructure of HA coatings. In a HA coating, there are two types of pores: (1) those that are within splats and (2) porosity between splats.

Pores within splats evolve from gas bubbles in a droplet and can be differentiated into open, closed, and through-thickness pores as described by Li et al. [98]. Open pores, which are either 1–2 μm or ~7 μm in diameter, appear when gas bubbles evaporate from the HA material. Closed pores arise when the highly viscous material of the splat freezes before the gas bubble can escape. Unlike open pores, which are only at the surface of the splats, through-thickness pores are oriented transverse through the splat thickness. All of the above pores within the splat architecture contribute to the porosity of the HA coating, which is, however, mainly defined by the interstices between the accumulation of splats.

Porosity that forms between splats may be correlated directly to the crystalline HA phase, i.e. the porosity of HA coatings increases with a larger amount of crystalline HA phase [89]. This phase differentiation arises because the crystalline HA splats are less viscous and therefore flatten less and are slow to cool. Hence, voids between these splats are not filled by viscous material, which may be differentiated from the case of an amorphous phase [89] (Fig. 9.16). Furthermore, it was found that the increase of less viscous amorphous phase decreases the surface roughness, and hence the coating is more smooth. A larger amount of amorphous phase, therefore, may be correlated to a decrease in coating porosity.

Other workers [137] arrived at similar conclusions concerning the influence of surface roughness on cell adhesion and proliferation. This case study found that the most rough HA disc surface, which was prepared by roughening with 180 grit SiC paper, enhanced the number of detached cells, the attachment strength, and the bone cell proliferation and activity.

In summary, bone cells need space between the coating splats to enable good anchoring, whereas pores that are too large may hinder cell growth in the coating.

Table 9.8 Thermo-physical properties of hydroxyapatite coatings (Non-marked values after Tsui et al. [104])

Property	Temperature (°C)	Value	Reference
Thermal conductivity [W × (m K)$^{-1}$]	–	0.013[a]	[23]
	10	0.72[b]	
	1079	2.16	
Specific heat [J × (kg K)$^{-1}$]	20–1027	766	
	100	700	[138]
Thermal diffusivity [cm^2 s^{-1}]	–	5.7×10^{-3}	[121, 139]
Thermal expansion [K^{-1}]	20	13.3	
	820	13.3	
Melting point [°C]		1,650	

[a]No temperature mentioned
[b]Marked as "low" temp

Furthermore, higher porosity may lead to lower mechanical properties and may negatively influence the long-term stability of the coating. The coating stability depends, as well, on factors such as the percentage ratio between the different phases and the coating thickness.

9.6.2 *Thermo-physical and Mechanical Properties*

The thermo-physical properties of HA coatings (Table 9.8) define the coating performance during the heating and cooling periods of the manufacturing process as well as under in vivo and in vitro behaviour.

A low thermal conductivity, as mentioned by Gross et al. (1998) [23], minimises chemical changes in the particles [23] and, so, ensures stable phases. The negative thermal diffusivity value of HA coatings indicates the slow heat-dissipating properties of the material [121], which is essential for the HA splats to transform into a crystalline phase.

The coefficient for thermal expansion of HA 13.3×10^{-6} K^{-1} is greater than that of a typical orthopaedic alloy, i.e. 9×10^{-6} K^{-1} for Ti6Al4V [98]. Consequently, residual stresses evolve within the coating/substrate system, which may be modified by heat treatment after the plasma spray process. One shortcoming of this strategy to reduce residual stress is that structural changes in the coating and the implant metal may ensue.

Hydroxyapatite coatings differ widely in thickness, phase content, microstructure, and porosity, all caused by varying the plasma spray parameters and feedstock. These processing effects, in combination with non-standard measurement methods and conditions, lead to a range of values for the same mechanical property of HA coatings.

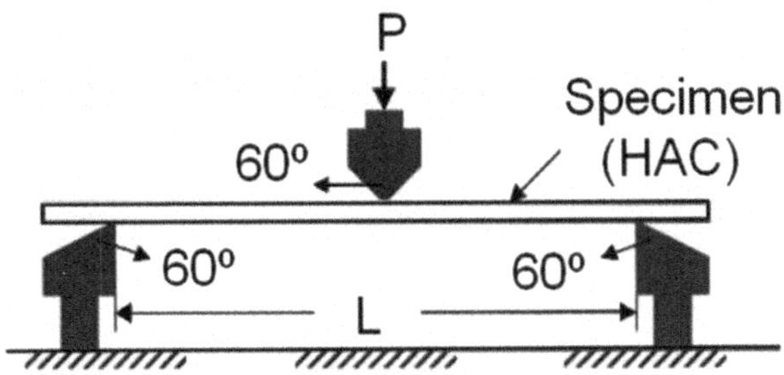

Fig. 9.17 Three-point-bending test for Young's modulus determination, after ASTM E-855 (Yang et al. [85]). "HAC" refers to the hydroxyapatite coating that is located on the top of the sample surface (Reprinted with permission. The copyright is held by the referenced source)

The Young's modulus of the coating was determined using a cantilever beam bend test [104] with an average value of 4.2 GPa for compression. This value is less than the average value of 20.3 GPa investigated [85] by means of a three-point bend test (Fig. 9.17). Other tests [140] have reached peak values of 60 GPa by using a microindentation test.

The study by Tsui et al. [104] indicated that the compression modulus was higher than that in tension. This structure/property effect was ascribed to microcracks and pores. Thus, under compression loading, cracks will be consolidated, and only the pores weaken the structure. Whereas if the coating is placed under tension, the strain will be influenced by cracks and pores and, therefore, will be more weak. Within the context of the orthopaedic application that operates under alternating stress cycles, the mechanical properties of a HA coating will lie between the two extreme strains, which reflects the true stresses imposed onto a coating in vitro.

Another mechanical property of interest is the Young's modulus that is an indicator of the coating stiffness. The modulus difference between the HA coating and the surrounding bone is about 20 GPa (Table 9.9). The corresponding high modulus mismatch between the implant metal (e.g. Ti6Al4V = 106 GPa [86]) and either the coating or the bone indicates that strains develop at these interfaces. These differences in stiffness lead to dissimilar deformations that cause stress. The net result is that degeneration of the bone matrix may occur at the coating–bone interface. That is, there may be degradation of bonding at the coating–implant interface that arises, fundamentally, from the modulus mismatch.

The bond strength determination includes the adhesive and the cohesive attachment properties of the coating. Tensile bond tests are prepared by using adhesives to fix a dummy support to the specimen assembly. If this adhesive penetrates through cracks and pores to the coating–implant interface, then non-representative higher bond strengths are measured [104]. This experimental concern explains the large range of values reported for the bond strengths, ranging from 9 MPa [104] up to 29 and 31 MPa [85]. Other reasons for these differences can be attributed to variations in spray parameters, feedstock, and heat treatment of the coating.

Table 9.9 Mechanical properties of hydroxyapatite coatings. (Non-marked values after Tsui et al. [104])

Property	Value	References
Young's modulus [GPa]	41.5–60.1[a]	[140]
	15.6–25[b]	[85]
Tension	0.50–3.42[c]	
Compression	3.17–5.20[c]	
Flexural	3.72–4.31[c]	
Elastic limit [MPa]	50	
Bonding strength [MPa]	4.15–13.92[c]	
	21–29[b]	[85]
	15.8–31.5[a]	[140]
Interfacial shear strength [MPa]	11.70–19.66[d]	[141]
Interfacial fracture toughness [MPa $m^{1/2}$]	0.28–1.08[c]	
	0.6–1.0	[86]
	0.6–1.41	[142]
Poisson's ratio	0.3	
Density [g/cm^3]	2.9	[86]
	2.82–2.89[c]	
Roughness R_a [μm]	1.1–8.1[e]	

[a]Nanostructure tests
[b]Time-dependent in vivo test
[c]Dependent on thermal spray parameters
[d]Time-dependent in vitro test
[e]Dependent on thermal spray parameters and coating thickness

Figure 9.18 depicts the experimental configurations employed to measure the adhesion of coatings. Interfacial fracture toughness describes the ability to resist crack initiation and propagation; a higher fracture toughness indicates that the material is less brittle. Values of fracture toughness are in the range of around 1 $MPam^{1/2}$. Variations may be explained by different surface roughnesses and feedstock particle sizes, which both have a strong influence on the coating adhesion [104].

Hardness is a mechanical property of a HA coating that depends on the phase ratio [89]. The amorphous phase and calcium oxide influence the hardness, which decreases with increasing amorphous phase and increases with increasing CaO.

The mechanical properties of any thermal spray coating are contingent on internal stresses since these influence the long-term behaviour (Table 9.10). Tsui et al. [104] investigated the relationship between Young's modulus and quenching stress. If the quenching stress increases, for example, due to varying plasma spray parameters, less microcracks appear in the coating since these are a sign of relaxation. Fewer microcracks, however, also imply an increase of the Young's modulus, because fewer defects in the form of voids are present in the coating.

Furthermore, Tsui et al. examined residual stresses in the implant metal and the HA coating (Fig. 9.19). The stress in the metal changes from tensile towards compressive when reaching the coating interface. This is caused by the large

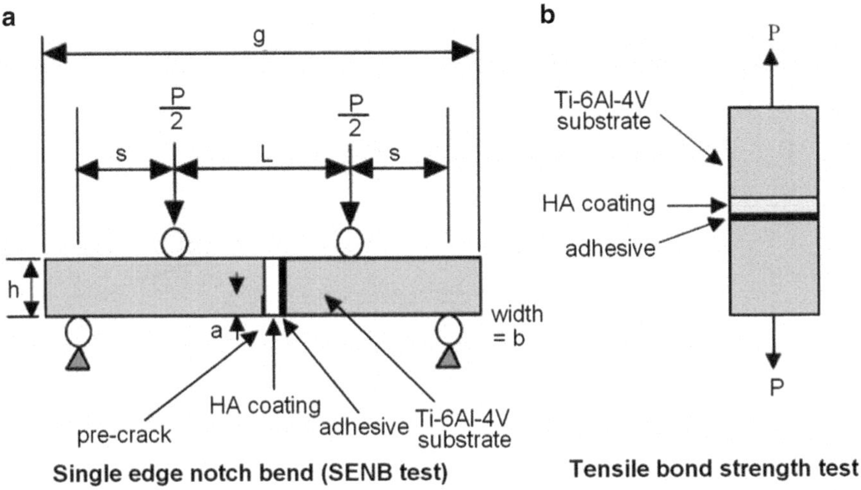

Fig. 9.18 Adhesion measurement with (**a**) single-edge notch bend test and (**b**) tensile bond test (Tsui et al. [104]. Reprinted with permission. The copyright is held by the referenced source)

Table 9.10 Stress properties of hydroxyapatite coatings (Non-marked values after Tsui et al. [104])

Property	Value	References
Coating stress (average) [MPa]	21–41[a, b]	
Quenching stress [MPa]	15–23[a]	
Residual stress [MPa]	33–44[b]	
	−21.2 to −44.2[c]	[85]
Residual strain [%]	−0.115 to −0.127[c]	[85]

[a]Properties depend on plasma spray power and gas mixture
[b]Coating on a Ti6Al4V alloy
[c]Time-dependent in vivo test. A negative value indicates a compressive stress

differences of the thermal expansion coefficients [104], i.e. HA = 13.3×10^{-6} K^{-1} and Ti6Al4V = 9×10^{-6} K^{-1}. The larger coefficient of HA leads to a greater expansion than the metal and compressive stresses evolve at the implant–coating interface. Stress in the coating was determined to be always tensile and increased slightly with the distance from the metal surface, which correlated well with the respective Young's moduli.

Other investigators [143] found a greater Young's modulus for the crystalline phase than the amorphous one. The amorphous phase is located mainly at the coating–metal interface, and, therefore, Young's modulus increases with coating thickness since the amount of crystalline phase also increases.

Time-dependent studies of HA coatings in simulated body fluid [85] showed a significant decrease of the residual stress from 44 to 21 MPa within four weeks

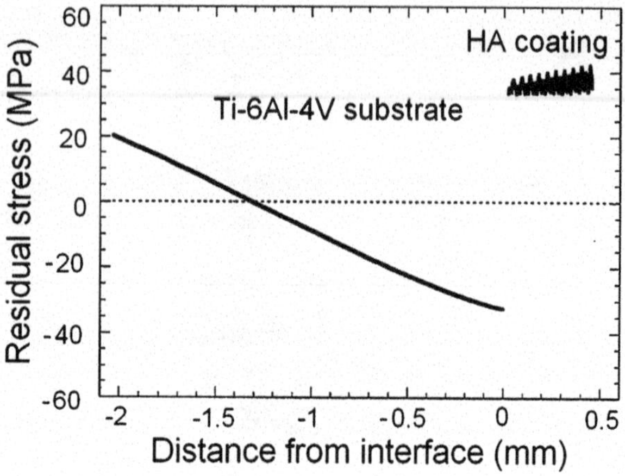

Fig. 9.19 Residual stresses within the implant–metal and the HA coating (Tsui et al. [104]. Reprinted with permission. The copyright is held by the referenced source)

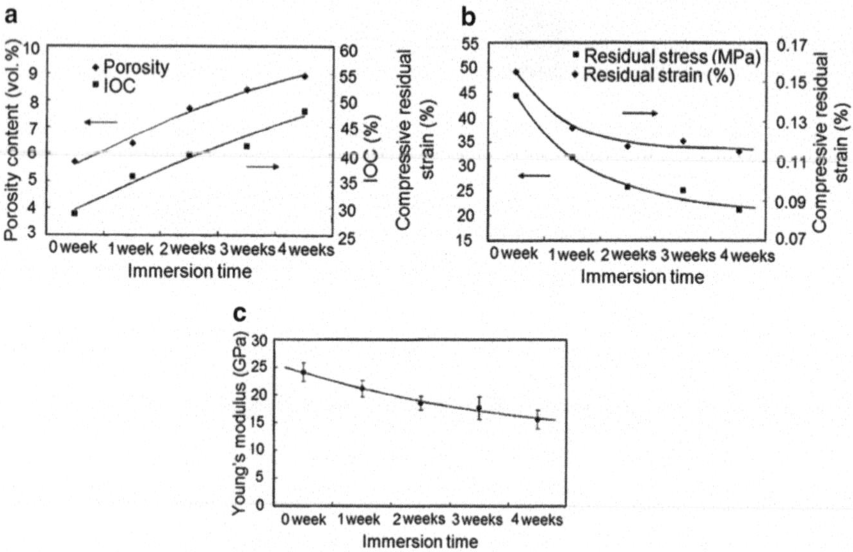

Fig. 9.20 Development of the HA coating properties over 4 weeks in simulated body fluid: (**a**) Young's modulus, (**b**) porosity, and (**c**) compressive residual stress and strain (Yang et al. [85]. Reprinted with permission. The copyright is held by the referenced source)

(Fig. 9.20). Furthermore, a relationship between porosity, Young's modulus, and residual stress was determined. The porosity increased linearly over time. Thus, the Young's modulus decreased in a complementary fashion, as did the residual stress that reflected a decrease in strain. A physical explanation is that regions of the HA coating dissolve when exposed to physiological media, which causes an increase in porosity. This morphological change reduces the residual stress and strain as well as a decrease of the Young's modulus. This study does not consider the possible increase of strength of the coating–bone system when bone starts to grow inside the coating structure. Such bone growth would reflect the natural bone modelling and remodelling processes and be expected to regenerate some stability.

9.6.3 Coating Thickness

The mechanical and resorption properties of the HA coating are related to the coating thickness since there will be phase changes. Several investigators [144, 145] examined the influence of the coating thickness on the shear strength. The results showed higher shear strength for a 50 μm coating than for a 200 μm thick coating. Another study on sheep by Svehla et al. (2002) [146] showed a contrary result with an increase of shear stress with increasing coating thickness, especially over 100 μm.

Furthermore, all of these studies demonstrated that only coatings up to 150 μm thick exhibited failures, such as cracks, at the coating–bone interface. The 200 μm thick coating [144] featured additional failures within the coating and at the coating–implant interface. Therefore, these outcomes recommend the use of thinner coatings of 100 μm to minimise fatigue failure within the coating and, hence, to provide a better long-term performance.

The resorption of the coating in vivo has to be considered to ensure that sufficient coating provides a long-term grip of the bone to the implant when the dissolution process has ceased. The study of Svehla et al. [146] reports that the bone on-growth increases with increasing coating thickness up to 100 μm, with an equal amount of bone cells on a 150 μm thick coating.

Studies of the nature reported above have led to conventions for coating thickness. Coatings between 50 and 75 μm are commonly used for orthopaedic implants [40], whereas coatings for dental implants are at least 100 μm thick.

9.6.4 Phase Arrangement

The phase diagram (Fig. 9.2) indicates that HA only emerges under circumstances that are influenced strongly by the process temperature and the calcium oxide percentage in the feedstock powder [119]. Figure 9.21 shows the X-ray diffraction results from a HA coating that displays many calcium phosphate phases.

The calcium phosphate phases dissolve both in vivo and in vitro; however, the dissolution rate increases in the ranking order of crystalline hydroxyapatite $<$ β-tricalcium phosphate $<$ α-tricalcium phosphate $<$ amorphous hydroxyapatite $<$ tetracalcium phosphate [147]. Note that this ranking of the dissolution rates agrees with those presented in Sect. 9.2.1.3. The dissolution rate also relies on the morphology, roughness, surface area, porosity, and residual stresses of the coating [29]. Furthermore, dissolution depends strongly on the crystal size within

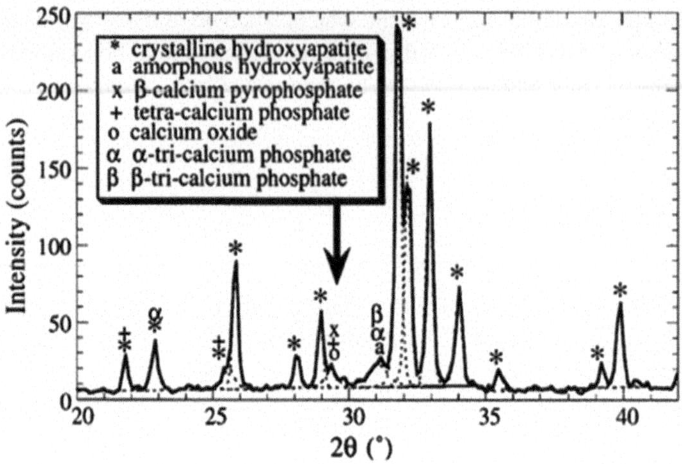

Fig. 9.21 Phases found in a plasma-sprayed HA coating (Tsui et al. [104]. Reprinted with permission. The copyright is held by the referenced source)

the coating; for example, it has been demonstrated that larger crystals led to a decrease of the dissolution rate of the coating [148].

A HA coating consists of an agglomeration of single splats. These splats are not homogenous but consist of a phase mix due to different heat and dehydroxylation parameters in the core and the shell of the droplets. Several authors [96, 105, 119] have developed models that describe the manner in which a single splat may consist of diverse phases.

Gross et al. (1998) [119] developed a model indicating that splat phases depend on the plasma flame temperature (Fig. 9.22), since this parameter regulates the viscosity of the splats and the degree of dehydroxylation. Following this model, crystalline, not dehydroxylated, HA can be found in the core of droplets and splats. The amorphous, highly dehydroxylated and fast-cooling phase develops at the metal surface, while oxyapatite, which cools down slower, is located near the outer splat surface. Higher temperatures lead to tricalcium and tetracalcium phosphates as well as to calcium oxide. Calcium oxide is not desirable due to its bio-incompatible properties.

Sun et al. (2003) [105] developed a model concerning the coating formation and the recrystallisation of the amorphous phase (Fig. 9.23). The model considers that during the solidification of the splat, some regions of the amorphous and stoichiometric phase (between the core and shell) recrystallise due to longer cooling times on the coating surface. Furthermore, this model considers that subsequent droplets influence the previous layers. That is, heat from the plasma flame and from the overlapping, new droplets melt the outer sections of the prior-formed splats. This process may lead to recrystallisation since the new splats decrease the cooling rate of the already deposited splats. Secondly, while the first-formed splats recrystallise, new OH- groups have time to infiltrate these regions and generate a crystalline phase out of a former amorphous phase.

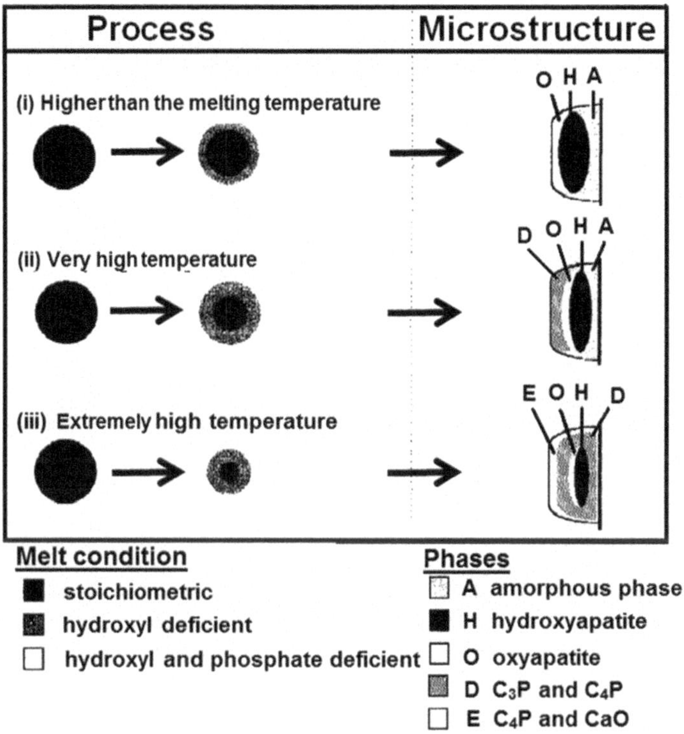

Fig. 9.22 Splat development model dependent on plasma flame temperature (Gross and Berndt [119]. Reprinted with permission. The copyright is held by the referenced source)

9.6.5 In Vitro Behaviour

The time-dependent in vivo behaviour of the coating is decisive for the functionality of the implant. ASTM F1609 [39] provides general conditions for the expected in vitro and in vivo behaviour of calcium phosphate coatings. Several studies have investigated coating performance in vitro in animal tests and in human patients.

Kim et al. performed an in vitro study (2004) [149] to investigate the mechanism for the development of a natural apatite-like bone matrix onto an artificial HA substrate. Sintered HA was soaked into simulated body fluid (aka "SBF"; Table 9.11) and examined before the soaking process and 3, 6, 9, 12, 24, 48, 72, and 120 h after remaining in the fluid. The zeta potential on the coating surface and the Ca/P ratio were analysed (Fig. 9.24) and a model developed (Fig. 9.25).

The HA coating shows a negative surface potential when placed into the SBF. This enables the positive calcium ions to interact with the HA, and a calcium-rich amorphous calcium phosphate (ACP) layer is formed. Therefore, the calcium–phosphate ratio increases, and the surface potential becomes positive, which attracts the negative phosphate ions of the SBF towards the HA surface.

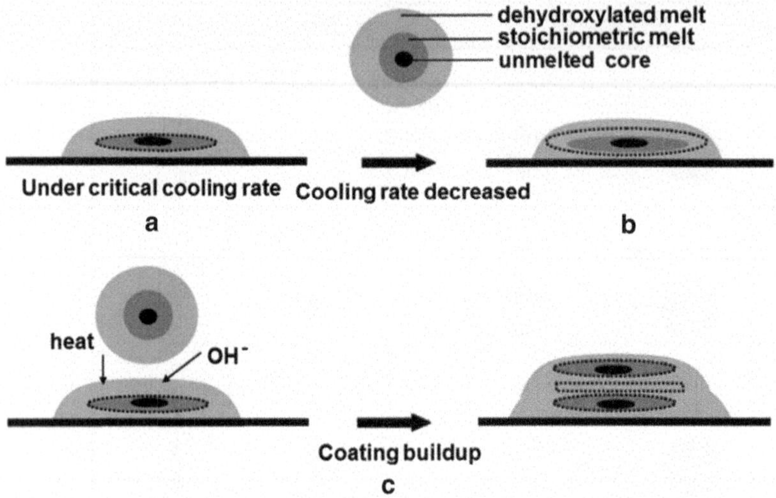

Fig. 9.23 The development of a HA coating during thermal spray deposition (Sun et al. [105]). (**a**) Crystalization of the stoichiometric melt. (**b**) Recrystallization of the dehydroxylated melt due to the decreased cooling rate during droplet solidification. (**c**) Recrystallization of the amorphous phase in the prior-formed splat due to heat from both the incoming droplet and the plasma flame and the re-hydroxylation during the coating buildup (Reprinted with permission. The copyright is held by the referenced source)

Table 9.11 Composition of simulated body fluid (*SBF*) in comparison with human blood plasma (After Khor et al. [150])

Ion	Ion concentration in SBF mM] (pH 7.40)	Ion concentration in blood plasma [mM]
Na^{+}	142.0	142.0
K^{+}	5.0	5.0
Mg^{2+}	1.5	1.5
Ca^{2+}	2.5	2.5
Cl^{-}	147.8	103.0
HCO_3^{-}	4.2	27.0
HPO_4^{2-}	1.0	1.0
SO_4^{2-}	0.5	0.5

This process evolves after 6–9 h of soaking time and creates a calcium-poor area in the HA that decreases the local Ca/P ratio and reduces the amount of surface HA. Subsequently, bone-like apatite forms from the crystallising calcium-poor ACP, with the incorporation of calcium and phosphate from physiological fluids. This apatite is equivalent to the natural bone matrix in terms of structure and composition. The apatite structure grows and integrates further calcium and phosphate from the host fluid. Kim et al. observed a needle-like morphology of the apatite crystals on the HA surface. The zeta potential stabilised to around −10 mV after 120 h of soaking in the SBF and the hydroxyapatite Ca/P ratio reverted almost to its original level of 1.67.

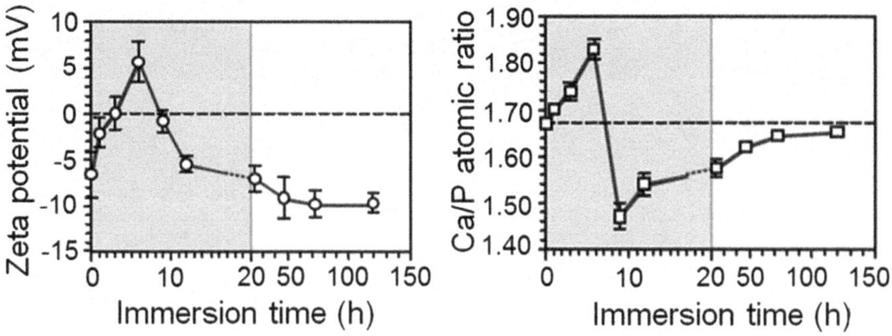

Fig. 9.24 Zeta potential and Ca/P ratio within immersion time in SBF (Kim et al. [149]. Reprinted with permission. The copyright is held by the referenced source)

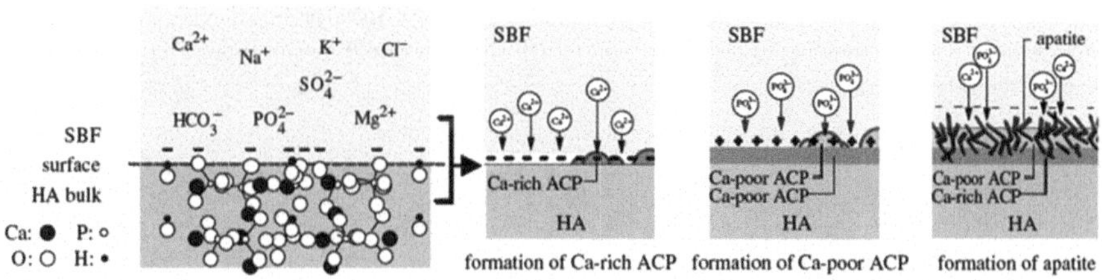

Fig. 9.25 Process of forming natural bone apatite on the HA coating (Kim et al. [149]. Reprinted with permission. The copyright is held by the referenced source)

The group around Weng [151] investigated the development of the bone-like apatite layer in SBF. The initial surface dissolution of HA was observed after 4 h as well as the appearance of cracks and fragmented splats. Whole splats vanished from the HA surface after a further two hours. After 12 h, the first granular layers of bone-like apatite, which initiated in the lower-level pore regions, propagated to the outermost regions of the coating surface. Finally, after 24 h of placement into the SBF, the whole HA surface was covered with a 2.5 μm thick layer of bone-like apatite. The dunelike surface became more smooth and thick. At day six, hillocks of more than 20 μm thickness were observed. The surface layer exhibited a netlike structure consisting of short micro-rods that were similar in morphology to other work [149].

Other studies [150] have confirmed these results where the in vitro behaviour of HVOF-sprayed HA coatings and splats was investigated. Coatings formed from 30 and 50 μm feedstock were soaked in SBF (Fig. 9.26). The surface of the 30 μm coating revealed full coverage with a precipitated layer after three days, while the more coarse 50 μm coating required 7 days to cultivate such a layer.

The investigations of Khor et al. also examined the phase changes in the coatings during incubation in SBF. Both coatings exhibited different phase ratios due to the different melt states of the splats caused by different feedstock sizes. Therefore, it can be explained that dissolution and phase changes emerge earlier in the coating

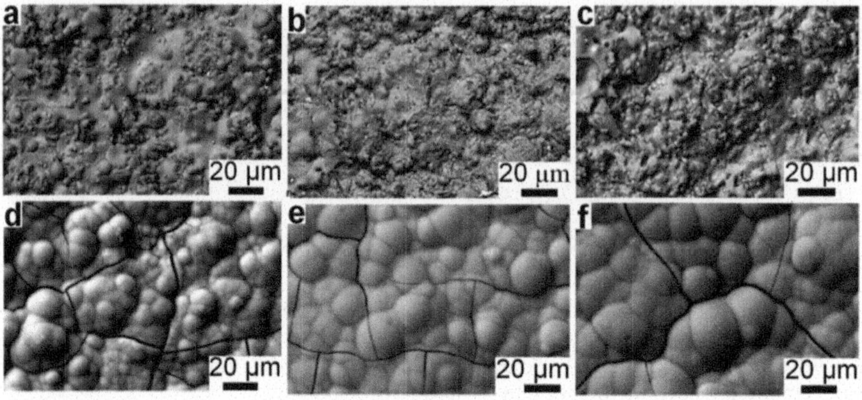

Fig. 9.26 Surface changes of coating formed from 30 μm feedstock after soaking in SBF for (**a**) 0 h, (**b**) 6 h, (**c**) 1 day, (**d**) 3 days, (**e**) 7 days, and (**f**) 14 days. A fully precipitated layer covers the surface after 3 days of incubation (Khor et al. [150]. Reprinted with permission. The copyright is held by the referenced source)

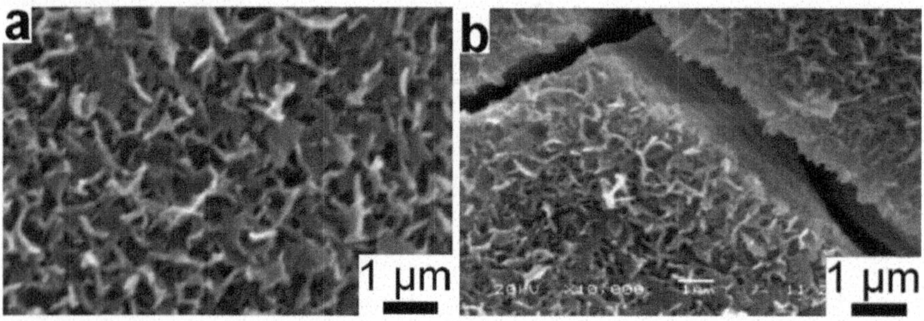

Fig. 9.27 Structure of (**a**) the precipitated layer and (**b**) a coating crack (Khor et al. [150]. Reprinted with permission. The copyright is held by the referenced source)

formed from more fine feedstock. Tetracalcium phosphate disappeared quickly, whereas the dissolution rate of α-tricalcium and β-tricalcium phosphate took 14 days in SBF. The amorphous phase was step-by-step replaced by a crystalline structure, which was visible as a precipitated layer on the coating surface and explained by the mechanism of Kim et al. (2004) [149]. This layer was identified as a bone-like HA with a bone-like crystalline structure (Fig. 9.27).

Khor et al. [150] examined the weight and calcium concentration changes in the coating (Fig. 9.28). The 30 μm coating revealed a weight decrease after 6 h of SBF immersion due to the initial dissolution of tetracalcium phosphate, tricalcium phosphate, and amorphous HA. The coating weight increased with the crystallisation of the amorphous phase and the formation of the precipitated layer. On the other hand, there was no weight decrease for the 50 μm coating, and it was speculated that the larger splat size presented lesser dissolution.

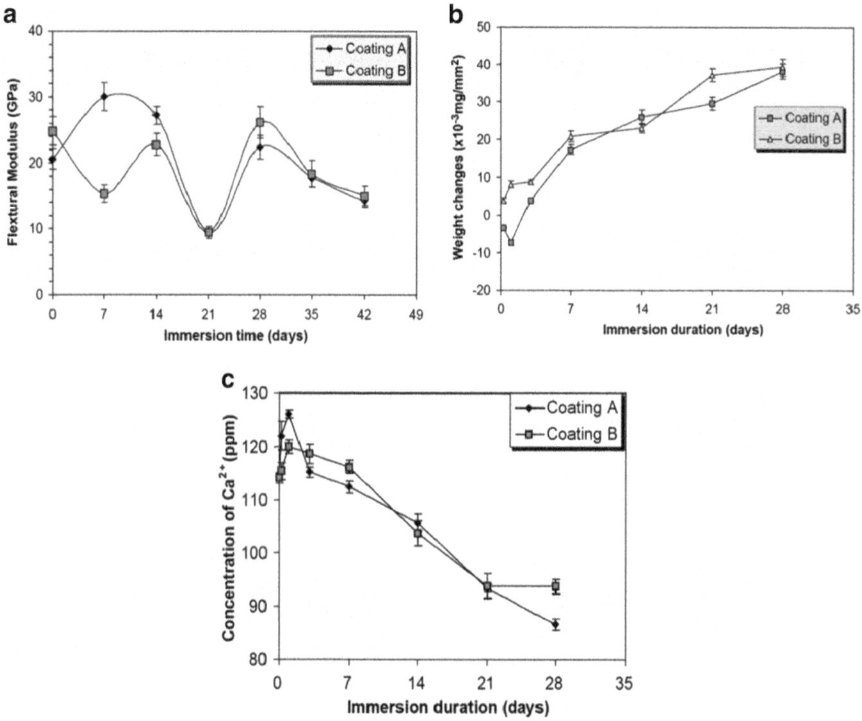

Fig. 9.28 Changes of the coating properties: (**a**) flexural modulus, (**b**) weight, and (**c**) calcium concentration within immersion time. Coating A is formed from feedstock of 30 μm, and coating B feedstock is 50 μm (Khor et al. [150]. Reprinted with permission. The copyright is held by the referenced source)

Furthermore, with incipient development of the bone-like apatite layer, the dissolution of the coating elements reduced but did not cease within the experimental time frame, and this was reflected by the non-linear trend of the results. Overall, (1) the dissolution rate of the 30 μm coating was much higher than the 50 μm coating, and (2) the 30 μm coating demonstrated a significantly faster development of the apatite layer. Therefore, there is a relationship between dissolution and the development of a bone-like layer.

The proposed development of calcium within the coating in the study of Khor et al. [150] is equivalent to the model developed by Kim et al. [149]. Within the first few hours, the calcium level in the coating increased by absorbing calcium from the fluid and deposited it as an amorphous phase on the coating [150]. Thereby the 30 μm coating assimilated more calcium than the 50 μm coating. This tendency reversed after the first few days, and the calcium concentration reduced since, now, the calcium was remodelled into the new bone-like apatite. Khor et al. also mention that further dissolution of calcium from regions of the coating remote from the surface may be realised through cracks. Both coatings started losing calcium around

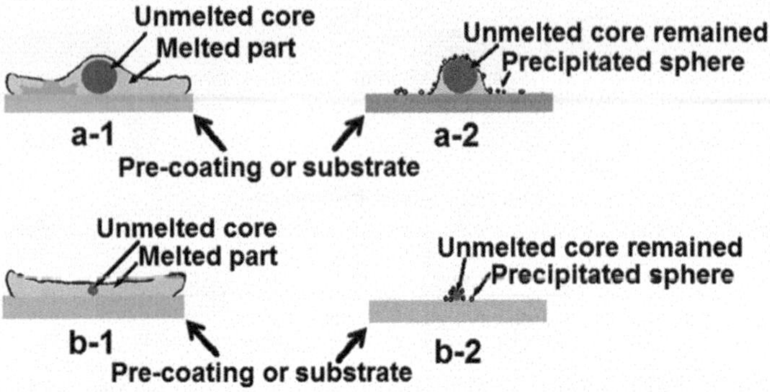

Fig. 9.29 Performance model of (*a*) half melted and (*b*) nearly fully melted splats. "-1" and "-2" indicate before and after exposure to the simulated body fluid, respectively (Khor et al. [150]. Reprinted with permission. The copyright is held by the referenced source)

the same time; however, the 30 μm coating commenced this process earlier by developing the apatite layer. Thus, there are indications of a relationship between the amount of calcium absorption in the first few hours and the ability to cultivate bone-like apatite early.

Khor et al. [150] used a three-point bend method to measure the Young's modulus of the HA coatings. The modulus of the 30 μm coating increased initially due to the rapid development of a dense bone-like apatite layer, whereas the modulus of the 50 μm coating declined because of the initial dissolution. Later, the 30 μm coating developed an apatite layer, and hence the modulus increased. Both coatings exhibited a drop in their moduli around the 21st day, which was proposed to be a result of further stress reduction due to dissolution and crack formation in the coating. The modulus increased with further growth of the apatite layer and stabilised at about 15 GPa.

A mechanistic model has been presented [150] concerning the development of the splats and their influence on the formation of bone-like apatite layers (Fig. 9.29). The melted sections of a HA splat offers tricalcium and tetracalcium phosphate and amorphous HA. These phases exhibit high dissolution rates, whereas the unmelted splat centre consists of the original feedstock powder, i.e. crystalline HA that has a slower dissolution rate. It was observed that a mostly molten splat disappeared rapidly without the development of bone-like apatite. The remaining core, in contrast, offers a surface for development of an apatite layer, but dissolution is necessary. Consequently, an ideal coating will offer a mixture of fast-dissolving phases and crystalline structures, for instance, evolving from unmelted cores, to offer a foundation for bone-like apatite.

Despite the name "bone-like apatite", the developing apatite matrix shows a different phosphate structure and a lack of OH^- groups in comparison to naturally grown bone [151]. But, nevertheless, this matrix is sufficient to induce bone cells to be laid down and develop natural bone tissues on the frame of the bone-like apatite.

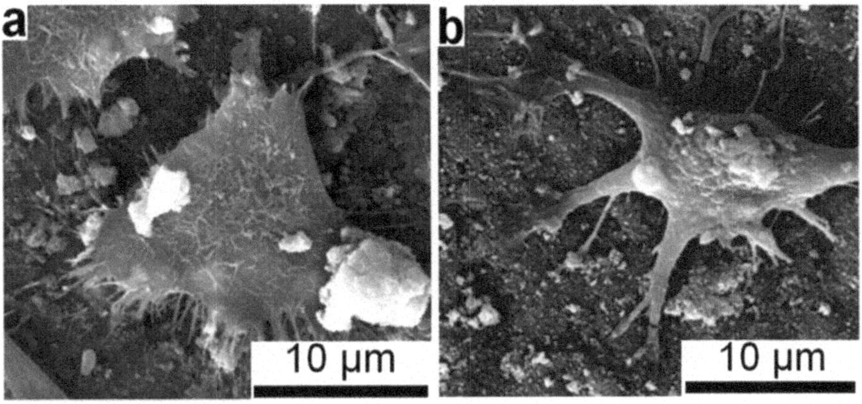

Fig. 9.30 Osteoblast cells on the (**a**) spherical and (**b**) rod-like coating surface. The cells on (**a**) demonstrated a bigger and faster growth (Zhao et al. [154]. Reprinted with permission. The copyright is held by the referenced source)

The influences of different coating properties on the bone growth mechanism have been demonstrated by in vitro and in vivo studies. For example, Lu et al. (1998) [152] demonstrated that the regenerated bone provided stable anchoring for the implant. The bone growth differs between regions within the bone itself: with the most new matrix material located in cortical bone, followed by cancellous bone and then the medullar region. Hara et al. (1999) [153] used mechanical tests to investigate the good bonding strength of the coating onto the implant.

As mentioned previously, the work by Deligianni et al. (2001) [137] showed the dependency of surface roughness for cell attachment and ingrowth. More rough coating surfaces revealed more attached bone-forming cells and higher bond strengths. Another investigation [154] revealed that the bone cell behaviour depends on the microstructure of the HA coating. The morphology of the spherical and rod-like nanocrystals was examined with respect to supporting cell growth and adhesion. A spherical structure activated cells to a greater degree and was the preferred crystal morphology (Fig. 9.30).

Ergun et al. (2008) [155] investigated the relationship between Ca/P ratio of nanostructured HA coatings and the adhesion of bone-forming cells. An increase in this ratio, i.e. an increase in the relative proportion of calcium, also increased the number of bone cells attached to the coating surface within a limited time frame (Fig. 9.31).

Other studies have also examined the influence of HA composition on the bioactive properties. It was found that β-tricalcium phosphate improved cell proliferation for HA coatings [55]. Furthermore, the effect of a higher ratio of β-TCP in the sintered coating increased the bond strength and fracture toughness of the coating [156]. These results show that fast cell proliferation is supported by rapidly dissolving phases such as β-tricalcium phosphate and amorphous HA. The cell response is also related to the specific porosity and average pore size, which are physical characteristics determined by the thermal spray manufacturing process.

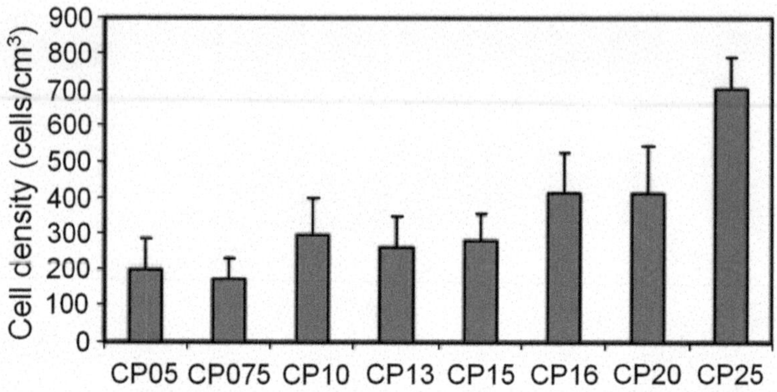

Fig. 9.31 Cell density on nanostructured HA coating differing in CA/P ratio (CP) (Ergun et al. [155]. Reprinted with permission. The copyright is held by the referenced source)

9.6.6 In Vivo Behaviour

The in vivo behaviour of HA coatings has also been studied so that relationships to clinical practice can be established. Long-term studies, such as the 15-year follow-up study by Epinette (2008) [157] or the research on 166 hips over 15 years by Capello et al. (2006) [158], demonstrated (1) a faster and more painless ingrowth of implants coated with HA and (2) better bone tissue modelling and remodelling quality. Other investigations [159, 160] showed no significant differences between the new coated implant and the older systems. Any inconsistencies arose due to (1) implant designs that were not compatible with the HA coating or (2) significant differences in the patient groups.

As described previously, the bone growth mechanism includes the dissolution of regions of the HA coating, as verified by post-mortem retrievals [161] or case studies [162], which showed that it was rare for the coating to totally dissolve within 4 years. The dissolution of the HA coating is the prime cause for concern against their use since any major material loss can lead to inferior properties such as bond strength and Young's modulus.

There are different mechanisms concerning the part or complete in vivo disappearance of HA coatings. Bauer (1995) [163] hypothesised methods of (1) dissolution, (2) resorption by bone cells as part of the natural modelling and remodelling processes, (3) delamination caused by bond failures, and (4) abrasion of the coating surface due to an inadequate initial fixation of the implant. Gross et al. (2002) [164] added to these mechanisms by including the loss of particles that may arise from (5) lamellae cracking due to residual stresses and (6) free crystalline debris caused by dissolution of the amorphous phase (Fig. 9.32).

The losses via (1) dissolution and (2) resorption are the necessary foundation for the support of bone growth. It is important that the coating thickness and the percentage of the more resilient crystalline HA are sufficient to ensure long-term existence. Provision of a high bond strength is achieved by means of the

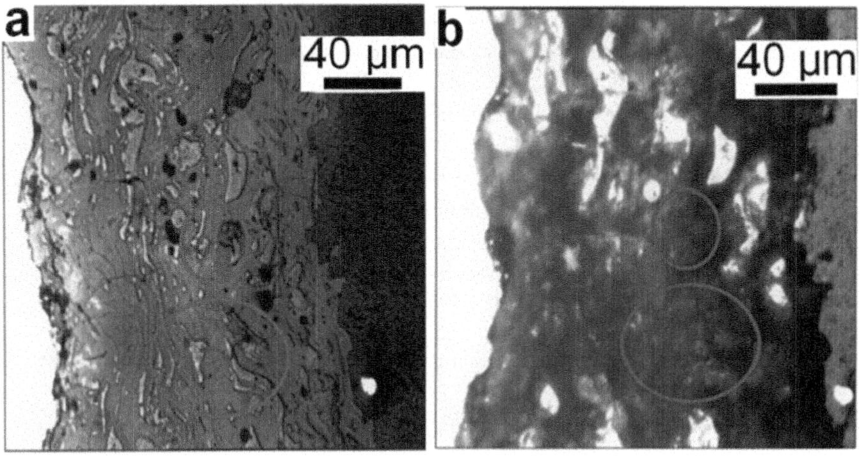

Fig. 9.32 HA coating (**a**) before and (**b**) after accelerated degradation (Gross et al. [164]. Reprinted with permission. The copyright is held by the referenced source)

manufacturing method and attaining the beneficial coating phases and structures. Any coating losses caused by abrasion during the clinical insertion procedure need to be reduced by appropriate surgical procedure. The particle debris that results from cracks and amorphous phase dissolution have not been sufficiently investigated but can be expected to cause only a small degree of coating loss.

Bloebaum et al. (1998) [165] examined the behaviour of macrophages with regard to HA coating debris. Particles no larger than the 30 μm diameter macrophages can be resorbed and degraded. Larger particles may be enclosed in the developing bone matrix, engulfed by giant cells or drift through to nearby tissue and, therefore, be transported to other regions of the body. Any transported particles can cause third-body wear as described in the study by Morscher et al. (1998) [166]. The HA particles are much harder than implant materials such as polyethylene. Therefore, any transported HA particles are likely to damage the PE surface and lead to failure of this implant. Furthermore, the high hardness of the ceramic coating debris can cause metallic debris to form within an articulated total joint replacement.

As well as potential damage of the bearing surface, there will be generation of polyethylene and metal debris due to friction. These particles have a biochemical influence of the surrounding tissue that can cause osteolysis due to allergic body reactions. Thus, macrophages and giant cells that try to ingest the metallic and polyethylene particles, but cannot digest them, die. Other cells encapsulate these dead cells and the particles, which leads to cell degeneration in this area. The overall negative outcome may be loosening and failure of the implant. The dissolution of HA coating particles is necessary to build up new bone, but the appearance of larger, independent coating particles must be avoided to reduce the possibility of third-body wear.

HA coatings were designed to enhance bone growth on in vivo implants during the first stage of the implantation so that primary stabilisation could be assured. These coatings for clinical purpose have been produced mainly by plasma spray methods to ensure the desired mechanical properties, phase ratios, and microstructures.

In vitro and in vivo, the HA coating responds to the physiological environment and forms an artificial, bone-like apatite, which provides the foundation for the bone cells to develop natural bone tissue. Regions of the coating, especially amorphous HA, tricalcium, and tetracalcium phosphate, dissolve to support bone growth mechanisms.

9.6.7 Optimisation of Hydroxyapatite Coating Characteristics

The studies suggest the preferred properties for a HA coating. The coating thickness should be between 50 and 100 μm to provide a balance between shear strength and shear strains. Furthermore, such a thickness offers sufficient coating material, even after partial dissolution, to build a foundation for long-term survival. It is important that the coating be composed of a certain percentage of crystalline HA so that the dissolution rate is reduced.

The amorphous phase should be located mainly at the coating surface where it can support the development of bone-like apatite. Crystalline, less fast-dissolving, HA should be regionally located towards the coating–implant surface to ensure long-term survival of the coating, as well as providing adequate bond strength. Some crystalline phases need to be mixed among the amorphous phase, so that bone-like apatite can appropriate a foundation when other phase components dissolve.

The Young's modulus of the amorphous phase is less than that of crystalline HA. Therefore, the progression of the Young's modulus profile across the metal implant to the coating and towards the bone tissue should be gradual with no abrupt stiffness discontinuities. The coating surface should exhibit a lower modulus than the coating–implant interface, since the Young's modulus of the bone is much lower than that of metal.

The phase of calcium oxide should be avoided since it has a very high dissolution rate that will lead to loosening of the implant. Higher ratios of β-TCP or the addition of other bone growth-stimulating materials may enhance the natural bone growth.

HA coatings on implants have the main aim to enhance bone growth. Therefore, the coating should provide several properties. The coating surface should provide sufficiently large pores so that bone-forming cells can infiltrate and, therewith, effectively connect natural bone with the implant. However, the pores should not be too large, since the bridging of wider spaces takes more time, while a fast ingrowth is preferred. A typical pore size of 50–100 μm is preferred. The coating surface should also support rapid bone ingrowth, and this can be beneficiated by using bone growth factors and adjusting the surface roughness to maximise interfacial contact without compromising mechanical integrity during the prosthesis insertion process.

The mechanical coating properties of density, Young's modulus and shear, and tensile strength should be in a range within the bone properties to avoid additional stress and hence material failure or bone resorption.

9.7 The Interface Between the Coating and Bone

9.7.1 *In Vivo Response*

A HA coating reacts in vivo with the surrounding body fluid. As a result, a bone-like apatite layer develops on the coating surface, which is the foundation for further bone matrix development.

Ducheyne et al. [167] investigated and summarised the events taking place on an in vivo HA coating (Fig. 9.33). The coating phases (1) dissolve at various rates. In return, the body fluid (2) precipitates on the ceramic, and (3) ion exchange between the two substances occurs. These modifications (4) within the coating surface continue, as well, into deeper layers, ending in the crystallisation of the calcium-poor amorphous calcium phosphate and the development of a bone-like apatite layer [149]. The ion changes in the body fluid near the coating surface (5) influence the activity of bone-forming cells. The osteoblasts either (6) deposit on the coating surface or (7) deposit within the coating. Depending on the environmental conditions, the cells will then deposit either (a) mineral or (b) organic substances. Later, activated by (8) chemotaxis (via chemical impulses that are activated by cell movement) osteoprogenitor cells, preosteoblasts, (9), settle on the coating surface and proliferation starts (10). Cell differentiation into osteoblasts and the formation of extracellular matrix take place.

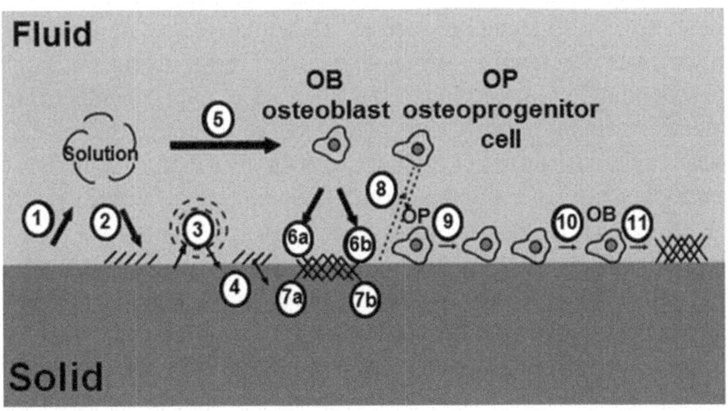

Fig. 9.33 Schematic diagram of events taking place on an in vivo HA coating (Ducheyne et al. [168]. Reprinted with permission. The copyright is held by the referenced source)

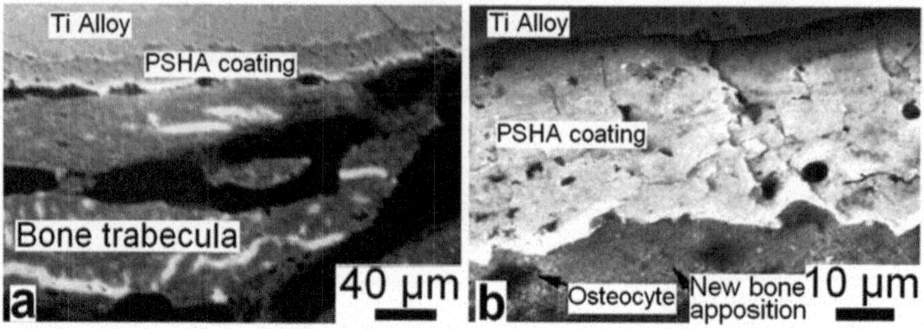

Fig. 9.34 ESEM micrograph of a plasma-sprayed HA-coated Ti alloy after 10-day implantation in tibia and femur of dogs. (**a**) Trabecular bone developing on parts of the coating surface. (**b**) A higher-resolution image of (**a**) (Porter et al. [31]. Reprinted with permission. The copyright is held by the referenced source)

Hence, the natural bone modelling process starts, which will soon be followed by remodelling mechanisms; as indicated by (11) in Fig. 9.33. Furthermore, Ducheyne and Qiu (1999) [168] pointed out that different in vivo mechanisms influence the bone growth process on HA coatings.

9.7.2 *Modelling and Remodelling Processes*

Different studies have investigated the bone-forming cell behaviour and the long-term bone growth. Porter et al. (2002) [31] observed early bone growth and bone cell activity on some parts of the HA coating surface after 10 days in vivo (Fig. 9.34). They found collagen fibrils, an indicator for the beginning of the bone matrix formation, directly bonded onto the coating surface. Typical apatite crystals were found in other areas of the coating surface. This study shows mineral and organic deposition that was described by Ducheyne et al. [168]. All regions, where bone tissue started bonding on the coating, showed a transition of minerals from HA into the bone matrix. In addition, early osteocytes were found in the interface, including their lacunae (cavities), as a result of the bone-forming process on the HA coating.

Six months after in vivo implantation, Hemmerle et al. (1997) [169] noticed complete bone on-growth of the HA coating. Two types of tissue were found at the coating–bone interface: (1) crystallised, afibrillar and acellular tissue, covering the coating itself, and (2) a bone-like mineralised matrix, which had developed on top of the first growth layer (Fig. 9.35a). Both phases support the model [168] where mineralisation on the coating surface is followed by cell activities on top of this.

Hardy et al. (1991) [170] examined hip stems in autopsies after an average of 6-month implantation time. The coating was totally covered by natural bone matrix. Depending on the precise location in the femur, the bone tissue consisted of a thick layer of cancellous bone, followed by the cortex (Fig. 9.35b, c, d). Some parts of the

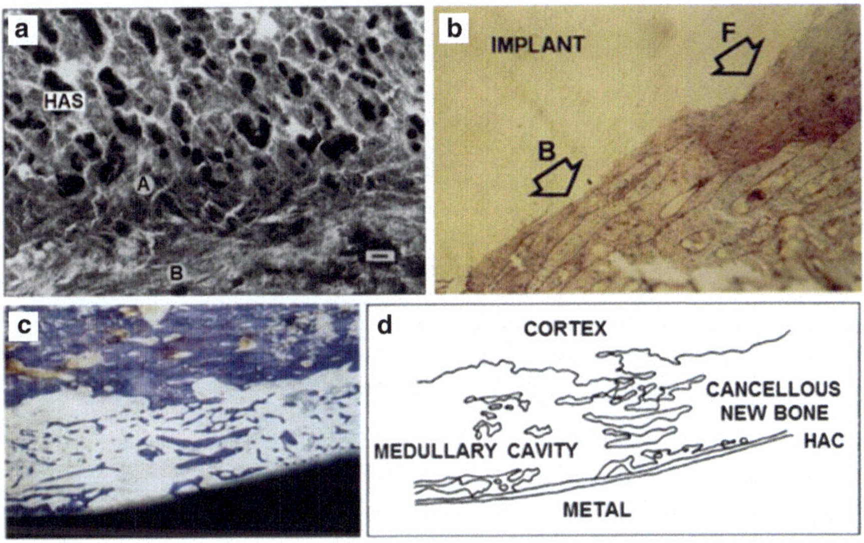

Fig. 9.35 HA coating–bone interface after six month. (**a**) Acellular and afibrillar mineralisation of coating periphery (A) and mineralised bone-like tissue (B) (Hemmerle et al. [169]). (**b**) After prosthesis removal, fibrous tissue "F" is observed between the bone and implant in the proximal, uncoated area. Region B shows that there is less fibrous tissue where the HA coating begins. (Masson's trichrome × 20) (**d**) shows a diagram of features revealed in (**c**), which is a longitudinal section of the calcar. The gap between the calcar femorale and the implant is filled with cancellous new bone (Toluidine blue × 170) (Hardy et al. [170]) (Reprinted with permission. The copyright is held by the referenced sources)

cancellous bone revealed greater amounts of stromal tissue, which are the remains of the initial bone-growing phase, before final bone matrix development took place. The development of two different tissues was detected at the intersection between the coated and uncoated implant surface. Cancellous bone was observed on the coated area of the implant. However, only loose fibrous matrix was present on the metal surface (Fig. 9.35b) at those locations where the coating terminated. This evidence of bone growth supports the beneficial properties of HA coatings.

Porter et al. [171] revealed via autopsy the long-term behaviour of HA coatings on titanium stems. It was observed that bone matrix bonded on the entire coating after 8.5 months. Furthermore, they detected parts of the mineralised HA coating within the newly developed bone and osteocytes within the young bone tissue as a result of the bone modelling process. In addition, Porter et al. identified that the new bone matrix had not only grown inside the HA coating pores in some regions but also all through the coating until it reached the metal surface (Fig. 9.36a). The same observation of bone on-growth and bone ingrowth was determined by Dippel et al. (1998) [172] in their in vivo studies (Fig. 9.36b).

Thus, several studies have observed (1) good bone growth along the coating surface, (2) rapid and highly dense cell activity, and (3) good bonding of bone onto the HA coating.

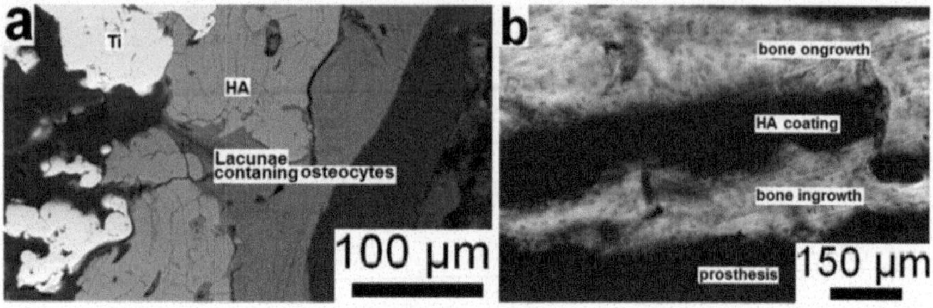

Fig. 9.36 Bone growth on and within hydroxyapatite coating on the implant surface (**a**) after 8.5 month, by Porter et al. [171], and (**b**) after 18 month, by Dippel et al. [172] (Reprinted with permission. The copyright is held by the referenced sources)

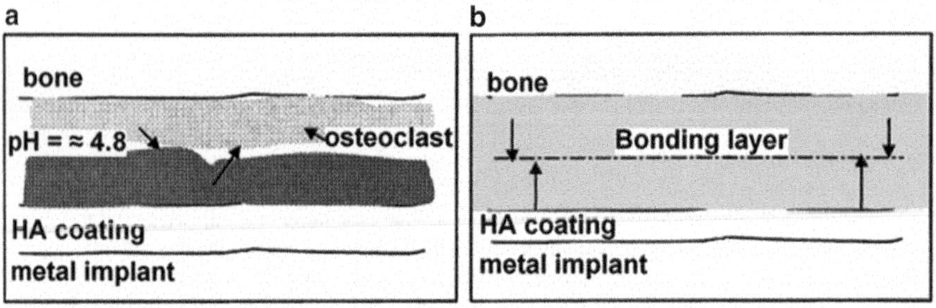

Fig. 9.37 A schematic that depicts bone remodelling. (**a**) Osteoclasts reduce pH to fasten the resorption of HA in bone and, therefore as well, in the coating. (**b**) Bidirectional growth leads to development of a bonding layer (Sun et al. [40]. Reprinted with permission. The copyright is held by the referenced source)

After the first bone modelling, remodelling processes change the coating–bone interface. Sun et al. (2001) [40] described this process by means of a model (Fig. 9.37). The new bone matrix encloses osteoclasts that resorb normal bone so that the bone forms in response to the mechanical needs. In this process, the normal pH of around 7.4 is adjusted to pH 4.8, which leads to faster resorption of carbonated HA in bone as well as the HA coating (Fig. 9.37a). The newly developed bone on the coating grows towards the older, original bone matrix, while that one grows towards the coating. This bidirectional growth will lead to a bonding layer (Fig. 9.37b), which ordains the coating for good long-term in vivo performance and stability.

9.7.3 Interactions at the Implant–Coating Interface

Modern metal implants are fabricated from stainless steel or titanium and its alloys. Ti6Al4V is one of the special alloys that has found wide application. These metals have been proved over the last few decades under clinical conditions. The addition of HA, and particularly the coating manufacturing process, has an influence on the metal surface, which has been investigated in several studies to improve the long-term capability of prostheses.

Nelea et al. (2007) [173] examined the interface between a titanium alloy (Ti5Al2.5Fe) and sputtered HA coating. The interface between HA and the alloy developed TiO_2 during the coating process. The oxidation of titanium happens in several stages, from TiO to oxide-deficient phases until the stable TiO_2 phase is formed [173]. The layer of TiO_2 acts as a barrier against further oxidation. The occurrence of titanium dioxide provides unambiguous evidence of oxidation processes during the coating application of HA. The diffusion and accumulation of titanium and TiO_2 was observed in the coating most close to the metal substrate and was defined as the newly developed interface. The oxidation and diffusion processes as well as interface layer location, depth, and composition depended on the coating process parameters of temperature, heating duration, and the gas environment.

The oxidation of titanium may take place via three mechanisms during the sputtering process. The titanium may diffuse into the HA due to the elevated temperature of the sputtering process, whereupon uptake of oxygen from the amorphous phase, which tends to be located in the deeper layers of the coating, takes place. Secondly, the oxygen from the amorphous phase may diffuse into the metal surface and lead to titanium oxidation. Thirdly, oxygen from the working gas of the sputtering process can be absorbed by the HA coating and diffuse towards the metal base. These mechanistic diffusion and oxidation processes have been observed by Nieh et al. (2001) [174].

Other coating studies [175, 176] employed a pulsed laser method under a water atmosphere to deposit HA coatings onto Ti6Al4V. The naturally formed oxide on Ti6Al4V developed into a thick interface layer when exposed to the coating application conditions. Raman spectroscopy revealed different types of oxidised titanium over the time, for example, TiO_{2-x} and amorphous Ti_2O_3. The oxidation process was explained under three mechanisms [175]: (1) The oxygen within the HA coating can be a source for oxygen, (2) oxygen from the water atmosphere may diffuse through the coating to the metal surface, and (3) the HA coating may perform as a barrier and hinder oxygen diffusion towards the Ti6Al4V. The first two models provide explanations for the growth of the oxidised interface layer after application of HA coating layers.

The mechanism concerning the HA acting as a barrier to oxygen was based on the observation of decreasing O/Ti ratios in the upper layers of the interface over longer heat treatment periods. This specific statement opposes that of other studies [173]. However, there is some agreement that the behaviour of the coating and the interface layer depends on heat treatment, environmental gas, the phase components, and their ratios.

The interface layer between the pulsed laser deposited HA coating and Ti6Al4V metal has been investigated [176] in detail with secondary ion mass spectroscopy (SIMS), scanning electron microscopy (SEM), X-ray diffraction (XRD), Raman spectroscopy, and X-ray photoelectron spectroscopy (XPS) (Fig. 9.38). The distance intervals between the sampling points were about 0.5 μm.

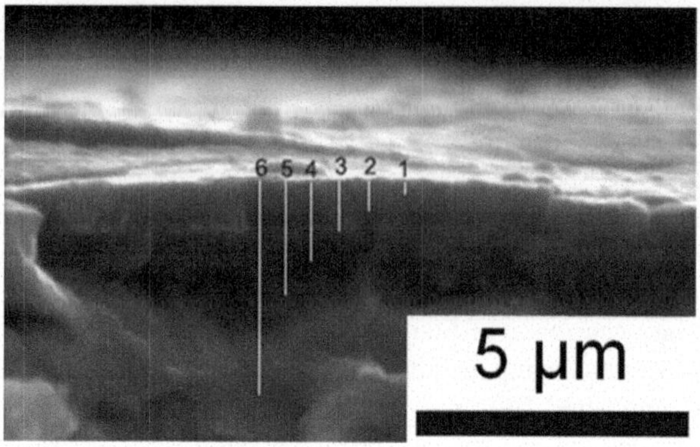

Fig. 9.38 SEM cross section of HA coating, interface, and titanium alloy with mark-ups of SIMS points 1–6 (Fernández-Pradas et al. [176]. Reprinted with permission. The Copyright is held by the referenced source)

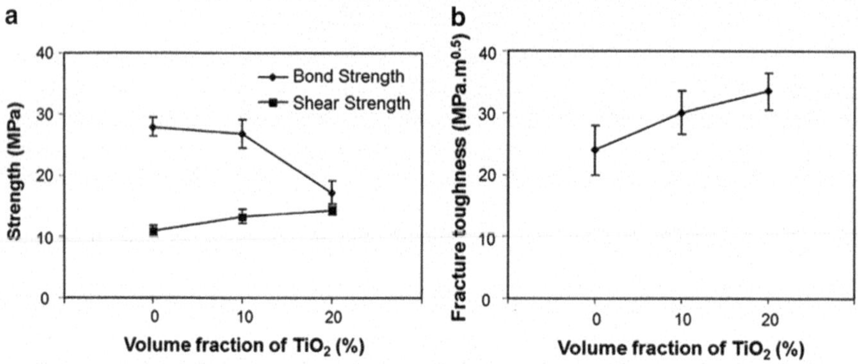

Fig. 9.39 Hydroxyapatite-TiO_2 coating. (**a**) Strength and (**b**) fracture toughness (Li et al. [177]. Reprinted with permission. The copyright is held by the referenced sources)

The precise details of this fundamental research are outside the scope of this current chapter. The summary comments show that the surface of the titanium alloy exhibited a thin layer of titanium oxide before the application of the HA coating. An oxide layer of $TiO_{2\text{-}x}$ developed on top of the metal surface during the coating application process. Amorphous Ti_2O_3 appeared at the interface between the oxide layer and HA coating, which indicates that less oxygen diffused towards the alloy rather than away from it. This supports the theory that HA coatings may act as an oxygen barrier.

Li et al. (2002) [177] examined the influence of titanium dioxide on the mechanical properties of plasma-sprayed HA coatings (Fig. 9.39). HA–TiO_2 coatings were formed by adding regulated amounts of TiO_2 to the feedstock. In addition to the typical HA coating phases and titanium oxide, $CaTiO_3$ was found; indicating a reaction between the two feedstock constituents. The investigation of the mechanical properties of this coating revealed an increase of the Young's modulus, in conformity with expectations when adding a material with a higher modulus. However, the Young's modulus decreased with an increase in the titanium volume percentage due to the influence of newly developed multiphases. The same phases also attributed to a lower bond strength.

As well, the properties of titanium dioxide influenced the shear strength. The low coefficient of thermal expansion decreased the composite coefficient of the coating and reduced stresses at the coating–metal interface, thereby improving the shear strength. Furthermore, the addition of TiO_2 improved the fracture toughness by increasing the bonding between the splats due to beneficial chemical reactions. The addition of 10 vol.% of titanium dioxide improved the mechanical properties of the HA coating. Thus, the development of an intermediate layer of TiO_2 and HA may not necessarily weaken the metal-coating system.

9.7.4 Engineering Models for Coating–Implant Interactions

HA is used extensively in dental surgery; for example, Hedia (2007) [178] examined the influence of a graded Young's modulus on the von Mises stresses of HA-coated dental implants. The two-dimensional model simulated the load force under chewing conditions with a refined finite mesh at the coating–bone interface. The von Mises stresses within the coating were examined under two coating parameters: (1) a singular Young's modulus throughout the coating and (2) a graded modulus that was 110 GPa at the coating apex and 2 GP at the coating root that was located in the bone.

HA, as it is used for medical coatings, is a complex, orthotropic material composed of different phases that exhibits different mechanical properties and in vivo behaviour. The HA interfaces, both at the bone and metal locations, influence the long-term performance of the coating. An artificial bone-like apatite layer is formed at the bone–coating interface via chemical processes, which stimulates the contact and activity of bone-developing cells. Regions of the coating dissolve during this process by means of bone modelling and remodelling procedures. There is a synergy between weakening of the coating in terms of Young's modulus and bond strength but at the same time intimate contact with the bone that is the foundation for stabilisation and fixation of the implant.

An intermediate layer with oxidised metal elements and coating particles develops during the coating application process by thermal spray deposition. The influence of this process and the layer itself has not been detailed in the literature. In some cases, this layer does not always occur for HA coatings.

Several finite element models have examined coatings under special load conditions [179–181]. These models are all based on the principle of unified, isotropic coating layers that do not, for example, distinguish between microstructural features such as porosity and the different arrangements and ratios of amorphous and crystalline HA. Thus, the outcomes of such studies need to be treated with caution.

Another aspect concerning the finite element studies is that the temporal changes in the HA coatings, that is, the dissolution, modelling, and remodelling processes, have not been adequately addressed. There will be microstructural changes in terms of phase distribution, porosity, and cracking associated with these changes, all of which will influence the three-dimensional stress state of the coating–implant–body interactions. Neither macroscopic nor microscopic models have addressed these issues.

Thus, the above factors lead to failure between crystalline and amorphous HA splats in clinical coatings when the inherent stresses are sufficiently high. Splat delamination may result and give rise to the HA coating failures that have been reported in the literature [163].

9.8 Concluding Remarks

Hydroxyapatite-coated prostheses have demonstrated clinical success. However, there is still much to learn concerning their optimisation and functionality from the perspective of a fundamental mechanistic understanding. Further studies, for example, could investigate the changes of stress in the coating under various crystallinity and porosity levels and how dissolution changes the three-dimensional structure of the coating over time.

Another study could deal with the reliance of the dissolution rate and its influence on the microstructure–performance relationship. In this study, the fundamental building block of a thermal spray HA coating would be assessed. That is, the intrinsic splat structure of the coating would be used as a metric to examine the HA structure layer-by-layer. An arrangement as described in Table 9.12 could be adopted for such an analysis. Thereby the bone layer would be designed as a simple plate with a bonded contact to the coating surface. The bone material parameters could be chosen [182] with a Young's modulus for new bone of 5 GPa and a Poisson's ratio of 0.3.

Some recommendations for HA coatings can be provided:

1. The coating porosity should not be too high since the pores are a main location for high stresses, which could lead to the failure of splat adhesion with the possible result of coating delamination. However, a certain porosity, especially at the coating surface, is necessary for the adhesion of bone-forming cells onto the coating.

Table 9.12 Possible dependencies for a bone growth study

	Ratio[a]				
	1:1	1.5:1	2:1	2.5:1	3:1
Bone appearance week	1	1	2	2	3
Bone layer growth rate per week [%]	90	75	65	50	40

[a]The ratio refers to a ratio of crystalline splats to amorphous splats summed over the three topmost coating layers. The week refers to the dissolution week for the initial appearance of a thin bone layer

2. A higher amount of crystalline splats at the coating bottom will ensure a better transition of stress between the coating and metal implant. This will lead to longer-lasting adhesion between both components and, therewith, support the long-term in vivo performance of a HA-coated implant.
3. Amorphous splats should be located, preferably, at the coating surface. Low stresses in these splats will support a bone modelling and remodelling process better than either (1) high stresses within crystalline splats or (2) the stress peaks that may appear at the interfaces between amorphous and crystalline splats. Furthermore, more rapid dissolution of amorphous splats enhances growth of bone tissue on and into the coating.
4. Some crystalline splats should be located in the vicinity of the coating surface since these splats provide a base for bone-forming cells. The amorphous HA is replaced as it dissolves in vivo.
5. The crystallisation rate between the different layers throughout the coating should change constantly: from mostly crystalline at the bottom towards mostly amorphous at the surface. Thus, large differences in crystallisation of neighbouring layers should be avoided since splats with different material properties cause stress jumps within the coating. Any large discontinuities in stress could result in delamination of splats or the coating architecture.

Acknowledgments Mr. Md. Fahad Hasan thanks the Swinburne University of Technology for the provision of a postgraduate research scholarship that has enabled this research to be performed. Ms. Tietz performed this work while she was a student visiting Australia. The authors thank the academic administrators at the Swinburne University of Technology in Australia and the University of Rostock in Germany who facilitated this cooperation. As well, CCB thanks Professor Besim Ben-Nissan for his constant encouragement and support in this exciting area over some 25 years. He has been truly inspirational.

References

1. Lysaght MJ, O'Loughlin JA (2000) Demographic scope and economic magnitude of contemporary organ replacement therapies. ASAIO J 46(5):515–521
2. Ratner BD, Hoffman AS, Schoen FJ, Lemons JE (eds) (1996) Biomaterials science: an introduction to materials in medicine. Academic, San Diego
3. Balani K, Anderson R, Laha T, Andara M, Tercero J, Crumpler E, Agarwal A (2007) Plasma-sprayed carbon nanotube reinforced hydroxyapatite coatings and their interaction with human osteoblasts in vitro. Biomaterials 28(4):618–624
4. Hench LL (1998) Bioceramics. J Am Ceram Soc 81(7):1705–1727
5. Li P, De Groot K (1993) Calcium phosphate formation within sol-gel prepared titania in vitro and in vivo. J Biomed Mater Res 27(12):1495–1500
6. Locardi B, Pazzaglia UE, Gabbi C, Profilo B (1993) Thermal behaviour of hydroxyapatite intended for medical applications. Biomaterials 14(6):437–441
7. Ong JL, Lucas LC (1994) Post-deposition heat treatments for ion beam sputter deposited calcium phosphate coatings. Biomaterials 15(5):337–341
8. Liu RF, Xiao XF, Lin LY, Ni J, Chen GY (2004) Study on the bonding strength and thermal stability of electrodeposition HA/TiO_2 composite coating. Chin J Inorg Chem 20(2):225–230

9. Myoui A, Tamai N, Nishikawa M, Araki N, Nakase T, Akita S, Yoshikawa H (2004) Three-dimensionally engineered hydroxyapatite ceramics with interconnected pores as a bone substitute and tissue engineering scaffold. In: Yaszemski MJ, Trantolo DJ, Lewandrowski KU, Hasirci V, Altobelli DE, Wise DL (eds) Biomaterials in orthopedics. Marcel Dekker, New York, pp 287–300
10. Albee FH (1920) Studies in bone growth: triple calcium phosphate as a stimulus to osteogenesis. Ann Surg 71(1):32–39
11. Geros L, Geros RZ (1993) Dense hydroxyapatite. In: Hench LL, Wilson J (eds) An introduction to bioceramics. World Scientific, River Edge, NJ, USA, pp 139–180
12. Schneider SJ Jr (1991) Ceramics and glasses. ASM International, Materials Park
13. Dumbleton J, Manley MT (2004) Hydroxyapatite-coated prostheses in total hip and knee arthroplasty. J Bone Joint Surg 86(11):2526–2540
14. Chou L, Marek B, Wagner WR (1999) Effects of hydroxylapatite coating crystallinity on biosolubility, cell attachment efficiency and proliferation in vitro. Biomaterials 20(10):977–985
15. De Groot K, Geesink R, Klein CP, Serekian P (1987) Plasma sprayed coatings of hydroxylapatite. J Biomed Mater Res 21:1375–1381
16. Beevers CA, McIntyre DB (1946) The atomic structure of fluorapatite and its relation to that of tooth and bone material. Miner Mag 27:254–257
17. Sudarsanan K, Young RA (1969) Significant precision in crystal structural details: holly springs hydroxyapatite. Acta Crystallographica B (Struct Crystallogr Crystal Chem) B25:1534–1543
18. Elliot JC, Mackie PE, Young RA (1973) Monoclinic hydroxyapatite. Science 180:1055–1057
19. Haverty D, Tofail SAM, Stanton KT, McMonagle JB (2005) Structure and stability of hydroxyapatite: density functional calculation and rietveld analysis. Phys Rev B Condens Matter Mater Phys 71(9):1–9
20. Ravaglioli A, Krajewik A (1992) Bioceramics: materials, properties, applications. Springer, Dordrecht
21. Lacout JL (1992) Calcium phosphates as bioceramics. In: Muster D (ed) Biomaterials–hard tissue repair and replacement. Elsevier Science, Amsterdam, pp 81–95
22. White AA, Kinloch IA, Windle AH, Best SM (2010) Optimization of the sintering atmosphere for high-density hydroxyapatite–carbon nanotube composites. R Soc Interface 7(Suppl 15):S529–S539
23. Gross KA, Berndt CC, Stephens P, Dinnebier R (1998) Oxyapatite in hydroxyapatite coatings. J Mater Sci 33(15):3985–3991
24. Fang Y, Agrawal DK, Roy DM (1994) Thermal stability of synthetic hydroxyapatite. In: Hydroxyapatite and related materials. CRC Press, Boca Raton
25. Nicholson JW (2002) The chemistry of medical and dental materials. Royal Society of Chemistry, Cambridge, UK
26. Lee JH (2012) Tensegrity-inspired nanocomposite structures. PhD thesis, Georgia Institute of Technology, August 2012. See https://smartech.gatech.edu/bitstream/handle/1853/44839/Lee_JiHoon_201208_phd.pdf. Accessed 22 Nov 2013
27. Zanello LP, Zhao B, Hu H, Haddon RC (2006) Bone cell proliferation on carbon nanotubes. Nano Lett 6(3):562–567
28. Heimann RB (2006) Thermal spraying of biomaterials. Surf Coat Technol 201(5):2012–2019
29. Sun L, Berndt CC, Khor KA, Cheang HN, Gross KA (2002) Surface characteristics and dissolution behavior of plasma-sprayed hydroxyapatite coating. J Biomed Mater Res 62(2):228–236
30. Ducheyne P, Beight J, Cuckler J, Evans B, Radin S (1990) Effect of calcium phosphate coating characteristics on early post-operative bone tissue ingrowth. Biomaterials 11(8):531–540
31. Porter AE, Hobbs LW, Benezra Rosen V, Spector M (2002) The ultrastructure of the plasma-sprayed hydroxyapatite-bone interface predisposing to bone bonding. Biomaterials 23:725–733

32. Terner LL, Moskowitz D, Van Alsten RL (1979) European Patent EP 0005632 A2 Plasma spray coating composition, method of coating articles and articles coated with the composition. 28 November 1979. See http://www.google.com/patents/EP0005632A2. Accessed 22 Nov 2013
33. Liao C-J, Lin F-H, Chen K-S, Sun J-S (1999) Thermal decomposition and reconstitution of hydroxyapatite in air atmosphere. Biomaterials 20(19):1807–1813
34. Sridhar TM, Kamachi Mudali U, Subbaiyan M (2003) Sintering atmosphere and temperature effects on hydroxyapatite coated type 316L stainless steel. Corros Sci 45(10):2337–2359
35. Yang Y, Kim KH, Agrawal CM, Ong JL (2004) Interaction of hydroxyapatite-titanium at elevated temperature in vacuum environment. Biomaterials 25(15):2927–2932
36. Lazić S, Zec S, Miljević N, Milonjić S (2001) The effect of temperature on the properties of hydroxyapatite precipitated from calcium hydroxide and phosphoric acid. Thermochimica Acta 374(1):13–22
37. Huiskes R (1993) Mechanical failure in total hip arthroplasty with cement. Curr Orthop Biomech 7:239–247
38. Levingstone TJ (2008) Optimization of plasma sprayed hydroxyapatite coatings. PhD thesis, Dublin City University, Ireland
39. Anonymous (2008) ASTM F1609 – 08 standard specification for calcium phosphate coatings for implantable materials. American Society for Testing and Materials, West Conshohocken
40. Sun L, Berndt CC, Gross KA, Kucuk A (2001) Material fundamentals and clinical performance of plasma-sprayed hydroxyapatite coatings: a review. J Biomed Mater Res A 58(5):570–592
41. Anonymous, ASTM F1185-03 (2003) Standard specification for composition of ceramic hydroxyapatite for surgical implants. ASTM International, West Conshohocken
42. Anonymous (2000) BS ISO 13779-2:2000, International Organisation for Standards Implants for Surgery-Hydroxyapatite. Part 2: Coatings of Hydroxyapatite.
43. Taylor MP (1994) Assessment of plasma-sprayed hydroxyapatite coatings. PhD thesis, University of Birmingham, Birmingham
44. Cheang P, Khor KA (1995) Thermal spraying of hydroxyapatite (HA) coatings: effects of powder feedstock. J Mater Process Technol 48(1–4):429–436
45. Martin RB, Burr DB, Sharkey NA (1998) Skeletal tissue mechanics. Springer, New York
46. Anonymous (2013) Encyclopaedia Britannica, Compact bone: human bone structure. http://www.britannica.com/EBchecked/topic/129490/compact-bone. Britannica
47. Wick D (2005) Biomechanical basics of sports movements. Spitta Verlag, Balingen
48. Zhu K, Greenfield H, Xueqin D, Fraser DR (2001) Improvement of bone health in childhood and adolescence. Nutr Res Rev 14:119–151
49. Schlichting K, Schell H, Kleemann RU, Schill A, Weiler AW, Duda GN, Epari DR (2008) Influence of scaffold stiffness on subchondral bone and subsequent cartilage regeneration in an ovine model of osteochondral defect healing. Am J Sports Med 36(12):2379–2391
50. Meyers MA, Chen P-Y, Lin AY-M, Seki Y (2008) Biological materials: structure and mechanical properties. Prog Mater Sci 53:1–206
51. Wang X, Shen X, Li X, Agrawal CM (2002) Age-related changes in the collagen network and toughness of bone. Bone 31(1):1–7. Erratum in: Bone, 2003, 32(1):107
52. Robinson RA, Elliott SR (1957) The water content of bone. I. The mass of water, inorganic crystals, organic matrix and 'CO_2 space' components in a unit volume of dog bone. J Bone Joint Surg 39(1):167–188
53. Patton HD, Fuchs AF, Hille B, Scher AM, Steiner R (1989) Textbook of physiology, 21st edn. W.B. Saunders Company, Philadelphia, p 1596
54. Ball M, Grant DM, Lo WJ, Scotchford CA (2008) The effect of different surface morphology and roughness on osteoblast-like cells. J Biomed Mater Res A 86(3):637–647
55. Ng AM, Tan KK, Phang MY, Aziyati O, Tan GH, Isa MR, Aminuddin BS, Naseem M, Fauziah O, Ruszymah BH (2008) Differential osteogenic activity of osteoprogenitor cells on HA and TCP/HA scaffold of tissue engineered bone. J Biomed Mater Res 85A:301–312

56. Karsenty G, Kronenberg HM (2003) Postnatal bone growth – growth plate, modeling and remodeling. In: Glorieux FH, Pettifor JM, Jüppner H (eds) Pediatric bone: biology and diseases. Elsevier, London, pp 119–133
57. Ott SM (2002) Histomorphometric analysis of bone remodeling. In: Boleziian JP, Raisz LG, Gideon GA (eds) Principles of bone biology. Academic Press, San Diego, pp 303–320
58. Landis WJ, Librizzi MG, Dunn MG, Silver FH (1995) A study of the relationship between mineral content and mechanical properties of turkey gastrocnemius tendon. J Bone Min Res 10:859–867
59. Rho J-Y, Tsui TY, Pharr GM (1997) Elastic properties of human cortical and trabecular lamellar bone measured by nanoindentation. Biomaterials 18:1325–1330
60. Reilly DT, Burnstein AH, Frankel VH (1974) The elastic modulus of bone. J Biomech 7:271–275
61. Bloebaum RD, Skedros FG, Vajda EG, Bachus KN, Constantz BR (1997) Determining mineral content variations in bone using backscattered electron imaging. Bone 20(5):485–490
62. Grosland NM, Goel VK, Lakes RS (2001) Techniques and applications of adaptive bone remodeling concepts. In: Leondes C (ed) Biomechanical systems – techniques and applications: musculoskeletal models and techniques. CRC Press, Boca Raton
63. Jäger I, Fratzl P (2000) Mineralized collagen fibrils: a mechanical model with a staggered arrangement of mineral particles. J Biophys 79:1737–1746
64. Anonymous ASTM standard C633-01: standard test method for adhesion or cohesive strength of flame-sprayed coatings, American Society for Testing and Materials, West Conshohocken
65. Osborn JF (1985) The biomaterial hydroxylapatite ceramic – basics and clinical application. Quintessenz Verlag, Dordrecht
66. Osborn JF (1987) The biological benefit of ceramic hydroxylapatite coatings for a titanium femur implant – first histological evaluations of a human explants (Die bilogische Leistung der Hydroxylapatitkeramikbeschichtung aud dem Femurschaft einer Titanendoprothese – erste histologische auswertung eines Humanexplanates). Biomed Technik 32:177–183 (in German)
67. Monarcho MR, Constant G (1985) Spraying techniques for apatite coatings. Couches Minces Vide 40:305–308
68. Anonymous (2001) http://www.handbookofmineralogy.org/pdfs/hydroxylapatite.pdf "Hydroxylapatite", Mineral Data Publishing
69. Bongio M, van den Beucken JJ, Nejadnik MR, Leeuwenburgh SC, Kinard LA, Kasper FK, Mikos AG, Jansen JA (2011) Biomimetic modification of synthetic hydrogels by incorporation of adhesive peptides and calcium phosphate nanoparticles: in vitro evaluation of cell behavior. Eur Cells Mater 22:359–376
70. Aydin E, Planell JA, Hasirci V (2011) Hydroxyapatite nanorod-reinforced biodegradable poly(l-lactic acid) composites for bone plate applications. J Mater Sci Mater Med 22(11):2413–2427
71. Li TT, Lee JH, Kobayashi T, Aoki H (1996) Hydroxyapatite coating by dipping method and bone bonding strength. J Mater Sci Mater Med 7:355–357
72. Russell SW, Luptak KA, Suchicital CTA, Alford TL, Pizziconi VB (1996) Chemical and structural evolution of sol-gel-derived hydroxyapatite thin films under rapid thermal processing. J Am Ceram Soc 79(4):837–842
73. Seema K, Uma B, Suchita K (2012) Transformations in sol-gel synthesized nanoscale hydroxyapatite calcined under different temperatures and time conditions. J Mater Eng Perform 21(8):1737–1743
74. Singh VK, Reddy BR (2012) Synthesis and characterization of bioactive zirconia toughened alumina doped with HAp and fluoride compounds. Cerami Int 38(7):5333–5340
75. Yankee SJ, Pletka BJ, Luckey HA, Johnson WA (1990) Process for fabricating HA coatings for biomedical applications, thermal spray research and applications. In: Third annual thermal spray conference. ASM International, Materials Park, pp 433–438

76. Li H, Khor KA, Chow V, Cheang P (2007) Nanostructural characteristics, mechanical properties and osteoblast response of spark plasma sintered hydroxyapatite. J Biomed Mater Res 82A:296–303
77. Blalock TL, Bai X, Narayan R, Rabiei A (2008) Effect of substrate temperature on mechanical properties of calcium phosphate coatings. Appl Biomater Pt B 85B:60–67
78. Drevet R, Fauré J, Benhayoune H (2012) Thermal treatment optimization of electrodeposited hydroxyapatite coatings on TI6Al4v substrate. Adv Eng Mater 14(6):377–382
79. Jamesh M, Kumar S, Sankara Narayanan TSN (2011) Electrodeposition of hydroxyapatite coating on magnesium for biomedical applications. J Coat Technol Res 9(4):495–502
80. Chen F, Lam WM, Lin CJ, Qiu GX, Wu ZH, Luk KDK, Lu WW (2007) Biocompatibility of electrophoretical deposition of nanostructured hydroxyapatite coating on roughen titanium surface: In vitro evaluation using mesenchymal stem cells. J Biomed Mater Res B Appl Biomater 82(1):183–191
81. Johnson S (2005) Pulsed laser deposition of hydroxyapatite thin films. Master's thesis, Georgia Institute of Technology, January 2005. See https://smartech.gatech.edu/. Accessed 22 Nov 2013
82. Thian ES, Huang J, Ahmad Z, Edirisinghe MJ, Jayasinghe SN, Ireland DC, Brooks RA, Rushton N, Best SM, Bonfield W (2008) Influence of nanohydroxyapatite patterns deposited by electrohydrodynamic spraying on osteoblast response. J Biomed Mater Res 85A:188–194
83. Lin CK, Berndt CC (1994) Measurement and analysis of adhesion strength for thermally sprayed coatings. J Therm Spray Technol 3(1):75–104
84. Khor KA, Gu YW, Pan D, Cheang P (2004) Microstructure and mechanical properties of plasma sprayed HA/YSZ/Ti-6Al-4V composite coatings. Biomaterials 25(18):4009–4017
85. Yang YC, Chang E, Lee SY (2003) Mechanical properties and Young's modulus of plasma sprayed hydroxyapatite coating on Ti substrate in simulated body fluid. J Biomed Mater Res 67A:886–899
86. Sun L, Berndt CC, Gross KA (2001) Characterization and mechanical properties of flame sprayed hydroxyapatite/polymer composite coatings. In: Berndt CC, Khor KA, Lugscheider EF (eds) Thermal spray 2001: new surfaces for a millennium. ASM International, Materials Park
87. Khor KA, Li H, Cheang P (2003) Characterization of bone-like apatite precipitated on high velocity oxy-fuel (HVOF) sprayed calcium phosphate deposits. Biomaterials 24:769–775
88. Balani K, Chen Y, Harimkar SP, Dahotre NB, Agarwal A (2007) Tribological behavior of plasma-sprayed carbon nanotube-reinforced hydroxyapatite coating in physiological solution. Acta Biomater 3(6):944–951
89. Mancini CE, Berndt CC, Sun L, Kucuk A (2001) Porosity determinations in thermally sprayed hydroxyapatite coatings. J Mater Sci 36(16):3891–3896
90. Kweh SWK, Khor KA, Cheang P (2002) An in vitro investigation of plasma sprayed hydroxyapatite (HA) coatings produced with flame-spheroidized feedstock. Biomaterials 23(3):775–785
91. Chawla V, Sidhu BS, Puri D, Prakash S (2007) State of art: plasma sprayed nanostructured coatings: a review. Mater Forum 32:137–143
92. Ding C, Liu X, Zheng X (2003) Biocompatibility of plasma-sprayed biomedical coatings. Mater Sci Forum 439:30–33
93. Pawlowski L (2008) The science and engineering of thermal spray coatings. Wiley, Chichester
94. Anonymous (2013) DC plasma modelling, Centre for Advanced Coating Technologies, University of Toronto. http://www.mie.utoronto.ca/labs/cact/Research/DCPlasma/DCPlasma.html
95. Davis JR (2004) Handbook of thermal spray technology. ASM Thermal Spray Society, Materials Park
96. Deram V, Minichiello C, Vannier R-N, Le Maguer A, Pawlowski L, Murano DD (2003) Microstructural characterizations of plasma sprayed hydroxyapatite coatings. Surf Coat Technol 166:153–159

97. Narayanan R, Seshadri SK, Kwon TY, Kim KH (2008) Review: calcium phosphate-based coatings in titanium and its alloys. J Biomed Mater Res B Appl Biomater 85B:279–299
98. Li H, Khor KA, Cheang P (2004) Thermal sprayed hydroxyapatite splats: nanostructures, pore formation mechanisms and TEM characterization. Biomaterials 25(17):3463–3471
99. Zhao L, Bobzin K, Ernst F, Zwick J, Lugscheider E (2006) Study on the influence of plasma spray processes and spraying parameters on the structure and crystallinity of hydroxylapatite coatings (Untersuchung des EInflusses der Spritzverfahren und -paramter auf die Schichtstruktur und -kristallinität von Hydroxylapatit). Mat-wiss u Werkstofftechn 37(6):516–520 (in German)
100. Gordon England Independent metallurgist and consultant to the Thermal Spray Coating Industry, Plasma spray process. http://www.gordonengland.co.uk
101. Montavon G, Sampath S, Berndt CC, Herman H, Coddet C (1995) Effects of vacuum plasma spray processing parameters on splat morphology. J Therm Spray Technol 4(1):67–74
102. Cizek J, Khor KA, Prochazka Z (2007) Influence of spraying conditions on thermal and velocity properties of plasma sprayed hydroxyapatite. Mater Sci Eng C 27(2):340–344
103. Guessasma S, Montavon G, Coddet C (2005) Velocity and temperature distributions of alumina-titania in-flight particles in the atmospheric plasma spray process. Surf Coat Technol 192(1):70–76
104. Tsui YC, Doyle C, Clyne TW (1998) Plasma sprayed hydroxyapatite coatings on titanium substrates – Part 1: mechanical properties and residual stress levels. Biomaterials 19(22):2015–2029
105. Sun L, Berndt CC, Grey CP (2003) Phase, structural and microstructural investigations of plasma sprayed hydroxyapatite coatings. Mater Sci Eng A 360(1–2):70–84
106. Yang CY, Wang BC, Chang E, Wu JD (1995) The influences of plasma spraying parameters on the characteristics of hydroxyapatite coatings: a quantitative study. J Mater Sci Mater Med 6(5):249–257
107. Quek CH, Khor KA, Cheang P (1999) Influence of processing parameters in the plasma spraying of hydroxyapatite/Ti-6Al-4V composite coatings. J Mater Process Technol 89–90:550–555
108. Funk W, Goebe F (1985) Bond strength optimization of plasma-sprayed Cr2O3 layers by factorial two-level experiments. Thin Solid Films 128:45–55
109. Fauchais P (2004) Understanding plasma spraying. J Phys D Appl Phys 37(9):R86–R108
110. Leung K, Heberlein J, Pfender E (1995) Particle trajectory control with the use of different carrier gases, thermal spray science and technology. In: Berndt CC, Sampath S (eds) 8th national thermal spray conference. ASM International, Materials Park
111. Lacefield WR (1993) Hydroxylapatite coatings. In: Hench LL, Wilson J (eds) An introduction to bioceramics. World Scientific Publishing Company, Singapore
112. Mawdsley JR, Su YJ, Faber KT, Bernecki TF (2001) Optimization of small-particle plasma-sprayed alumina coatings using designed experiments. Mater Sci Eng A 308(1–2):189–199
113. Kweh SW, Khor KA, Cheang P (2000) Plasma-sprayed hydroxyapatite (HA) coatings with flame-spheroidized feedstock: microstructure and mechanical properties. Biomaterials 21:1223–1234
114. Lu YP, Li ST, Zhu RF, Li MS (2002) Further studies on the effect of stand-off distance on characteristics of plasma sprayed hydroxyapatite coating. Surf Coat Technol 157(2–3):221–225
115. Tsui YC, Doyle C, Clyne TW (1998) Plasma sprayed hydroxyapatite coatings on titanium substrates. Part 2: optimisation of coating properties. Biomaterials 19(22):2031–2043
116. Khor KA, Li H, Cheang P (2004) Significance of melt-fraction in HVOF sprayed hydroxyapatite particles, splats and coatings. Biomaterials 25(7–8):1177–1186
117. Anonymous (2013) High velocity oxygen fuel thermal spray process. http://www.gordonengland.co.uk/. Gordon England – Independent Metallurgist and consultant to the Thermal Spray Coating Industry
118. Anonymous (2013) HVOF/AF. http://www.metal-monster.com/HVOF_HVAF.html. Metal-Monster Ltd., North Shore 2013, Metal-Monster, 2013

119. Gross KA, Berndt CC (1998) Thermal processing of hydroxyapatite for coating production. J Biomed Mater Res 39:580–587
120. Li H, Khor KA, Cheang P (2002) Properties of heat-treated calcium phosphate coatings deposited by high-velocity oxy-fuel (HVOF) spray. Biomaterials 23:2105–2112
121. Gross KA, Berndt CC, Herman H (1998) Amorphous phase formation in plasma-sprayed hydroxyapatite coatings. J Biomed Mater Res 39(3):407–414
122. Weng J, Liu X-G, Li X-D, Zhang X-D (1995) Intrinsic factors of apatite influencing its amorphization during plasma-spray coating. Biomaterials 16(1):39–44
123. Overgaard S, Bromose U, Lind M, Bünger C, Søballe K (1999) The influence of crystallinity of the hydroxyapatite coating on the fixation of implants. J Bone Joint Surg 81(B):725–731
124. Yamada M, Shiota M, Yamashita Y, Kasugai S (2007) Histological and histomorphometrical comparative study of the degeneration and osteoconductive characteristics of alpha- and beta-tricalcium phosphate in block grafts. J Biomed Mater Res B Appl Biomater 82B:139–148
125. de Bruijn JD, Bovell YP, van Bitterwijk CA (1994) Structural arrangements at the interface between plasma sprayed calcium phosphates and bone. Biomaterials 15(7):543–550
126. Roy RK (2001) Design of experiments using the Taguchi approach: 16 steps to product and process improvement. Wiley, New York
127. Barrentine LB (1999) An introduction to design of experiments. American Society for Quality, Milwaukee
128. Antony J (2003) Design of experiments for engineers and scientists. Butterworth-Heinemann, Oxford
129. Anonymous (2013) Design of experiments (DOE), http://www.moresteam.com/toolbox/t408.cfm. Accessed 22 Nov 2013
130. Anonymous (2013) JMP software, DOE. http://www.jmp.com/capabilities/DOE.shtml. SAS Institute Inc. Accessed 22 Nov 2013
131. Lin BT, Jean MD, Chou JH (2007) Using response surface methodology for optimizing deposited partially stabilized zirconia in plasma spraying. Appl Surf Sci 253(6):3254–3262
132. Li JF, Liao H, Normand B, Cordier C, Maurin G, Foct J, Coddet C (2003) Uniform design method for optimization of process parameters of plasma sprayed TiN coatings. Surf Coat Technol 176(1):1–13
133. Steeper TJ, Varacalle DJ, Wilson GC, Riggs WL, Rotolico AJ, Nerz J (1993) A design of experiment study of plasma-sprayed alumina-titania coatings. J Therm Spray Technol 2(3):251–256
134. Dyshlovenko S, Pierlot C, Pawlowski L, Tomaszek R, Chagnon P (2006) Experimental design of plasma spraying and laser treatment of hydroxyapatite coatings. Surf Coat Technol 201(5):2054–2060
135. Dyshlovenko S, Pawlowski L, Roussel P, Murano D, Le Maguer A (2006) Relationship between plasma spray operational parameters and microstructure of hydroxyapatite coatings and powder particles sprayed into water. Surf Coat Technol 200(12–13):3845–3855
136. Kuroda S, Clyne TW (1991) The quenching stress in thermally sprayed coatings. Thin Solid Films 200(1):49–66
137. Deligianni DD, Katsala ND, Koutsoukos PG, Missirlis YF (2001) Effect of surface roughness of hydroxyapatite on human bone marrow cell adhesion, proliferation, differentiation and detachment strength. Biomaterials 22(1):87–96
138. Gross KA, Gross V, Berndt CC (1998) Thermal analysis of amorphous phase in hydroxyapatite coating. J Am Ceram Soc 81(1):106–112
139. Kijima T, Tsutsumi M (1979) Preparation and thermal properties of dense polycrystalline oxyhydroxyapatite. J Am Ceram Soc 62(9–10):455–460
140. Li H, Khor KA (2006) Characteristics of the nanostructures in thermal sprayed hydroxyapatite coatings and their influence on coating properties. Surf Coat Technol 201:2147–2154
141. Chang CK, Wu JS, Mao DL, Ding CX (2001) Mechanical and histological evaluations of hydroxyapatite-coated and noncoated Ti6Al4V implants in tibia bone. J Biomed Mater Res 56:17–23

142. Filliaggi MJ, Coombs NA, Pilliar RM (1991) Characterization of the interface in the plasma-sprayed HA coating/Ti-6Al-4V implant system. J Biomed Mater Res 25:1211–1229
143. Zhang C, Leng Y, Chen J (2001) Elastic and plastic behaviour of plasma sprayed hydroxyapatite coatings on Ti-6Al-4V substrate. Biomaterials 22:1357–1363
144. Wang BC, Lee TM, Chang E, Yang CY (1993) The shear strength and the failure mode of plasma sprayed hydroxyapatite coating to bone: the effect of coating thickness. J Biomed Mater Res 27:1315–1327
145. Yang CY, Wang BC, Lee TM, Chang E, Chang GL (1997) Intramedullary implant of plasma-sprayed hydroxyapatite coating: an interface study. J Biomed Mater Res 36(1):39–48
146. Svehla M, Morberg P, Bruce W, Zicat B, Walsh WR (2002) The effect of substrate roughness and hydroxyapatite coating thickness on implant shear strength. J Arthroplasty 17(3):304–311
147. Ducheyne P, Radin S, King L (1993) The effect of calcium phosphate ceramic composition and structure on in vitro behaviour: I. dissolution. J Biomed Mater Res 27(1):25–34
148. Zhang Q, Chen J, Feng J, Cao Y, Deng C, Zhang X (2003) Dissolution and mineralization behaviours of HA coatings. Biomaterials 24:4741–4748
149. Kim T-M, Himeno T, Kawashita M, Kokubo T, Nakamura T (2004) The mechanism of biomineralization of bone-like apatite on synthetic hydroxyapatite: an in vitro assessment. J R Soc Interface 1:17–22
150. Khor KA, Li H, Cheang P, Boey SY (2003) In vitro behavior of HVOF sprayed calcium phosphate splats and coatings. Biomaterials 24:723–735
151. Weng J, Liu Q, Wolke JG, Zhang X, de Groot K (1997) Formation and characteristics of the apatite layer on plasma-sprayed hydroxyapatite coatings in simulated body fluid. Biomaterials 18:1027–1035
152. Lu JX, Gallur A, Flautre B, Anselme K, Descamps M, Thierry B, Hardouin P (1998) Comparative study of tissue reactions to calcium phosphate ceramics among cancellous, cortical and medullar bone sites in rabbits. Biomed Mater Res 42:357–367
153. Hara T, Hayashi K, Nakashima Y, Kanemaru T, Iwamoto Y (1999) The effect of hydroxyapatite coating on the bonding of bone to titanium implants in the femora of ovariectomised rats. J Bone Joint Surg 81B:705–709
154. Zhao Y, Zhang Y, Ning F, Guo D, Xu Z (2007) Synthesis and cellular biocompatibility of two kinds of HAP with different nanocrystal morphology. J Biomed Mater Res B Appl Biomater 83B:121–126
155. Ergun C, Liu H, Webster TJ, Olcay E, Yilmaz S, Sahin FC (2008) Increased osteoblast adhesion on nanoparticulate calcium phosphates with higher Ca/P ratios. J Biomed Mater Res 85A:236–241
156. Ni S, Lin K, Chang J, Chou L (2008) Beta-$CaSiO_3$/beta-$Ca_3(PO_4)_2$ composite materials for hard tissue repair: in vitro studies. J Biomed Mater Res 85A:72–82
157. Epinette JA, Manley MT (2008) Uncemented stems in hip replacement – hydroxyapatite or plain porous: does it matter? Based on a prospective study of HA Omnifit stems at 15-years minimum follow-up. Hip Int 18(2):69–74
158. Capello WN, D'Antonio JA, Jaffe WL, Geesink RG, Manley MT, Feinberg JR (2006) Hydroxyapatite-coated femoral components: 15-year minimum followup. Clin Orthop Relat Res 453:75–80
159. Camazzola D, Hammond T, Gandhi R, Davey JR (2009) A randomized trial of hydroxyapatite-coated femoral stems in total hip arthroplasty: a 13-year follow-up. J Arthroplasty 24(1):33–37
160. Yoon KS, Kim HJ, Lee JH, Kang SB, Seong NH, Koo KH (2007) A randomized clinical trial of cementless femoral stems with and without hydroxyapatite/tricalcium-phosphate coating: an 8- to 12-year follow-up study. J Arthroplasty 22(4):504–508
161. Tonino AJ, Therin M, Doyle C (1999) Histology and histomorphometry around five components retrieved at post mortem. J Bone Joint Surg 81B(Br):148–154
162. Buma P, Gardeniers JW (1995) Tissue reactions around a hydroxyapatite-coated hip prosthesis. Case report of a retrieved specimen. J Arthroplasty 10(3):389–395
163. Bauer TW (1995) Hydroxyapatite: coating controversies. Orthopedics 18:885–888

164. Gross KA, Ray N, Rokkum M (2002) The contribution of coating microstructure to degradation and particle release in hydroxyapatite coated prostheses. J Biomed Mater Res B Appl Biomater 63(2):106–114
165. Bloebaum RD, Lundeen GA, Bachus KN, Ison I, Hofmann AA (1998) Dissolution of particulate hydroxyapatite in a macrophage organelle model. J Biomed Mater Res 40(1):104–114
166. Morscher EW, Hefti A, Aebi U (1998) Severe osteolysis after third-body wear due to hydroxyapatite particles from acetabular cup coating. J Bone Joint Surg 80B(Brit):267–272
167. Ducheyne P, Bianco P, Radin S, Schepers E (1993) Bioactive materials: mechanisms and bioengineering considerations. In: Ducheyne P, Kokubo T, van Blitterswijk CA (eds) Bone bioactive biomaterials. Reed Healthcare Communications, Leiderdorp, The Netherlands, pp 1–12
168. Ducheyne P, Qiu Q (1999) Bioactive ceramics: the effect of surface reactivity on bone formation and bone cell function. Biomaterials 20:2287–2303
169. Hemmerle J, Cuisinier FJG, Schultz P, Voegel J–C (1997) HRTEM study of biological crystal growth mechanisms in the vicinity of implanted synthetic hydroxyapatite crystals. J Dent Res 76(2):682–687
170. Hardy DC, Frayssinet P, Guilhem A, Lafontaine MA, Delince PE (1991) Bonding of hydroxyapatite-coated femoral prostheses: histopathology of specimens from four cases. J Bone Joint Surg 73B:732–740
171. Porter AE, Taak P, Hobbs LW, Coathup MJ, Blunn GW, Spectord M (2004) Bone bonding to hydroxyapatite and titanium surfaces on femoral stems retrieved from human subjects at autopsy. Biomaterials 25:5199–5208
172. Dippel B, Mueller RT, Pingsmann A, Schrader B (1998) Composition, constitution and interaction of bone with hydroxyapatite coatings determined by FT Raman microscopy. Biospectroscopy 4:403–412
173. Nelea V, Morosanu C, Bercu M, Mihailescu IN (2007) Interfacial titanium oxide between hydroxyapatite and TiAlFe substrate. J Mater Sci Mater Med 18:2347–2354
174. Nieh TG, Jankowski AF, Koike J (2001) Processing and characterization of hydroxyapatite coatings on titanium produced by magnetron sputtering. J Mater Res 16(11):3238–3245
175. Fernández-Pradas JM, García-Cuenca MV, Clèries L, Sardin S, Morenza JL (2002) Influence of the interface layer on the adhesion of pulsed laser deposited hydroxyapatite coatings on titanium alloy. Appl Surf Sci 195:31–37
176. Fernández-Pradas JM, García-Cuenca MV, Morenza JL (2005) Analysis of the interface between a pulsed laser deposited calcium phosphate coating and a titanium alloy substrate. Appl Phys Mater Sci Process 80(2):325–331
177. Li H, Khor KA, Cheang P (2002) Titanium dioxide reinforced hydroxyapatite coatings deposited by high velocity oxy-fuel (HVOF) spray. Biomaterials 23:85–91
178. Hedia HS (2007) Effect of coating thickness and it's material on the stress distribution for dental implants. J Med Eng Technol 31(4):280–287
179. Fogarassy P, Cofino B, Millet P, Lodini A (2005) Residual stress in hydroxyapatite coating: nonlinear analysis and high-energy synchrotron measurements. IEEE Trans Biomed Eng 52(7):1161–1166
180. Zhang XS, Revell PA, Evans SL, Tuke MA, Gregson PJ (1999) In vivo biocompatibility and mechanical study of novel bone-bioactive materials for prosthetic implantation. J Biomed Mater Res 46(2):279–286
181. Thompson JI, Gregson PJ, Revell PA (1999) Analysis of push-out test data based on interfacial fracture energy. J Mater Sci Mater Med 10(12):863–868
182. Aoki H, Ozeki K, Ohtani Y, Fukui Y, Asaoka T (2006) Effect of a thin HA coating on the stress/strain distribution in bone around dental implants using three-dimensional finite element analysis. Bio Med Mat Eng 16:157–169

Chapter 10
Bioactive Composites Reinforced with Inorganic Glasses and Glass–Ceramics for Tissue Engineering Applications

Alexandre A. Barros, Álvaro J. Leite, Ricardo A. Pires, João F. Mano, and Rui L. Reis

Abstract Bioactive composites, prepared by the combination of glasses or glass–ceramics with natural or synthetic polymers or blends, have been extensively exploited in bone tissue engineering. Their bioactive character is usually derived from the glass or glass–ceramic phase and is one of the most relevant properties to generate bone bonding. Herein we focus on the development of bioactive composite structures that target tissue engineering applications, with special emphasis on bone regeneration. Some concepts, e.g., bioactivity and biocompatibility, are initially introduced, followed by a description of the synthetic approaches that have been reported for the preparation of bioactive inorganic glasses or glass–ceramics. Different strategies to compound these inorganic particles with polymeric phases are detailed, spanning from conventional methodologies and wet spinning to rapid prototyping. Finally, a series of systems that have been developed for bone tissue engineering are described (including injectable systems, 3D scaffolds, membranes, and biomimetic layer-by-layer structures), as well as their in vitro biological response.

Keywords Bioactive composites • Glass–ceramics • Bioactivity • Biomaterials • Tissue engineering

---

A.A. Barros • Á.J. Leite • R.A. Pires • J.F. Mano (✉) • R.L. Reis
3B's Research Group – Biomaterials, Biodegradables and Biomimetics, University of Minho, Headquarters of the European Institute of Excellence on Tissue Engineering and Regenerative Medicine, AvePark, 4806-909 Taipas, Guimarães, Portugal

ICVS/3B's – PT Government Associate Laboratory, Braga, Guimarães, Portugal
e-mail: jmano@dep.uminho.pt

B. Ben-Nissan (ed.), *Advances in Calcium Phosphate Biomaterials*, Springer Series in Biomaterials Science and Engineering 2, DOI 10.1007/978-3-642-53980-0_10,

10.1 Introduction

Autografts have been considered as the gold standard for bone reconstructive surgeries because of its high performance and no risk for transfer of diseases or rejection (problematic in the allografts) [1]. However, there are several problems related with this procedure, such as the limited amount of available material and donor site morbidity [1–3]. Thus, the development of alternatives has been highly relevant for bone reconstructive surgery. In this context, the tissue engineering concept was introduced during the 1980s [4]. Since then, the bone tissue has been one of the most investigated tissues to regenerate or repair [5].

Current challenges in bone tissue engineering involve the development of scaffold biomaterials which provides local environment that enhances the recruitment of endogenous progenitor cells, improving the healing process and tissue regeneration [6]. In addition, the ideal bone tissue engineering construct should be readily available, easily adaptable to the site in terms of size and shape, mechanically strong, and biodegradable [7, 8]. Moreover, the biomaterial should be biocompatible (i.e., giving an appropriate response under the biological medium) and present bioactivity (i.e., able to generate a calcium phosphate layer onto its surface).

The weak fixation of the biomaterials within the bone structure is one of the major reasons that impair the use of scaffolds in load-bearing sites. The lack of interfacial adhesion between the implant and bone, which results in a fibrous capsule surrounding the implant which allows micromotion to occur, causes pain to the patient and space for wear particles to accumulate, ultimately contributing to the failure of the implant. To overcome this problem, a series of strategies has been developed to generate bioactive fixation. Under this concept, an interfacial bonding between the implant and the bone tissue is promoted through the coating of the biomaterial with a biologically active hydroxyapatite layer. As bone is also highly mineralized (by hydroxyapatite), this bioactive fixation forms a bond at the implant–bone interface with strength equal to or greater than the bone itself.

In this context, the bioactivity of a specific biomaterial gains significant relevance within bone tissue engineering. In fact, a large number of biomaterials are not bioactive, and several methods have been proposed to induce this property [9]. A widely established strategy to promote bioactivity is the incorporation of glass or glass–ceramic inorganic particles. These particles are usually produced with the inclusion of calcium and phosphate groups in order to feed the biomaterial with the main constituents of hydroxyapatite. In the first years of development, bioactive glass coatings onto metals and ceramics were being proposed to avoid the formation of capsules of fibrous tissue surrounding the implants [10]. Nowadays it is common their incorporation into composite systems, where polymers can act as a continuous medium for their immobilization [11]. Additionally, the biodegradation of the polymeric phase has been also considered as critical within a bone tissue engineering perspective, in order to allow new bone to be formed while the composite degrades [12].

In the following sections, we will give an overview on the most important topics related with composites containing bioactive glasses or glass–ceramics, including some concepts that are relevant in this field; synthetic approaches to the production of glass/glass–ceramic particles; their processing in combination with biodegradable polymer to generate composite structures that combine biocompatibility, bioactivity, and biodegradability; and the capacity to promote new bone formation.

10.2 Biocompatibility and Bioactivity in Bone Tissue Engineering

Biocompatibility is defined as the ability of a material to give an appropriate response to a specific biological application [13]. In addition to effectiveness, the materials used in biomedical devices must also be safe. In this sense, biocompatibility may be generally regarded as the ability of a material to interact with living cells/tissues or a living system by not being toxic and injurious or causing immunological reactions while performing or functioning appropriately [14].

The evaluation of the biocompatibility of biomaterials involves a detailed characterization (e.g., bulk and surface chemical composition, density, porosity, mechanical and degradation properties) and extensive biological testing, first at the in vitro level, then in in vivo animal models, and ultimately in human clinical trials [15].

The first biomaterials were based on the concept of bioinertness. Under this approach, the development of a material that would not react with the surrounding tissues was targeted. Nowadays, bioactive materials are preferred, where bioactivity is defined as "the ability of the material to induce the formation of an interfacial bonding between the implant and living tissues, without the formation of a fibrous capsule separating the biomaterial and the tissue." In the case of the bioactive glasses, various in vitro and in vivo studies show that a series of interfacial reactions occur that leads to the formation of an apatite layer on the glass surface responsible for bone bonding [16, 17].

The formation of an apatite layer is governed by a complex set of steps that start on the immobilization of calcium and phosphate ions in the surface of the biomaterial forming a biologically active hydroxycarbonate apatite. This layer evolves to form different calcium phosphate phases until it generates hydroxyapatite or hydroxyapatite-like coatings [18, 19] with their characteristic cauliflower morphology (Fig. 10.1).

In a bone tissue engineering perspective, bioactivity can be categorized into class A, when the biomaterial presents osteoproduction (bone growth in the bulk of the biomaterial) and osteoconduction (stimulation of bone growth at the interface), and class B, when it only presents osteoconduction [18].

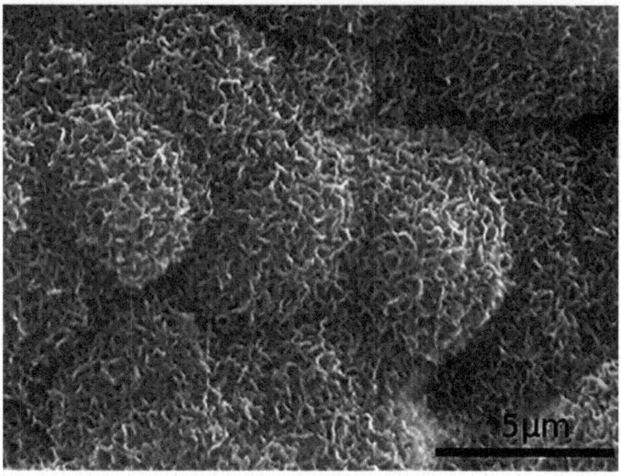

Fig. 10.1 Typical cauliflower morphology of hydroxyapatite when deposited on the surface of a bioactive biomaterial (Reprinted from Ref. [20], Copyright 2007, with permission from Elsevier)

In vitro bioactivity test evaluates the ability of the biomaterial to form an apatite surface layer when in contact with simulated body fluid (SBF), a solution that presents ionic concentrations similar to human blood plasma [21, 22].

After the initial description of this methodology, a series of modifications have been proposed in the composition of SBF. One of the most relevant is mSBF that presents ionic concentrations equal to the human plasma, with the exception of HCO_3^-, whose concentration was reduced to the level of saturation of calcite [23]. This type of approach is also used as a surface modification methodology, generating an apatite coating that enhances the bioactivity of the biomaterial [24]. Other modifications to the SBF solution have been reported, the use of higher ion concentrations (e.g., 1.5 × SBF, 5.0 × SBF, among many others) to reduce the time frame of the apatite deposition are common [24, 25].

The use of SBF or SBF-like solutions is one of most commonly used approaches to test the bioactivity of a biomaterial. However, the different steps of this methodology should be carefully controlled, and the conclusions that one can take from such a characterization are not consensual [19, 26].

10.3 Synthesis and Preparation of Bioactive Composite Systems

10.3.1 Bioactive Inorganic Particles and Their Synthesis

Bioactive inorganic particles (glasses or glass–ceramics) are usually composed of silicates or phosphosilicates (as network formers) combined with different proportions of glass modifiers, e.g., sodium oxide (Na_2O) and calcium oxide (CaO), among others. They have been studied for more than 40 years and are characterized by their bioactivity and unique bone bonding properties, which are usually related to their surface chemistry. A landmark on the development of these systems was the work of Hench et al. [27]. They showed that the bioglass 45S5 (with a general composition $0.461SiO_2:0.026P_2O_5:0.269CaO:0.244Na_2O$) is able to promote the formation of a calcium phosphate layer on its surface within a time frame of 30 days. This glass composition is one of the most studied ones [27–29]. The concentration of SiO_2 in the glass/glass–ceramic structure seems to be a critical parameter that governs the bonding of the material to living tissue [27]. It has been proven that glass formulations that present fast bonding not only to bone but also to soft tissues are prepared with 45–52 % (by weight) of SiO_2 [30]. Glasses with a SiO_2 content ranging from 55 to 60 % react more slowly and do not bind to soft tissues. Compositions with >60 % of SiO_2 do not bond to bone and are considered as bioinert [27, 31]. Additionally, bioactive glasses have been demonstrated to stimulate the growth and maturation of osteoblasts [31–33]. Most of these materials degrade naturally, similarly to other synthetic substitutes, such as calcium phosphates (CaPs). The degradation products are, usually, metabolized by the body and excreted through the urine [34].

The brittle behavior and weak mechanical properties observed in bioactive glasses are the major difficulties associated with their use in biomedical applications. The bending strength of most bioactive glasses is in the range of 40–60 MPa, which is not enough for load-bearing applications, while their modulus is between 30 and 35 GPa, very close to that of cortical bone. The combination of biodegradable polymers with bioactive glasses has been proposed to produce biodegradable products that show high levels of bioactivity and also improve some of their mechanical properties as compared to conventional glasses [35–37].

Bioactive glasses and glass–ceramics can be obtained by melting at high temperatures followed by casting into a mold or splat quenching. An alternative approach for glass synthesis is the sol–gel route [29, 38, 39]. Both strategies are detailed in the following sections.

10.3.1.1 Melt-Based Approach

Bioactive inorganic particles can be synthesized by different methodologies, and the melt-quenching approach is one of the most traditional and straightforward routes. Under this procedure, the glass precursors (e.g., silica, phosphates, carbonates, etc.) are mixed in a mortar, transferred to a crucible, and fired to temperatures able to melt the whole mixture that can go up to 1,600 °C or higher, depending on the formulations [16, 40–44]. The homogeneous mixture is then splat quenched into ice water or onto a metal plate maintained at room temperature. This process allows the chemical structure to be frozen [13, 45]. Depending on the starting materials, the heating process can be done stepwise, namely, 300 °C if the starting materials contain ammonia in their chemical structure (e.g., sodium ammonium hydrogenophosphate) and/or 650 °C if the starting materials are carbonates (e.g., calcium carbonate). These thermal treatments allow the release of by-products, such as ammonia or CO_2 that diffuse through the precursors and are released from the mixture [40–42]. Bioactive glasses prepared by melting are usually denser and do not contain any remnants of organic components or water; nevertheless, melt-derived bioactive glasses have a limited surface area, being one of their main disadvantages when in contact with the biological tissues or fluids [46, 47]. The high temperature used in the fabrication of these inorganic particles through the conventional melt-based process does not allow the incorporation of bioactive organic molecules/materials (e.g., proteins, growth factors, genes, hormones, etc.) during the fabrication process.

10.3.1.2 Sol–Gel Approach

Advances in sol–gel processing technology allowed the manufacture of a new generation of bioactive glasses overcoming some of the drawbacks of the melt-based approach (e.g., high processing temperatures) [48]. This low-temperature process dispenses the use of Na_2O in bioactive glass compositions (the main role of this component in the glass compositions is related to the lowering of the glass melting temperature) and allows incorporating polymers and organic molecules to make less brittle hybrid materials [11]. Also, sol–gel route allows a wider range of bioactive compositions for a better response to specific clinical applications, permits the easier control of its morphology and chemical composition, enables an easier design of the material's morphology (powders, monoliths, nanoparticles, gels), and generates materials with high specific surface area, osteoconduction properties, degradability, and nanoporosity [35, 45–47, 49]. In fact, the main physical differences between melt and sol–gel-derived glasses are that the latter ones tend to have inherent nanoporosity, whereas melt-based glasses are denser. The nanoporosity can result in improved cellular response due to the nanotopography that might reach a surface area 100× higher than for similar compositions produced through the melt-based approach [50, 51]. This property increases the solubility of the glass, which is important in a bioactivity perspective [11]. This characteristic is confirmed by in vitro (in SBF) and in vivo studies that report a higher bioactivity and degradability of the sol–gel-derived glasses when compared to the melt-derived ones [51].

The sol–gel route essentially forms and assembles nanoparticles of silica at room temperature. It is a synthetic route where a solution containing the glass compositional precursors (e.g., alkoxides or metal chlorides) undergoes hydrolysis and condensation reactions to form a gel either in water or in an organic solvent. A typical silicate precursor is tetraethyl orthosilicate (TEOS), while common precursors for calcium and phosphate groups are calcium nitrate tetrahydrate and triethyl phosphate, respectively [11, 52]. Adding water or a water/alcohol mixture to TEOS promotes the hydrolysis of the alkoxide functionality generating silicic acid. The addition of an acid or a base as a catalyst allows the silicic acid to condense into a network of silica-based gel through the release of water molecules. Depending on the experimental conditions and compositions, these two steps might

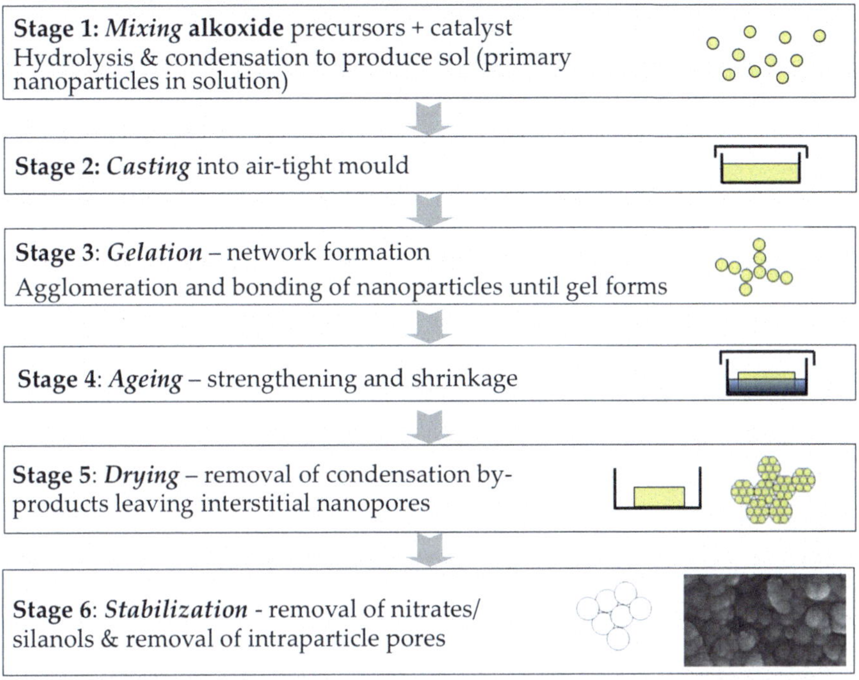

Fig. 10.2 A flow chart of the acid-catalyzed sol–gel process used to synthesize bioactive glasses, including schematics of the evolution of the gel and its nanoporosity (Reprinted from Ref. [11], Copyright 2013, with permission from Elsevier)

occur simultaneously [53]. At the initial time frame of the silicic acid condensation, a sol is generated. The subsequent agglomeration of the particles that constitute the sol forms the gel. This gelation step proceeds slowly. Complete cross-linking of the silicate network is achieved during the ageing step [53, 54]. A procedure can be adapted to generate glass particles and not a 3D glass structure (e.g., Fig. 10.2). In this approach the experimental conditions are manipulated to inhibit the agglomeration of the particles generated in the initial steps of the procedure [55, 56]. Typical bioactive compositions can be binary systems, e.g., SiO_2-CaO; ternary systems, e.g., SiO_2-CaO-P_2O_5; or quaternary systems, e.g., SiO_2-CaO-Na_2O-P_2O_5 [52, 57, 58]. The silanol group is critical for the bioactivity of the glass. In addition, gel-derived bioactive glasses may contain high-energy silicate ring structures, which further activate the material reactivity [12, 14, 15].

Microparticles, monoliths, or foams are usually produced using acidic catalysis (Fig. 10.2) [11]. Using this methodology, the primary nanoparticles (with diameters around 2 nm) present in the sol coalesce and condensation (polymerization) occur, forming Si–O–Si bonds. The nanoparticles coarsen, coalesce, and bond together, forming a gel network of assembled nanoparticles [59]. The gel is dried and is heated at temperatures above 700 °C to produce a nanoporous bioactive glass [11].

As water and alcohol evaporate during drying, they generate an interconnected porous network. The pores are formed in the interstices between the coalesced nanoparticles [59], and their size depends on the precursors used, the glass composition, and the pH of the reaction [60]. Pore diameters are typically in the range of 1–30 nm [52].

If the synthesis is carried out under basic conditions, submicrometer particles are formed [61]. Compared with micron-sized bioactive ceramic particles, nano-sized particles have a higher specific surface area and can form a tighter interface with the polymer matrix in a composite formulation [62–65]. Furthermore, reducing the size of the particles would not only accelerate the formation of a bioactive hydroxyapatite surface layer but also provide more active sites for osteoblast attachment, enhancing their proliferation and differentiation, as well as tissue growth [66, 67]. Also, they exhibit, to some extent, similar nanoarchitecture as the physiological bone [68]. Work on the fabrication of bioactive glass nanoparticles (BG-NPs) by the sol–gel route has been reported [55, 65, 69]. Hong et al. obtained ternary BG-NPs (SiO_2-CaO-P_2O_5) by the combination of two strategies, sol–gel and coprecipitation approaches. The mixture of precursors was hydrolyzed in an acidic environment and condensed in alkaline condition, and the resultant particles were collected by freeze-drying [62]. Briefly, the sol–gel synthesis procedure comprised as follows: mixture of TEOS, $Ca(NO_3)_2$, ethanol, and water; addition of citric acid (catalyst) to adjust solution pH at 1–2; vigorous agitation to promote the hydrolysis of the silica precursor; adding drop by drop the resultant sol into a $(NH_4)_2HPO_4$ solution under vigorous agitation; continuously adding ammonia into the solution to maintain the pH at 10–11; separating the particles by centrifugation; and the collection after freeze-drying. After calcination at 700 °C, it was possible to obtain particles with an average diameter of around 20–40 nm [62]. It was found that both binary and ternary BG-NPs prepared by this method exhibit bioactive features [70]. Formulations, morphologies, and sizes of BG-NPs could be tailored by varying the production conditions and the feeding ratio of the reagents [56, 71]. For instance, Chen et al. investigated the effects of the experimental conditions on the morphology of BG-NPs of the system SiO_2–CaO–P_2O_5, and they found that the use of lactic acid decreased the size of the BG-NPs [72].

The sol–gel versatility allows the incorporation of different ions to the glass structure (e.g., Zn^{2+}, Mg^{2+}, Ag^{+}, etc.) in order to improve the glass functionality and bioactivity [43]. El-Kady et al. produced silver-doped BG-NPs that showed antibacterial activity against different types of bacteria. This type of particles could be used to minimize the occurrence of bacterial infections generated by the implantation of bone tissue engineering scaffolds [73].

The sol–gel technique has been also applied in the synthesis of a variety of bioactive monolithic and particulate glasses (e.g., Fig. 10.3). However, a high-temperature calcination step is required to eliminate organic remnants, the processing is relatively time consuming, and it is difficult to obtain defects-free bioactive glass monoliths with diameters above 1 cm. Defects are mainly due to the shrinkage that occurs during drying. For particles, vapor stresses through the interconnected pore

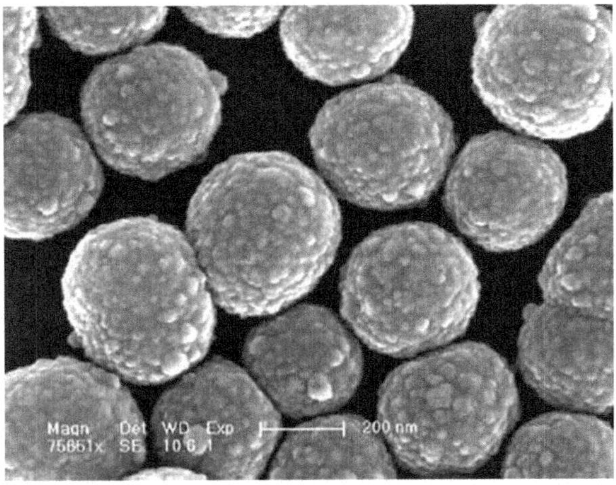

Fig. 10.3 Bioactive silica-based particles prepared through the sol–gel route (Reproduced from Ref. [76] by permission of John Wiley & Sons Ltd.)

network are small, and the path of evaporation is short, although, for monolithic objects, the path from the center of the monolith to the surface is long, and the drying stresses can introduce fracture [11, 74]. The enumerated drawbacks of the sol–gel route, allied with the low cost of the melting procedure makes this latter route dominant in the commercial production of bioactive glasses [75].

10.3.2 Natural-Based Polymeric Phases/Composites and Their Processing

The combination of bioactive inorganic particles with natural-based polymers generated a family of bioactive composites with a wide range of applications, from structural implants to tissue engineering scaffolds [74, 77]. These composites combine the flexibility of polymers with the stiffness, strength, and bioactive character of the inorganic glass fillers. So far, most of the published work on this class of composites has been carried out using conventional (micron-size) inorganic particles as fillers (or coatings) [77, 78]. However, the capacity to produce nano-sized particles/fibers allowed the development of bionanocomposites through the combination of nano-reinforcements and biodegradable polymers of different origins. These bionanocomposites have been explored, for example, as porous scaffolds for bone tissue engineering applications or membranes with potential applications in the dental field [79–81].

These types of bioactive composite structures can be produced using different methodologies, namely, melt-based ones (which requires the use of a thermoplastic polymer), wet chemistry approaches, or rapid prototyping. These three main processing methodologies will be further detailed in the next sections.

10.3.2.1 Conventional Melt-Based Methodologies

Conventional melt-based processing techniques (e.g., extrusion, injection molding, compression molding, fused deposition molding, etc.) are based on the melting of a particular polymer in order to shape it or mix it with different reinforcements [82]. In this perspective, non-thermoplastic materials are not possible to be processed using these methodologies. Most of the natural-based biodegradable polymers are not thermoplastic, limiting their melt-based processing [83, 84]. Researchers have overpassed this limitation through the combination of natural-based polymers with thermoplastic polymers [85]. Under this approach, different polymeric blends, able to be processed using melt-based technologies, were developed (e.g., blends of starch and synthetic polymers and blends of chitosan and aliphatic polyesters) [86–92].

Thermoplastic polymers or blends have been used as matrices for the production of glass-/glass–ceramic-based composite systems [93–98]. Most of the published work targeted their use in bone tissue engineering. The inorganic phases are introduced to enhance the bioactivity of the material, while some of the mechanical properties are improved [96].

Melt-based processing using blowing agents or compression molding followed by particulate leaching has been used to obtain porous inorganic/organic biodegradable composites [99, 100]. It is also worth to highlight that physical blowing agents, such as supercritical CO_2 or water, have been shown to be effective on developing porous glass-/glass–ceramic-based composites for bone tissue engineering applications [101]. In fact, porosity is a critical parameter when complete bone regeneration is targeted. It allows the cell colonization in the bulk of the biomaterial and, subsequently, new bone production.

10.3.2.2 Wet-Spinning Approaches

Wet spinning is a phase inversion technique allowing the production of polymer fibers through an immersion–precipitation process. In the methodology, a solution of polymer is continually spun through a spinneret leading to the formation of a polymeric filament. The spun occurs into a coagulation bath composed of a poor solvent (non-solvent) or a non-solvent–solvent mixture with respect to the polymer being processed. A homogeneous solvated filament, composed of polymer, solvent, and possible additives, solidifies because of polymer desolvation, caused by solvent–non-solvent exchange [102]. The essential feature in wet spinning is the transfer of solvent from the polymer to the coagulating bath. The major drawbacks that limit the rate of wet spinning are usually related with the need for sufficient time for coagulation to occur, the dependence on the rate of solvent diffusion, and the considerable viscous drag of the coagulating baths [102].

Through the assembly of the thin wet-spun fiber meshes, it is possible to fabricate 3D networks of fiber meshes. This methodology imparts flexibility to the manufacturing process, allowing the design of scaffolds with properties that can be adjusted depending on the targeted site (e.g., thicker scaffolds for the long bones or membrane-like scaffolds for the maxilla regions) [103, 104]. It has been reported that the combination of wet-spun chitosan fibers with bioglass enhances the material bioactivity and promotes osteoblast proliferation and ALP activity [105]. Wet-spinning technologies also enable to create hybrid materials with high levels of organization and avoid the thermal degradation of natural origin polymers compared to other techniques, such as the melt spinning [103]. Wet spinning has been used for the production of wet-spun fibers for drug release [106] and polymeric scaffolds for tissue engineering applications [104, 107].

10.3.2.3 Rapid Prototyping

Rapid prototyping is based on an approach that combines computer science and manufacturing technologies. The main advantage of these techniques is their ability to produce complex structures using a computer-aided design (CAD) model [13]. Currently, different rapid prototyping techniques are used for biomedical applications and can be classified as (1) laser-based, (2) nozzle-based, and (3) printer-based systems [108].

Laser-based systems benefit from the photopolymerization pathway as a basis to fabricate cross-linked polymeric scaffolds. This type of processing methodology has been also employed to develop 3D scaffolds constructed solely with bioactive glasses [109]. In this approach a CO_2 laser is used to soften or melt the glass particles that are injected to the targeted position by means of a nozzle. The processed particles bind to the substrate at the position where they interact with the laser radiation. These 3D constructs exhibit a higher crystallization degree than their parent glass powder precursors. They maintain their bioactive character after processing, although the rate of apatite formation when immersed in SBF is slower [109].

The main limitation of the nozzle-based techniques is that the resolution is determined by the nozzle size, which makes it difficult to design and fabricate scaffolds in the micron- or nano-size. The well-known processing of (pre)-polymers by pressure exerted on extrusion/dispensing units supports the second category of rapid prototyping systems. Under this approach, the production of bioactive glass–polycaprolactone (PCL) composites is achieved by stereolithography, through the printing of PCL–glass mixtures and cross-linking of methacrylated PCL. The resulting 3D constructs are bioactive, being able to generate an apatite layer upon immersion in SBF. Additionally, the constructs revealed to be non-cytotoxic towards fibroblasts, inducing an increase in cell activity when the bioactive glasses were added up to a concentration of 20 % [110].

The printer-based systems combine powder beds and the deposition of a binder that fuses the particles, or directly depositing material using inkjet technology [108, 111, 112]. It has been used to process biodegradable polymeric scaffolds for tissue engineering applications [13]. This process prints a binder onto a surface in a sequential layered way. The processing parameters such as the speed, flow rate, and drop position can be computer controlled to produce complex 3D scaffolds.

Several recent research works have been reported on the fabrication of 3D scaffolds using highly bioactive mesoporous glasses as starting materials. For example, Yun et al. reported the synthesis of ordered bioactive 3D glass scaffolds exhibiting a hierarchical porosity composition using a combination of sol–gel, double polymers templating, and rapid prototyping techniques [113]. The resulting scaffolds presented three lengths of porosity: mesopores (2–50 nm), macropores (>50 nm), and giant pores (30–100 μm) [114]. The in vitro tests revealed that the bioactive behavior of mesoporous bioactive glasses was preserved because a carbonate hydroxyapatite layer was formed onto the material surface after 24 h of immersion in SBF [108, 115].

The processing of alginate–glass composites has also been achieved using 3D printing, with the inclusion of mesoporous bioactive glass particles in a concentration up to 50 % (w/w). The addition of glass particles to the alginate phase induced an increase on its compressive strength and stiffness. Only the compositions with high glass content (30 and 50 %) exhibited apatite formation onto the composite structure upon SBF immersion. The glass particles were also loaded with dexamethasone prior to the processing of the composite. Its release profiles showed that the glass particles have the capacity to exhibit sustained delivery properties within the glass–alginate system. The authors also report the formation of apatite particles when the constructs were cultured with human bone marrow stem cells for 7 days [116]. The use of other bioactive agents, such as growth factors, can also be incorporated into the scaffolds during the printing process, although the maintenance of their stability depends strongly on the experimental conditions [112].

10.4 Applications of Bioactive Composites Within Bone Tissue Engineering

10.4.1 Injectable Systems

Some injectable systems composed by the combination of polymers and bioactive inorganic particles have been proposed for bone tissue engineering [71]. However, one of the main difficulties in the injection of such suspensions of a solid phase is the filter-press effect responsible for a variation of the solid/liquid ratio during the injection that eventually hampers the injection flow through the creation of a backpressure in the syringe [117]. The injectability is related to the viscosity of the suspension, in particular the solid/liquid ratio and the suspension stability [43]. A number of additives have been used to improve the injectability.

Another drawback is the washout phenomenon, which corresponds to the disaggregation or dispersion of the paste during or after its placement. This event is not intrinsic to the material and is related to the viscosity of the medium in which the paste is injected. It has been shown that the viscosity of the paste has to be higher than that of the target medium to avoid dispersion from the administration zone [7, 43, 118]. Calcium phosphate-based cements have been extensively explored in this form; they generate apatite following the setting and hardening reactions. The key advantages of these cements are their self-setting properties and the possibility to apply them within a minimum invasive surgery framework.

Injectable systems have been proposed as new tissue engineering strategies to deliver cells and bioactive agents (encapsulated in a biodegradable matrix) through minimally invasive procedures. Couto et al. combined a chitosan–β-glycerophosphate salt formulation with sol–gel-derived BG-NPs to prepare bioactive thermo-responsive hydrogels for orthopedic reconstruction and regenerative medicine applications [71]. The size and spherical shape of the particles guarantee the efficient injection of these systems through small-gauge needles into the bone defects. The system presented a gelation point around 36.8 °C, being suitable for intracorporal application. It was also observed that the gelation temperature could be manipulated through the increase of the chitosan deacetylation degree. Upon immersion in SBF, the composites containing BG-NPs induced the formation of bone-like apatite clusters that were well integrated in the organic structure. The density of the apatite precipitates increased with increasing BG-NP content and soaking time in SBF. Despite more research is required to fully validate the use of such systems in the bone regeneration context, this osteoconductive injectable biodegradable system has a large unexplored potential in bone tissue engineering [71].

10.4.2 3D Scaffolds

3D porous composite scaffolds can induce the ingrowth of cells to the desired shape and may facilitate the vascularization of new tissue [119]. Composites found in nature contain an inorganic phase embedded in an organic matrix, usually assembled in a complex and hierarchical structure [120]. Biomimetic osteoconductive nanocomposites may be obtained by combining bioactive glass/ceramics with a polymeric matrix [74].

One approach to combine scaffolds with bioactive glasses is the use of highly porous glass scaffolds coated with polymer, such as poly(DL-lactide) (PDLLA) or poly(3-hydroxybutyrate) (PHB) [121, 122]. Chen et al. used PDLLA to coat a bioglass foam with 90 % porosity with pore diameter between 500 and 700 μm [122]. The thin coating resulted in an improved work of fracture [122]. However, these types of coatings can mask the surface of bioactive glass scaffolds generating a non-bioactive surface. This drawback significantly decreases the effectiveness of polymer-coated scaffolds in terms of osteoconductivity and osteoinductivity. The long-term effectiveness of the coating is also under concern since its degradation lead to a brittle glass–ceramic scaffold [96].

Foams produced by thermally induced phase separation are promising bioglass containing composites for bone regeneration [123]. In this case, the biodegradable polymer is dissolved in dimethyl carbonate, and the particulate glass fraction is added. The mixture is quenched in liquid nitrogen and lyophilized. PDLLA foams containing 40 % (w/w) of bioactive glass have been produced with tubular pores (with 100 μm of diameter) with interconnectivity between 10 and 50 μm and porosities up to 97 %. The thin pore walls allow the bioactive particles to be exposed. Despite the high porosity, the pore and interconnectivity sizes are too low to allow the cells to colonize the interior of the scaffold, while the high percentage of porosity (and thin pore walls) contributes to low mechanical resistance [124].

The addition of bioglass particles to a biodegradable polymeric matrix is a typical approach to generate conventional composite systems. Polymers, such as polylactic acid (PLA), polyglycolic acid (PGA), and their copolymers (PLGA), have been utilized as matrices. These systems have been used clinically for the past years [77]. The incorporation of bioglass in these polymeric matrices (e.g., PLGA) can increase the stiffness and compressive strength of the composite. However, in some cases, the addition of a glass phase can be detrimental. For example, composite systems based on the compounding of PDLLA with bioactive glass particles (with particle size between 50 and 125 μm) were produced using twin-screw extrusion, and, as the glass content was increased, the bending, torsional, and shear strengths of the composite decreased [96]. Moreover, it is still difficult to match the degradation rate of the polymer with that of the glass.

The development of nanocomposites using nanoparticles dispersed in a polymeric matrix has the potential to improve the interaction with the host tissue/cells [125, 126]. Sol–gel-derived BG-NPs have also been introduced into freeze-cast gelatin–chitosan foams resulting in pore sizes in the range of 150–300 μm [127]. Their mechanical strength was augmented with the reduction of the composite porosity. Bioactive glass–collagen–phosphatidylserine scaffolds (including 65 wt% of the sol–gel-derived 58S glass) were produced with 75 % of porosity and with pore sizes up to 300 μm. They exhibited a compressive strength of 1.5 MPa. However, pore interconnectivity was low [128].

Hong et al. combined PLLA and sol–gel-derived BG-NPs [65]. The porous PLLA/BG-NP scaffolds were prepared by a thermal-induced phase separation method [55]. They found that increasing the amount of BG-NPs into the PLLA matrix altered the morphology and porosity of the scaffolds. The addition of BG-NPs to the PLLA matrix induced an increase of both compressive modulus and strength of the scaffolds. In vitro tests revealed that these composites (prepared with different proportions of BG-NPs) are bioactive. The addition of BG-NPs increased the water uptake of the scaffolds, especially at a low BG-NP loading, and also greatly affected the degradation rate of the PLLA matrix [55].

The correct dispersion of bioactive glasses in a polymeric matrix is dependent on the interfacial bonding and the compatibility between both phases. The BG-NP/PLLA composite system was studied by Liu et al. [129] to evaluate strategies to overcome these dispersion and compatibility drawbacks. The authors prepared BG-NPs via the sol–gel route and grafted low-molecular-weight PLLA in the particle surface using a diisocyanate. They were able to homogeneously disperse the modified particles within the PLLA matrix, improving both the nucleating rate and degree of crystallization of the composite. The grafting modification induced an increase on the tensile strength, tensile modulus, and impact energy of the composites by increasing the phase compatibility. Thus, this strategy can be used to prepare composite structures able to be employed in bone tissue engineering at load-bearing sites. In vitro bioactivity tests compared pure PLLA scaffolds and BG-NP/PLLA nanocomposite [129]. The results demonstrated that BG-NP containing composites had a higher capacity to induce the formation of an apatite layer on the scaffold surface. The culture of bone marrow stromal cell onto these composites revealed that BG-NP particles facilitate the attachment and proliferation of stem cells onto the surface of the scaffolds [129].

Nonetheless, it is important to notice that when bioactive glass particles are combined with a polymer matrix, most of the cells are only in contact with the polymeric phase. Additionally, some particles might protrude from the surface through a process difficult to control [96].

10.4.3 Membranes and Layer-by-Layer Structures

Composite membranes have been also developed for dental applications and bone tissue engineering. Specifically, in guided tissue/bone regeneration, membranes are used as barriers to prevent the invasion of the faster-growing soft tissue cells into the defect site and to regenerate periodontal ligament, cementum, and bone.

Membranes generated by the combination of chitosan and bioglass [130, 131] or BG-NPs [81] (the ternary SiO_2-CaO-P_2O_5 and quaternary SiO_2-CaO-P_2O_5-MgO systems) have been prepared by solvent casting. Under this approach a polymeric solution containing the inorganic filler is poured onto a vessel and left to dry at room temperature to generate the membranes [81]. The membranes prepared with the composite formulations presented an improved mechanical performance and excellent apatite forming ability compared to pure chitosan membranes [81, 130–132]. The combination of BG-NPs and chitosan increased the composite stiffness [132], while the metabolic activity of periodontal ligament cells (hPDL) and stem cells cultured on these membranes was enhanced with the addition of BG-NPs. In addition, an increase in the hPDL proliferation when they were cultured onto the composite membranes was observed [132]. The addition of BG-NPs promoted greater cell matrix mineralization by both types of cells. Thus, the chitosan/BG-NP membranes could have potential to be used as a temporary guided tissue regeneration membrane in periodontal regeneration. They could act as barrier membranes to prevent the invasion of the periodontal defects by soft tissues since these membranes were non-cytotoxic and did not present early degradation [132].

Nonetheless, the application of these materials for periodontal regeneration requires the contact of the two sides of the membranes with distinct biological environments in which only one of the sides is in contact with a region where osteointegration is targeted. Thus, composite membranes were developed to present distinct properties in both sides. One of the sides was designed to be a barrier to soft tissue invasion by blocking the migration of epithelial cells [130, 131, 133]. The other side of the membrane was formulated to promote bone growth. In this way, biocompatible and biodegradable composite membranes were produced through the combination of PDLLA and bioglass particles, featuring an asymmetric bioactivity and a good integration between the polymeric and inorganic phases. These membranes were prepared using an adjusted solvent casting method, which promoted the nonuniform distribution of the inorganic component along the membrane thickness. Only the bioglass-rich side of the membrane induced the precipitation of bone-like apatite in SBF, indicating that this biomaterial exhibit asymmetric osteoconductive properties [80, 133]. Their mechanical properties were also evaluated, and a clear plasticization effect of water was detected as well as an increase in stiffness. SaOs-2 cells attached on both sides and proliferated during 7 days of culture [80]. Results with both human bone marrow stromal cells and hPDL cells revealed an improved cell adhesion and proliferation and stimulated cell differentiation, mineralization, and production of extracellular matrix and calcium nodules, suggesting the positive effect of adding the bioactive microparticles into the PDLLA matrix [133]. The results indicate that the proposed asymmetric PDLLA/bioglass membranes have potential to be used in guided bone tissue regeneration therapies.

Luz et al. used micro-contact printing to pattern mineralizable elements onto a membrane [134]. Freestanding chitosan membranes were used, and circular motifs containing BG-NPs were printed on them using previously inked PDMS stamps. The bioactive character of the BG-NP spots allowed the nucleation and growth of apatite, highly localized in the patterned regions of the chitosan membranes. Results showed that L929 cells replicated the initial inorganic pattern preferring the environment created by the BG-NPs rather than migrating to chitosan. With this simple micro-contact printing approach, it was proved that it is possible to control the cellular interactions with a bioactive substrate at the microscale level. Successful patterning of fibroblasts is an indication of the versatility of the developed system. This approach allows the spatial control of the biomaterials' properties at the microscale and could be potentially used for skin, vascular, articular, and bone tissue engineering. Additionally, these systems can also be used under cocultures systems or to develop substrates able to confine cells in specific regions [134].

Finally, Couto et al. developed a biodegradable multilayer coating, through the sequential deposition of a polycation (chitosan) and an anionic element (BG-NPs) [135]. Quartz crystal microbalance (QCM-D) study revealed that this methodology could be used to produce nanostructured multilayers upon increasing the number of layer-by-layer cycles [135]. The hypothesis of this concept was that such robust coatings could also induce the formation of apatite upon immersion in SBF [135]. The proposed method could be also employed in the coatings of substrates with complex geometries, including scaffolds for bone tissue engineering, and, thus, constitutes a new technological solution to improve osteoconductivity of a variety of implants for orthopedic applications [135].

10.5 Future Trends

During the past years the development of bioactive composite systems has been mainly focused on the incorporation of different inorganic mechanical reinforcements, which are also able to improve the bioactivity of the composites. The inorganic particles can be also used for the controlled delivery of bioactive agents, such as anti-inflammatory drug or proteins that promote different biological events (e.g., growth factors).

The decoration of the composite surface with bioactive molecules is being extensively studied in tissue engineering. A strong investment in the exploitation of grafting of different peptides, antibodies, or proteins that are able to induce stem cell recruitment, proliferation, and differentiation both in the surface and in the bulk of the 3D constructs is expected.

At the initial years of development, it was given a strong effort on materials science and engineering, although the science in this field is evolving into a more multidisciplinary approach, where materials science and biology are combined to create methodologies and biomaterials able to promote complete bone regeneration.

Acknowledgments We acknowledge the financial support of the EU 7th Framework Programme (FP7/2007–2013) under grant agreement no. REGPOT-CT2012-316331-POLARIS. RAP and AJL acknowledge the Portuguese Foundation for Science and Technology (FCT) for their postdoc (BPD/39333/2007) and PhD (BD/73174/2010) grants, respectively.

References

1. Bauer TW, Muschler GF (2000) Bone graft materials – an overview of the basic science. Clin Orthop Relat Res 371:10–27
2. Summers BN, Eisenstein SM (1989) Donor site pain from the ilium – a complication of lumbar spine fusion. J Bone Jt Surg-Br 71(4):677–680
3. Konduru S, Findlay G (2009) Anterior cervical discectomy: to graft or not to graft? Br J Neurosurg 23(1):99–103
4. Skalak R, Fox CF (1988) Tissue engineering. Liss, New York
5. Langer R, Vacanti JP (1993) Tissue engineering. Science 260(5110):920–926
6. Ohtsuki C, Kamitakahara M, Miyazaki T (2009) Bioactive ceramic-based materials with designed reactivity for bone tissue regeneration. J R Soc Interface 6(Suppl 3):S349–S360
7. Rajzer I, Castano O, Engel E, Planell JA (2010) Injectable and fast resorbable calcium phosphate cement for body-setting bone grafts. J Mater Sci-Mater Med 21(7):2049–2056
8. Link DP, van den Dolder J, Jurgens WJFM, Wolke JGC, Jansen JA (2006) Mechanical evaluation of implanted calcium phosphate cement incorporated with PLGA microparticles. Biomaterials 27(28):4941–4947
9. Alves NM, Leonor IB, Azevedo HS, Reis RL, Mano JF (2010) Designing biomaterials based on biomineralization of bone. J Mater Chem 20(15):2911–2921
10. Hench LL, Splinter RJ, Allen WC, Greenlee TK (1971) Bonding mechanisms at the interface of ceramic prosthetic materials. J Biomed Mater Res 5(6):117–141
11. Jones JR (2013) Review of bioactive glass: from Hench to hybrids. Acta Biomater 9(1):4457–4486

12. Salgado AJ, Coutinho OP, Reis RL (2004) Bone tissue engineering: state of the art and future trends. Macromol Biosci 4(8):743–765
13. Ducheyne P, Healy KE, Hutmacher DE, Grainger DE, Kirkpatrick CJ (2011) Comprehensive biomaterials. Elsevier, Boston
14. Bhatia SK (2010) Biomaterials for clinical applications. Springer, New York
15. Hench LL (1998) Bioceramics. J Am Ceram Soc 81(7):1705–1728
16. Wren AW, Cummins NM, Coughlan A, Towler MR (2010) The effect of adding organic polymers on the handling properties, strengths and bioactivity of a Ca-Sr-Zn-Si glass polyalkenoate cement. J Mater Sci 45(13):3554–3562
17. Hench LL, Jones JR, Sepulveda P (2002) Bioactive materials for tissue engineering scaffolds. In: Polak JM, Hench LL, Kemp P (eds) Future strategies for tissue and organ replacement. World Scientific Publishing Company, Singapore
18. Hench LL (1998) Bioactive materials: the potential for tissue regeneration. J Biomed Mater Res 41(4):511–518
19. Bohner M, Lemaitre J (2009) Can bioactivity be tested in vitro with SBF solution? Biomaterials 30(12):2175–2179
20. Boesel LF, Cachinho SCP, Fernandes MHV, Reis RL (2007) The in vitro bioactivity of two novel hydrophilic, partially degradable bone cements. Acta Biomater 3(2):175–182
21. Kokubo T, Kushitani H, Sakka S, Kitsugi T, Yamamuro T (1990) Solutions able to reproduce in vivo surface-structure changes in bioactive glass–ceramic a-W3. J Biomed Mater Res 24(6):721–734
22. Reis RL, Neves NM, Mano JF, Gomes ME, Marques AP, Azevedo HS (2008) Natural-based polymers for biomedical applications. Woodhead Publishing Ltd, Cambridge
23. Oyane A, Kim HM, Furuya T, Kokubo T, Miyazaki T, Nakamura T (2003) Preparation and assessment of revised simulated body fluids. J Biomed Mater Res Part A 65A(2):188–195
24. Song WH, Jun YK, Han Y, Hong SH (2004) Biomimetic apatite coatings on micro-arc oxidized titania. Biomaterials 25(17):3341–3349
25. Barrere F, van Blitterswijk CA, de Groot K, Layrolle P (2002) Influence of ionic strength and carbonate on the Ca-P coating formation from SBFx5 solution. Biomaterials 23(9):1921–1930
26. Kokubo T, Takadama H (2006) How useful is SBF in predicting in vivo bone bioactivity? Biomaterials 27(15):2907–2915
27. Ogino M, Ohuchi F, Hench LL (1980) Compositional dependence of the formation of calcium-phosphate films on bioglass. J Biomed Mater Res 14(1):55–64
28. Bakry AS, Tamura Y, Otsuki M, Kasugai S, Ohya K, Tagami J (2011) Cytotoxicity of 45S5 bioglass paste used for dentine hypersensitivity treatment. J Dent 39(9):599–603
29. Rahaman MN, Day DE, Sonny Bal B, Fu Q, Jung SB, Bonewald LF, Tomsia AP (2011) Bioactive glass in tissue engineering. Acta Biomater 7(6):2355–2373
30. Wilson J, Pigott GH, Schoen FJ, Hench LL (1981) Toxicology and biocompatibility of bioglasses. J Biomed Mater Res 15(6):805–817
31. Hench LL (2006) The story of bioglass (R). J Mater Sci-Mater Med 17(11):967–978
32. Bielby RC, Pryce RS, Hench LL, Polak JM (2005) Enhanced derivation of osteogenic cells from murine embryonic stem cells after treatment with ionic dissolution products of 58S bioactive sol–gel glass. Tissue Eng 11(3–4):479–488
33. Bielby RC, Christodoulou IS, Pryce RS, Radford WJP, Hench LL, Polak JM (2004) Time- and concentration-dependent effects of dissolution products of 58S sol–gel bioactive glass on proliferation and differentiation of murine and human osteoblasts. Tissue Eng 10(7–8): 1018–1026
34. Lai W, Garino J, Ducheyne P (2002) Silicon excretion from bioactive glass implanted in rabbit bone. Biomaterials 23(1):213–217
35. Burdick JA, Mauck RL (2010) Biomaterials for tissue engineering applications: a review of the past and future trends. Springer, New York
36. Hatton PV, Hurrell-Gillingham K, Brook IM (2006) Biocompatibility of glass-ionomer bone cements. J Dent 34(8):598–601

37. Niederauer G, Kieswetter K, Leatherbury NC, Greenspan DC (2002) Biodegradable implant material comprising bioactive ceramic. US patent 6344496
38. Fu Q, Saiz E, Rahaman MN, Tomsia AP (2011) Bioactive glass scaffolds for bone tissue engineering: state of the art and future perspectives. Mater Sci Eng C 31(7):1245–1256
39. Nayak JP, Kumar S, Bera J (2010) Sol–gel synthesis of bioglass-ceramics using rice husk ash as a source for silica and its characterization. J Non-Cryst Solids 356(28–30):1447–1451
40. Pires RA, Abrahams I, Nunes TG, Hawkes GE (2009) The role of alumina in aluminoborosilicate glasses for use in glass-ionomer cements. J Mater Chem 19(22):3652–3660
41. Pires RA, Abrahams I, Nunes TG, Hawkes GE (2006) Multinuclear magnetic resonance studies of borosilicate glasses for use in glass ionomer cements: incorporation of CaO and Al2O3. J Mater Chem 16(24):2364–2373
42. Pires R, Abrahams I, Nunes TG, Hawkes GE (2004) Non-random cation distribution in sodium-strontium-phosphate glasses. J Non-Cryst Solids 337(1):1–8
43. Wren A, Clarkin OM, Laffir FR, Ohtsuki C, Kim IY, Towler MR (2009) The effect of glass synthesis route on mechanical and physical properties of resultant glass ionomer cements. J Mater Sci-Mater Med 20(10):1991–1999
44. De Barra E, Hill RG (1998) Influence of alkali metal ions on the fracture properties of glass polyalkenoate (ionomer) cements. Biomaterials 19(6):495–502
45. Goller G, Demirklran H, Oktar FN, Demirkesen E (2003) Processing and characterization of bioglass reinforced hydroxyapatite composites. Ceram Int 29(6):721–724
46. Arcos D, Vallet-Regí M (2010) Sol–gel silica-based biomaterials and bone tissue regeneration. Acta Biomater 6(8):2874–2888
47. Wood D, Hill R (1991) Glass ceramic approach to controlling the properties of a glass-ionomer bone-cement. Biomaterials 12(2):164–710
48. Hench LL (1999) Bioactive glasses and glass-ceramics. Bioceramics 293:37–63
49. Luz GM, Mano JF (2011) Preparation and characterization of bioactive glass nanoparticles prepared by sol–gel for biomedical applications. Nanotechnology 22(49):494014
50. Lei B, Chen XF, Wang YJ, Zhao NR, Du C, Fang LM (2010) Surface nanoscale patterning of bioactive glass to support cellular growth and differentiation. J Biomed Mater Res Part A 94A(4):1091–1099
51. Sepulveda P, Jones JR, Hench LL (2001) Characterization of melt-derived 45S5 and sol–gel-derived 58S bioactive glasses. J Biomed Mater Res 58(6):734–740
52. Li R, Clark AE, Hench LL (1991) An investigation of bioactive glass powders by sol–gel processing. J Appl Biomater 2(4):231–239
53. Hench LL, West JK (1990) The sol–gel process. Chem Rev 90(1):33–72
54. Dowling AH, Fleming GJP (2011) The influence of poly(acrylic) acid number average molecular weight and concentration in solution on the compressive fracture strength and modulus of a glass-ionomer restorative. Dent Mater 27(6):535–543
55. Hong Z, Reis RL, Mano JF (2009) Preparation and in vitro characterization of novel bioactive glass ceramic nanoparticles. J Biomed Mater Res Part A 88A(2):304–313
56. Hong ZK, Merino EG, Reis RL, Mano JF (2009) Novel rice-shaped bioactive ceramic nanoparticles. Adv Eng Mater 11(5):B25–B29
57. Saravanapavan P, Jones JR, Pryce RS, Hench LL (2003) Bioactivity of gel-glass powders in the CaO-SiO2 system: a comparison with ternary (CaO-P_2O_5-SiO_2) and quaternary glasses (SiO_2-CaO-P_2O_5-Na_2O). J Biomed Mater Res Part A 66A(1):110–119
58. Siqueira RL, Peitl O, Zanotto ED (2011) Gel-derived SiO_2-CaO-Na_2O-P_2O_5 bioactive powders: synthesis and in vitro bioactivity. Mater Sci Eng C 31(5):983–991
59. Lin S, Ionescu C, Pike KJ, Smith ME, Jones JR (2009) Nanostructure evolution and calcium distribution in sol–gel derived bioactive glass. J Mater Chem 19(9):1276–1282
60. Valliant EM, Turdean-Ionescu CA, Hanna JV, Smith ME, Jones JR (2012) Role of pH and temperature on silica network formation and calcium incorporation into sol–gel derived bioactive glasses. J Mater Chem 22(4):1613–1619

61. Labbaf S, Tsigkou O, Muller KH, Stevens MM, Porter AE, Jones JR (2011) Spherical bioactive glass particles and their interaction with human mesenchymal stem cells in vitro. Biomaterials 32(4):1010–1018
62. Hong ZK, Reis RL, Mano JF (2008) Preparation and in vitro characterization of scaffolds of poly(L-lactic acid) containing bioactive glass ceramic nanoparticles. Acta Biomater 4(5):1297–1306
63. Kothapalli CR, Shaw MT, Wei M (2005) Biodegradable HA-PLA 3-D porous scaffolds: effect of nano-sized filler content on scaffold properties. Acta Biomater 1(6):653–662
64. Roco MC (1999) Nanoparticles and nanotechnology research. J Nanoparticle Res 1(1):1–6
65. Hong ZK, Zhang PB, Liu AX, Chen L, Chen XS, Jing XB (2007) Composites of poly(lactide-co-glycolide) and the surface modified carbonated hydroxyapatite nanoparticles. J Biomed Mater Res Part A 81A(3):515–522
66. Wheeler DL, Stokes KE, Hoellrich RG, Chamberland DL, McLoughlin SW (1998) Effect of bioactive glass particle size on osseous regeneration of cancellous defects. J Biomed Mater Res 41(4):527–533
67. Ducheyne P (1999) Effect of bioactive glass particle size on osseous regeneration. J Biomed Mater Res 46(2):301–303
68. Liu H, Webster TJ (2007) Nanomedicine for implants: a review of studies and necessary experimental tools. Biomaterials 28(2):354–369
69. Hong Z, Liu A, Chen L, Chen X, Jing X (2009) Preparation of bioactive glass ceramic nanoparticles by combination of sol–gel and coprecipitation method. J Non-Cryst Solids 355(6):368–372
70. Luz GM, Leite AJ, Neto AI, Song WL, Mano JF (2011) Wettable arrays onto superhydrophobic surfaces for bioactivity testing of inorganic nanoparticles. Mater Lett 65(2):296–299
71. Couto D, Hong Z, Mano JF (2009) Development of bioactive and biodegradable chitosan-based injectable systems containing bioactive glass nanoparticles. Acta Biomater 5(1):115–123
72. Chen XF, Lei B, Wang YJ, Zhao N (2009) Morphological control and in vitro bioactivity of nanoscale bioactive glasses. J Non-Cryst Solids 355(13):791–796
73. El-Kady AM, Ali AF, Rizk RA, Ahmed MM (2012) Synthesis, characterization and microbiological response of silver doped bioactive glass nanoparticles. Ceram Int 38(1):177–188
74. Boccaccini AR, Erol M, Stark WJ, Mohn D, Hong ZK, Mano JF (2010) Polymer/bioactive glass nanocomposites for biomedical applications: a review. Compos Sci Technol 70(13):1764–1776
75. Zhang D, Vedel E, Hupa L, Ylanen H, Hupa M (2005) In vitro characterization of bioactive glasses. Bioceramics 17(284–286):481–484
76. Hong ZK, Luz GM, Hampel PJ, Jin MS, Liu AX, Chen XS, Mano JF (2010) Mono-dispersed bioactive glass nanospheres: preparation and effects on biomechanics of mammalian cells. J Biomed Mater Res Part A 95A(3):747–754
77. Rezwan K, Chen QZ, Blaker JJ, Boccaccini AR (2006) Biodegradable and bioactive porous polymer/inorganic composite scaffolds for bone tissue engineering. Biomaterials 27(18):3413–3431
78. Gomes FO, Pires RA, Reis RL (2013) Aluminum-free glass-ionomer bone cements with enhanced bioactivity and biodegradability. Mater Sci Eng C 33(3):1361–1370
79. Fernandes EM, Pires RA, Mano JF, Reis RL (2013) Bionanocomposites from lignocellulosic resources: properties, applications and future trends for their use in the biomedical field. Prog Polym Sci. doi:10.1016/j.progpolymsci
80. Caridade SG, Merino EG, Martins GV, Luz GM, Alves NM, Mano JF (2012) Membranes of poly(DL-lactic acid)/bioglass (R) with asymmetric bioactivity for biomedical applications. J Bioact Compat Polym 27(5):429–440
81. Luz GM, Mano JF (2010) New composite membranes containing bioactive glass-ceramic nanoparticles and chitosan for biomedical applications. Adv Mater Forum 636–637:31–35
82. Tadmor Z, Gogos CG (2006) Principles of polymer processing. Wiley, New Jersey

83. Mano JF, Silva GA, Azevedo HS, Malafaya PB, Sousa RA, Silva SS, Boesel LF, Oliveira JM, Santos TC, Marques AP, Neves NM, Reis RL (2007) Natural origin biodegradable systems in tissue engineering and regenerative medicine: present status and some moving trends. J R Soc Interface 4(17):999–1030
84. Kramschuster A, Turng L-S (2013) Fabrication of tissue engineering scaffolds. Handbook of biopolymers and biodegradable plastics. William Andrew Publishing, Boston
85. Babu R, O'Connor K, Seeram R (2013) Current progress on bio-based polymers and their future trends. Prog Biomater 2(1):8
86. Reis RL, Cunha AM, Fernandes MH, Correia RN (1997) Treatments to induce the nucleation and growth of apatite-like layers on polymeric surfaces and foams. J Mater Sci-Mater Med 8(12):897–905
87. Demirgoz D, Elvira C, Mano JF, Cunha AM, Piskin E, Reis RL (2000) Chemical modification of starch based biodegradable polymeric blends: effects on water uptake, degradation behaviour and mechanical properties. Polym Degrad Stab 70(2):161–170
88. Neves NM, Kouyumdzhiev A, Reis RL (2005) The morphology, mechanical properties and ageing behavior of porous injection molded starch-based blends for tissue engineering scaffolding. Mater Sci Eng C 25(2):195–200
89. Oliveira JT, Correlo VM, Sol PC, Costa-Pinto AR, Malafaya PB, Salgado AJ, Bhattacharya M, Charbord P, Neves NM, Reis RL (2008) Assessment of the suitability of chitosan/polybutylene succinate scaffolds seeded with mouse mesenchymal progenitor cells for a cartilage tissue engineering approach. Tissue Eng A 14(10):1651–1661
90. Duarte ARC, Mano JF, Reis RL (2010) Enzymatic degradation of 3D scaffolds of starch-poly-(ε-caprolactone) prepared by supercritical fluid technology. Polym Degrad Stab 95(10):2110–2117
91. Santos MI, Unger RE, Sousa RA, Reis RL, Kirkpatrick CJ (2009) Crosstalk between osteoblasts and endothelial cells co-cultured on a polycaprolactone–starch scaffold and the in vitro development of vascularization. Biomaterials 30(26):4407–4415
92. Ghosh S, Gutierrez V, Fernández C, Rodriguez-Perez MA, Viana JC, Reis RL, Mano JF (2008) Dynamic mechanical behavior of starch-based scaffolds in dry and physiologically simulated conditions: effect of porosity and pore size. Acta Biomater 4(4):950–959
93. Jukola H, Nikkola L, Gomes ME, Chiellini F, Tukiainen M, Kellomäki M, Chiellini E, Reis RL, Ashammakhi N (2008) Development of a bioactive glass fiber reinforced starch–polycaprolactone composite. J Biomed Mater Res B Appl Biomater 87B(1):197–203
94. Kellomäki M, Niiranen H, Puumanen K, Ashammakhi N, Waris T, Törmälä P (2000) Bioabsorbable scaffolds for guided bone regeneration and generation. Biomaterials 21(24):2495–2505
95. Leonor IB, Sousa RA, Cunha AM, Reis RL, Zhong ZP, Greenspan D (2002) Novel starch thermoplastic/bioglass((R)) composites: mechanical properties, degradation behavior and in-vitro bioactivity. J Mater Sci-Mater Med 13(10):939–945
96. Niemela T, Niiranen H, Kellomaki M, Tormala P (2005) Self-reinforced composites of bioabsorbable polymer and bioactive glass with different bioactive glass contents. Part 1: Initial mechanical properties and bioactivity. Acta Biomater 1(2):235–242
97. Niiranen H, Pyhalto T, Rokkanen O, Kellomaki M, Tormala P (2004) In vitro and in vivo behavior of self-reinforced bioabsorbable polymer and self-reinforced bioabsorbable polymer/bioactive glass composites. J Biomed Mater Res Part A 69A(4):699–708
98. Thompson ID, Hench LL (1998) Mechanical properties of bioactive glasses, glass-ceramics and composites. Proc Inst Mech Eng Part H-J Eng Med 212(H2):127–136
99. Correlo VM, Boesel LF, Pinho E, Costa-Pinto AR, Alves da Silva ML, Bhattacharya M, Mano JF, Neves NM, Reis RL (2009) Melt-based compression-molded scaffolds from chitosan–polyester blends and composites: morphology and mechanical properties. J Biomed Mater Res Part A 91A(2):489–504
100. Ghosh S, Viana JC, Reis RL, Mano JF (2008) Development of porous lamellar poly(l-lactic acid) scaffolds by conventional injection molding process. Acta Biomater 4(4):887–896

101. Mathieu LM, Bourban PE, Månson JAE (2006) Processing of homogeneous ceramic/polymer blends for bioresorbable composites. Compos Sci Technol 66(11–12):1606–1614
102. Puppi D, Piras AM, Chiellini F, Chiellini E, Martins A, Leonor IB, Neves NM, Reis RL (2011) Optimized electro- and wet-spinning techniques for the production of polymeric fibrous scaffolds loaded with bisphosphonate and hydroxyapatite. J Tissue Eng Regen Med 5(4):253–263
103. Leonor IB, Rodrigues GT, Gomes ME, Reis RL (2011) In situ functionalization of wet-spun fibre meshes for bone tissue engineering. J Tissue Eng Regen Med 5(2):104–111
104. Tuzlakoglu K, Pashkuleva I, Rodrigues MT, Gomes ME, van Lenthe GH, Muller R, Reis RL (2010) A new route to produce starch-based fiber mesh scaffolds by wet spinning and subsequent surface modification as a way to improve cell attachment and proliferation. J Biomed Mater Res Part A 92A(1):369–377
105. Tuzlakoglu K, Reis RL (2007) Formation of bone-like apatite layer on chitosan fiber mesh scaffolds by a biomimetic spraying process. J Mater Sci-Mater Med 18(7):1279–1286
106. Denkbas EB, Seyyal M, Piskin E (2000) Implantable 5-fluorouracil loaded chitosan scaffolds prepared by wet spinning. J Membr Sci 172(1–2):33–38
107. Zhang XF, Hua H, Shen XY, Yang Q (2007) In vitro degradation and biocompatibility of poly(L-lactic acid)/chitosan fiber composites. Polymer 48(4):1005–1011
108. Yeong W-Y, Chua C-K, Leong K-F, Chandrasekaran M (2004) Rapid prototyping in tissue engineering: challenges and potential. Trends Biotechnol 22(12):643–652
109. Comesana R, Lusquinos F, del Val J, Lopez-Alvarez M, Quintero F, Riveiro A, Boutinguiza M, de Carlos A, Jones JR, Hill RG, Pou J (2011) Three-dimensional bioactive glass implants fabricated by rapid prototyping based on CO2 laser cladding. Acta Biomater 7(9):3476–3487
110. Elomaa L, Kokkari A, Narhi T, Seppala JV (2013) Porous 3D modeled scaffolds of bioactive glass and photocrosslinkable poly(epsilon-caprolactone) by stereolithography. Compos Sci Technol 74:99–106
111. Billiet T, Vandenhaute M, Schelfhout J, Van Vlierberghe S, Dubruel P (2012) A review of trends and limitations in hydrogel-rapid prototyping for tissue engineering. Biomaterials 33(26):6020–6041
112. Hoque ME, Chuan YL, Pashby I (2012) Extrusion based rapid prototyping technique: an advanced platform for tissue engineering scaffold fabrication. Biopolymers 97(2):83–93
113. Yun HS, Kim SH, Khang D, Choi J, Kim HH, Kang M (2011) Biomimetic component coating on 3D scaffolds using high bioactivity of mesoporous bioactive ceramics. Int J Nanomedicine 6:2521–2531
114. Yun HS, Kim SE, Hyun YT, Heo SJ, Shin JW (2007) Three-dimensional mesoporous-giantporous inorganic/organic composite scaffolds for tissue engineering. Chem Mater 19(26):6363–6366
115. Xie B, Parkhill RL, Warren WL, Smay JE (2006) Direct writing of three-dimensional polymer scaffolds using colloidal gels. Adv Funct Mater 16(13):1685–1693
116. Luo YX, Wu CT, Lode A, Gelinsky M (2013) Hierarchical mesoporous bioactive glass/alginate composite scaffolds fabricated by three-dimensional plotting for bone tissue engineering. Biofabrication 5(1):1–13
117. Provenzano MJ, Murphy KPJ, Riley LH (2004) Bone cements: review of their physiochemical and biochemical properties in percutaneous vertebroplasty. Am J Neuroradiol 25(7):1286–1290
118. Temenoff JS, Mikos AG (2000) Injectable biodegradable materials for orthopedic tissue engineering. Biomaterials 21(23):2405–2412
119. Griffith LG (2002) Emerging design principles in biomaterials and scaffolds for tissue engineering. Repar Med Grow Tissues Organs 961:83–95
120. Luz GM, Mano JF (2010) Mineralized structures in nature: examples and inspirations for the design of new composite materials and biomaterials. Compos Sci Technol 70(13):1777–1788
121. Bretcanu O, Chen Q, Misra SK, Boccaccini AR, Roy I, Verne E, Brovarone CV (2007) Biodegradable polymer coated 45S5 bioglass-derived glass-ceramic scaffolds for bone tissue engineering. Glass Technol-Eur J Glass Sci Technol Part A 48(5):227–234

122. Chen QZ, Boccaccini AR (2006) Poly(D, L-lactic acid) coated 45S5 bioglass (R)-based scaffolds: processing and characterization. J Biomed Mater Res Part A 77A(3):445–457
123. Maquet V, Boccaccini AR, Pravata L, Notingher I, Jerome R (2004) Porous poly(alpha-hydroxyacid)/bioglass (R) composite scaffolds for bone tissue engineering. I: preparation and in vitro characterisation. Biomaterials 25(18):4185–4194
124. Blaker JJ, Maquet V, Jerome R, Boccaccini AR, Nazhat SN (2005) Mechanical properties of highly porous PDLLA/bioglass (R) composite foams as scaffolds for bone tissue engineering. Acta Biomater 1(6):643–652
125. Marelli B, Ghezzi CE, Mohn D, Stark WJ, Barralet JE, Boccaccini AR, Nazhat SN (2011) Accelerated mineralization of dense collagen-nano bioactive glass hybrid gels increases scaffold stiffness and regulates osteoblastic function. Biomaterials 32(34):8915–8926
126. Misra SK, Ansari T, Mohn D, Valappil SP, Brunner TJ, Stark WJ, Roy I, Knowles JC, Sibbons PD, Jones EV, Boccaccini AR, Salih V (2010) Effect of nanoparticulate bioactive glass particles on bioactivity and cytocompatibility of poly(3-hydroxybutyrate) composites. J R Soc Interface 7(44):453–465
127. Peter M, Binulal NS, Nair SV, Selvamurugan N, Tamura H, Jayakumar R (2010) Novel biodegradable chitosan-gelatin/nano-bioactive glass ceramic composite scaffolds for alveolar bone tissue engineering. Chem Eng J 158(2):353–361
128. Xu CX, Su PQ, Chen XF, Meng YC, Yu WH, Xiang AP, Wang YJ (2011) Biocompatibility and osteogenesis of biomimetic bioglass-collagen-phosphatidylserine composite scaffolds for bone tissue engineering. Biomaterials 32(4):1051–1058
129. Liu AX, Hong ZK, Zhuang XL, Chen XS, Cui Y, Liu Y, Jing XB (2008) Surface modification of bioactive glass nanoparticles and the mechanical and biological properties of poly(L-lactide) composites. Acta Biomater 4(4):1005–1015
130. Caridade SG, Merino EG, Luz GM, Alves NM, Mano JF (2010) Bioactivity and viscoelastic characterization in physiological simulated conditions of chitosan/bioglass (R) composite membranes. Adv Mater Forum 636–637(Pt 1 and 2):26–30
131. Caridade SG, Merino EG, Alves NM, Mano JF (2012) Bioactivity and viscoelastic characterization of chitosan/bioglass (R) composite membranes. Macromol Biosci 12(8):1106–1113
132. Mota J, Yu N, Caridade SG, Luz GM, Gomes ME, Reis RL, Jansen JA, Walboomers XF, Mano JF (2012) Chitosan/bioactive glass nanoparticle composite membranes for periodontal regeneration. Acta Biomater 8(11):4173–4180
133. Leal AI, Caridade SG, Ma JL, Yu N, Gomes ME, Reis RL, Jansen JA, Walboomers XF, Mano JF (2013) Asymmetric PDLLA membranes containing bioglass (R) for guided tissue regeneration: characterization and in vitro biological behavior. Dent Mater 29(4):427–436
134. Luz GM, Boesel L, del Campo A, Mano JF (2012) Micropatterning of bioactive glass nanoparticles on chitosan membranes for spatial controlled biomineralization. Langmuir 28(17):6970–6977
135. Couto DS, Alves NM, Mano JF (2009) Nanostructured multilayer coatings combining chitosan with bioactive glass nanoparticles. J Nanosci Nanotechnol 9(3):1741–1748

Chapter 11
Development of Skeletal Drug Delivery System Based on Apatite/Collagen Composite Cement

Makoto Otsuka

Abstract Since bone resorption and formation occur repeatedly within the functional units referred to as bone multicellular units, uncoupling between bone resorption by osteoclasts and bone formation by osteoblasts causes an absolute decrease in the amount of bone in osteoporosis. For that reason, it is necessary to fully understand the remodeling characteristics of bone grafts by osteoclasts and osteoblasts to high-bioactive materials. We have, therefore, prepared hydroxyapatite (HAp) and collagen composites to improve bioaffinity through the interaction between materials and bone cells for applications in drug delivery devices. Apatite/collagen composite cements could be applied to artificial bone drug delivery systems without drug inactivation caused by high pressure and those that exhibit long-term slow drug release in vitro and high in vivo biocompatibility in osteoporosis model rats. On the other hand, geometrical structure of pores in implantable artificial bone has been proven successful in bone generation, since bone-related cells can be cultured more readily in interconnected porous materials, such as coral-modified implant made by calcium phosphate. Interconnective pores in coral-like material are therapeutically effective in bone regeneration within the body through the introduction of bone cells and capitally blood vessels as a scaffold for bone cells to spread and proliferate. The interconnective porous biomaterials are, therefore, developed based on self-setting apatite/collagen composite cement as materials with enhanced biocompatibility and drug delivery capability. Since the drug release rate from the composite device could be controlled by various geometrical factors, the relationship between drug-release rate and number of the macropores was investigated by in vitro dissolution test. Bioaffinity of the interconnective porous biomaterials of apatite/collagen composite cement was examined in rat models using X-ray computed tomography.

M. Otsuka (✉)
Faculty of Pharmacy, Research Institute of Pharmaceutical Science, Musashino University, 1-1-20 Shinmachi, 202-8585 Nishi-Tokyo, Tokyo, Japan
e-mail: motsuka@musashino-u.ac.jp

B. Ben-Nissan (ed.), *Advances in Calcium Phosphate Biomaterials*, Springer Series in Biomaterials Science and Engineering 2, DOI 10.1007/978-3-642-53980-0_11,

Keywords Apatite cement • Apatite/collagen composite • Biocompatibility • Drug delivery • Nanostructure • Cell scaffold

11.1 Introduction

In order to develop highly bioactive bone materials, it is vital that the characteristics of bone graft remodeling by osteoclasts and osteoblasts are fully understood. Since bone resorption and formation occur repeatedly in the functional units called bone multicellular units, which maintain the dynamic equilibrium of mineral density in normal bone [1], uncoupling between bone resorption by osteoclasts and bone formation by osteoblasts causes an absolute decrease in the amount of bone in osteoporosis. Bioactive ceramics with excellent bioaffinity, such as hydroxyapatite (HAp), β-tricalcium phosphate, and bioglass ceramics, are developed and can directly connect with bone [2]. However, the materials currently used as artificial bones possesses characteristics that are inadequate when compared to natural bone such as their brittle nature and poor mechanical strength. The material could also remain in the bone for an extended period because their chemical composition and geometrical structure are very different from natural bone and they exhibit lower bioaffinity [2].

On the other hand, a HAp/collagen composite with a nanostructure which is similar to natural bone was realized by Miyamoto et al. [3] and Kikuchi et al. [4, 5] and they reported that apatite and collagen were self-organizing and formed nanostructure composites by a simultaneous titration coprecipitation method and concluded that the molecular interaction between apatite and collagen induced formation of nanostructure particles, which has similar characteristics and biocompatibility to natural bone. John et al. [6] prepared apatite/collagen composite by using collagen sponge and investigated its suitability for bone repair applications. The results indicated that the bio-mimic materials had significantly high bioaffinity with natural bone after implantation and the molecular level structure of HAp/collagen composites is a very important factor for the biocompatibility of artificial bone in vivo. We have, therefore, developed self-setting HAp/collagen composite cement to improve bioaffinity by enhancing the interaction between the composites and bone cells for applications in drug delivery and cell scaffold devices [7].

11.2 Artificial Bone Cements Based on Self-Setting Apatite/Collagen Composite Cements (AC)

11.2.1 Physicochemical Prosperities of the AC

To develop an artificial self-setting bone cement with almost the same chemical formulation (80 % HAp and 20 % collagen) as natural bone, the AC was prepared

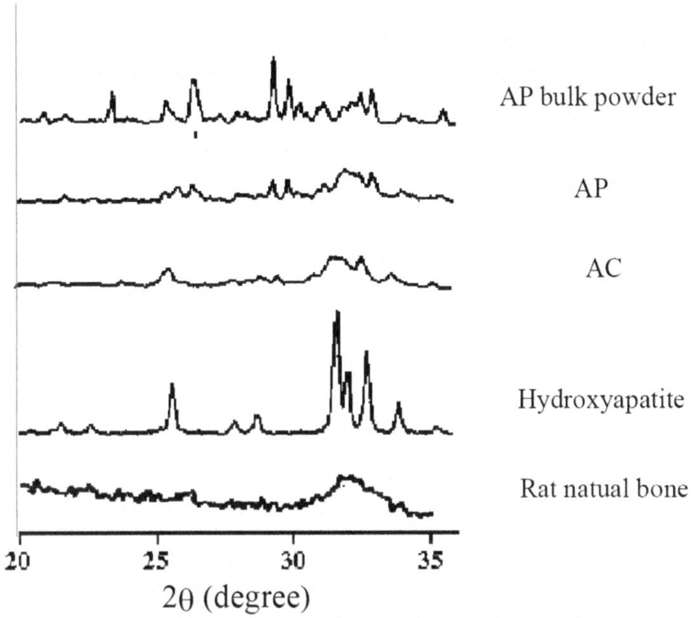

Fig. 11.1 X-ray diffraction profiles of self-setting apatite cement bulk powder (AP) and self-setting apatite/collagen composite cement (AC)

as follows: firstly, self-setting apatite cement bulk powder (AP) consisting of an equimolar mixture of tetracalcium phosphate (TECP, $Ca_4(PO_4)_2O$) and dicalcium phosphate dihydrate (DCPD, $CaHPO_4{\cdot}2H_2O$) was prepared by grinding in an agate vibration mixer mill [8–10]. The AC bulk powder was obtained by grinding the AP powder with 20 % type I bovine collagen in the vibration mixer mill. The AP or AC bulk powder (0.500 g) was mixed homogeneously with 0.20 mL of 11 mM phosphoric acid. The final paste was poured into a plastic mold and stored at 37 °C and 100 % relative humidity for 24 h.

The X-ray powder diffraction (XRD) profiles of the sample cements (Fig. 11.1) were measure to evaluate the test material characteristics as an index of bioaffinity. The fresh fixed AP cements showed typical diffraction peaks of HAp at $2\theta = 31.8$ and 32.8° with additional peaks at $2\theta = 28.9$ and 29.5° due to TECP and at $2\theta = 26.5°$ due to DCPD. The XRD results indicated that the majority of metastable calcium phosphates, DCPD and TECP, transformed into low-crystallinity HAp, but some parts of DCPD and TECP did not transform and remained in the cements. In contrast, the XRD profiles of AC had broad peaks at 31–33° due to bone-like HAp and no peaks due to TECP and DCPD (Fig. 11.1). The results also suggested that crystalline transformation of AP is accelerated by the addition of collagen and mechanical treatment. The transformed apatite structure in the AC was similar to natural bone apatite with low crystallinity reported by Kikuchi et al. [4], because the bone-like nano-apatite crystals precipitated out on collagen matrices during setting

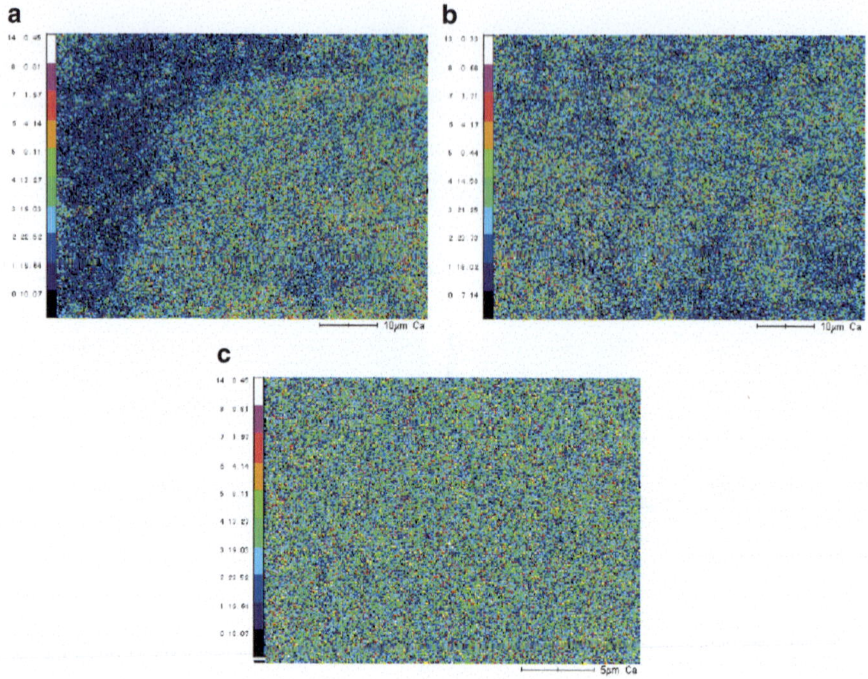

Fig. 11.2 Effects of grinding on element dispersibility of the AC by electron probe microanalyzer

time after mixing the solution. Chhettry et al. [8] reported the relationship between crystallinity and solubility of bone-like carbonated apatite and demonstrated that natural bone apatite had low crystallinity and high solubility. Therefore, the apatite in the AC might have high solubility and high biocompatibility.

Scanning electron microscopy (SEM) and electron probe microanalyzer (EPMA) were performed to characterize element dispensability in the AC [7]. The SEM of AC without grinding showed a rough surface and large particles (more than 20 μm particles in diameter), indicating that the cement was a heterogeneous system. In contrast, AC with grinding showed a smooth surface consisting of particles less than 1–2 μm in diameter.

The natural bone had a smooth surface with cracks. The result of mapping of calcium by EPMA suggested that there are calcium rich and less part in the AC without grinding (Fig. 11.2a). The calcium ion distribution in the AC (Fig. 11.2b) was more homogeneous than that in the AC without grinding, and the calcium ion homogeneity was almost the same as that of natural bone (Fig. 11.2c). These results indicated that AC without grinding had a heterogeneous structure in which collagen and calcium phosphates were not mixed uniformly. On the other hand, calcium and phosphates were dispersed homogeneously at the nanoscale in the cement as well as in the natural bone.

The result indicated that the raw materials of the apatite cement, such as DCPC and TECP, were micronized by mechanical energy during grinding in the vibration

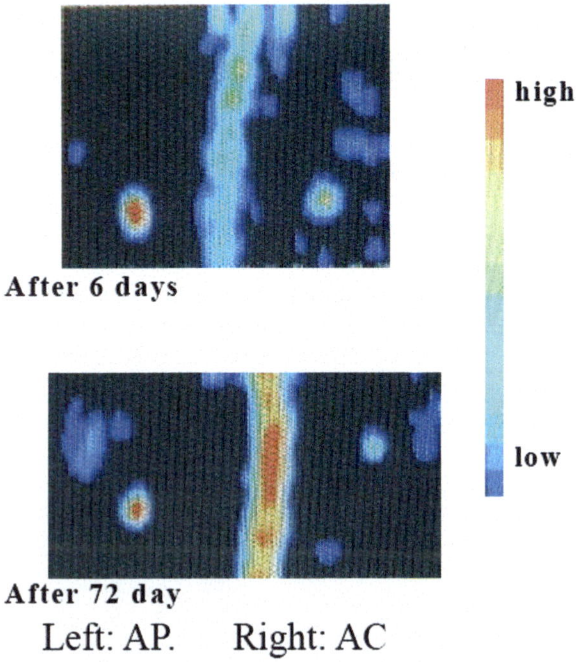

Fig. 11.3 Microradiogram of implanted AP and AC cements in rats by DEXA

mill and distributed into collagen matrices. Then, the micronized DCPD and TECP dissolved and recrystallized to nanoparticle apatite on collagen matrices. Since apatite formation of cement was catalyzed on collagen matrices, almost 100 % of calcium phosphate might be transformed to apatite.

11.2.2 Biodegradation of the AC in Rats

AC cements were implanted into the backs of rats and the density measured using bone mineral densitometry. Microradiograms of the AP and AC (Fig. 11.3) were measured by dual energy X-ray absorptiometry after implant in the rats, and the cement mineral content (BMC) was evaluated based on the microradiograms. The BMC of the implanted cements decreased with time, indicating that the cement was gradually bioabsorbed. Bioabsorption rates of the implanted cements (Fig. 11.4a) were dependent on the quality of cement (cement formulation). The BMCs of both of the AC and AP decrease over time, and the BMC of the AC was found to be significantly lower than that of the AP.

The effect of grinding on the BMC of the implanted cements (Fig. 11.4b) revealed the concentration of BMC decreases over time regardless of whether grinding was performed. The concentration of BMC in AC without grinding was always found to be lower than that of the AC.

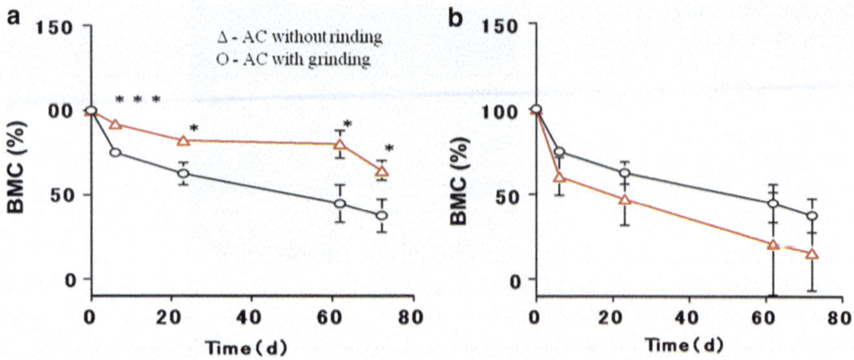

Fig. 11.4 Effects of cement formulation on the BMC of AP and AC cements by DEXA

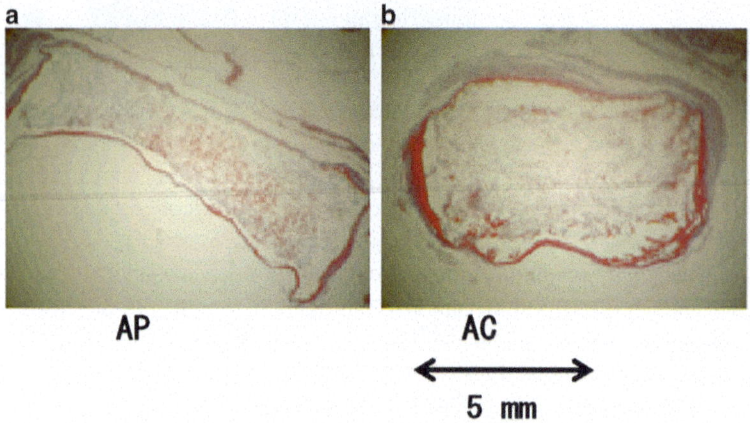

Fig. 11.5 Cross-section micrographs of (**a**) AP and (**b**) AC cements after 72 days of implantation

The results of the AP and AC suggested that the biodegradation rate was dependent on the cement quality and geometrical structure, and the rate can be shown as AP < AC < AC without grinding. The biodegradation rate of the AP was found to be the slowest as it is composed entirely of pure inorganic material. On the contrary, by having a nanoscale heterogeneous structure consisting of 80 % apatite and 20 % collagen, the AC without grinding had the highest biodegradation rate (Fig. 11.2a, d). The decreasing BMC behavior of the AC was found to be between those of the AP and the AC without grinding. This is mainly due to a decrease in the particle size of the cement and bone-like cells penetrating into the cement after implantation.

Figure 11.5 shows the micrographs of the cross section of the demineralized sample cement blocks after 72 days of implantation in soft tissue. The AP (Fig. 11.5a) kept its original diameter (6 mm) in soft tissues after implantation. A slight reduction in thickness was also observed as the organic components have penetrated into the cement. The data from the in vivo experiment showed shrinkage in the diameter of AC by approximately 30 %, while an increase in thickness was recorded (Fig. 11.5b). In contrast, AC without grinding (data not shown) was totally absorbed and no traces of the cement were discovered in the soft tissues.

These results indicated that the BMC changes and their bioaffinity were significantly dependent on the quality of apatite and the nano-geometrical structure in the cement. The biodegradation rate of the AC could be controlled by the cement formulation and the geometrical structure.

11.3 Drug Delivery System Based on Apatite/Collagen Composite Cements

In order to develop bone regenerative artificial bone systems, it is necessary that bone growth factors are loaded in bioactive artificial bone matrices and slowly releases through time. Shiraki et al. [9] reported that metacarpal bone mineral density was increased in osteoporosis through the administration of menatetrenone, vitamin K_2 (VK2, anti-osteoporosis drug). They indicated that VK2 prevented trabecular bone loss and the occurrence of bone fractures [10] in osteoporosis. Therefore, the VK2 is selected as a model drug and loaded in the bone cement matrices to develop a drug delivery system.

11.3.1 Therapeutic Effect of Drug Delivery System of the AC on Bone Mass in the Rats

Apatite/collagen composite cements loaded with bone growth factors is believed to have a better biocompatibility than simple artificial bone implants. The effects of anti-osteoporosis drug on bone mass were investigated in the osteoporosis rats. The AC cement bulk powder was prepared by grinding 80 % AP with 20 % collagen for 20 min. After that, the bulk powder (0.500 g) of the AP or AC was mixed homogeneously with 0.20 mL of 11 mM phosphoric acid, then 10 mg of VK2 powders were mixed, and the final paste was poured into a plastic mold and stored at 37 °C and 100 % relative humidity for 24 h. Three types of the drug delivery devices were developed [7]:

1. APK – VK2 loaded in the AP
2. ACPK – VK2 loaded in the AC without grinding
3. ACGK – VK2 loaded in the AC with grinding

After the VK2-loaded devices were implanted in the osteoporosis rats, the BMC was measured as index of biodegradation rate. Figure 11.6 shows the effects of VK2 on BMC of apatite/collagen cements implanted in osteoporosis rats. The BMC profile of the ACGK was significantly higher than those of the ACPK and

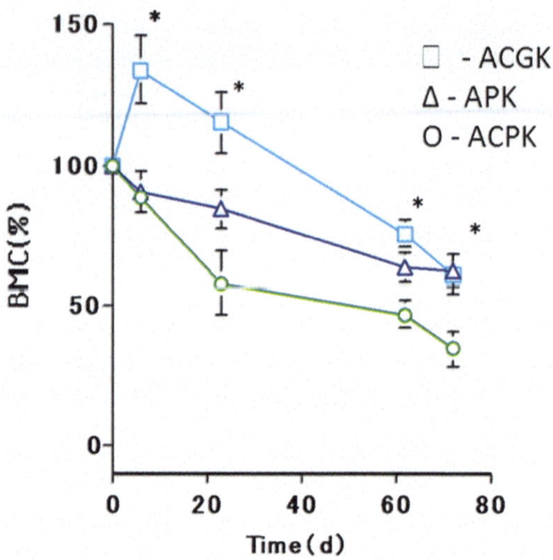

Fig. 11.6 Effects of cement formulation on BMC of AP and AC cements containing VK2

APK. On the other hand, the microstructure of ACGK was significantly different from APK, and that difference was drastically affected by the duration of the experimental. For ACGK, the amount of BMC reached its peak at day 7. ACPK and APK recorded the highest and slowest degradation rates of BMC, respectively. At day 21, the amount of BMC present can be shown as ACGK > APK > ACPK.

The micrographs of the cross sections of the apatite/collagen cements containing VK2 taken after 72 days of implantation were shown in Fig. 11.7. After implantation, it was discovered that the APK cement had undergone deformation but there are no evidence to suggest penetration of organic components into the cement material (Fig. 11.7a). Likewise for the ACPK cement with a reduction in diameter but an increase in thickness, the shape of the ACGK cement had been completely distorted after 72 days (Fig. 11.7b).

The BMC result of the cements loaded with VK2 suggests that their formulation has a significant effect on the rate of biodegradation. After 72 days, the ACGK cement recorded an increase in BMC, which was also higher than the ACPK cement (Fig. 11.6). The organic components had penetrated deeply into the center of the ACGK (Fig. 11.7b). These results suggested that the changes in BMC were more dynamic for the ACGK than the ACPK cement. As shown in the X-ray diffraction results, grinding the apatite/collagen composite cement can lead to a crystalline structure that is more or less the same as natural bone; this could have an influence on the release of bone growth factors such as VK2 and the regeneration and absorption of bone during the experimental period.

The BMC profile of AC suggests the quick release of VK2 may encourage organic components to penetrate the ACPK cement and stimulate the activity of the surrounding cells. Observations made from the ACPK micrographs revealed organic components had penetrated into the cement and causing the shape the cement to totally deform. On the other hand, a complete absorption of AC was observed.

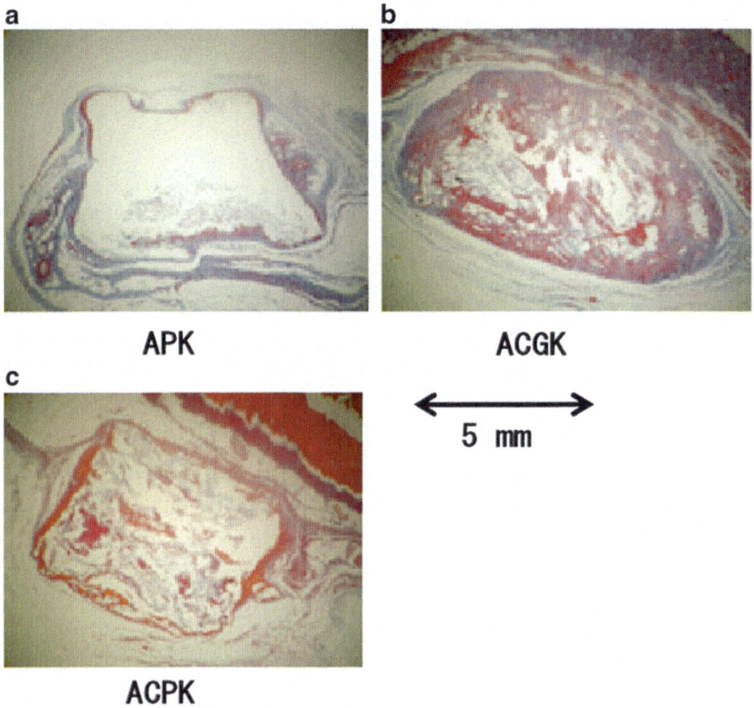

Fig. 11.7 Cross-section micrographs of (**a**) APK, (**b**) ACGK, and (**c**) ACPK cement after 72 days of implantation

On the contrary, the biodegradation profile of APK was almost identical to the AP, and the organic components did not penetrate deeply into the cement. These phenomena suggested that both mineral absorption and precipitation were induced by the organic components and VK2 in the APK cement. Nonetheless, only absorption was observed on the AP cement. The AP and APK cements were composed almost entirely of inorganic components, and the formulation and geometrical structures of the cement are different to natural bone; as a result bone growth factors might be not affected in the formation of bone.

11.4 Skeletal Bone Cell Scaffold Based on Apatite/Collagen Composite Cements

The geometrical structure of pores in implantable artificial bone affects bone regeneration, since bone-related cells grow and proliferate more effectively in interconnected porous materials, such as coral-modified implants made of calcium phosphate and porous β-TCP ceramics. Interconnective pores in coral-like materials

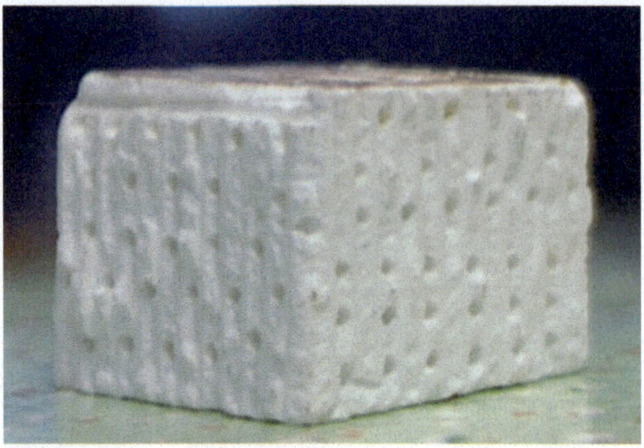

Fig. 11.8 Photograph of ACP block

are therapeutically effective for bone regeneration in the body through the introduction of bone cells and blood vessels [11, 12]. Notably, interconnective porous biomaterials are useful as a scaffold for bone cell cultures for implant. Kuboki et al. [13] discovered the various types of interconnective voids, and pores in artificial bone enhanced the transition from artificial material to natural bone. These voids played a key role in stimulating tissue invasion and biocompatibility. Based on the test results, it can be suggested that continuous voids supported the formation of new bone by allowing the bone cells and/or tissues to penetrate into the voids more readily and the growth of new blood vessels commences.

11.4.1 Biodegradation of Scaffold Based on Apatite/Collagen Composite Cements with Interconnective Macropores in Rats

Since artificial bones are fabricated with favorable properties using apatite/collagen composite with connective voids, these devices could be utilized as a bone cell scaffold to culture bone marrow extracted from patients for bone regenerative medicine. Artificial bone cement with interconnecting pores as a cell scaffold device was therefore prepared based on the AC cement and its biocompatibility investigated after implantation into rats.

The ACP blocks were prepared as follows [14]: cement bulk powders were mixed homogeneously with 25 mM phosphoric acid to form a paste and poured into a mold (10 × 10 × depth mm) containing an organized stainless steel needlelike male dies 600 μm in diameter. The mold is then stored and hardened at 37 °C and 100 % relative humidity for 24 h. The cement blocks with voids were obtained after removing the pins as shown in Fig. 11.8. The APN and ACN blocks were used to harden the AP and AC cement pastes in the mold (10 × 10 × depth mm) without pins, respectively.

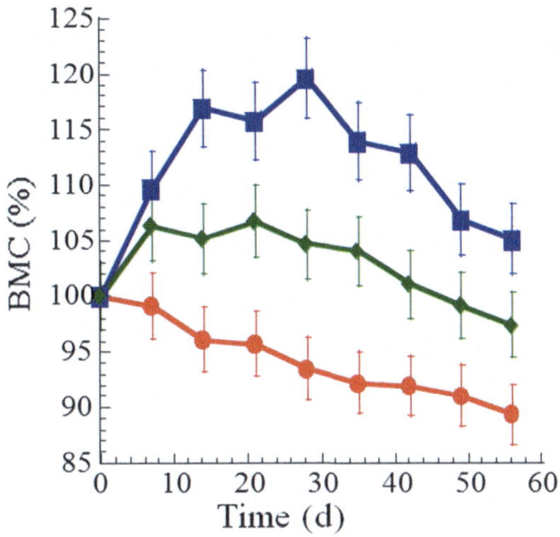

Fig. 11.9 Plot of time versus changes in BMC of cement blocks implanted in rats (■, ACC; ♦, ACN; •, APN)

The XRD result indicated that the calcium phosphates from ACN, ACC, and APN transformed into biological HAp with no peak due to the presence of raw materials, as previously reported [7]. The result of scanning electron microscopy with electron probe microanalyzer revealed the ACC cement has a smooth surface with particles less than 1–2 μm in size and is similar to natural bone [15]. It was also discovered that the geometrical structure of the implants has an effect on the behavior of their biological absorption. The microporosities of the APN and ACN measured using mercury porosimetry were found to be around 40 %, similar to the value previously published [14]. Therefore, the total porosity of the ACC cement was calculated to be approximately 64 % by combining the micro- and macropores which are 40 % and 23 %, respectively.

After the artificial bone blocks (ACN, ACC, and APN) were implanted subcutaneously in female SD rats, their BMC profiles were determined by dual energy X-ray absorptiometry (Fig. 11.9). The analysis revealed the BMC of ACC increased rapidly to around 120 % after 28 days but dropped to 105 % after 56 days. A similar trend was also observed for the ACN cement as their BMC rose to approximately 110 % after weeks 1–3 and at day 56 the BMC was around 98 %. In contrast, the BMC of APN decreased steadily throughout the entire experiment, and at day 56 the BMC was recorded to be approximately 90 % (Fig. 11.9).

The bone mineral density (BMD) of the implanted blocks were also measured and the results showed the density of ACC increased to around 108 % after 42 days and then declined significantly (Fig. 11.10). A gradual decrease was observed for the ACN cement during a 6-week period, and at the end of day 42, the BMD was approximately 92 %. Moreover, the BMD of APN remained unchanged during the first 4 weeks of the experiment but then the BMD steadily decreases and by day 56 it was around 94 %.

Based on these results, it is clear that the cement system will ultimately determine the changes in the BMD profile. During the latter stages of the experiment, a

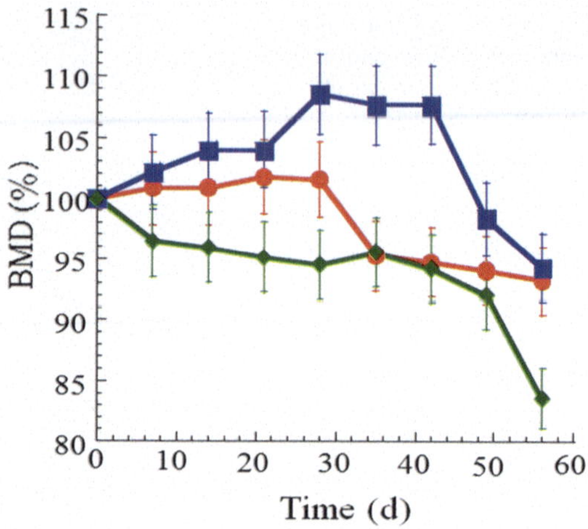

Fig. 11.10 Plot of time versus the changes in BMD of cement blocks implanted in rats. ■, ACC; ♦, ACN; •, APN

decrease in the BMC and BMD was observed with all the implanted blocks, 40–56 days due to the abdomen, and phagocytized on the surface of macropores by osteoclast-like cells bearing the same resemblance as bone remodeling. Photographs of removed implants also indicated that the deformation of the cement blocks can be considered as an indication of biological activity, the order of activity being ACC > ACN > APN. The results of deformation were consistent with the decrease in BMC after 40–56 days.

11.5 Drug Release from Biodegradable Apatite/Collagen Composite Cements with Interconnective Macropores

To improve biocompatibility, three-dimensional perforated porous apatite/collagen composite cement (ACC) with drug delivery capability was developed. It can be hypothesized that this will be a powerful tool in controlling bone regeneration if we can control the release of bone growth factors during cell culture [16].

11.5.1 Controlled In Vitro Drug Release from Skeletal Bone Cell Scaffold by Interconnective Macropores

The ACC device with drug delivery capability was prepared as follows: the AC cement paste containing an apatite cement bulk powder, 20 % type I bovine collagen, and 3 % indomethacin (IMC) bulk powder was poured into the mold (10.0 × 10.0 × 7.5 mm) to generate interconnective macropores (0, 20, 40, and 60 stainless needles) and stored at 37 °C and 100 % relative humidity for 24 h. The X-ray diffraction and FT-IR results of the cement blocks suggested that

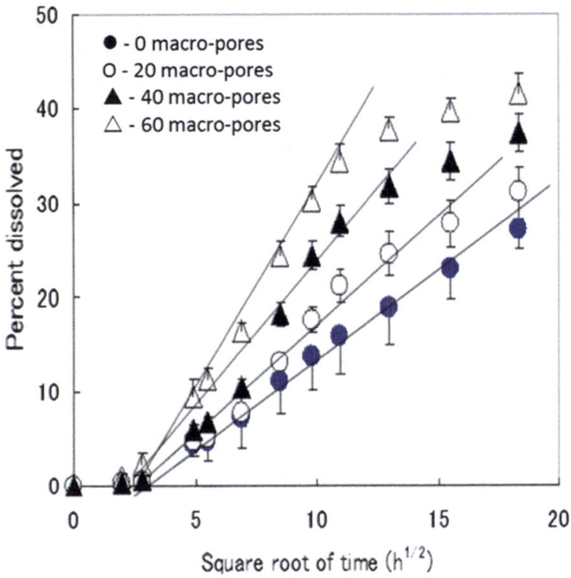

Fig. 11.11 Effects of interconnective macropores on in vitro release of IMC from ACC devices

its characteristics and biocompatibility are comparable to natural bone, and the application of the device as a biodegradation composite for bone repair can be anticipated [14].

To investigate the drug release capability of the ACC devices, tests were carried out in 25 mL of simulated body fluid (SBF) at a pH level of 7.25. The in vitro release of IMC from ACC with 20, 40, and 60 perforated pores in SBF after 336 h was 6.34 ± 0.48, 6.99 ± 0.46, 8.41 ± 0.61, and 9.34 ± 0.51 mg, respectively. By increasing the number of macropores, the release rate of IMC from ACC devices also increased. Since the drug release rate-limiting step of the release from unerosible-homogeneous drug-loaded matrix system was basically the drug diffusion process in the micropores in the matrix, the drug release from the planar surface matrix systems follows the Higuchi equation (Eq. 11.1):

$$M_t = A\sqrt{C_s \frac{D_i \varepsilon}{\tau} (2C_d - \varepsilon C_s)\, t} \qquad (11.1)$$

where M_t is the amount of drug released after time t, A is surface are of the device, D is the diffusion coefficient of the drug, C_s is the solubility, C_d is the concentration of drug in the matrix, τ is the tortuosity, and ε is the porosity.

The in vitro IMC release data from ACC with various numbers of macropores were used to plot IMC release against the square root of time (Fig. 11.11). Since the same cement formulation was used for all the ACC devices, the geometrical microstructure (micropore structure) was almost identical for all the devices, and the diffusion parameters of all ACC, such as porosity, drug concentration in the matrices, and pore tortuosity, were almost equal. The only exception is the surface

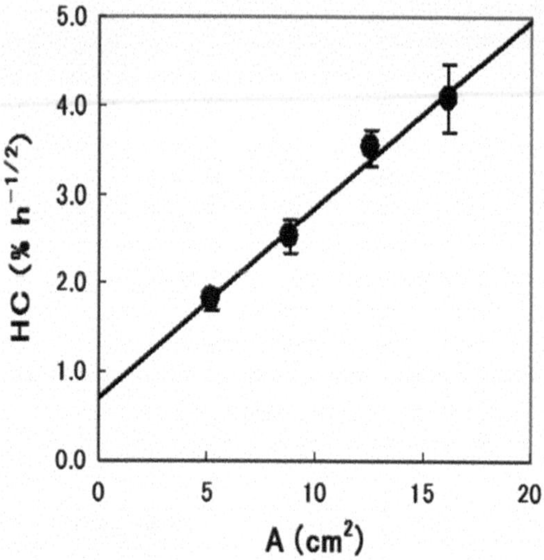

Fig. 11.12 Higuchi-type plot for the in vitro release of IMC from ACC in SBF

area of the devices relative to the geometrical macrostructure of ACC. Therefore, Higuchi equation (Eq. 11.1) can be simplified to form an equation where the surface area of macropores is taken into account as the surface area (A) of the device, and drug release rate of the ACC devices can be manipulated by controlling the value of A (Eq. 11.2):

$$M_t = A \bullet K \bullet \sqrt{t} \tag{11.2}$$

where K is a constant.

The linear relationship between HC and A of ACC as shown in Fig. 11.12 suggested the adequateness of Eq. 11.3, and value of K is derived from the slope of the graph. The results therefore suggest the rate of drug release can be controlled by number of macropores for culturing bone cells:

$$K = \sqrt{C_s \frac{D_i \varepsilon}{\tau} (2C_d - \varepsilon C_s)} \tag{11.3}$$

11.5.2 In Vitro Bone Cell Activity Responsive Drug Release from Biodegradable Apatite/Collagen Bone Cell Scaffold with Interconnective Macropores

As osteoclasts reabsorb bone matrices by exuding acid into the microenvironmental area under the cells [17], it is thus necessary to understand the remodeling of bone grafts by osteoclasts and osteoblasts in order to produce effective implantable apatite cement to deliver drugs to areas affected by osteoporosis.

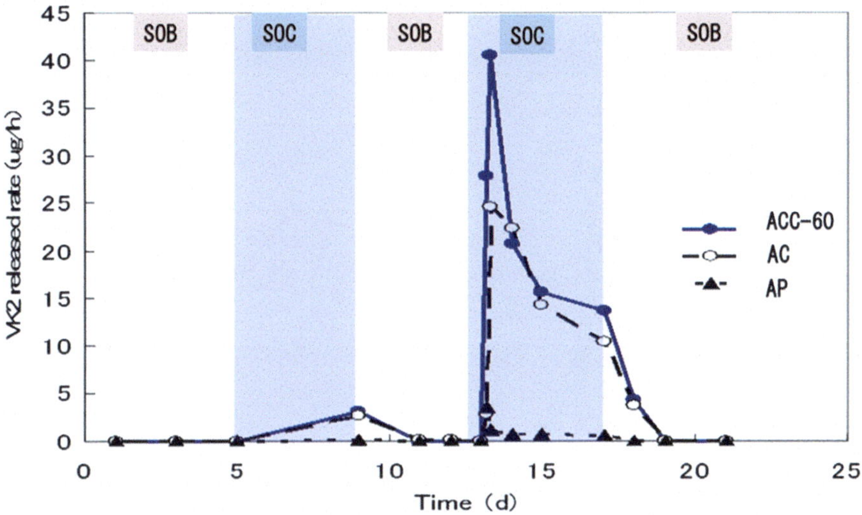

Fig. 11.13 Effects of dissolution mediums on VK2 release from the AP, AC, and ACC cements

Since the crystalline structure of AC was almost the same as natural bone [7], the material was phagocytized at the surface of macropores by bone-like cells, similar to the remodeling of bone.

Therefore, the rapid bioabsorption of AC may be considered to be similar to the biological action of active bone cells [7]. In order to clarify the rule of osteoclasts during drug release from the apatite/collagen nano-composite, we investigated the influence of the dissolution medium on the drug release capabilities of the device based on a physicochemical model for nanoscale bio-interface between bone matrices and bone cells.

The ACP0, ACP20, ACP40, and ACP60 were obtained as follows: the AC cement paste containing an apatite cement bulk powder, 20 % type I bovine collagen, and 2.5 % VK2 bulk powder was cast in the mold (10.0 × 10.0 × 7.5 mm) to make interconnective macropores (0, 20, 40, and 60 stainless needles) and stored at 37 °C and 100 % relative humidity for 24 h. The X-ray diffraction and FT-IR results suggested that the samples had similar characteristics to natural bone [16].

To clarify the role of bone remodeling in the drug delivery system based on HAp matrices, a physical in vitro dissolution model was established. The drug release profile was investigated in an SBF solution with a pH of 7.25 to simulate osteoblast-like conditions (SOB) and in an acetate buffer with a pH of 4.5 to simulate osteoclast-like conditions (SOC) [16].

Figure 11.13 shows the effect of the dissolution medium on the release of VK2 from AP, AC, and ACC60. It was discovered that virtually no drugs were being released from AC block and ACC-60 in SOB, but the situation was quite the opposite in SOC with significant improvements in the drug release rates. The drug

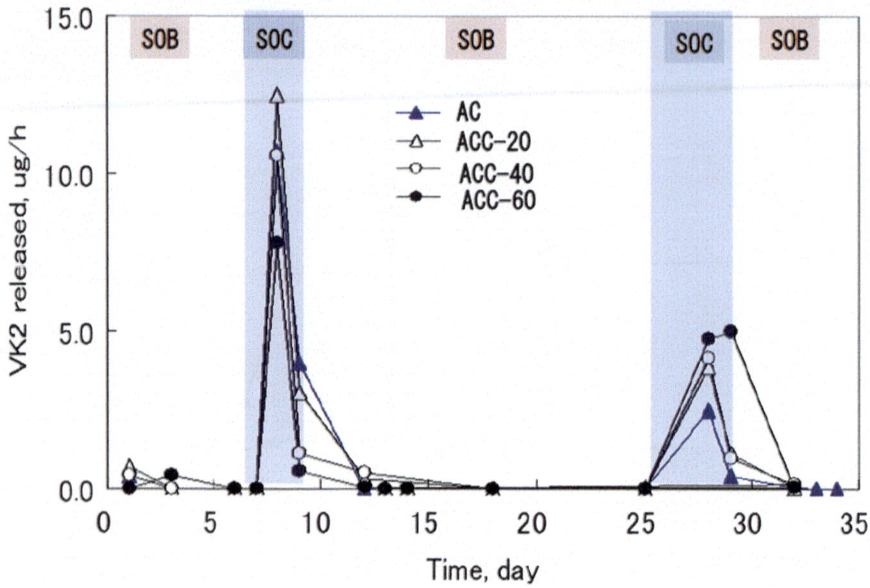

Fig. 11.14 Effects of dissolution medium on the ACC cement with different numbers of macropores

release and calcium phosphate dissolution results suggested that the HAp matrices in the device were dissolved in SOC, and the drug release was accelerated with increasing porosity. In SOB, however, the device was covered with precipitated HAp particles and inhibiting the release of drugs from micropores. The drug release from AC and ACC blocks were dependent on the dissolution medium. However, this is not the case for the AP block.

The drug release from the ACC and AC blocks in SOC was accelerated by the increase in porosity due to the dissolution of HAp matrices, as the biomimetic device had large pores up to 1 μm in size (Fig. 11.13), which could be connected between apatite and collagen matrices. In SOB, on the other hand, the devices were covered with small amounts of fine HAp particles, which inhibited drug release. The drug release results for the AP block revealed that the drug particles did not link together and were encapsulated in the cement matrices.

The relationship between macropore numbers of ACC block and the dissolution medium responses to VK2 release is shown in Fig. 11.14. Based on the drug release profiles, it can be hypothesized that the rate of drug release is dependent on the dissolution medium, and the results were repeated twice in SOC. For ACC, the maximum drug release rate in SOC was more or less proportional to the number of macropores.

Significant deformation of the ACC block was believed to be caused by a repeatable drug release in SOC and SOB (Fig. 11.14). The phenomena might be related to the bone cell activities and the responses to drug release from the cement device, given that the in vitro drug release experiments can be thought of as a physicochemical model for the remodeling of bone matrices by osteoblast and osteoclast cells. Perforated pores of the devices may possibly be used to control the release of drugs and could be utilized as a bone cell scaffold.

Acknowledgments The author would like to deeply thank Prof. William I. Higuchi, University of Utah for his great leadership to our international collaboration research. The author thanks Professor Hiroyuki Ohshima, Tokyo University of Science, and Dr. Atsuo Ito, NIAIST, for their scientific advice. The author thanks Mr. Ryuhei Hirano, Mr. Hideyuki Hamada, Mr. Hidenori Nakagawa, and Mr. Tomoaki Kuninaga for their experimental works.

References

1. Baron R, Vignery A, Horowitz M (1987) Lymphocytes, macrophages and the regulation of bone remodeling. In: Peck WA (ed) Bone and mineral research. Annual Elsevier, Amsterdam, pp 209–279
2. Aoki H (1994) Medical applications of hydroxyapatite. Ishiyaku EuroAmerica Inc., Tokyo, p 156
3. Miyamoto Y, Ishikawa K, Takechi M, Toh T, Yuasa T, Nagayama M, Suzuki K (1998) Basic properties of calcium phosphate cement containing atelocollagen in its liquid or powder phases. Biomaterials 19:707–715
4. Kikuchi M, Itoh S, Ichinose S, Shinomiya K, Tanaka J (2001) Self-organization mechanism in a bone-like hydroxyapatite/collagen nanocomposite synthesized in vitro and its biological reaction in vivo. Biomaterials 22:1705–1711
5. Itoh S, Kikuchi M, Koyama Y, Takakuda K, Shinomiya K, Tanaka J (2002) Development of an artificial vertebral body using a novel biomaterial, hydroxyapatite/collagen composite. Biomaterials 23:3919–3926
6. John A, Hong L, Ikada Y, Tabata Y (2001) A trial to prepare biodegradable collagen-hydroxyapatite composites for bone repair. J Biomater Sci Polym 12:89–705
7. Otsuka M, Kuninaga T, Otsuka K, Higuchi WI (2006) Effect of nanostructure on biodegradation behaviors of self-setting apatite/collagen composite cements containing vitamin K_2 in rats. J Biomed Mater Res B App Biomater 79B:176–184
8. Chhettry A, Wang Z, Hsu J, Fox JL, Baig AA, Barry AM, Zhuang H, Otsuka M, Higuchi WI (1999) Metastable equilibrium solubility distribution of carbonated apatite as function of solution composition. J Colloid Int Sci 218:57–67
9. Shiraki M, Shiraki Y, Aoki C, Miura M (2000) Vitamin K2 (menatetrenone) effectively prevents fractures and sustains lumbar bone mineral density in osteoporosis. J Bone Miner Res 15(3):515–521
10. Shiomi S, Nishiguchi S, Kubo S, Tamori A, Habu D, Takeda T, Ochi H (2002) Vitamin K2 (menatetrenone) for bone loss in patients with cirrhosis of the liver. Am J Gastroenterol 97(4):978–981
11. Delloye C, Cnockaert N, Cornu O (2003) Current concepts review, bone substitutes, an overview. Acta Orthop Belg 69:1–8
12. Miyai T, Ito A, Tamazawa G, Matsuno T, Sogo Y, Nakamura C, Yamazaki A, Satoh T (2008) Antibiotic-loaded poly-ε-caprolactone and porous β-tricalcium phosphate composite for treating osteomyelitis. Biomaterials 29:350–358
13. Kuboki Y, Jin Q, Kikuchi M, Mamood J, Takita H (2002) Geometry of artificial ECM: sizes of pores controlling phenotype expression in BMP-induced osteogenesis and chondrogenesis. Connect Tissue Res 43:529–534

14. Otsuka M, Nakagawa H, Otsuka K, Ito A, Higuchi WI (2013) Effect of geometrical structure on the in vivo quality change of a three-dimensionally perforated porous bone cell scaffold made of apatite/collagen composite. J Biomed Mater Res B Appl Biomater 101B(2):338–345
15. Otsuka M, Nakagawa H, Ito A, Higuchi WI (2010) Effect of geometrical structure on drug release rate of a three-dimensionally perforated porous apatite/collagen composite cement. J Pharm Sci 99(1):286–292
16. Otsuka M, Hirano R (2011) Bone cell activity responsive drug release from biodegradable apatite/collagen nano-composite cements, – in-vitro dissolution medium responsive vitamin K2 release colloids and surfaces B. Biointerfaces 85(2):338–342
17. Väänänen HK, Zhao H, Mulari M, Halleen JM (2000) The cell biology of osteoclast function. J Cell Sci 113(Pt 3):377–381

Chapter 12
Nanocrystalline Apatite-Based Biomaterials and Stem Cells in Orthopaedics

Feza Korkusuz, Muharrem Timuçin, and Petek Korkusuz

Abstract Nanocrystalline apatite-based biomaterials and stem cells are emerging research fields in orthopaedic surgery and traumatology that have the potential of improving quality of life of the elderly and enhance health-related socio-economic challenges. Nanocrystalline apatite-based biomaterials and especially calcium phosphate nano-biomaterials exploit new physical, chemical and biological properties that have the possibility to increase surface area and improve tissue integration. Stem cells of adult origin decrease inflammation, increase vascularity and are able to replace degenerated tissue cells during the process of regeneration. The bone is the only human tissue that regenerates. Musculoskeletal disorders including osteoporotic fractures and osteoarthritis decrease quality of life in the elderly and cause severe burden on economics. Nanocrystalline calcium phosphate bioceramics have the ability to prevent or treat osteoporotic fractures when combined with stem cells. These biomaterials may also be used for drug delivery purposes to treat bone infections when combined with stem cell as they can assist in treating osteoarthritis. Current research challenges are trying to overcome the toxicity and carcinogenesis with these cells and nanomaterials. Long-term stability of these cells and materials is another challenge for these materials. This chapter deals with nanocrystalline calcium phosphate bioceramics and mesenchymal stem cells.

F. Korkusuz, M.D. (✉)
Department of Sports Medicine, Hacettepe University Faculty of Medicine, Sihhiye, Ankara 06100, Turkey
e-mail: feza.korkusuz@hacettepe.edu.tr

M. Timuçin, Ph.D.
Department of Metallurgical and Materials Engineering, Middle East Technical University, Çankaya, Ankara 06800, Turkey
e-mail: timucin@metu.edu.tr

P. Korkusuz, M.D., Ph.D
Department of Histology and Embryology, Hacettepe University Faculty of Medicine, Sihhiye, Ankara 06100, Turkey
e-mail: petek@hacettepe.edu.tr

B. Ben-Nissan (ed.), *Advances in Calcium Phosphate Biomaterials*, Springer Series in Biomaterials Science and Engineering 2, DOI 10.1007/978-3-642-53980-0_12,

Keywords Bone regeneration • Stem cells • Nanocrystalline hydroxyapatite • Calcium phosphate • Bioceramics

12.1 Introduction

Medical materials also named as "biomaterials" are used alone or in combination with cells and signalling molecules to engineer and regenerate missing or injured tissues and organs [1]. Metals such as stainless steel, cobalt chromium and titanium alloys and various ceramics and polymers were successfully used to replace musculoskeletal tissues for decades. In fact, in early civilisations of Mesopotamia and Egypt, medical materials called "implants" were used to restore missing teeth and defects of bones. Material is the matter from which a thing is or can be made, and a biomaterial is defined as a biological or synthetic substance which can be introduced into body tissue as part of an implanted medical device or used to replace an organ and/or bodily function. Nanomaterial is a material having particles or constituents of nanoscale dimensions or one that is produced by nanotechnology. Bioceramics are non-metallic synthetic grafts used to regenerate and/or replace bones and joints [2–4]. Annually, 3–5 % of the world's population will have some form of medical implants inserted into their body. Fifty percent of these implants are used to replace degenerated joints and restore fractured bones. Although metals are the most commonly used implants, their longevity is limited and they need to be revised due to loosening. Studies to improve metallic implants mechanical and surface properties are advancing their clinical outcome. Particle disease [5] however is a leading cause of total joint revision procedures with no approved drug therapy to prevent or inhibit osteolysis. To prevent this disease, a new quest has emerged to investigate the possibility of using non-metallic implants including ceramics and polymers. Nanocrystalline apatite-based biomaterials were developed for biomedical applications [6–8]. We have produced and characterised various apatite-based biomaterials of micro- and nano-size to be used in bone regeneration. We replaced trace amount of calcium with trace elements in some of our formulations to better stimulate bone formation. This chapter covers our last 20 years of experience on apatite-based bioceramics and their interaction with cells and tissues.

12.2 Production of Nanocrystalline Apatite-Based Biomaterials

In the last 30 years, a class of oxidic inorganic compounds containing calcium and phosphorus in their structure has evolved into a variety of synthetic bone substitutes owing to the fact that the inorganic portion of the natural bone resembles closely the hydrated calcium phosphate compound known as hydroxyapatite. This compound is commonly represented by the formula $Ca_{10}(HPO_4)_6(OH)_2$ and is referred to as HAp in the literature. Chemically, the bone apatite is distinguished from synthetic HAp by a deficiency of calcium in its constitution and incorporation of a variety of ions such as Na^+, K^+, Mg^{2+}, Zn^{2+}, Sr^{2+}, Si^{4+}, F^- and $CO_3{}^{2-}$ in trace quantities, i.e. <1 %. These entities play important roles on the behaviour and the performance of the skeletal bone.

The synthetic mineral HAp was found to possess a multitude of useful biological properties which renders it as an indispensible material for replacement and repair of the natural bone tissue in the human body. It has excellent biocompatibility and bioactivity [9]. However, the resorption rate in the body is rather low. A second calcium phosphate compound, known as tricalcium phosphate, designated as TCP, also displayed desirable biological properties with faster resorption. Therefore, for adjustable resorption and remodelling, HAp and TCP can be combined in a biphasic composite with different proportions. The ratio of Ca to P in HAp is 1.67; this is very close to that in the natural bone. The formula for TCP is $3CaO{\cdot}P_2O_5$, hence its Ca to P ratio is lower.

Various techniques have been developed for synthesising calcium phosphate compounds mentioned above. The methods for producing HAp or TCP, and their combinations, results in fine ceramic powders with controlled chemical purity. The powders are then used to manufacture customised grafting materials for specific clinical applications. The grafts may be in the form of powder, granules or bulk ceramics sintered following the compaction of the powder in a suitable die. In bulk form, the sintered ceramic may be manufactured with desired pore architecture so that it mimics the natural bone in the body. Recently, HAp and TCP combined with biocompatible polymers are used for the production of various types of scaffolds. Another potential application is the coating of the surfaces of metallic or ceramic implants with thin layers of HAp or TCP in order to produce a biocompatible interface between the implant and the soft tissue.

The chemical route for obtaining HAp or TCP powder is based on an acid-base reaction which results in the precipitation of a solid precursor from aqueous solution. For this purpose the solution of a calcium salt of known molarity is combined by stirring with a solution containing phosphate ions of known strength in a reactor under controlled temperature and pH conditions [10–13]. By observing correct stoichiometry a solid precursor of the desired calcium phosphate compound is formed. This slurry is aged and then the precursor is separated from the liquor by centrifugal filtration and repeated washings. The cake so obtained is calcined at temperatures above 700 °C in order to arrive at the calcium phosphate powder of interest. The formation of HAp or TCP throughout the chemical process can be described by the following ionic reactions:

$$10Ca^{2+} + 6PO_4{}^{3-} + 2OH^- \rightarrow Ca_{10}(PO_4)_6(OH)_2 \tag{12.1}$$

$$3Ca^{2+} + 2PO_4{}^{3-} \rightarrow 3CaO \cdot P_2O_5 \tag{12.2}$$

A novel approach in chemical synthesis of nanocrystalline HAp powder has been reported [14] in which the application of microwave irradiation during the process resulted in spherulitic HAp particles which exhibited long-term flow ability even after 3 years of storage in non-hermetically sealed containers. Still another novelty was the use of sol-gel technique for the synthesis of ultrafine HAp powders [15–17]. In general, the amorphous precursors of the sol-gel route were found to crystallise to HAp at lower temperatures, but the products suffered from carbonate inclusions.

In a solid-liquid reaction approach [18, 19], the calcium phosphate compound was synthesised by reacting a dilute phosphoric acid solution with an aqueous slurry of $Ca(OH)_2$, again under controlled temperature and pH. The resulting mass is then dried by heating, and then the precursor was calcined in a muffle furnace to obtain the CaP powder. The advantage of this process was that all participating ions were preserved in the solid mass, minimising the compositional variations, but the powder particle size would be coarser.

Although HAp possesses desirable biocompatibility, its medical applications were reported to be limited due to poor mechanical properties and inefficacy in its osseo-behaviour. For example, low tensile strength and low fracture toughness have been the major causes which inhibited the use of HAp ceramics in load bearing applications. One way of enhancing the strength and osseointegration is to use siliconised HAp. Silicon (Si) was incorporated in the HAp structure by partial replacement of the phosphorus as described in the following formula [20, 21]:

$$Ca_{10}(PO_4)_{6-x}(SiO_4)_x(OH)_{2-x} \tag{12.3}$$

In a review on the synthesis of silicon substituted HAp and α-TCP [22], it was reported that silicon tends to inhibit grain growth in CaP materials resulting in finer microstructure, which constitute the basis for improved strength. In addition, it has been found that silicon played a significant role on the bone and the cartilage systems. The increased bioactivity and apposition were attributed to a number of different factors such as transformation of the material surface to a biologically equivalent apatite, increased solubility of the material and a more electronegative surface, all encouraging enhanced biomimetic precipitation on the surface.

12.2.1 Combining with Trace Elements

The calcium phosphate powders and ceramics used in our bone substitution studies included pure HAp, HAp+TCP composites, Si- and/or Sr-doped HAp and HAp+wollastonite composites. As defined recently [23], we used the acid-base reaction technique for manufacturing powders of HAp containing Si and trace elements for biomedical purposes. The HAp powder modified with Si was produced by partial substitution of trace elements for P in the molecular formula of HAp.

The Si addition was made to the $Ca(OH)_2$ slurry in the form of an organometallic solution of Si known as TEOS. The formula of HAp modified by silicon was $Ca_{10}(PO4)_5{\cdot}5(SiO_4)_{0.5}(OH)_{1.5}$. Trace elements were added to the Ca site of the HAp in an amount of 250, 500 and 1,000 ppm. An equivalent amount of Ca was reduced in the $Ca(OH)_2$ suspension. The HAp powder which contained trace elements and Si as co-dopants had 250, 500 and 1,000 ppm of trace element and 0.5 atom of Si in the molecular formula.

Wollastonite is a calcium silicate compound formulated as $CaSiO_3$. Wollastonite has osteoconductive properties by its own [24]. Wollastonite was added to HAp in order to produce HAp-wollastonite composites in this study. Synthetic wollastonite was manufactured by the reaction of an intimate mixture of $CaCO_3$ and SiO_2 powders in accordance with the following reaction:

$$CaCO_3 + SiO_2 \rightarrow CaSiO_3 \qquad (12.4)$$

This reaction was carried out at 1,250 °C for a total duration of 72 h. The formation of wollastonite was verified by X-ray diffraction (XRD) analysis.

A frit was introduced into HAp-wollastonite powder mixtures to facilitate sintering of the compacts. Frit had a chemical composition on weight percent basis as 5.5 % Na_2O, 12.1 % CaO, 11.8 % Al_2O_3 and 60.6 % SiO_2.

12.2.2 Characterisation

12.2.2.1 X-Ray Diffraction Analysis (XRD)

X-ray diffraction analysis is used for material characterisation and to determine the crystal structure of nanocrystalline apatite-based biomaterials. Crystallographic descriptions of trace elements incorporated into the HAp composites are carried out according to the Joint Committee on Powder Diffraction and Standards (JCPDS, HA, 09-0432).

12.2.2.2 Porosity Test

Pore formation in ceramics causes attachment and proliferation of osteoblasts. Pore formation in the composites is tested according to the standard test method for water absorption, bulk density, apparent porosity and apparent specific gravity of fired whiteware products (ASTM C 373-88). For obtaining porosity firstly, weight of ceramics (W_{dry}) is measured before placing them into water. After 24 h of immersion in water, weight of suspended samples (W_{susp}) was measured. The composites are placed onto paper towel for wiping out of the water from the surface and saturated weights (W_{sat}) are measured. In the present study, xylene was used as immersion liquid instead of water.

The results of the test are expressed by using the formula given below:

$$d_{bulk} = W_{dry} \times 0.861 / \left(W_{sat} - W_{susp}\right) \tag{12.5}$$

where d_{bulk} is the bulk density of the ceramic and 0.861 is the density of xylene.

The following formulae were used for obtaining sintered density in terms of percentage of the theoretical density (%TD) and the percentage porosity (%P):

$$d_{bulk}/d_{th} \times 100 = \%TD \tag{12.6}$$

$$100 - \%TD = \%P \tag{12.7}$$

The theoretical density of hydroxyapatite was taken as 3.156 g/cm^3.

12.2.2.3 Scanning Electron Microscopy (SEM)

The scanning electron microscope equipped with an X-ray microanalysis system was used for imaging higher magnifications of the material. SEM examinations are performed on broken surfaces after coating materials with a gold layer by the sputter coating equipment.

12.3 Bone Structure and Function

The bone itself is a composite consisting of HAp nanorods embedded into a collagen matrix. It is a protein matrix strengthened basically with calcium and phosphate. Mostly type I collagen and cells form its organic component where minerals establish its inorganic phase. The bone is a metabolically active vascular tissue that has the capability to regenerate.

Bones are categorised as long, short, flat and irregular according to their shapes. Long bones are separated into parts according to their functions. The outer shell that is named as the *cortex* (Fig. 12.1) is thicker and the middle part that contains the bone marrow that is named as the *medulla* (Fig. 12.2) is narrower at the center of the long bone. This is the narrow shaft of bone called the *diaphysis*. The areas next to the diaphysis and towards the endings of the bone are named as *metaphysis*. The cortex becomes narrower and the medulla is wider in the metaphysis. Blood circulation and metabolic activity is higher in the metaphysis related to its structure, whereas the diaphysis is stronger but metabolically less active. The metaphysis ends at the *physis* which is of cartilage named also as the *growth plate* in children and growing adolescent. Longitudinal growth of bones occurs from the physis, whereas transverse growth occurs from the *apophysis*. The physis and apophysis calcify at the end of the growth period. The area from the physis to the end of the bone

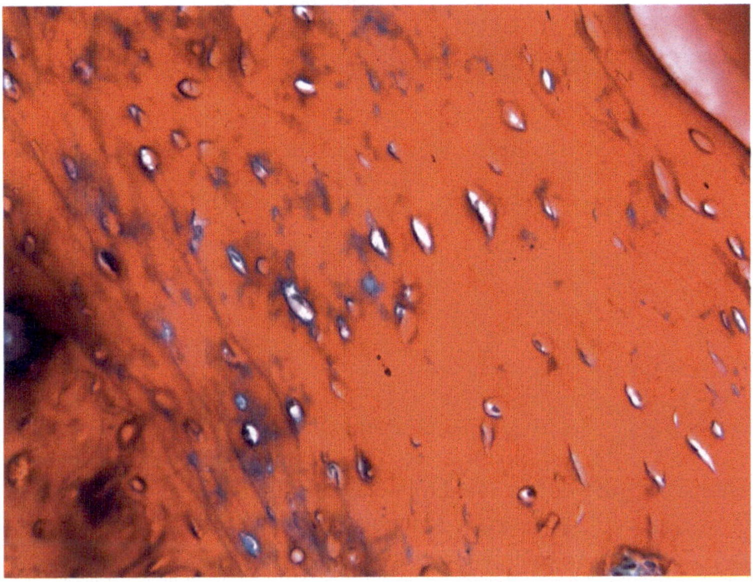

Fig. 12.1 Cortical bone

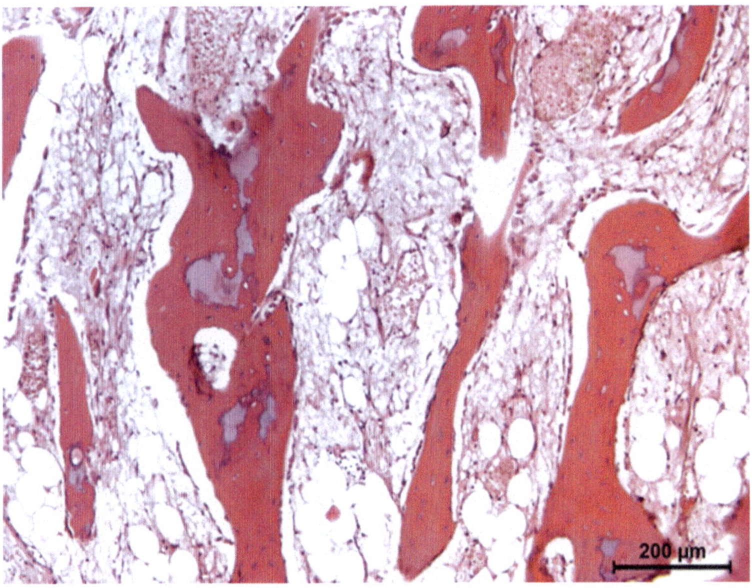

Fig. 12.2 Cancellous bone

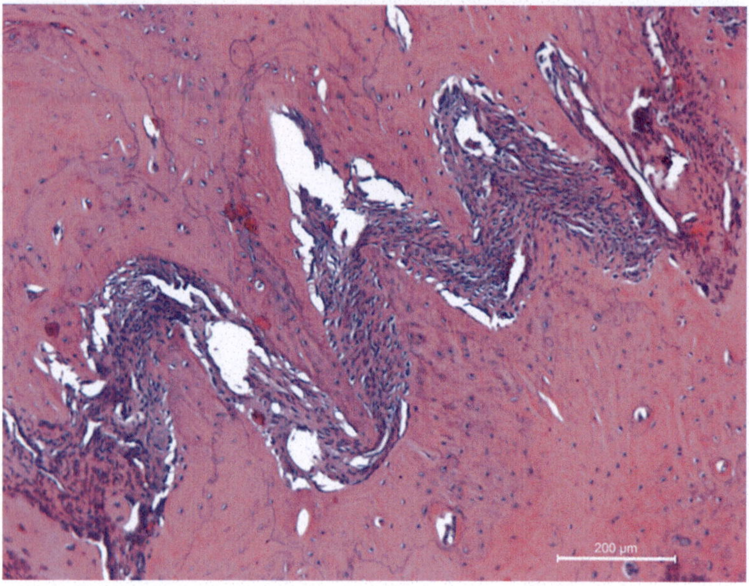

Fig. 12.3 Flat bones of the cranium connect each other with connective tissue

is named as the *epiphysis*. Almost each long bone ends with *articular cartilage* constituting a joint that allows movement. Samples to short bones are the ones at the wrist and ankle joints. These bones are tightly packed with ligaments allowing essential but limited motion. Bones of the cranium (Fig. 12.3) are typical flat bones and bones of the spine are examples of irregular bones.

Bones protect internal organs from outer powers. They allow movement as all muscles attach to them. Bones produce new blood cells in their bone marrow and the bone marrow is one of the most well-known sources of mesenchymal stem cells. The bone also serves as the depot of minerals and trace elements. For example. calcium is stored in bones and when needed it is released from there by certain hormones.

Mechanical properties of bone are important for protection and movement functions. The minerals that constitute the inorganic part of the bone attain strength that can indirectly be measured by dual energy X-ray absorptiometry (DXA) [25]. An alternative technology named *vibration analysis* is assessed to quantify bone strength recently [26]. The organic part of the bone is mainly of collagen type 1. This component gives elasticity to the bone. Due to its unique composition of organic and inorganic components, the bone is as strong as steel but lighter. As the bone is a living tissue, cells regularly exchange its components. This turnover of organic and inorganic parts of the bone is characterised as homeostasis. As one part of the bone is broken down (catabolised), it is regenerated (anabolised) immediately in children and adults. With ageing and due to the genetic code of individuals, the breaking down of the bone by *osteoclasts* turns to be faster than new bone production by *osteoblasts*, leading to a condition of brittle bone.

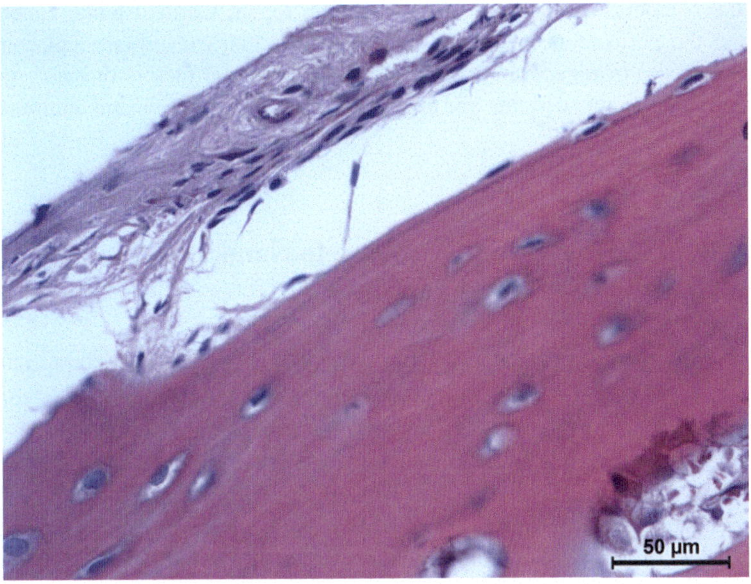

Fig. 12.4 The periosteum

Osteoporosis is defined as loss of bone mineral density (BMD) and deterioration of bone microarchitecture leading to low quality of the bone that may end up with fractures [27]. From the mechanical point of view, whenever the organic component is removed the bone becomes brittle. When the inorganic component is removed the bone becomes highly elastic but it cannot bear weight. The balance of the bone is maintained by its cells through various internal and external stimulators. Bone morphogenic proteins (BMP) which are mostly members of the transforming growth factor (TGF) beta family are the most important signalling molecules that act on bone cell proliferation and differentiation. BMPs are also important in bone growth and regeneration. Systemic growth factors, neural mediators [28] and physical, electrical and magnetic stimulators are proposed to mediate bone formation and regeneration through BMPs [29].

When the unity of the bone is interrupted by a fracture, the initial stage of response will be inflammation. The skin of the bone that is called the *periosteum* (Fig. 12.4) prevents the leakage of blood into other tissues. The so-called haematoma entrapped in the periosteum will short after play a major effect in regeneration. The necrotic tissue at the fracture ends is resorbed by osteoclasts when internal or external fixation is attained. This is followed by the repair of blood cells and appearance of osteoblast. Osteoblasts repair the injured bone, whereas the haematoma is calcified by these cells. After initial healing is achieved, osteoblasts will reshape the bone working together with osteoclasts. This final stage of repair is named as regeneration as the original tissue is reconstructed. Osteocytes are the cells of bone tissue that are responsible of communication. In case of injury, these cells invite the osteoclasts and osteoblasts to initiate repair. Cortical bone, cancellous bone and the periosteum have cells and mediators that can initiate and continue with the process of regeneration. Still the most important factors that take role in bone regeneration are adequate and appropriate blood circulation and attainment of stability.

12.4 Stem Cells and Cell Response to Nanocrystalline Apatite-Based Biomaterials

Mesenchymal stem cells (MSCs) have the potential to convert to osteoblasts when essential [30, 31]. These cells are frequently used together with natural or synthetic matrices to regenerate the bone [31]. Apatite-based biomaterials are currently used in non-weight-bearing bone sites as osteoconductive materials. In a recent study, we were able to produce 300 and 500 nm nano-HAp powder clusters (Figs. 12.5 and 12.6) by heating them up to 300 °C and 1,000 °C, respectively. When these nano-HAp powder clusters were combined with MSCs in culture, they attached (Fig. 12.7) and proliferated well (Fig. 12.8) on the surface of the clusters.

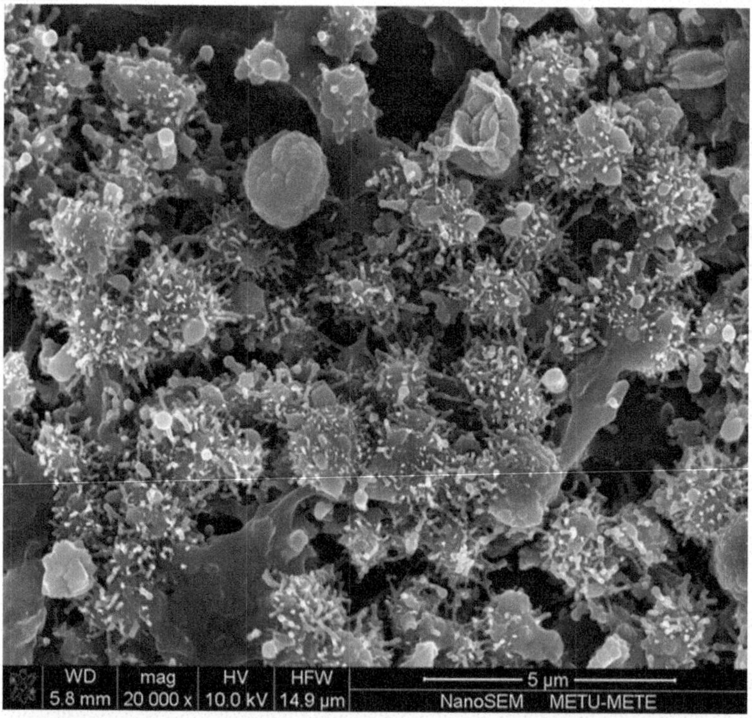

Fig. 12.5 Scanning electron micrographs on 300 and 500 nm nano-HAp powder clusters

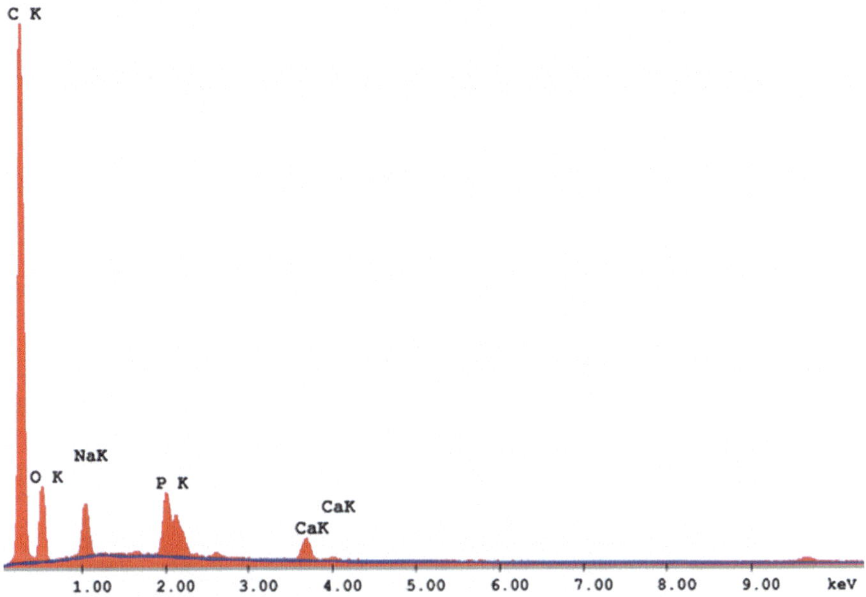

Fig. 12.6 XRD of nano-HAp powder clusters

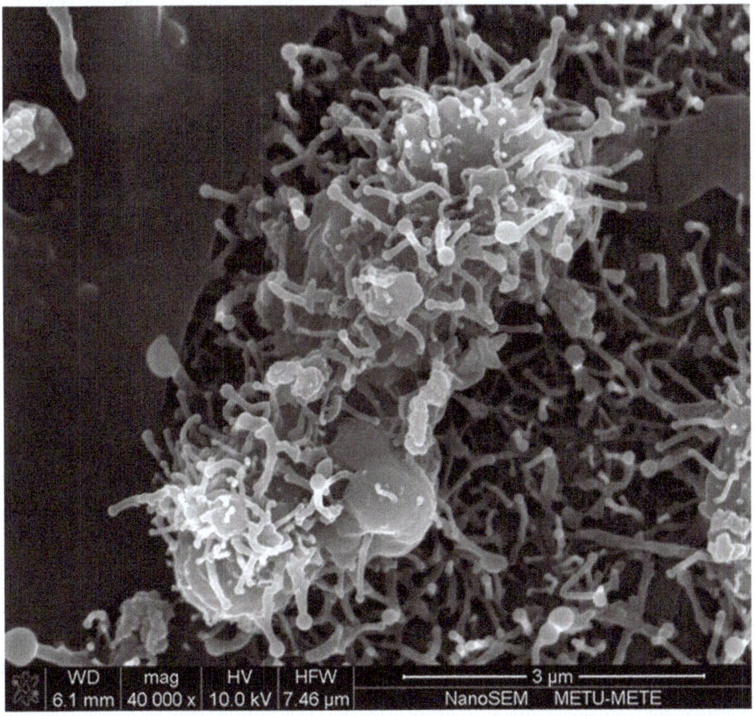

Fig. 12.7 MCSs attached on nano-HAp powder clusters

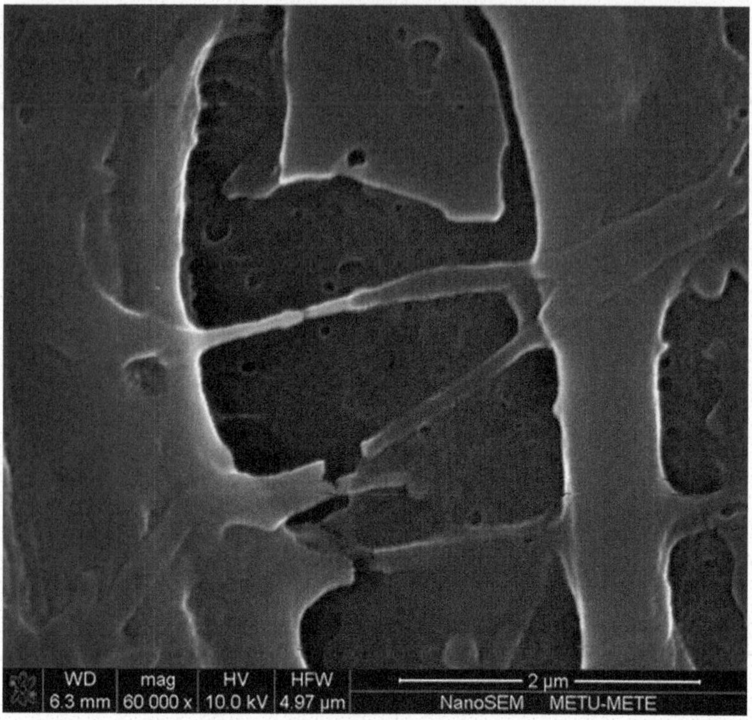

Fig. 12.8 Proliferation and extracellular matrix formation of MSCs on nano-HAp powder clusters

Attachment and proliferation of MSCs on nano-HAp was assessed using a real-time cell electronic system (Fig. 12.9).

Transmission electron microscopy (Fig. 12.10) and scanning electron microscopy (Fig. 12.11) revealed that the nano-HAp was biocompatible. Cells grew and exhibited their extracellular matrix on the nano-HAp powder clusters (Fig. 12.12). Over a period of time, all the nano-HAp powder clusters were covered with the extracellular matrix of MSCs (Fig. 12.13).

12.5 Tissue Response to Nanocrystalline Apatite-Based Biomaterials

Synthesis of nanocrystalline apatite-based biomaterials is recently well studied [32–34]. As nano-HAp is a relatively new material, few in vivo studies were carried out [35]. Our recent clinical experience with trace element-containing HAp [23] revealed that the basic material that we used to produce our nano-HAp powders was Acceptable.

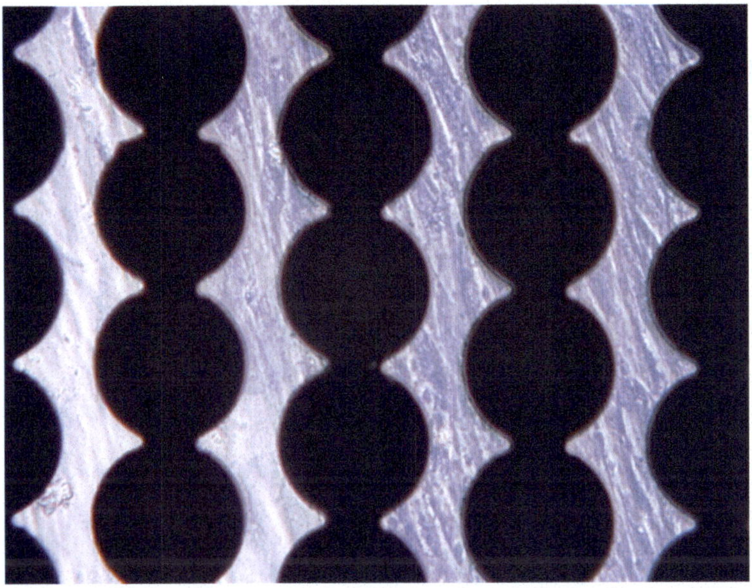

Fig. 12.9 MSCs growing on nano-HAP ceramic powder clusters in a real-time cell electronic system

Fig. 12.10 Transmission electron microscopy of MSCs implanted on nano-HAp powder clusters revealed their biocompatibility

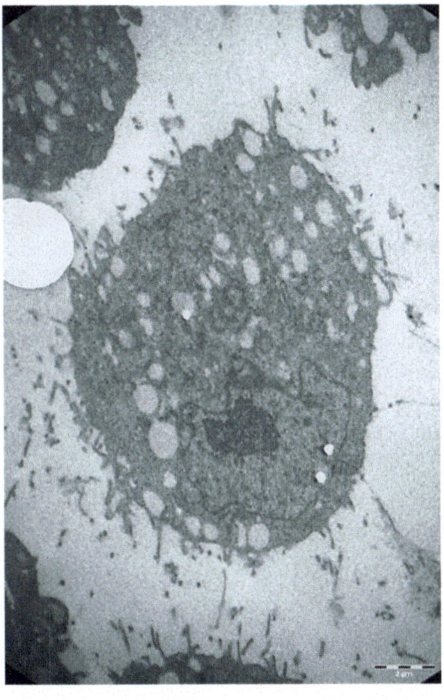

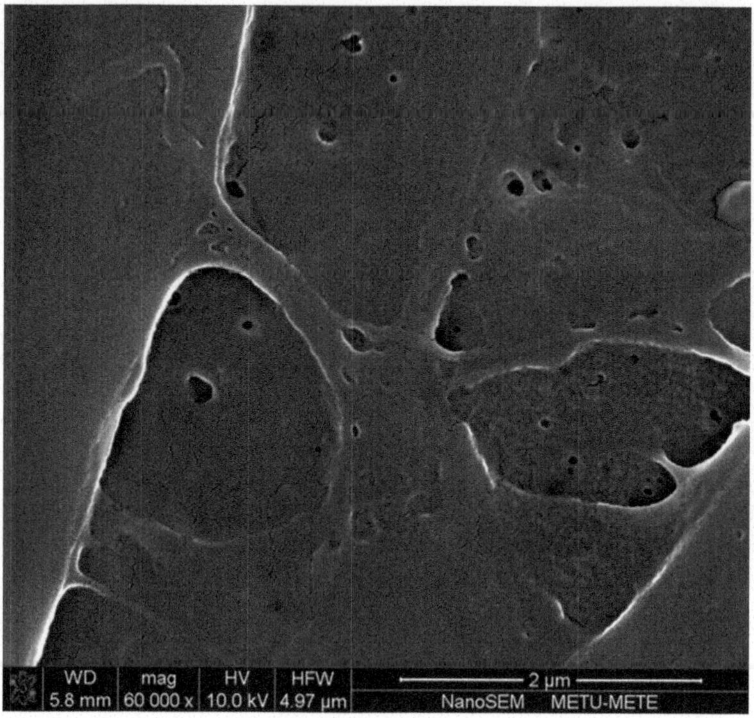

Fig. 12.11 Scanning electron microscopy of MSCs implanted on nano-HAp powder clusters revealed that they exhibited growth and extracellular matrix production

12.6 Growth Factor and Drug Delivery

Growth factors, cells and scaffolds are essential components of regenerative medicine. As stated previously, BMPs are used to regenerate the bone alone or in combination with cells and scaffolds [36]. BMP-2-loaded nanoparticles combined with fibrin presented potent effects of MSCs during bone regeneration [36]. Such composites were also efficient in regenerating mandibular defects [37]. Nano-HAp combined with poly(lactide-co-glycolide) promoted MSC adhesion and osteogenic differentiation recently [38]. What we discovered from our studies were in line with these recent findings. Nano-HAp can be combined with polymers to slow down the release of growth factors and antibiotics. Nano-HAp can also be used to attach MSC that will be delivered to the bone.

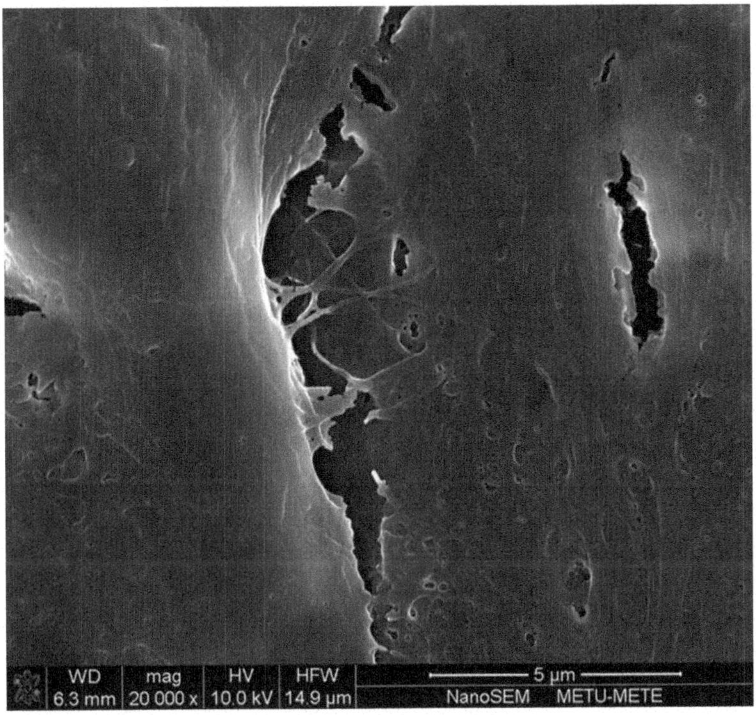

Fig. 12.12 MSCs immediately covered the nano-HAp ceramics

12.7 Implant Surface Coatings

Integration of implants into the bone largely depends on surface properties. Nano-HAp coating had potential benefits to enhance implant osseointegration in rats [39]. A recent review assessed the effectiveness of coating orthopaedic implants with nano-HAp [40–42]. Trace elements such as Mg and Sr can be dropped on to the nano-HAp coating of implants [39]. We concur with the idea that expanding the surface area of the bone-implant interface will aid better osseointegration.

In conclusion, our findings with nano-HAp powders revealed that this biomaterial is biocompatible and allows MSC attachment and proliferation. Attached cells produce the extracellular matrix, and they may aid implant integration and/or release of BMP or antibiotics.

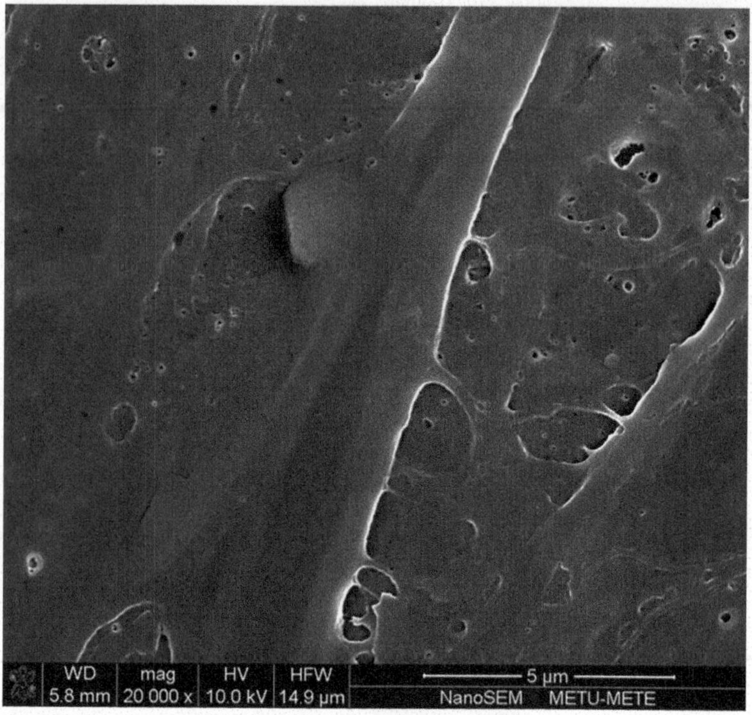

Fig. 12.13 In about 1–2 weeks, all nano-HAp surfaces were covered with the extracellular matrix of the MSCs

Acknowledgements Authors thank Duygu Uçkan Çetinkaya MD, PhD, and Sevil Arslan MSc of Hacettepe University Faculty of Medicine, PediSTEM Stem Cell Research Center, for their contribution to MSC studies.

References

1. Amini AR, Laurencin CT, Nukavarapu SP (2012) Bone tissue engineering: recent advances and challenges. Crit Rev Biomed Eng 40(5):363–408
2. Korkusuz F, Tomin E, Yetkiner DN, Timuçin M, Öztürk A, Korkusuz P (2011) Synthetic bone grafts. TOTBID Dergisi 10:134–142
3. Korkusuz F, Senköylü A, Korkusuz P (2003) Hard tissue-implant interactions-2: bone-ceramic and bone-polymer interactions. Eklem Hastalik Cerr (formerly J Arthroplast Arthrosc Surg) 14:109–125
4. Demirkiran H (2012) Bioceramics for osteogenesis, molecular and cellular advances. Adv Exp Med Biol 760:134–147
5. Beck RT, Illingworth KD, Saleh KJ (2012) Review of periprosthetic osteolysis in total joint arthroplasty: an emphasis on host factors and future directions. J Orthop Res 30(4):541–546
6. Catledge SA, Fries MD, Vohra YK, Lacefield WR, Lemons JE, Woodard S, Venugopalan R (2002) Nanostructured ceramics for biomedical implants. J Nanosci Nanotechnol 2(3–4):293–312

7. Cazalbou S, Eichert D, Ranz X, Drouet C, Combes C, Harmand MF, Rey C (2005) Ion exchanges in apatites for biomedical application. J Mater Sci Mater Med 16(5):405–409
8. Dorozhkin SV (2010) Nanosized and nanocrystalline calcium orthophosphates. Acta Biomater 6(3):715–734
9. Suchanek W, Yoshimura M (1998) Processing and properties of hydroxyapatite-based biomaterials for use as hard tissue replacement implants. J Mater Res 13(1):97–117
10. Hayek E, Newesely H (1963) Pentacalcium monohydroxyorthophosphate. Inorg Synth 7:63–65
11. Tas AC, Korkusuz F, Timucin M, Akkas N (1997) An investigation of the chemical synthesis and high-temperature sintering behaviour of calcium hydroxyapatite (HA) and tricalcium phosphate (TCP) ceramics. J Mater Sci Mater Med 8:91–96
12. Choi D, Kumta PN (2006) An alternative chemical route for the synthesis and thermal stability of chemically enriched hydroxyapatite. J Am Ceram Soc 89(2):444–449
13. Morales JG, Burgues JT, Boix T, Fraile J, Clemente RR (2001) Precipitation of stoichiometric hydroxyapatite by a continuous method. Cryst Res Technol 36(1):15–26
14. Sarig S, Kahana F (2002) Rapid formation of nanocrystalline apatite. J Cryst Growth 237–239:55–59
15. Layrolle P, Ito A, Tateishi T (1998) Sol-gel synthesis of amorphous calcium phosphate and sintering into microporous hydroxyapatite bioceramics. J Am Ceram Soc 81(6):1421–1428
16. Varma HK, Babu SS (2005) Synthesis of calcium phosphate bioceramics by citrate gel pyrolysis method. Ceram Int 31:109–114
17. Agrawal K, Singh G, Puri D, Prakash S (2011) Synthesis and characterization of hydroxyapatite powder by sol-gel method for biomedical application. J Miner Mater Char Eng 10(8):727–734
18. Akao M, Aoki H, Kato K (1981) Mechanical properties of sintered hydroxyapatite for prosthetic applications. J Mater Sci 16:809–812
19. Vakıfahmetoglu C, Park J, Korkusuz F, Ozturk A, Timucin M (2009) Production and properties of apatite-wollastonite ceramics for biomedical applications. Interceram 58(2–3):86–90
20. Gibson IR, Best SM, Bonfield W (1999) Chemical characterisation of silicon substituted hydroxyapatite. J Biomed Mater Res 44(4):422–428
21. Gibson IR, Best SM, Bonfield W (2002) Effect of silicon substitution on the sintering and microstructure of hydroxyapatite. J Am Ceram Soc 85(11):2771–2777
22. Pietak AM, Reid JW, Stott MJ, Sayer M (2007) Silicon substitution in the calcium phosphate bioceramics. Biomaterials 28:4023–4032
23. Izci Y, Seçer HI, Ilica AT, Karaçalioglu O, Onguru O, Timuçin M, Korkusuz F (2012) The efficacy of bioceramics for the closure of burr-holes in craniotomy: case studies on 14 patients. J Appl Biomater Funct Mater 11:e187–e196. doi:10.5301/JABFM.2012.9252
24. Lin K, Zhai W, Ni S et al (2005) Study of the mechanical property and in vitro biocompatibility of CaSiO3 ceramics. Ceram Int 31:323–326
25. Arpınar P, Şimsek B, Sezgin OC, Birlik G, Korkusuz F (2005) Correlation between mechanical vibration analysis and dual energy X-ray absorptiometry (DXA) in the measurement of in vivo human tibial bone strength. Technol Health Care 13:107–113
26. Bediz B, Özgüven HN, Korkusuz F (2010) Vibration measurements predict the mechanical properties of human tibia. Clin Biomech 25:365–371
27. Atik OS, Gunal I, Korkusuz F (2006) Burden of osteoporosis. Clin Orthop Relat Res 443:19–24
28. Muratli HH, Korkusuz F, Korkusuz P, Bicimoglu A, Ercan ZS (2007) Bosentan, a non-specific endothelin antagonist, stimulates fracture healing. Biomedical engineering: application. Basis Commun 19:37–46
29. Chen G, Deng C, Li YP (2012) TGF-β and BMP signaling in osteoblast differentiation and bone formation. Int J Biol Sci 8:272–288
30. Steinert AF, Rackwitz L, Gilbert F, Nöth U, Tuan RS (2012) Concise review: the clinical application of mesenchymal stem cells for musculoskeletal regeneration: current status and perspectives. Stem Cells Transl Med 1:237–247

31. Dominici M, Le Blanc K, Mueller I, Slaper-Cortenbach I, Marini FC, Krause DS, Deans RJ, Keating A, Prockop DJ, Horwitz EM (2006) Minimal criteria for defining multipotent mesenchymal stromal cells. The International Society for Cellular Therapy position statement. Cytotherapy 8:315–317
32. Vandecandelaere N, Rey C, Drouet C (2012) Biomimetic apatite-based biomaterials: on the critical impact of synthesis and post-synthesis parameters. J Mater Sci Mater Med 23:2593–2606
33. Zhou H, Lee J (2011) Nanoscale hydroxyapatite particles for bone tissue engineering. Acta Biomater 7:2769–2781
34. McMahon RE, Wang L, Skoracki R, Mathur AB (2013) Development of nanomaterials for bone repair and regeneration. J Biomed Mater Res B Appl Biomater 101:387–397
35. Chen Y, Chen H, Shi J (2013) In vivo bio-safety evaluations and diagnostic/therapeutic applications of chemically designed mesoporous silica nanoparticles. Adv Mater 25:3144–3176
36. Park KH, Kim H, Moon S, Na K (2009) Bone morphogenic protein-2 (BMP-2) loaded nanoparticles mixed with human mesenchymal stem cell in fibrin hydrogel for bone tissue engineering. J Biosci Bioeng 108:530–537
37. Li J, Li Y, Ma S, Gao Y, Zuo Y, Hu J (2010) Enhancement of bone formation by BMP-7 transduced MSCs on biomimetic nano-hydroxyapatite/polyamide composite scaffolds in repair of mandibular defects. J Biomed Mater Res A95:973–981
38. Lock J, Nguyen TY, Liu H (2012) Nanophase hydroxyapatite and poly(lactide-co-glycolide) composites promote human mesenchymal stem cell adhesion and osteogenic differentiation in vitro. J Mater Sci Mater Med 23:2543–2552
39. Cheng Z, Guo C, Dong W, He FM, Zhao SF, Yang GL (2012) Effect of thin nano-hydroxyapatite coating on implant osseointegration in ovariectomized rats. Oral Surg Oral Med Oral Pathol Oral Radiol 113:e48–e53
40. Fox K, Tran PA, Tran N (2012) Recent advances in research applications of nanophase hydroxyapatite. ChemPhysChem 13:2495–2506
41. Yamada M, Ueno T, Tsukimura N, Ikeda T, Nakagawa K, Hori N, Suzuki T, Ogawa T (2012) Bone integration capability of nanopolymorphic crystalline hydroxyapatite coated on titanium implants. Int J Nanomedicine 7:859–873
42. Roy M, Bandyopadhyay A, Bose S (2011) Induction plasma sprayed Sr and Mg doped nano hydroxyapatite coatings on Ti for bone implant. J Biomed Mater Res B Appl Biomater 99:258–265

Chapter 13
Marine Structures as Templates for Biomaterials

Besim Ben-Nissan and David W. Green

Abstract During the last two decades, "learning from nature" has given us new directions for the use of natural organic and inorganic skeletons, drug delivery devices, new medical treatment methods initiating unique designs and devices ranging from nano- to macroscale. These materials and designs have been instrumental to introduce the simplest remedies to vital problems in regenerative medicine, providing frameworks and highly accessible sources of osteopromotive analogues, scaffolds and drug delivery device proteins. This is exemplified by the biological effectiveness of marine structures such as corals and shells and sponge skeletons, extracts of spongin and nacre, sea urchin, sea snails and *Foraminifera*. Organic matrix and inorganic marine skeletons possess a habitat suitable for proliferating added mesenchymal stem cell populations and promoting clinically acceptable bone formation. A wide range of applications of these marine structures and their conversion methods are covered by excellent review papers and chapters. In this chapter based on our research, published work and book chapters, we aim to cover the nature, morphology and the use of some of these structures for tissue engineering, bone grafts, drug delivery and specific extracts such as proteins for regenerative medicine.

Keywords Marine structures • Nacre • Coral • Sponges • Sea urchin • Protein • Bone grafts • Drug delivery

---

B. Ben-Nissan (✉)
School of Chemistry and Forensic Science, Faculty of Science, University of Technology, Broadway, Ultimo, PO BOX 123, Sydney, NSW 2007, Australia
e-mail: b.ben-nissan@uts.edu.au

D.W. Green
School of Chemistry and Forensic Science, University of Technology, PO BOX 123, Broadway, Sydney, NSW, Australia

Faculty of Dentistry, The University of Hong Kong, Hong Kong, China

B. Ben-Nissan (ed.), *Advances in Calcium Phosphate Biomaterials*, Springer Series in Biomaterials Science and Engineering 2, DOI 10.1007/978-3-642-53980-0_13,

13.1 Introduction

Just after the "general relativity theory" was published, Eduard, Einstein's younger son, asked "how come he was so famous". He smiled and remarked that "When a blind beetle crawls over the surface of a curved branch, it doesn't notice that the track it has covered is indeed curved"; he quietly added to that, "I was lucky enough to notice what the beetle didn't notice".

The term "learning from nature" or "biomimetics" has been a very promising and satisfactory concept that allows us to improve the efficiency and the functionality of an engineering design or device. Nature has been the most inspiring creative engineering source in the human history. Throughout history we have been trying to learn to mimic nature's designs to develop application for solving problems either in our daily life, in engineering, in science or most recently in medicine with unique designs and approaches.

Nature can teach us in many ways on how to build structures, design architectures and fabricate materials and substances with exemplary high performance for many functions. The study of biomimetics and marine structures has provided approaches for generating unique inorganic scaffolds and organic materials for use in regenerative medicine with the potential to outperform conventional advanced man-made functional materials. The way natural systems allocate energy for different functions can instruct us on how to best optimise the design of materials and structures with minimum energy use and with molecular or nano-level control. For example, both bone formation and resorption depend on the same principles.

The essence of better performing natural materials compared to their synthetic counterparts is to give more attention to design and optimisation, the property of self-assembly, approach to the problems with mixed laminated and/or mixed organic–inorganic composites and control and repair of fracture. The building functions of organisms make use of "bottom-up" chemical processes over many length scales.

By harnessing these processes including many nanoscale ones, we have the potential to generate "living materials" that adapt and respond to their surroundings [1]. There is now greater appreciation and understanding of the significance of bio-inspired and nanoscale approaches than ever before to the generation of new medical materials and devices. The structural component of tissue engineering is the most amenable to this type of analysis alongside the increased sophistication of materials chemistry and new nanofabrication methods to provide exceptional biomimetic solutions.

This review is based on many published book chapters and papers that cover only a small fraction of an enormous range and richness of marine structures. This chapter outlines the development and progress of biomimetic approaches in regenerative medicine and provides worked examples from our own research and fellow researchers specifically on inorganic natural nano- and microporous structures.

13.2 Biomimetics and Evolution

The translation of products from nature into technology is fundamental and the most powerful and successful way of resolving technological and scientific problems. Natural history collections are a unique and rich source of practical ideas and solutions for the initial stages of tissue reassembly in artificial culture. Studying the chemistry, the evolution of tissues and organs, their function and design is an undiscovered route to provide elements that can be used to reconstruct tissues in the simplest and most practical way possible. We can even use fossilised organisms as good models for providing new materials. While nature cannot produce the perfect designs, it can generate the most ideal, optimised and functional adaptive ones.

Biological structures and biomaterials have evolved by natural selection over many millions of years of strict conditioning, smoothing out trade-offs between conflicting demands and limitations of an environment in order to maximise fitness. These conflicts are omnipresent but can be partially resolved to generate extremely well-functioning materials. The end results are biomaterials with compromises that exhibit high levels of performance made with minimum use of energy.

The evolution of tissues by natural selection provides us with a view of how different strategies of development have been harnessed by organisms according to function. As a result we should be able to provide simplified assembly strategies to recreate functional approximations of every human tissue.

One of the most fascinating bio-inspired approaches is to directly use cells and organisms to grow biomaterials and grow them to our specifications and requirements literally in the beaker or test tube [2]. This can be achieved by judicious modulation of the growing environment. Single-celled organisms such as diatoms, Foraminifera and coccolithophores are a convenient starting point as they are the most rudimentary and elementary organisms to grow and support in artificial culture and provide enough utility for proving this approach as practically beneficial. Diatoms are of great interest for the development of new strategies in nanotechnology and molecular assembly as they provide modes of construction at these scales that could benefit the development of new generation biomedical devices such as miniature biosensors. Diatoms have even been described as "natural-born lithographers" in recognition of the technique [3]. Sussman is exploiting the mechanisms of patterning by diatoms to use in patterning microchips. Others have suggested using them as drug-eluting modules because of their beneficial microscopic size and reticulated internal pore structure [4]. Growing materials with living cells integrated during synthesis and construction is an attractive proposition. In this way the directed evolution may be possible with specific organisms that rapidly reproduce so that many thousands of generations are produced in short experimental periods. Protocols are well established now for the mass production of new proteins using a combination of site random mutagenesis followed by high-throughput screening [5].

Synthetic tissue biology is a newly emerging discipline which seeks to engineer tissues and form them into complex biological assemblages [6]. One approach in this endeavour is to reverse engineer biological materials, tissues, organs or systems to "decipher" how they are put together and how they operate at highest level of detail. It can be suggested that it can revolutionise the concepts and approach for re-engineering biological systems.

Synthetic biology for forming multicellular tissues uses the most advanced methods available for building extracellular environments to direct morphogenesis of cells and tissues. In another way cells are designed and constructed with novel functions and coaxed into multicellular organisations.

In the vast diversity of nature, there are countless identifiable "ground" plans about how to construct and organise cells and tissues into organs. Matter joins together in an evolution by natural selection which has consistently originated assembly rules and design solutions that have been conserved and reapplied in organisms throughout the gradual ascendency and emergence of new forms of life.

13.3 Biomaterial Synthesis and Production

A century ago, artificial devices were made from materials as diverse as gold and wood and were developed to a point where they could replace various components of the human body. These materials are capable of being in contact with bodily fluids and tissues for prolonged periods of time, "whilst eliciting little, if any, adverse reactions". When these synthetic materials are placed within the human body, the tissues react towards the implant in a variety of ways. The mechanism of tissue interaction at a nanoscale level is dependent on the response to the implant surface. As such, three terms for description of a biomaterial, representing the tissue responses, have been defined by Hench and West, in 1990, as bioinert, bioresorbable and bioactive [7].

Based on the acceptance of the importance of tissue–implant interactions on the nanoscale, quite extensive development of nanotechnology in science and engineering has taken place during the last two decades. This does not come as a surprise, considering that functional nanostructured materials have the capability of being adapted and integrated into a range of engineering and biomedical devices. This is because most biological systems, including viruses, membrane and protein complex, exhibit natural nanostructures. The microstructure and properties of these new generation nanostructured materials depend on the synthesis method as well as on the processing routes. Hence it is of extreme importance to select the most appropriate technique for the preparation of materials with desired designs and property combinations.

Synthesis techniques commonly used for the production of inorganic materials such as advanced ceramics include a range of solid state, liquid state and gaseous ionic state processing methods. Wet chemical processing techniques such as co-precipitation and sol–gel have been commercially employed to obtain nanoparticles, nanocoatings and nanostructured solid blocks and shapes. In modern ceramic technology pressing is accomplished by placing the powder into a die and applying pressure to achieve compaction. Hot pressing (HP) and hot isostatic pressing (HIP) are the most commonly used methods for the production of bioceramics. HIP can induce the higher densities and small grain structures required for good mechanical properties, whereby heat and pressure are applied simultaneously and the pressure is applied from all directions via a pressurised gas such as helium or argon. Flat plates or blocks and non-uniform components are relatively easily produced using HP or HIP.

Sol–gel processing is unique in that it can be used to produce different forms, such as powders, platelets, coatings, fibres and monoliths of the same composition, merely by varying the chemistry, viscosity and other factors of a given solution [8]. The advantages of the sol–gel technique are numerous: it is of the nanoscale; it results in a stoichiometric, homogeneous and pure product, owing to mixing on the molecular scale; high purity can be maintained as grinding can be avoided; it allows reduced firing temperatures due to its small particle sizes with high surface areas; it has the ability to produce uniform fine-grained structures; it allows the use of different chemical routes (alkoxide or aqueous-based); and it is easily applied to complex shapes with a range of coating techniques. Shrinkage up to a number of coatings, depending on the chemistry, is fairly uniform perpendicular to the substrate and the coatings can dry rapidly without cracking. However, shrinkage becomes an important issue in monolith ceramic production [8].

Most biomaterials aimed to be used within the physiological environment require appropriate surface finish to allow soft or hard tissue attachment without any adverse reaction. In addition biomaterials for hard tissue attachment need similar chemical composition of bone. Hard tissues of nearly all animals include calcium and phosphate ion combinations as calcium phosphate compounds with a variety of minerals. The structure of the bone consists of nano-to-micron range interconnected pores. To emulate and produce these intricate designs synthetically is difficult or in some instances nearly impossible due to the restrictions in resolution of the currently used production techniques although new generation 3D printing techniques might be one of the most recent techniques to achieve this difficult task in the near future.

On the other hand, nature has the answer to these intricately fine porous structures: some marine structures by their virtue of natural need contain excellent interconnected pores and architectures that can encounter and solve the problems mentioned above. They have very fine nanometre to a few hundred micron range interconnected pores and excellent mechanical properties. In addition most are made of or contain inorganic materials such as calcium carbonate and calcium phosphates with a range of minerals containing Mg, Sr and Si that helps to improve the properties of hard tissues after implantation. The organic matter within the marine skeletons (although small) contains a range of materials such as proteins with very promising possible medical applications [9].

13.4 The Inorganic Matter and Proteins

The marine environment is uniquely rich in structures with highly functional architectures with interconnected open pores, which offer high mechanical strength and chemical compositions suitable for use as is or converted to materials appropriate for human implantation.

Currently an increasing number of compounds and materials are being identified from marine organisms such as calcium carbonates to proteins and applied to medical applications. In this regard, marine species have been a valuable resource for the discovery of novel active pharmaceuticals [9].

In applications for tissue engineering, coral skeletons and converted coralline apatites are exquisite examples [10]. They have demonstrated substantial clinical success as templates for tissue reconstruction. This has spurred on researchers to look at other skeletons with better mechanical and/or biological properties. These unique 3-dimensional marine structures supported growth and enhanced differentiation of stem cell progenitors into bone cells unlike standard carbonate frameworks that do not induce stem cell differentiation.

These marine materials and designs have been instrumental to introduce the simplest remedies to vital problems in regenerative medicine, providing frameworks and highly accessible sources of osteopromotive analogues and mineralising proteins. This is exemplified by the biological effectiveness of marine structures (including corals and shells and sponge skeletons) to house self-sustaining musculoskeletal tissues and to the promotion of bone formation by extracts of spongin. Biological molecules that pivotal to the regulation and guidance of bone morphogenesis and particularly the events in mineral metabolism and deposition were the first molecular components established for calcification, morphogenesis and wound healing. It emerges that bone morphogenic protein (BMP) molecules, the main cluster of bone growth factors for human bone morphogenesis, are secreted by endodermal cells into the developing skeleton. Signalling proteins, TGF-β and Wnt-prime targets in bone therapeutics are present in early marine sponge development. Furthermore, ready-made organic and inorganic marine skeletons possess a habitat suitable for proliferating added mesenchymal stem cell (MSC) populations and promoting clinically acceptable bone formation [11].

13.5 Marine Skeletons

Using natural skeletons in a direct way as a scaffold for growing cells into tissue emerged for making new bone tissue, as a product of hydrothermal processing [12]. Transformed coral (converted to calcium phosphates) has been the primary source of natural skeletons for bone tissue engineering because of its chemical, crystallographic and structural complementarity to native human bone [13]. For the same reasons, since then, researchers have made use of invertebrate marine skeletons of hydrozoans, cuttlefish [14], marine sponges [1], nacre sea shell and echinoderm spines [15] as templates with optimal ranges of pore sizes, channels and structural networks for organising and nourishing the growth of human tissues as a prelude to transplantation into the patient. In other developments whole natural skeletons (without conversion to HAp) have been used as templates for carrying biomolecules. Accordingly diatom skeletons have been tethered with active biomolecules such as an antibody to be used in immunodiagnostics [16]. Mollusc shells are a fascinating model for understanding the complexities of biomineralisation such as the control and regulation of protein–mineral interactions [17].

Considerable research efforts have been focused on the development of efficient and cost-effective methods to produce calcium phosphate with apatite structure from biogenic natural materials. These include hydroxyapatite (HAp), tricalcium phosphate (both α- and β-TCP), tetracalcium phosphate (TTCP) and octacalcium phosphate (OCP). Different natural materials composed of calcium carbonate and possessing unique architecture like coral [10, 18–20], sea urchins [21, 22], pearl [23], nacre [24], Mediterranean mussel [25], sea and land snails [26] and cuttlefish [14] have been reported to have potential to be used or produced as calcium phosphate materials for biomedical applications. Past research shows that we have so far identified candidate biomatrices in nature, with varied chemical homologies and structural analogies to human extracellular matrices and whole tissues. The utility of selected species of these marine animals has been applied to the regeneration of human bone and cartilage. However, their full utility in these tissues and other tissues has yet to be harnessed and fully exploited.

13.6 Marine Shells (Nacre)

Unlike any other biomaterial, nacre from the pearl oyster, *Pinctada maxima*, is able to induce osteogenesis and bone formation from latent osteoprogenitors along an endochondral pathway, consisting of a cartilage tissue intermediary phase [27].

The outer nacreous layer of a particular species of mollusc shell is an unlikely and unexpected source of biomaterial for engineering new bone. In the absence of synthetic chemistry, natural biomaterials were widely used by physicians from ancient civilisations of India, China, Egypt and Central America, and it was the ancient Mayans who discovered the unique property of nacre to heal seamlessly onto living human bone without causing harm. The scientific basis of fusion with bone was first uncovered by Lamghari and Lopez. Under closer scrutiny nacre was found to activate skeletal cells, induce bone formation and provide structural support in a clinical trial [28, 29].

Nacre has been tested in human, sheep and rabbit models [28, 29]. In human patients fresh woven bone bonds itself throughout the nacre implant, augmented by the heightened activities of osteoblasts and osteoclasts. While nacre is stably tolerated in vivo, its degradation and resorption is limited, and this could hinder its use within calcified tissue requiring rapid self-renewal [28, 29]. Although somehow controversial in definition according to nacre researchers, the "water-soluble matrix fraction" (WSM) of nacre directly induces bone formation [30]. Molecules from nacre matrix have been shown to decrease bone resorption by acting on osteoclast metabolism [31]. The available evidence suggests that mobile signal transmitters involved in the biological control of mineralisation (as an initiator and inhibitor of calcium carbonate crystallisation at the mineralising growing front) dissolved into solution induced differentiation of surrounding latent osteoprogenitor cells [32]. The reason why nacre directly induces human cells to form new bone is best explained by the idea that "a signalling" biomolecule involved in regulating cell-mediated biomineralisation is common to both vertebrate bone tissue and nacre. These biomolecules must have been, therefore, conserved by evolutionary selection pressures.

The so-called osteopromotive effect, as measured by ALP expression, of nacre is also commensurate with treatment with dexamethasone, at least in fibroblasts. Size exclusion HPLC of the water-soluble matrix has uncovered protein fractions rich in glycine and alanine, with specific biochemical effects on human fibroblasts that modulate cell differentiation and proliferation [33]. Peptides are prevalent in the nacre matrix. Particular individual fractions have been shown to give rise to specific responses from cultured osteoblast cells. Protein fractions with low molecular weight (less than 1 kDa), for example, upregulated ALP secretion, whereas high molecular weight fraction reduced ALP secretion. Detailed sequencing of water-soluble proteins using proteomics offers enhanced characterisation of nacre matrix proteins. Nacre WSM was also shown to increase the secretion of a key inhibitor of apoptosis, cytoplasmic Bcl-2, and has an influence on rat calvarial osteoblast maintenance and survival. Low molecular weight fractions were recently found to increase expression of collagen type I and the osteogenic associated mRNA expression of osteopontin and Runx-2 [34].

Further detailed characterisation of the bioactive LMW molecules has led to the identification of 110 molecules in the 70–100 Da range comprising of glycine-enriched peptides with structural similarities and high affinities for each other. A highly defined matrix protein with a 10 kDa size named as p10 has specifically demonstrated an increase in human fibroblast cell ALP expression [35] lending greater hope that the osteogenic signal molecules can be isolated in their vital functional form. A soluble p60 protein conglomerate extracted from decalcified nacre possesses sufficient bioactivity on 3T3 and MSC to induce the secretion of mineral nodules. Some of the specific biomolecular mechanisms and associations between the signal molecules and cellular processes are being gradually uncovered. Some biomineralisation researchers are doubtful that nacre proteins are the primary cause of osteoinduction. In a study by Liao et al. [36], nacre failed to stimulate an in vivo osteogenic response, although bone-to-nacre apposition and bonding did occur directly. Liao et al. suggested that nacre provided a favourable surface chemistry, rich in phosphorus, favourable to osteoclast and osteoblast recruitment, attachment and matrix synthesis [36]. In an in vivo ectopic bone environment, surface modified nacre was found not to be osteoinductive and osteoconductive within demineralised bone matrix, but its integration and fusion with bone was

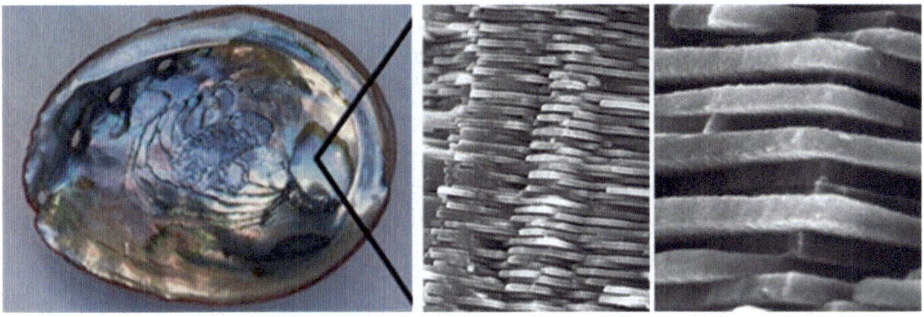

Fig. 13.1 Nacre microstructure showing platelike structure containing calcium carbonate platelets and protein interface helping good fracture toughness

better than non-nacre controls. In another study Kim et al. [37] investigated the role of interfacial properties on the biocompatibility of nacre and specifically its unique bone-bonding ability. Kim and colleagues concluded that the organic matrix is what makes nacre bond to bone so well, as it creates a favourable surface charge for optimal biological associations. When implanted the organic matrix of nacre is thought to generate a new interfacial microenvironment that forms many functional associations with the surrounding tissue leading to a better bone bonding than bioceramic implants without an organic matrix. According to Shen et al. the osteogenic responses to nacre particles and pearl proceeded much faster following soaking in a simulated body fluid (SBF) that generates a HAp-rich layer on the particles [23]. The WSM was implicated in the formation of this HAp layer and the augmented cell responses.

Taken altogether nacre provides an appropriate tissue-compatible physical platform which slowly elute unique peptides that initiate and drive bone formation. In addition nacre—due to its organic content and platelike design—is mechanically tough (fracture toughness equivalent to titanium), non-immunogenic and rapidly biodegradable, without eliciting detrimental physiological effects (Fig. 13.1). These characteristics of nacre offer us a unique substrate for delivery of a functional (possibly osteopromotive) agent to sites of bone loss in quantities that lead to rapid bone repair and regeneration.

13.7 Marine Skeletal Proteins in Regenerative Medicine

It has already been shown that coral and marine sponge skeletons can support self-sustaining musculoskeletal tissues and that extracts of spongin collagen and nacre seashell organic matrices promote bone mineralisation. Use of ready-made organic and inorganic marine skeletons is one of the simplest potential remedies to major problems hindering the future development of regenerative orthopaedics such as providing a richness of framework designs and now a potentially rich, accessible source of osteopromotive analogues and biomineralisation proteins. This should not be surprising given that the pivotal biomineralisation proteins, which orchestrate bone morphogenesis, are also found in the earliest calcifying marine organisms. In support of this notion, it has emerged that BMP molecules— the main cluster of bone growth factors for human bone morphogenesis—are secreted by endodermal cells into the developing skeleton. In addition, the regenerative signalling proteins are also present in early marine sponge development and instrumental to stem cell activation in Cnidarians. Based on this match between vertebrate and invertebrate main developmental proteins, we have published the nature and extent of this evolutionary relatedness and use it to support the development of a new strategy, which is to my selected marine origin organic matrices for novel metabolic signalling and structural proteins/peptides and protein analogues to apply in regenerative orthopaedics, particularly when using adult stem cells [9, 38]. To support this we showed the early-stage evidence gathered in our own laboratory the presence of fibrinogen fragments and early osteopromotive effects of a coral organic matrix extract on stem cells [39]. In practice the discovery of new osteo-promotive and osteo-accelerant protein analogues will require the use of traditional chromatography techniques, osteoactivity assays to hone in on potential proteins of significance and advanced proteomic tools to provide accurate sequencing, determine the mechanisms and molecular pathways involved in osteoactivation and determine the efficiency and effectiveness of marine skeleton-derived protein modulation of the stem cell (MSC) proteome. As more analogues are discovered using proteomic tools, skeletal organic matrices may have ever-increasing utility for regenerative orthopaedics [9].

13.7.1 Marine Sponge Skeletons

Marine sponges possess the most primitive form of extant tissue but share much in common with multicellular tissues which have apparently conserved many features evolved by these first multicellular organisms [40]. Morphological and biochemical similarities exist between marine sponge and vertebrate extracellular matrix (ECM) alluding to fundamental rules of organisation evolved first by marine sponges. Three collagen types have so far been identified from marine sponge. All sponges are composed of 22 nm thin collagen fibrils with highly ordered periodic banding. Although the collagen ultrastructure is relatively simple compared to vertebrate collagens, amino acid sequences and genome organisation are similar. Collagen fibrils are secreted in bundles in a similar manner to vertebrates. Similarly collagen fibrils are closely associated with proteoglycans which, in mammalian tissue blueprint, shape and form at long range scales. Fibronectin, dermatopontin and tenascin polypeptides are also found in marine sponge collagen fibres and cross-react with antibodies raised against vertebrate analogues highlighting their common origins. Some sponge species possess an analogue of type IV collagen found in vertebrate basement membrane collagens [41]. The organisation of collagen fibrils is analogous to collagen type XIII which sticks cells to surfaces. It is with

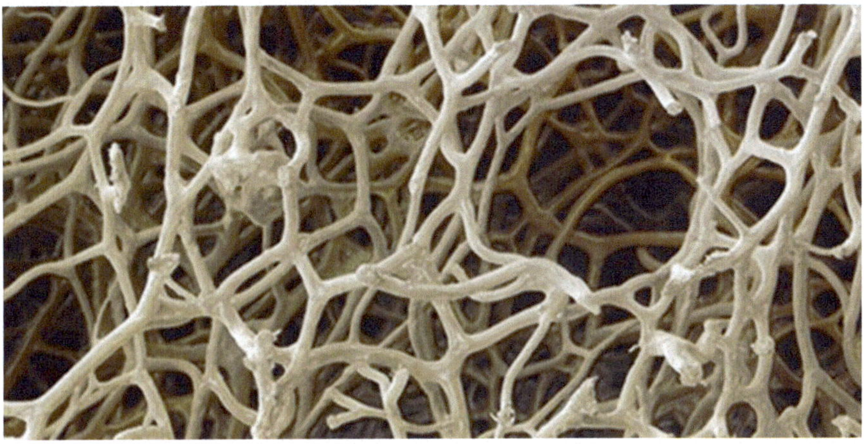

Fig. 13.2 Sponge interconnected lattice-like structure

these properties (fibronectin and cell adherent collagens) that collagenous marine sponges represent a significant potential for future development as bioactive tissue engineering scaffolds.

At present, marine sponges are extensively exploited for novel biological compounds as potential treatments for cancer tumours, leukaemia and inflammation. Marine sponges are also a source of collagen for cosmetics [40] and dermatological preparations [42]. In total 50 % of all marine-derived materials are sourced from a wide spectrum of marine sponges. Collagenous marine sponge skeletons are incredibly soft, strong, highly absorbent and elastic, resistant to high temperatures and bacterial attack. Such properties make them highly suited for surgical procedures. The exact conditions to grow marine sponges at a large enough scale for commerce are being investigated by a number of researchers. Some have established aquatic pilot farms for the cultivation of selected bath sponge species. Marine sponges are sufficiently adaptable for commercial scale production. Another aim for cultivating marine sponges is to extract medically important secondary metabolites in much larger quantities than is possible from collections made by conventional bio-prospecting. The superior optimised structural design of silica marine sponges has been alluded to and which provides useful lessons for construction of man-made frameworks with minimal starting materials for maximum strength [43, 44]. They reported on the structural properties of biosilica observed in the hexactinellid sponge Euplectella sp. Consolidated, nanometre-scaled silica spheres are arranged in well-defined microscopic concentric rings glued together by organic matrix to form laminated spicules. The assembly of these spicules into bundles, effected by the laminated silica-based cement, results in the formation of a macroscopic cylindrical lattice-like structure reinforced by diagonal ridges. It can be added that there is, therefore, considerable mechanical benefit to specific arrangements of structural elements at many different hierarchies of scale (Fig. 13.2).

It has been suggested that the 3D topology and specific surface features of hydrozoans instigated faster cell adhesion, proliferation and differentiation [45]. More needs to be done to determine the exact mechanism of action between material and cell. Collagenous marine sponges fulfil the potential of a clinically relevant scaffold for a range of tissues including bone and cartilage. The fibre-bonded meshwork of sponges provides conduits for cell guidance alongside spaces for rapid tissue infiltration and infilling. It has been discovered that the collagenous composition of the fibres promotes attachment of all human cell types. The unique layered ultrastructure may explain the high wettability and adsorption of growth factors onto the collagen fibres which infuse into attached cells and promote their activities.

Collagenous marine sponges fulfil the potential of a clinically relevant scaffold for a range of tissues including bone, cartilage, fat connective, liver and kidney. Tissue formation within 4 weeks in vivo was shown to be both extensive (completely filling the entire sponge implant) and well developed with the quality and structure of tissue being equivalent to immature bone and neocartilage [13].

The fibre-bonded meshwork provides conduits for cell guidance alongside spaces for rapid tissue infiltration and infilling. The unique layered ultrastructure may explain the high wettability and adsorption of growth factors onto the collagen fibres which infuse into attached cells and promote their activities [1].

13.7.2 Echinoderm Skeletal Elements

Sea urchin skeletal plates are punctured by a very regular series of pores. Approximately three quarters of the pores are exits for tube feet (200 μm pore diameters at the spine bases to 600 μm pore diameters for the tube feet in Centrostephanus nitidus), while the remainder are channels connected to the reproductive and alimentary systems and are very much larger to accommodate larger throughputs of fluid (1,000–2,000 μm pore diameter). Hydrothermal processing of echinoderm structures transforms the chemical and mechanical properties with equivalence to human bone. Echinoderm skeletons are constructed from a unique, intricately shaped, 3D, single crystalline meshwork with a topological structure in which every internal pore and channel is in direct contact with all others (periodic minimal surface). This property is likely to facilitate mass transfer and tissue development [46]. Studies using the replamine form technique for replicating perforate echinoderm structural elements generate promising hard tissue replacements to bone, as well as candidate prostheses for blood vessels and trachea. In this context the skeletal ossicles from the sea star (Pisaster giganteus) have been investigated. They provide an ideal architecture together with physical and chemical properties conducive to bone restoration [15].

The sea urchin spicule is a composite of organic and inorganic materials that the animal synthesises using the most readily available elements in seawater. The fully formed spicule is composed of a single crystal with an unusual morphology in 3D.

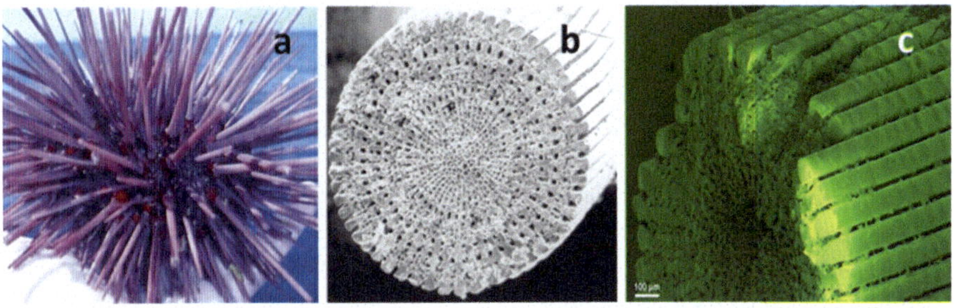

Fig. 13.3 Sea urchin structure showing the arrangements of the spikes: (**a**) general overall structure, (**b**) cross section of a single spike (spicule), and (**c**) enlarged spicule surface

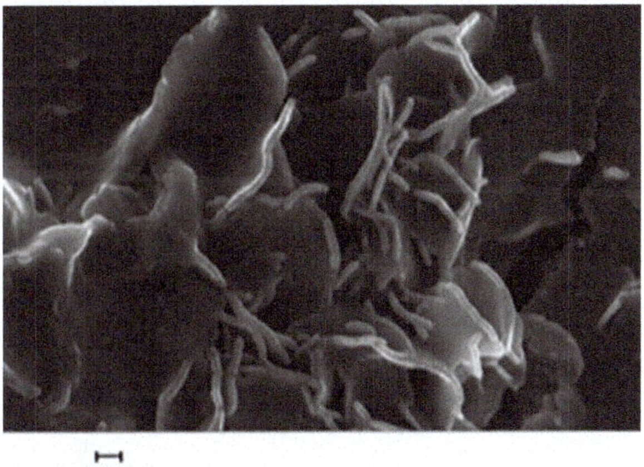

Fig. 13.4 Pseudo-platelike structure of amorphous (sol–gel-developed) calcium phosphate that transforms to fully crystalline plate nano-hydroxyapatite above 300 °C (scale 200 nm)

It has no facets and forms a starlike shape. To achieve such unusual morphologies, sea urchin and other marine organisms deposit a disordered amorphous mineral phase first and then let it slowly transform into a crystal with neatly aligned into a lattice with a specific and regular orientation while maintaining their general morphology. This is a unique transformation from amorphous to ordered crystalline structure—at room temperature—that needs to be clearly observed and understood for directional growth in future biomaterials. The sea urchin spicule is formed inside a clump of specialised cells and begins as the animal lays down a single crystal of calcite, from which the rest of the spicule is formed (Fig. 13.3). Starting from the crystalline centre, three arms extend at 120° from each other. The three radii are initially 40–100 nm-sized amorphous calcium carbonate but slowly convert to calcite. Mechanism as yet not clearly understood but might be through ordered precipitation and growth mechanism at known crystallographic orientations of calcite or aragonite.

Similar transformation from amorphous structure to crystalline form can be observed in a sol–gel-developed hydroxyapatite where the amorphous hydroxyapatite transforms to crystalline nanoplatelets by a thermally activated process (Fig. 13.4) without any large morphological change. In order to simulate the amorphous to crystalline transformation, we have developed a novel method to produce single-phase, nano-sized, platelike, mixed A–B type carbonate-containing apatite (CAH) similar to bone apatite for effective bone tissue integration [47]. The methodology emulates biomineralisation, where topotactic transition from OCP to HAp.

The synthetic process developed involves formation of thin (1–1.4 nm) layered calcium phosphonate by a self-assembly process. At the early stages, the phosphonate-derived apatite shows slightly curved platelike-shaped amorphous apatite which converts to crystalline form with significant changes to both a- and c-axes as function of temperature. The thermal decomposition of these layered amorphous structures leads to formation of highly crystalline well-organised platelike carbonated apatite [47, 48]. The overall carbonate content varies from 4 to 6.4 wt%, within the temperature range of 500–700 °C. This carbonate content corresponds well with the amount found in mammalian hard tissues.

Although sea urchin transformation is carried out at ambient temperatures, this analogue transition in sol–gel-derived synthetic HAp shows a platelike morphological change of amorphous but near platelike-shaped apatite to perfectly crystalline platelike apatite with thermal activation from room temperature to 300 °C (Fig. 13.4).

13.7.3 Coral Skeletons

Natural coral exoskeletons have been used widely as a bone replacement in orthopaedic, maxillofacial, dental and neurosurgery owing to their combination of good mechanical properties, open and interconnected porosity and ability to form chemical bonds with bone and soft tissues in vivo [49, 50]. Infect corals have the best mechanical properties of the porous calcium-based ceramics and resorb at a rate equivalent to host bone formation (Fig. 13.5).

The beginning of the coral life cycle starts with the polyps which absorbs the calcium ions and carbonic acid present in the seawater to produce the calcium carbonate in the form of aragonite crystals. The remaining composition consists of trace elements of magnesium, strontium, fluorine and phosphorus in the phosphate form [51]. Once implanted in the human body, these elements play a critical role in the bone mineralisation process and in the activation of key enzymes associated with bone remodelling cells. Strontium has been shown to contribute to the mineralisation process by stimulating osteoblasts while inhibiting osteoclasts [52]. Similarly, fluorine helps bone formation through similar stimulatory effect on osteoblast proliferation. Magnesium is also long known to be beneficial in bone remodelling as it has been shown to increase the mechanical properties of newly formed bone [53].

The organic composition has an important part to play in coral biocompatibility. The abundance, conformation and composition of the organic matrices are responsible for successful biological integration of natural coral with human host [38].

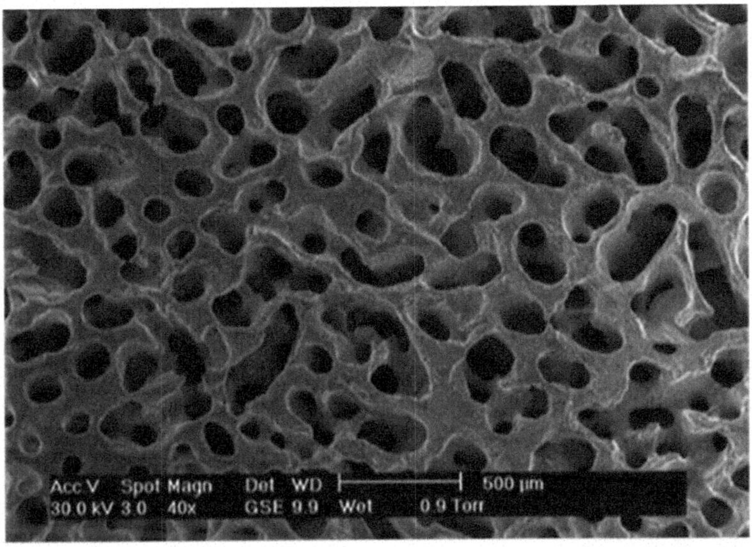

Fig. 13.5 Coralline apatite converted by hydrothermal process showing interconnected porous structure

Use of coral skeletons for general routine orthopaedic surgery and tissue engineering has been so far limited to external fixation devices as they are inappropriate for strictly load-bearing applications due to their calcium carbonate structure with high dissolution rates. Sol–gel coating technologies can be used to enhance the strength of corals, and this enables them to be used at more skeletal locations [50, 54]. Corals offer great opportunities to tissue engineering of bone either in their natural form or as hybridised synthetic forms. Coral skeleton combined with in vitro expanded HBMSC increased osteogenesis more than those obtained with scaffold alone or scaffold with fresh marrow [39]. In vivo large animal segmental defect in both orthopaedic and maxillofacial surgery led to complete recorticalisation and formation of medullary canal with mature lamellar cortical bone and onlay graft for contour augmentation of the face giving rise to clinical union in a high number of cases [55, 56]. Structural and biomineralisation studies of coral can be used to inform the development of new advanced functional materials because of the unique nanoscale organisation of organic tissue and mineral as highlighted by Ehrlich et al. [20]. At a macrostructural level, the deep-sea bamboo coral exhibited bone-like biochemical and mechanical properties. A specialised collagen matrix (acidic fibrillar) serves as a model for future potential tissue engineering applications. The matrix supported both osteoblast and osteoclast growth, and the exceptional bio-elastomeric properties of the collagen matrix (gorgonin) of this coral make it potentially suitable for blood vessel implants. Quinones cross-link and harden the collagenous gorgonin proteins and closely resemble human keratin. The mechanism by which gorgonin is synthesised and interacts with the process of mineralisation may provide lessons for the generation of a synthetic-collagen-like material [20].

13.8 Drug Delivery and Marine Structures

Slow or targeted drug delivery system is a system that is capable of releasing a preloaded pharmaceutical agent to a targeted site at a specific rate and most importantly at a therapeutically relevant concentration. The main aim of this type of system compared with conventional drug intake (injection or tablet) is to facilitate the local and specific area delivery, dosage and duration control and hence appropriate active drug delivery while causing minimal side effects. While technological advancement has produced innovative and refined drug delivery systems, the fundamental basis that defines what a drug delivery system remains unchanged. The therapeutic advantages of these systems can be attributed to many underlining factors: predictability of release rate and minimised drug concentration, thereby reducing any possible adverse systemic effect. Prolonged duration of drug therapy such as the need for frequent re-dosing has been problematic in many global applications of drugs such as the treatment protocol of malaria in Africa. Many factors are considered in the development of drug delivery systems in accordance to the desired application. This includes the agent to be carried, the administration route, the material used, the degradation rate, the loading efficiency, the physical and chemical properties of the material, the practicality for large-scale production, toxicity, among other parameters.

Many materials such as ceramics, polymers, alginate and polysaccharides have shown potential advantages as drug delivery systems [57]. However, marine materials such as coral exoskeletons and marine shells show a better promise due to their easy conversion to calcium phosphates, intricate interconnected pores and their controllable dissolution rates.

The pore size and interconnectivity of the coral pores are a critical factor in the rate of coral as a bone graft and slow drug delivery material. Moreover, the uniform porosity of the exoskeletons provides a more constant drug loading and therefore providing a more predictable drug release rate of which both are crucial factors that directly impact the effectiveness of the drug delivery system. Natural structures although not perfect often exhibit intricate morphologies that justify the efforts for biomimetic approach.

13.9 Foraminifera and Drug Delivery

During an overseas summer break, I have noticed that the sand that I was walking on the beach looked as perfect spheres and showed intricate structure (Fig. 13.6). I brought some to our laboratories, and after XRD analysis I noticed that it was not silica sand but calcium carbonate. After proper characterisation, we identified it as a marine structure belonging to the *Foraminifera* family. *Foraminifera* are abundant and are found in all marine environments, but different species exist with different

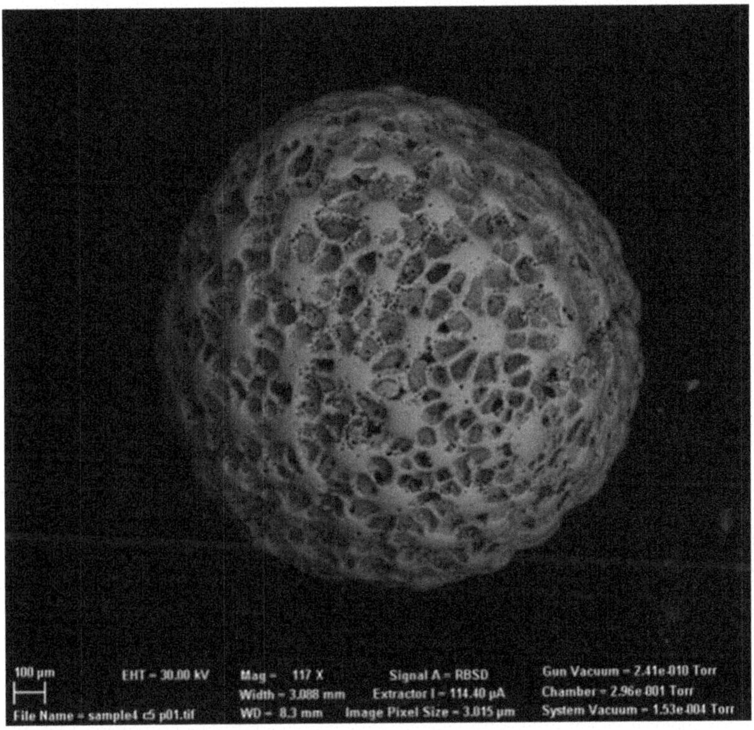

Fig. 13.6 Foraminifera macrostructure

shapes depending on their environment. *Foraminifera* are single-celled organisms with shells consisting of multilayer inner chambers commonly divided and added during its growth.

Prior to any marine material can be used as a drug delivery material, it must first undergo a rigorous process to test the composition, purity, morphology and suitability for drug loading and its slow dissolution without any adverse effect to the patient. Unless specifically protein and organic matter is required to be extracted, prior to sterilisation of calcium carbonate material, any residual organic constituents are removed by immersing in solution of sodium hypochlorite and then drying at about 100 °C [58].

During slow drug delivery studies, spherical and star-shaped shells floresianus (Foraminifera) from the coral beach sand of the Great Barrier Reef, Australia, and Okinawa, Japan, were collected. The microspherical samples were intact and measured 0.5–1.5 mm in diameter (Fig. 13.6). These shells or more appropriately microspheres possess unique interconnected porous structures that have evolved to circulate seawater and collect light for the mutual benefit of symbiotic algal cells that reside inside the shell. Microcomputed tomography (μ-CT) and scanning electron microscopy (SEM) imaging confirmed that shells were internally permeated by a 3D

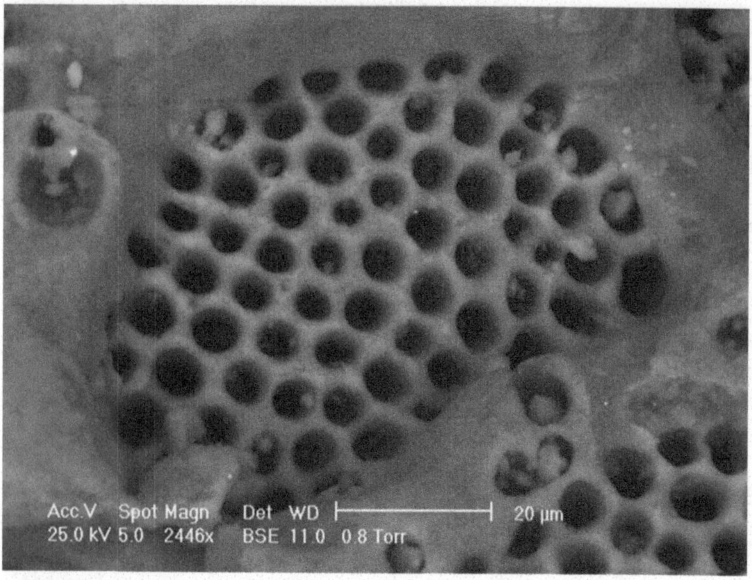

Fig. 13.7 Enlarged microstructure showing interconnected 5 μm porous structure

network of microscopic interconnected channels measuring 1–10 μm in diameter. Between the micropores surface of the solid spine area was made of calcium carbonate platelets consisting nano- and meso-pores (Fig. 13.7).

It was necessary to hydrothermally convert these microsphere shells into more stable, highly crystalline β-tricalcium phosphate (β-TCP) and/or HAp using the methods developed and published earlier [10]. In certain circumstances of drug delivery applications, TCP presents the more ideal composition compared with other calcium phosphates.

Chemical conversion of foraminifer's shells to HAp (microspheres) did not change the original untransformed structure making it available for adsorption of candidate drug compounds and to allow new bone cell penetration into the micropores. This was demonstrated in animal trials [59–61].

Constructs that are generated in this manner provide many distinct advantages for tissue engineering as a physical template and devices for controlled release of BMP, water-soluble proteins (WSP), genes and growth factors. Since the chemistry occurs at room temperature and consists of an aqueous phase, biological molecules can be safely incorporated during synthesis.

Natural spheres loaded with drugs can spontaneously degrade and progressively release entrapped biological contents introduced during synthesis. The release profile shows relatively slow, local release of drugs such as bisphosphonate, gentamicin and simvastatin from micro- and macrospheres for extended periods [62, 63].

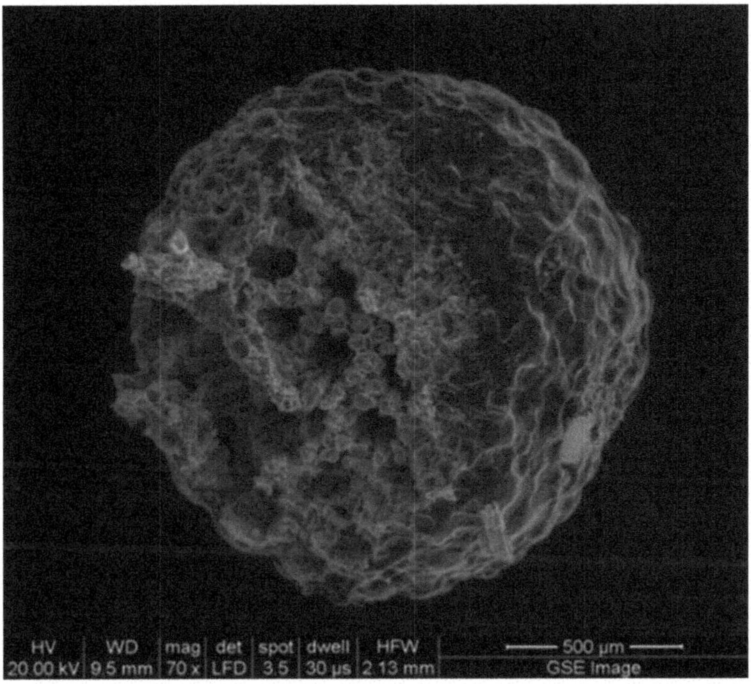

Fig. 13.8 Foraminifera microsphere during dissolution studies showing dissociation of the calcium phosphate and other loaded pharmaceuticals and minerals

Due to the pore architecture, these microspheres within the physiological environment can dissolve and supply both calcium and phosphate ions and any other beneficial ions and the drugs incorporated to the immediate tissues. Foraminifera after dissolution is shown in Fig. 13.8.

13.10 Stem Cell Regulation

There is also growing realisation that the composition of a scaffold material is vitally important to organise stem cell activities as they are dependent on the extracellular fabric for life support and to guide their subsequent evolution and development [38, 59]. Re-creation of the native stem cell environment where stem cells normally reside (such as bone marrow) and are protected, managed and stabilised as self-renewing undifferentiated cells and given instruction on how to regulate the rate of progenitor and successor cell production is an active research area.

Marine structures such as Foraminifera, coral skeletons and converted coralline apatites have demonstrated substantial clinical success as a template for tissue reconstruction. This has spurred on researchers to look at other skeletons with better mechanical properties such as hydrozoans as unique potential candidates for tissue engineering of mineralised tissues [45]. The unique 3-dimensional structure supported growth and enhanced differentiation of stem cell progenitors into bone cells unlike standard carbonate frameworks that do not induce stem cell differentiation. It can be suggested that the 3D topology and specific surface features of hydrozoans induce faster cell adhesion, proliferation and differentiation.

13.11 Concluding Remarks

In nature, structures possess enviable properties such as complexity, sophistication and miniaturisation that are not (as yet) possible to fabricate in the laboratory. However, we are gradually inventing ways of replicating nature to produce similar levels of sophistication albeit to a limited extent. We are only able to recreate microscopic structures and surfaces with some level of biomimetic detail. This has been particularly true for the replication of both bio-organic and inorganic structures. One versatile approach has been to use biological microstructures as templates for the reproduction of inorganic structures with identical features. They have clear significance to the production of replacements for calcified tissues. This is achieved by using techniques in biomineral inspired materials chemistry. The concept is to exploit the consecutive developmental pathway of systems that nature employs to make skeletons from molecules into micro- and macroscopic structures. The process in inorganic fabrication is analogous to building a house. It begins with supramolecular pre-organisation, interfacial recognition, vectorial regulation and chemical transformation lending to multilevel processing. These processes are developed within confined reaction spaces directed in their formation by the templates themselves. The continual multiplication of these nano-assemblies builds up into the emergence of morphology and macroscale biomimetic forms.

In the near future, studies of the way natural materials are constructed and the way they adapt to their environment will enable us to produce an exciting array of self-responsive structures and materials for regenerative medicine and structural engineering applications. In nature biomaterials are made with immaculate resource and energy efficiency using common, readily available substrates through self-assembly into highly organised and structurally optimised hierarchies. This gives us the opportunity to produce structures with intricate shapes and architectures that are tailored to their functions and do not break down. The science and engineering have shown us how biomimetic approaches can yield promising outcomes for application in tissue engineering of skeletal tissues. Our work along is a part of ongoing research towards the design of clinically relevant scaffolds for regenerative medicine using a unique set of self-organising hierarchical structures including marine structures that are designed and synthesised according to biological principles of design.

There is a clear and present need for better tissue engineering scaffolds that possess more natural bio-responsive environments conducive to guiding the natural processes of regeneration which can be highly intricate and dynamic in space and time. Thus scaffolds must have intelligence designed into them to meet this biological challenge. We contend that there needs to be a step change to scaffold environments that are responsive whereby the synthesised biomatrix evolves in real time to meet the demands and optimisations of adaptive growth and regeneration of human tissues. As cells proliferate and differentiate, they alter their environment. Future advanced biomimetic scaffolds must be able to adapt to these changes and meet the ever-changing needs of developing tissues. Nature—although not perfect—uses simple chemistries, sound biological principles and formation of adequate structures with unique morphologies to distribute functional stress. Nanofabrication using combined biochemical, biological and biomechanical principles of assembly and design is still in its infancy. Use of this bio-inspired nanofabrication for tissue engineering is a unique approach that has enormous potential to improve scaffold design and tailor physico-chemical environments with an ability to micro-evolve. This is the next challenge: to grow materials with cells and promote their regulation of material synthesis.

Marine structures constantly adapt their composition, growth and hence function to dynamically changing environmental conditions and have the ability for self-repair when adaptation fails or is too slow. Advanced functional materials with these characteristics would see enormous benefit to engineering industries and biomedicine. At a time when we are concerned about air pollution, global climate change, consuming less energy and using fewer and sustainable resources, the design and fabrication of a new technology based on biomimetics is such an imperative.

Acknowledgments To write a chapter that involves a range of natural and synthetic materials and their discovery and development can only be achieved by taking into account a large number of research studies and related published papers. During the last two decades, a number of colleagues and past and present students contributed enormously in both research and their dissemination through publications. This chapter has been the collation of the ideas and published work that only touches the surface of the large contributions made during the years. There are a number of colleagues that we would like to thank: Dr. Joshua Chou who has been a very resourceful young researcher and contributed well in the drug delivery work. We would also like to acknowledge the contributions of Professors R. Vago, F.N. Oktar and R.M Conway and Drs. A. Milev, A. Choi, C. Chai, J. Russel and J. Hu and Mr I.J. Macha, which, without their contribution and timely visions, this chapter could not have been written.

References

1. Green D, Howard D, Yang XB, Kelly M, Oreffo ROC (2003) Natural marine sponge fibre skeleton: a biomimetic scaffold for human osteoprogenitor cell attachment, growth and differentiation. Tissue Eng 9:1159–1166
2. Parker AR, Martini N (2006) Structural colour in animals-simple to complex optics. Opt Laser Technol 38:315–322
3. Mock T, Samanta MP, Iverson V, Berthiaume C, Robison M, Holtermann K et al (2008) Whole-genome expression profiling of the marine diatom Thalassiosira pseudonana identifies genes involved in silicon bioprocesses. Proc Natl Acad Sci U S A 105(5):1579–1584

4. Green D, Ben-Nissan B (2008) Biomimetics: bio-inspired engineering of human tissue scaffolding for regenerative medicine. In: Tateishi T (ed) Biomaterials in Asia: in commemoration of the 1st Asian Biomaterials Congress. Tsukuba, Japan, pp 364–385
5. Kim ES (2008) Directed evolution: a historical exploration into an evolutionary experimental system of nanobiotechnology, 1965–2006. Minerva 46:463–484
6. Sia SK, Gillette BM, Yang GJ (2007) Synthetic tissue biology: tissue engineering meets synthetic biology. Birth Defects Res C 81(4):354–361
7. Hench LL, West JK (1990) The sol-gel process. Chem Rev 90:33–72
8. Ben-Nissan B, Choi AH (2006) Sol-gel production of bioactive nanocoatings for medical applications. Part I: an introduction. Nanomedicine 1(3):311–319
9. Green DW, Li G, Milthorpe B, Ben-Nissan B (2012) Adult stem cell coatings using biomaterials for regenerative medicine. Mater Today 15(1–2):61–68
10. Ben-Nissan B (2003) Natural bioceramic: from coral to bone and beyond. Curr Opin Solid State Mater Sci 7(4–5):283–288
11. Ben-Nissan B, Green DW (2013) Marine materials in drug delivery and tissue engineering: from natural role models, to bone regeneration and repair and slow delivery of therapeutic drugs, proteins and genes. In: Kim SK (ed) Marine biomaterials. Taylor & Francis/CSR Books. Boca Raton, FL, USA
12. Roy D, Linnehan S (1974) Hydroxyapatite formed from coral skeletal carbonate by hydrothermal exchange. Nature 247(438):220–222
13. Vago R, Plotquin D, Bunin A, Sinelnikov I, Atar D, Itzhak D (2002) Hard tissue remodeling using biofabricated coralline biomaterials. J Biochem Biophys Methods 50:253–259
14. Rocha JHG, Lemos AF, Agathopoulos S, Valero P, Kannan S, Oktar FN et al (2005) Scaffolds for bone restoration from cuttlefish. Bone 37(6):850–857
15. Martina M, Subramanyam G, Weaver JC, Hutmacher DW, Morse DE, Valiyaveettil S (2005) Developing macroporous bicontinuous materials as scaffolds for tissue engineering. Biomaterials 26:5609–5616
16. Townley HE, Parker AR, White-Cooper H (2008) Exploitation of diatom frustules for nanotechnology: tethering active biomolecules. Adv Funct Mater 18(2):369–374
17. Marin F, Luquet G (2004) Molluscan shell proteins. Comptes Rendus Palevol 3(6–7):469
18. Demers C, Hamdy C, Corsi K, Chellat F, Tabrizian M, Yahia L (2002) Natural coral exoskeleton as a bone graft substitute: a review. Biomed Mater Eng 12:15–35
19. Nowak D, Florek M, Nowak J, Kwiatek W, Lekki J, Zieba E et al (2005) Micro-spectrometric investigations of inorganic components of the black corals for biomedical applications. Key Eng Mater 284–286:297–300
20. Ehrlich H, Etnoyer P, Litvinov SD, Olennikova MM, Domaschke H, Hanke T et al (2006) Biomaterial structure in deep-sea bamboo coral (Anthozoa: Gorgonacea: Isididae): perspectives for the development of bone implants and templates for tissue engineering. Mater Werkst 37(6):552–557
21. Agaogullaria D, Kelb D, Gökçea H, Dumana I, Öveçoglua ML, Akarsubasic A et al (2012) Bioceramic production from sea urchins. Acta Phys Pol A 121(1):23–26
22. Samur R, Ozyegin L, Agaogullari N, Oktar FN, Agatopoulos S, Kalkandelen C et al (2013) Calcium phosphate formation from sea urchin (Brissus latecarinatus) via modified mechano chemical (ultrasonic) conversion method. Metallurgia 52(3):375–378
23. Shen Y, Zhu J, Zhang H, Zhao F (2006) In vitro osteogenic activity of pearl. Biomaterials 27:281–287
24. Bahar H, Yaffe A, Binderman I (2003) The influence of nacre surface and its modification on bone apposition: a bone development model in rats. J Periodontol 74:366–371
25. Macha IJ, Ozyegin LS, Chou J, Samur R, Oktar FN, Ben-Nissan B (2013) An alternative synthesis method for di calcium phosphate (monetite) powders from Mediterranean mussel (Mytilus galloprovincialis) shells. J Aust Ceram Soc 49(2):122–128
26. Kel D, Gökçe H, Bilgiç D, Ağaoğulları D, Duman I, Öveçoğlu ML et al (2012) Production of natural HA from land snails. Key Eng Mater 493:287–292

27. Lopez E, Vidal B, Berland S, Camprasse S, Camprasse G, Silve C (1992) Demonstration of the capacity of nacre to induce bone formation by human osteoblasts maintained in vitro. Tissue Cell 24:667–679
28. Lamghari M, Antonietti P, Berland S, Laurent A, Lopez E (2001) Arthrodesis of lumbar spine transverse processes using nacre in rabbit. J Bone Miner Res 16(12):2232–2237
29. Lamghari M, Berland S, Laurent A, Huet H, Lopez E (2001) Bone reactions to nacre injected percutaneously into the vertebrae of sheep. Biomaterials 22:555–562
30. Rousseau M, Lucilia PM, Almeida MJ, Milet C, Lopez E (2003) The water-soluble matrix fraction from the nacre of Pinctada maxima produces earlier mineralization of MC3T3-E1 mouse pre-osteoblasts. Comp Biochem Physiol B 135:1–7
31. Duplat D, Chabadel A, Gallet M, Berland S, Bedouet L, Rousseau M et al (2007) The in vitro osteoclastic degradation of nacre. Biomaterials 28(12):2155–2162
32. Westbroek P, Marin F (1998) A marriage of bone and nacre. Nature 392:861–862
33. Almeida MJ, Pereira L, Milet C, Haigle J, Barbosa M, Lopez E (2001) Comparative effects of nacre water-soluble matrix and dexamethasone on the alkaline phosphatase activity of MRC-5 fibroblasts. J Biomed Mater Res 57:306–312
34. Rousseau M, Boulzaguet H, Biagianti J, Duplat D, Milet C, Lopez E et al (2007) Low molecular weight molecules of oyster nacre induce mineralization of the MC3T3-E1. J Biomed Mater Res A 85A:487–497
35. Zhang C, Li S, Ma Z, Xie L, Zhang R (2006) A novel matrix protein p10 from the nacre of pearl oyster (Pinctada fucata) and its effects on both $CaCO_3$ crystal formation and mineralogic cells. Mar Biotechnol 8:624–633
36. Liao H, Mutvei H, Hammarstrom L, Wurtz T, Li J (2002) Tissue responses to nacreous implants in rat femur: an in situ hybridization and histochemical study. Biomaterials 23:2693–2701
37. Kim YM, Kim JJ, Kim YH, Rho JY (2000) Effects of organic matrix proteins on the interfacial structures at the bone-biocompatible nacre interface in vitro. Biomaterials 23:2089–2096
38. Green DW, Padula MP, Santos J, Chou J, Milthorpe B, Ben-Nissan B (2013) A therapeutic potential for marine skeletal proteins in bone regeneration. Mar Drugs 11(4):1203–1220
39. Green DW, Ben-Nissan B (2010) Biomimetic applications in regenerative medicine: scaffolds, transplantation modules, tissue homing device and stem cells. In: Amiji M, Tochilin V (eds) Handbook of materials for nanomedicine. Pan Stanford Publishing, Singapore
40. Swatschek D, Schatton W, Kellermann J, Muller WEG, Kreuter J (2002) Marine sponge collagen: isolation, characterization and effects on the skin parameters surface pH, moisture and sebum. Eur J Pharm Biopharm 53:107–113
41. Boute N, Exposito J-Y, Boury-Esnault N, Vacelet J, Noro N, Miyazaki K et al (1996) Type IV collagen in sponges, the missing link in basement membrane ubiquity. Biol Cell 88:37–44
42. Nicklas M, Schatton W, Heinemann S, Hanke T, Kreuter J (2009) Preparation and characterization of marine sponge collagen nanoparticles and employment for the transdermal delivery of 17b-estradiol-hemihydrate. Drug Dev Ind Pharm 35(9):1035–1042
43. Aizenberg J, Weaver JC, Thanawala MS, Sundar VC, Morse DE, Fratzl P (2005) Skeleton of Euplectella sp structural hierarchy from the nanoscale to the macroscale. Science 309(5732):275–278
44. Miserez A, Weaver JC, Thurner PJ, Aizenberg J, Dauphin Y, Fratzl P et al (2008) Effects of laminate architecture on fracture resistance of sponge biosilica: lessons from nature. Adv Funct Mater 18(8):1241–1248
45. Abramovitch-Gottlib L, Geresh S, Vago R (2006) Biofabricated marine hydrozoan: a bioactive crystalline material promoting ossification of mesenchymal stem cells. Tissue Eng 12(4):729–739
46. Aizenberg J, Hendler G (2004) Designing efficient microlens arrays: lessons from nature. J Mater Chem 14:2066–2072
47. Milev AS, Kannagara GSK, Ben-Nissan B, Wilson M (2004) Template directed synthesis of nanosized bone-like apatite. In: Schulte J (ed) Proceedings of the Asia Pacific nanotechnology forum 2003. World Scientific Publishing Co, Singapore, pp 87–92

48. Milev AS, Kannangara GSK, Ben-Nissan B (2003) Morphological stability of plate-like carbonated hydroxyapatite. Mater Lett 57(13–14):1960–1965
49. Vago R (2008) Beyond the skeleton. Cnidarian biomaterials as bioactive extracellular microenvironments for tissue engineering. Organogenesis 4(1):18–22
50. Ben-Nissan B (2004) Biomimetics and bioceramics. In: Reis RL, Weiner S (eds) Learning from nature how to design new implantable biomaterials: from biomineralization fundamentals to biomimetic materials and processing routes. Nato science series, vol 171, Springer, Dordrecht, pp 89–103
51. Stanley G (2003) The evolution of modern corals and their early history. Earth Sci Rev 60(3–4):195–225
52. Bonnelye E, Chabadel A, Saltel F, Jurdic P (2008) Dual effect of strontium ranelate: stimulation of osteoblast differentiation and inhibition of osteoclast formation and resorption in vitro. Bone 42(1):129–138
53. LeGeros R (1981) Apatites in biological systems. Prog Cryst Growth Charact Mater 41(1–2): 1–45
54. Choi AH, Ben-Nissan B (2007) Sol-gel production of bioactive nanocoatings for medical applications. Part II: current research and development. Nanomedicine 2(1):51–61
55. Papacharalambous S, Anastasoff K (1993) Natural coral skeleton used as onlay graft for contour augmentation of the face. A preliminary report. Int J Oral Maxillofac Surg 22(5):260–264
56. Leupold J, Barfield W, An Y, Hartsock L (2006) A comparison of ProOsteon, DBX, and collagraft in a rabbit model. J Biomed Mater Res B Appl Biomater 79(2):292–297
57. Bose S, Tarafder S (2012) Calcium phosphate ceramic systems in growth factor and drug delivery for bone tissue engineering: a review. Acta Biomater 8(4):1401–1421
58. Hu J, Russell JJ, Ben-Nissan B, Vago R (2001) Production and analysis of hydroxyapatite from Australian corals via hydrothermal process. J Mater Sci Lett 20(1):85–87
59. Chou J, Ito T, Bishop D, Otsuka M, Ben-Nissan B, Milthorpe B (2013) Controlled release of simvastatin from biomimetic β-TCP drug delivery system. PLoS One 8(1):e54676
60. Chou J, Ito T, Otsuka M, Ben-Nissan B, Milthorpe B (2013) Simvastatin-loaded β-TCP drug delivery system induces bone formation and prevents rhabdomyolysis in OVX mice. Adv Healthc Mater 2(5):678–681
61. Chou J, Green DW, Singh K, Hao J, Ben-Nissan B, Milthorpe B (2013) Adipose stem cell coating of biomimetic β-TCP macrospheres by use of laboratory centrifuge. Biores Open Access 2(1):67–71
62. Chou J, Ben-Nissan B, Green DW, Valenzuela SM, Kohan L (2011) Targeting and dissolution characteristics of bone forming and antibacterial drugs by harnessing the structure of microspherical shells from coral beach sand. Adv Eng Mater 13(1–2):93–99
63. Chou J, Valenzuela S, Bishop D, Ben-Nissan B, Milthorpe B (2012) Strontium- and magnesium-enriched biomimetic beta-TCP macrospheres with potential for bone tissue morphogenesis. J Tissue Eng Regen Med. doi:10.1002/term.1576

Chapter 14
Calcium Phosphate Derived from *Foraminifera* Structures as Drug Delivery Systems and for Bone Tissue Engineering

Joshua Chou, Jia Hao, Besim Ben-Nissan, Bruce Milthorpe, and Makoto Otsuka

Abstract Currently there is an urgent need to develop an appropriate slow drug delivery system to sustain the local and targeted release of the drug to increase therapeutic efficacy while reducing side effects. In this study, a novel drug delivery system by means of hydrothermally converting marine exoskeletons to β-tricalcium phosphate was investigated. The in vitro dissolution of key chemical compositional elements and the release of drugs such as simvastatin and antibiotics were measured. Coating of these *Foraminifera* shells with an apatitic bone cement material reduced the dissolution rate by 50 % compared with control samples. This study shows the potential applications of marine structure-derived calcium phosphates as efficient local drug delivery systems.

J. Chou (✉)
Faculty of Pharmacy, Research Institute of Pharmaceutical Science, Musashino University, 1-1-20 Shinmachi, 202-8585 Nishi-Tokyo, Tokyo, Japan

Faculty of Science, University of Technology, Sydney, NSW, Australia
e-mail: joshua@musashino-u.ac.jp

J. Hao
Oral Implantology and Regenerative Dental Medicine, Tokyo Medical and Dental University, Tokyo, Japan

B. Ben-Nissan
School of Chemistry and Forensic Science, Faculty of Science, University of Technology, Broadway, Ultimo, PO BOX 123, Sydney, NSW 2007, Australia
e-mail: b.ben-nissan@uts.edu.au

B. Milthorpe
Faculty of Science, University of Technology, Sydney, NSW, Australia

M. Otsuka
Faculty of Pharmacy, Research Institute of Pharmaceutical Science, Musashino University, 1-1-20 Shinmachi, 202-8585 Nishi-Tokyo, Tokyo, Japan
e-mail: motsuka@musashino-u.ac.jp

B. Ben-Nissan (ed.), *Advances in Calcium Phosphate Biomaterials*, Springer Series in Biomaterials Science and Engineering 2, DOI 10.1007/978-3-642-53980-0_14,

Keywords *Foraminifera* • Drug delivery • Calcium phosphates • Simvastatin • Antibiotics • Zinc

14.1 An Introduction to Drug Delivery Systems

Marine origin materials such as shells, corals, nacres and sponges also provide an abundant new source of inorganic material for drug delivery and tissue engineering applications. Research and development in this area has primarily focused on the applications of soft and hard tissue repair. However, the application of using marine shells as a carrier for drugs has remained relatively unexplored. This section discusses the advances on marine structures converted to calcium phosphate materials with relevance to drug delivery.

The field in the development of suitable biomaterials for drug delivery systems has been the focus of ongoing research since the 1940s when the first drug delivery system was developed to raise the drug concentration in blood plasma. Still the full replacement of living bone tissue techniques and materials is not available in clinical practice. In addition it is well known that the composition, anatomical structure and final function of culture-derived tissue do not accurately simulate the human archetype. To do this properly requires a support framework (scaffold) with features of an extracellular matrix, proteins to control development and potentiated cell types that reassemble into tissues. As of now scaffold-based tissue engineering is providing many useful structural environments where tissues can be reconstituted in their natural form and with normal functions. However, there are two outstanding issues that need to be addressed if tissues are to be regenerated fully in the laboratory. The first is to recreate a blood system within the developing tissue and provide adequate nutrition; this involves structures with interconnected right size porosity. The second is to simulate the delivery schedule of developmental proteins to cells for proliferation and differentiation into whole tissues. So far, clinical trials implementing these factors, in the regeneration of tissues, have not led to the anticipated results. The problem lies in the failure to recreate an interwoven cellular and molecular ecosystem made up of blood vessels, neurons, cells and regenerative biochemicals. This is a major necessity for proper tissue development.

This has led to a shift in approach towards fabricating materials and structures containing minerals and proteins, which are dispersed in controlled ways in scaffolds, to encourage endogenous repair, remodelling and regeneration. Tissue promoting proteins used in experimental and clinical regenerative therapies are expensive to produce. The production of proteins using recombinant technology is imperfect and that has made it difficult to make genuine native proteins with their entire set of evolved functions. Thus, there are good scientific reasons for developing relatively straightforward, low-cost alternatives that include structures with appropriate proteins and others. Marine invertebrates are one potential, unexamined source of structures that can be converted to calcium phosphates and select proteins with potential utility in strategies for regenerative medicine, in the laboratory, and possibly for the patient. They can further incorporate with a range of drugs that can be utilised as local drug delivery systems. In this current chapter we shall explain marine structures (specifically Foraminifera) that can be converted to calcium phosphates and can be loaded with a number of drugs used in tissue engineering.

14.1.1 Properties of Drug Delivery Systems

While technological advancements have produced innovative and refined drug delivery systems, the fundamental basis that defines what a drug delivery system remains unchanged. It is a system that is capable of releasing a preloaded bioactive agent to a targeted site at a specific rate and, most importantly, at a therapeutically relevant concentration. The main aim of this type of system compared with conventional drug intake is to facilitate the local specific area delivery, dosage and duration control and hence appropriate drug delivery while causing minimal side effects and no harm to the patient. The therapeutic advantages of these systems can be attributed to many underlining factors: predictability of release rate and minimised drug concentration thereby reducing any adverse systemic effect. Prolonged duration of drug therapy providing the need for frequent re-dosing and thus improving patient care and compliance has been problematic in many global applications of drugs such as the treatment protocol of malaria. Many factors are considered in the development of drug delivery systems in accordance to the desired application. This includes the agent to be carried, the administration route, the material used, the degradation rate, the loading efficiency, the physical and chemical properties of the material, the practicality for large-scale production, and toxicity, among other parameters.

14.1.2 Calcium Phosphate Materials for Drug Delivery Systems

Depending on the application, different materials with different properties can be employed to suite specific needs. One key factor that remains unchanged and one of the defining parameters to the success of the system is the property of the carrier material itself. One of the most commonly researched and used materials for drug delivery application is calcium phosphate compounds. The calcium phosphate family includes a series of derivatives that are distinguished by each material's degradation rate. Calcium phosphates such as tricalcium phosphate ($Ca_3(PO_4)_2$) (TCP) have a special relevance in drug delivery, as it is biocompatible without eliciting any inflammatory response or rejection by the body. While synthetic tricalcium phosphate compounds are readily available, they are still limited by the simplicity in their structural design, and focus has been centred on producing TCP compounds with uniform pores that are interconnected within the material. This allows for increased and more predictable drug loading and thus a more reliable release rate of the drug from the material.

The production of calcium phosphate compounds is well researched and established, which can include using calcium carbonate as a precursor material that undergoes a chemical exchange and transformation to calcium phosphate derivatives [1].

14.2 Marine-Based Calcareous Exoskeletons

The marine environment, with its enormous wealth of biological and chemical diversity [2, 3], represents an abundant and untapped source of useful natural structures awaiting discovery. While marine-derived chitosan, alginate and polysaccharides have shown potential advantages as drug delivery systems, coral exoskeletons can also be applied as an alternative material suitable for this task.

For over 30 years, coral exoskeletons have been extensively studied and used as bone grafts and where other marine structures have led to the development of pharmaceutics and their application in medicine [4–9].

Calcium carbonate (in the form of aragonite or calcite) can be found in many of the currently known marine organisms [10–12]. Each coral species possesses its unique architecture, namely, porosity, pore size and pore interconnectivity, microstructural composition and mechanical properties [13] that compliment key defining parameters of a drug delivery system. The pore size and interconnectivity of the coral pores are a critical factor in the rate of coral as a bone graft and slow drug delivery material. This interconnected porous network in coral exoskeletons can allow drugs to infiltrate to the centrum of the material [14]. Moreover, the uniform porosity of the exoskeletons provides a more constant drug loading, therefore providing a more predictable drug release rate of which both are crucial factors that directly impact the effectiveness of the drug delivery system. Biological structures often exhibit intricate morphologies that justify the efforts for biomimetic approach. Biomineralising organisms are natural manufacturers with which mankind only can try to compete possibly with limited success. There are a number of marine structures in addition to coral that has a unique structure. One class of marine structure belonging to the *Foraminifera* family has shown to be suitable for drug delivery applications. *Foraminifera* are abundant as fossils for the last 540 Ma and are found in all marine environments, but different species exists depending on the surrounding habitat. *Foraminifera* are single-celled organisms with shells consisting of multilayer inner chambers commonly divided and added during its growth.

14.2.1 Compositional Properties of Calcareous Exoskeletons

The beginning of the coral life cycle starts with the polyps which absorb the calcium ions and carbonic acid present in the seawater to produce the calcium carbonate in the form of aragonite crystals representing 97–99 % of the coral exoskeleton [15]. The remaining composition is made up of various elements and is dependent on the environment but mainly consists of trace elements of magnesium (0.05–0.2 %), strontium, fluorine and phosphorus in the phosphate form (0.02–0.03 %) [16, 17].

These elements that are composed in the coral exoskeleton structure are known to play a critical role in the bone mineralisation process and in the activation of key enzymes associated with bone remodelling cells. Strontium through extensive studies has shown to contribute to the mineralisation process by stimulating osteoblasts while inhibiting osteoclasts [18]. Similarly, fluorine, present 1.25–2.5 times more in coral than in the human bone, helps bone formation through similar stimulatory effect on osteoblast proliferation [15]. Magnesium is also beneficial in bone remodelling as it has been shown to increase the mechanical properties of newly formed bone [19]. Evidently, most of the elements in bone can be found in corals but they differ in their distribution.

14.2.2 Source of Supply, Quality Control and Sterilisation

One of the key limitations in the development of marine biopharmaceutics is with the key issues of purity and consistent supply. As previously stated *Foraminifera* are widely abundant and available commercially, thereby making it an attractive source of material for research and development. Before any marine material can be used as a carrier material, it must first undergo a rigorous process to control its quality from collection to manufacturing and to its final application. With increased sensitivity with modern screening techniques, studies can be performed to ensure that, within the limits of detection, no foreign entities or organic materials are left and that the material is of the highest quality. These studies can include optical, radiographic, chromatographic, spectrophotometric and biocompatibility analyses [17, 20]. Unless specifically protein and organic matter required, prior to sterilisation of calcium carbonate material, any residual organic constituents are removed by immersing in solution of sodium hypochlorite for at least 1 h then drying at about 100 °C followed by and not limited to ultrasound treatment [21].

14.2.3 Producing Calcium Phosphates from Calcareous Exoskeletons

It has been reported that marine-derived calcium carbonate exoskeletons possess fast degradation rate that may not be suitable for long-term drug therapy. However, it should be noted that this trait might potentially be useful for drug delivery applications that requires fast-acting and short-term therapy. To circumvent this limitation, several authors have shown the process of converting the calcium carbonate exoskeleton of coral to the more stable structure of calcium phosphates and its derivatives [21–23].

One of these processes is commonly referred to as the hydrothermal exchange conversion strategy that was developed by Roy and Linnehan in 1974 [24]. Simply,

Table 14.1 Ionic composition of Foraminifera before and after hydrothermal conversion to β-TCP

	Calcium (mg/g)	Phosphate (mg/g)	Strontium (mg/g)	Magnesium (mg/g)
Before conversion	17 ± 0.5	0	1.8 ± 0.05	30.6 ± 0.4
After conversion	17 ± 0.7	62 ± 9	2.1 ± 0.07	30.7 ± 0.2

this process exchanges the carbonate component of the coral for phosphate to produce calcium phosphates and its derivatives using high temperatures between 200 and 260 °C for 24–48 h following the reaction shown in Eq. (14.1):

$$10CaCO_3 + 6(NH_4)_2HPO_4 + 2H_2O \rightarrow Ca_{10}(PO_4)_6(OH)_2 + 6(NH_4)_2CO_3 + 4H_2CO_3 \tag{14.1}$$

The calcium to phosphate molar ratio can be adjusted accordingly to yield different forms of calcium phosphates. In certain circumstances of drug delivery applications, tricalcium phosphates (TCP) present the more ideal composition compared with other calcium phosphates. TCP has been extensively studied for use as bone grafts [25–28] and for drug delivery systems [29–32] owing to appropriate dissolution rate [33–35]. The hydrothermal conversion from calcium carbonate exoskeletons to TCP would require a Ca/P = 1.5. The time variant is an important factor as <24 h conversion would yield carbonated TCP while 48 h would complete the transformation [14]. Obviously this also depends on the size of the material converted.

Chemical compositional analysis of marine structures can be examined by various techniques including mass spectroscopy. Elemental quantification by inductively coupled plasma-mass spectroscopy (ICP) (Table 14.1) exhibits that the majority of the calcium, magnesium and strontium ions are preserved during this conversion process.

14.3 Drug Delivery Systems Based on Calcareous-Derived Calcium Phosphates

The therapeutic efficacy of any drug delivery system is dependent on how the drugs are loaded, how efficient are the drug loading and, most importantly, the release rate of the loaded drugs. Marine calcareous materials provide the ideal internal porous structure for drug loading, which this chapter will further discuss.

A key benefit in employing the use of hydrothermal exchange is the preservation of the structural integrity of the original material. The chemical composition has changed, but the structure remains intact as shown in Fig. 14.1. There exist a variety of strategies that can allow incorporation of pharmaceutics in this type of carrier material as illustrated in Fig. 14.2.

The most common and simplistic method of drug loading is through immersion of the carrier material in a concentrated solution containing the pharmaceutics for

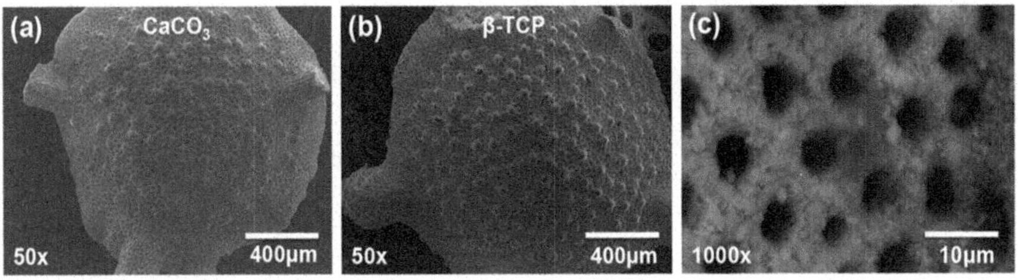

Fig. 14.1 Scanning electron micrographs showing (**a**) *Foraminifera* ($CaCO_3$) before conversion and (**b**) after hydrothermal conversion to β-TCP. The surface pores (**c**) are uniformly distributed and are approximately 5 μm in diameter

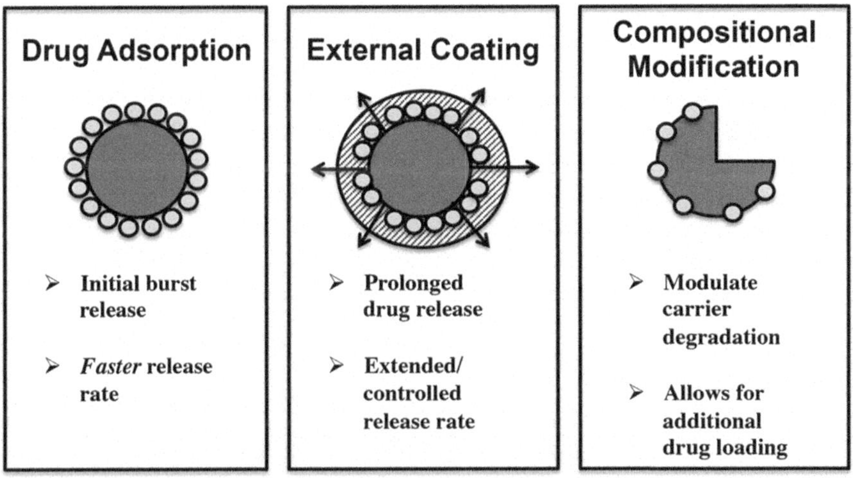

Fig. 14.2 Schematic summary detailing the strategies available for drug loading on carrier material such as calcareous-derived calcium phosphates

a period of time. These drugs are in turn adsorbed onto the surface and within the material, which will depend on the porosity of the carrier. The interconnected and uniformly porous network of the calcareous exoskeleton can provide a consistent and reliable drug loading as opposed to irregular porous materials. Once the system is placed in its intended environment, drugs will begin to be released into the surrounding environment initially through the surface of the carrier and as the pores are infiltrated through diffusion mechanism.

This characteristic can be observed by plotting a drug release plot based on the Higuchi Eq. (14.2), which the linearity of the graph will determine if the release is by diffusion through the matrix material:

$$M_t = A\sqrt{C_s \frac{D_i \varepsilon}{\tau}\left(2C_d - \varepsilon C_s\right)t} \quad (14.2)$$

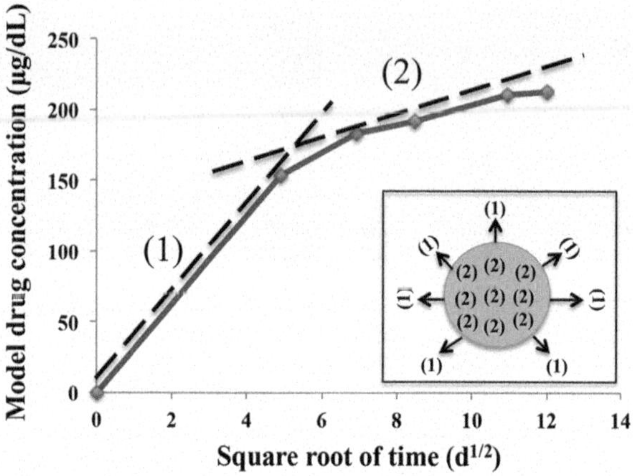

Fig. 14.3 Higuchi plot showing two phases of drug release: surface release slope (*1*) and drug diffusion release from the matrix material slope (2)

where M_t is the amount of drug release after time t, A is the matrix surface area, D is the diffusion coefficient of the drug, C_s is the solubility, C_d is the concentration of the drug in the matrix, τ is the tortuosity and ε is the porosity of the matrix. The release mechanism was demonstrated using a model drug incorporated with the calcareous-derived calcium phosphate material and plotting a subsequent drug release profile based on the Higuchi plot shown in Fig. 14.3.

The plot shows two phases of the drug released. The initial burst release was due to conventional release of drug from the surface of the carrier material as illustrated by slope (1). The second-order release profile shows a linear slope (2) in the Higuchi plot suggesting that the release of the drug from the matrix material is based on a drug diffusion process through the macro- and micropores of carrier. This provides an overview on the release mechanism profile from using these carrier materials and can allow further optimisation by controlling these release profiles.

14.3.1 Controlled Release of Bone Stimulatory Drug: Simvastatin

Bone repair and formation is a complex process that would require stimulatory compounds in the form of pharmaceutics, growth factors, proteins, etc., to assist in the regeneration process. In the case of osteoporosis, where there is an imbalance in bone remodelling process, the use of stimulants is even more crucial. The last few decades have witnessed the development of various bone stimulatory drugs like bisphosphonates and its derivatives and more recently simvastatin. In previous studies, simvastatin was successfully loaded with the *Foraminifera*-derived β-TCP (SV/β-TCP) with a 75 % loading efficiency. To control the release of simvastatin and control its release rate, an apatite coating was made around the β-TCP material (Ap/Sv/β-TCP) [36]. This reduced the release of simvastatin from 44 % down to 22 % which gave an approximately 50 % reduction in the release (Fig. 14.4).

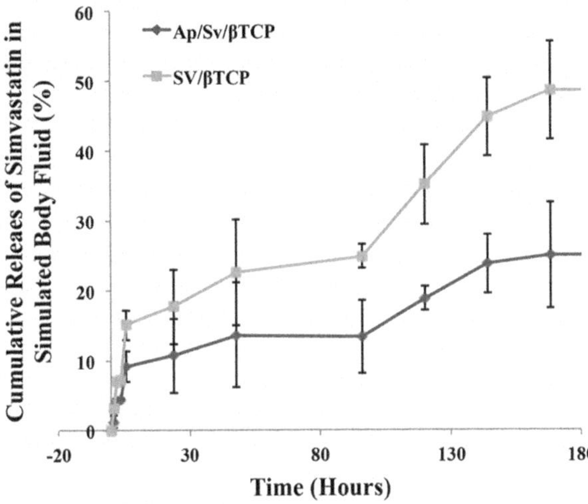

Fig. 14.4 The release of simvastatin in simulated body fluid over 7 days from β-TCP (SV/β-TCP) and apatite-coated β-TCP with simvastatin (Ap/Sv/β-TCP) showing a reduction of simvastatin release equal to approximately 50 %

This will allow a more prolong release of the drug into the local area thereby increasing the therapeutic efficacy of the system. This system was tested in an osteoporotic mice model where significant cortical and cancellous bone formation was observed in the localised area [37]. Furthermore, Ap/Sv/β-TCP produced significantly stronger bones compared with the experimental groups. This is thought to be the effect of slower local release of simvastatin, which again reinforces the potential benefits of using this drug delivery system. However, if the treatment is aimed for systemic applications such as osteoporosis, new strategies are needed to be developed. To assess the difference between local and systemic delivery in a separate study, Ap/Sv/β-TCP system was compared with direct injection of equal amount of simvastatin. The results over the 6-week experimental period showed that direct injection ignited severe localised muscle inflammation whereas the Ap/Sv/β-TCP showed no sign of any adverse effects [38].

This is again attributed to the slower controlled release of simvastatin within the range of therapeutic efficacy compared with direct injection of the drug. Depending on the application and the duration of the therapy required, the unique structures of *Foraminifera* could be adapted and modified to achieve the desired therapeutic effect.

14.3.2 Carrier for Antibiotic (Gentamicin) Against Methicillin-Resistant Staphylococcus aureus (MRSA)

Despite advances in hygiene management in surgical protocols, bacterial infections are still prevalent in modern surgeries. In second- or third-world operating theatres, the cases for infections are even higher. In orthopaedic surgery, *Staphylococcus aureus* (*S.aureus*) are the most common strain in the cause of infections. These

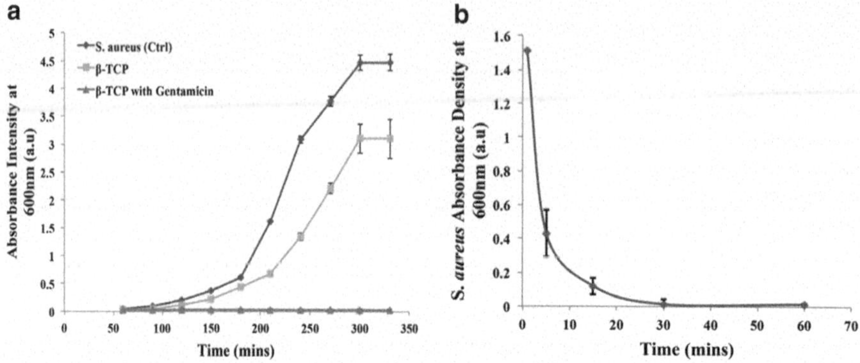

Fig. 14.5 Introducing the antibiotic (gentamicin)-loaded β-TCP Foraminifera to MRSA shows (**a**) inhibition on the growth of MRSA, and (**b**) time-delay introduction of the system shows prevention of MRSA growth after 30 min

infections generally go unnoticed till it is too late as the bacteria progressive proliferate and spread in the body. With bacteria evolving into superbugs and becoming ever more resistant to antibiotics, the use and application of antibiotics is even more crucial especially in the hospitals. PMMA loaded with antibiotics are widely used in orthopaedic surgeries as the treatment of choice. PMMA is not biodegradable and as such would require another surgery to remove it after its intended function. This would again risk the patient the chance of repeated infection. What is agreed upon scientists is the need for effective treatment and prevention systems against *S.aureus* and its kind ideally by a biodegradable carrier. With this aim in mind, foramina-derived β-TCP was loaded with gentamicin-sulphate antibiotic (GS-TCP) and evaluated to treat and/or prevent the occurrence of clinical strain methicillin-resistant *Staphylococcus aureus* (MRSA) in vitro [39]. The study showed that a single GS-TCP was capable of releasing antibiotics to prevent the growth of MRSA during its exponential growth phase.

Furthermore, a time-delayed study where GS-TCP was introduced to the MRSA at various times (5, 10, 15, 30, 60 and 1,440 (24 h) min) showed the negative presence of the MRSA thereby signifying the potential antibacterial efficacy of the GS-TCP (Fig. 14.5). Though this would still require further in vivo investigations and optimisation before it can be applied in a clinical setting, the results suggest that the carrier material can release antibiotics at a level that is therapeutically relevant in the prevention and treatment of MRSA and can be applied solely as an antibiotic treatment or implanted as a bone filler with antibiotic potential.

14.3.3 Synthetic Modification of β-TCP with Zinc

The previous two studies showed the potential of using *Foraminifera*-derived β-TCP as carriers for drugs, and it should be noted that β-TCP can be synthetically

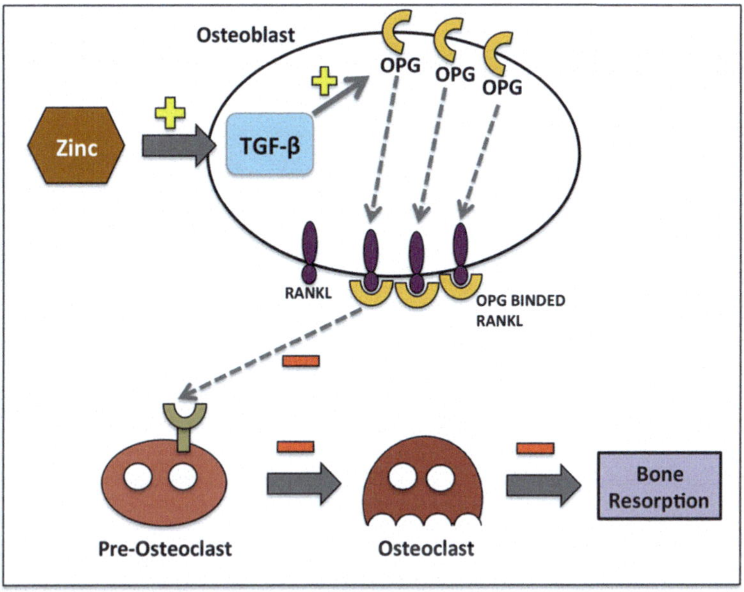

Fig. 14.6 The actions of zinc ions on the production of TGF-β in osteoblast cells which the increase in OPG production help reduce the maturation of osteoclast cells thereby limiting the cell's mode of action on bone resorption

modified to alter the chemical composition of the material thereby changing its biological properties. Trace elements, such as strontium and magnesium, that are involved in bone formation have been extensively studied and evaluated by incorporation into biomaterials for their ability to stimulate bone formation [18, 19]. This would require lengthy testing and optimisation to achieve the optimal therapeutic concentration adding to the production process as high concentration of these elements can initiate adverse effects. Natural calcareous exoskeletons like *Foraminifera* naturally possess both strontium and magnesium at small concentration within its natural composition, and so far studies have shown positive effect in vitro and in vivo. This had led to the motivation of further altering the chemical properties of the material in hope of increasing the stimulatory ability of these carriers.

Zinc, another trace element that is required in cell regulation, has also shown bone stimulatory effects and studies have linked zinc deficiency in osteoporotic patients [40, 41]. Zinc can promote bone growth [42] and inhibit bone resorption [43], along with antimicrobial resistance [44] which can impart multifunctionality in a drug delivery system. Zinc ions can act on various receptors of cells, but one of these actions is based on zinc's ability to increase the production of transforming growth factor-beta (TGF-β) in osteoblastic cells, which in turn increases the production of osteoprotegerin (OPG). This decreases the amount of RANKL that can bind to the RANK receptor of pre-osteoclast cells preventing its maturity and bone remodelling actions (Fig. 14.6).

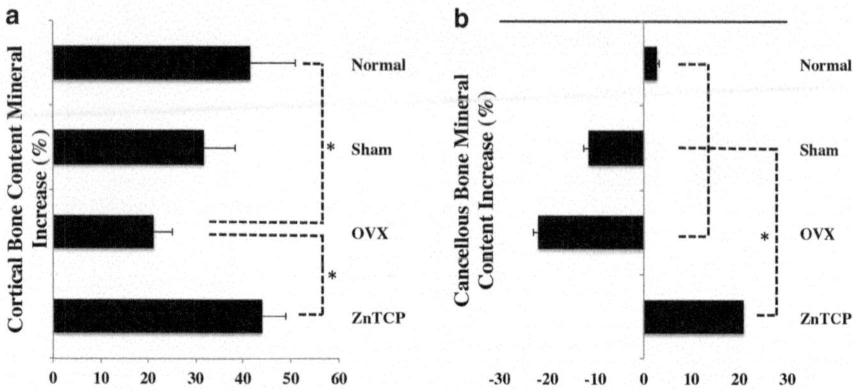

Fig. 14.7 Examination of the bone mineral content growth after 4 weeks shows (**a**) cortical bone to be significantly increase by the presence of Zn-TCP compared with OVX (ctrl), and (**b**) cancellous bone was also significantly stimulated by Zn-TCP compared with negative growth by OVX (ctrl). Asterisk sign represent $p < 0.05$, which was considered statistically significant

In recent studies, zinc ions were substituted into the β-TCP material and commonly referred to as zinc-tricalcium phosphate (Zn-TCP) [45]. This was achieved by adding zinc ions during the hydrothermal conversion process allowing zinc to be substituted into the lattice structure in place of the calcium ions. It should be cautioned that zinc at high concentration, like pharmaceutics, can exhibit adverse side effects. By incorporating key ions into the lattice structure of the material, the system can achieve further biological activities and allow the unfilled porous network to be incorporated with other compounds as a dual-drug delivery system.

14.3.4 Zn-TCP as a Drug Delivery System for Treatment of Osteoporosis

Osteoporosis is an elusive disease that would require a sustained treatment over an extended period. It is easy to recognise that any form of treatment would have to involve a multi-targeted approach, and this can be achieved through the development of multifunctional drug delivery systems. While previous studies have shown the effectiveness on the use of β-TCP in combination with simvastatin in the treatment of osteoporotic mice, it was thought that by increasing the stimulatory properties of the carrier material, it could provide a more effective form of treatment.

The Zn-TCP system was evaluated in an osteoporotic mice model for 4 weeks in which the system was implanted intramuscularly near the right femur bone. It should be noted that the purpose of this model is to observe if the stimulatory compounds released into the blood stream in the muscle can be delivered to needed areas, as osteoporosis is a systemic disease that affects the whole body. It is not anticipated that this will be used in a clinical setting. The results presented in Fig. 14.7 showed significant cortical and cancellous bone growth from Zn-TCP compared with the control groups near the localised right femur bone of the mice.

What is most noticeable is the cancellous bone growth where the osteoporotic group exhibit negative bone growth, which is consistent with the osteoporotic condition; Zn-TCP showed a significant cancellous bone growth of 20 %. The observed effect is currently limited to the localised long bone, and continued evaluation will investigate the long-term effect of the Zn-TCP system in a systemic applications. As a proof of concept, zinc was also directly injected into the osteoporotic mice at the same concentration of Zn-TCP. Over the experimental period, muscle deterioration and inflammation was observed at the site of injection confirming once again that highly localised dosage can elicit side effects whereas slow and controlled release systems are therapeutically more effective.

14.3.5 The Use of Zn-TCP for Other Bone Regeneration Applications

As previously mentioned, the key interest in the applications of natural calcareous precursor materials is in its unique porous structure that allows it to be exploited an appropriate carrier material, and as the mentioned studies have shown, this system shows promising stimulatory potential in promoting bone formation. However, the application of the use of *Foraminifera* is not limited to only delivering stimulatory compounds. Structures like these can also be applied or other bone tissue engineering applications such as fillers for bone defects or for bone augmentation applications. This section will highlight the use of this material for promoting bone formation in these areas.

14.3.5.1 Zn-TCP as Bone Filler Material for Defect Repair

One of the most common bone-related traumas is with bone fracture, which may be caused as a result of bone fragility from osteoporosis or simply from breakage. Under certain conditions, the repair of bone fractures will require the use of bone filler material based on calcium phosphate, which are widely used clinically while offering reliable results. With an ever-increasing healthcare costs and advancement in technologies, patients and society expect continual improvements related to healing rate and quality of treatment. To address this trend, Zn-TCP material developed was evaluated for fracture repair by implanting into a rat tibial defect model to observe the bone repair rate and quality as the defect healed compared with an empty control group [46]. As Fig. 14.8 illustrates, the bone mineral content (BMC) of the Zn-TCP was significantly higher compared with empty control and β-TCP starting 2 weeks after implantation. This trend continued until 8 weeks where the BMC level in the β-TCP reached the same level as Zn-TCP. This demonstrates the accelerated bone formation and healing of the defect site from the addition of zinc in the material

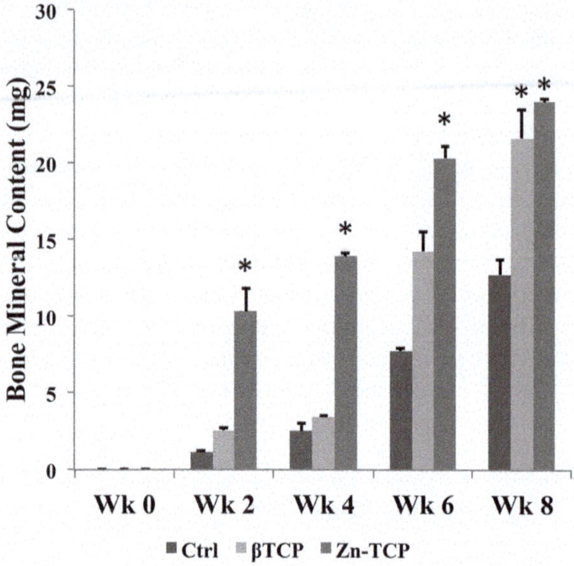

Fig. 14.8 Examination of the bone mineral content of Zn-TCP compared with empty control and β-TCP shows significant bone mineral formation starting at 2 weeks and continuing until 8 weeks where β-TCP had the same bone mineral level as Zn-TCP. Asterisk sign represent $p < 0.05$, which was considered statistically significant

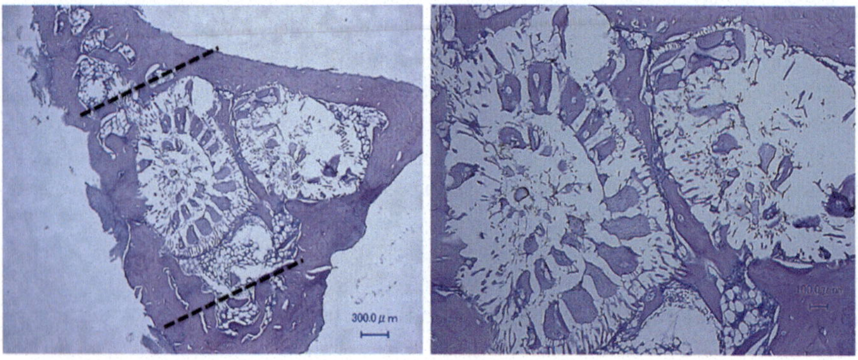

Fig. 14.9 Examination of the bone mineral content of Zn-TCP compared with empty control and β-TCP shows significant bone mineral formation starting at 2 weeks and continuing until 8 weeks where β-TCP had the same bone mineral level as Zn-TCP. *Dotted lines* illustrate the original defect made

compared with β-TCP. Histological slices shown in Fig. 14.9 showed that the defect in the Zn-TCP group was completely repaired and restoration of trabecular bone could be observed around the Zn-TCP material and from within. It is interesting to note that the structure of the internal porous chambers within the material was infiltrated with new bone formation and the presence of blood vessels within each of these chambers. This is illustrative on the importance of the porous structure of the implanted material in promoting faster bone formation and healing. The control group also showed repair of the defect, but trabecular bone formation was not

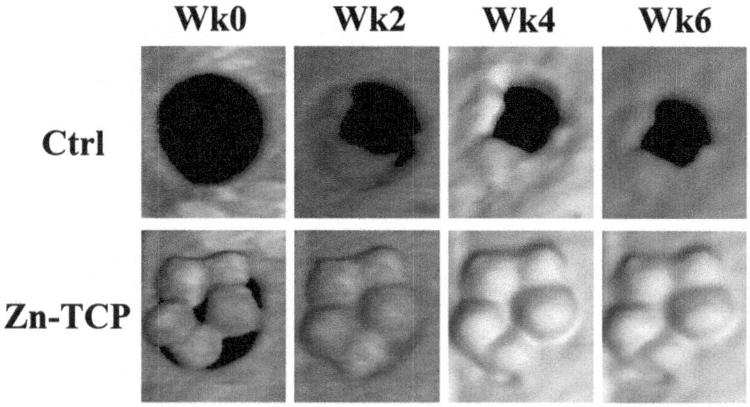

Fig. 14.10 Examination of the bone mineral content of Zn-TCP compared with empty control and β-TCP shows significant bone mineral formation starting at 2 weeks and continuing until 8 weeks where β-TCP had same bone mineral level as Zn-TCP

observed or very minimal. β-TCP group showed very similar new bone infiltration of the material within the material's porous chambers as shown previously the bone mineral content of both groups was closely similar after 8 weeks.

14.3.5.2 Zn-TCP as Bone Grafts for Bone Augmentation Procedures

The number of bone augmentation procedures in the dentistry field is rising significantly as the number of people requiring dental implants continues to increase. Before the implant can be inserted, the bone volume at the implant site must be enough to sustain the insert to allow successful bonding between the graft material and the surrounding bone. If the bone volume is not enough, bone augmentation procedures are carried out where commonly calcium phosphate-based bone grafts are used to promote bone growth over several months. This procedure is therefore time dependent where if the required bone volume can be achieved at a faster rate, it can potentially benefit the patient by reducing healing time and socio-economic costs. With this in mind, Zn-TCP was evaluated in a rat calvarial defect model to test the bone regenerative properties of the material. Figure 14.10 illustrates the progressive healing of the defect using x-ray micro-computed tomography to reconstruct the defect. These images confirm the results from the bone mineral content formation showing that the defect was closed at 2 weeks and the subsequent weeks that followed involved new bone formation within the material. In the control group after 6 weeks, a large proportion of the defect has yet regenerated. Examination of the bone mineral content presented in Fig. 14.11 shows Zn-TCP material was able to stimulate significant bone mineral growth compared with the empty control as early as 2 weeks, and this trend was observed for the duration of the experiment. It can be seen that the empty control group, without any graft material,

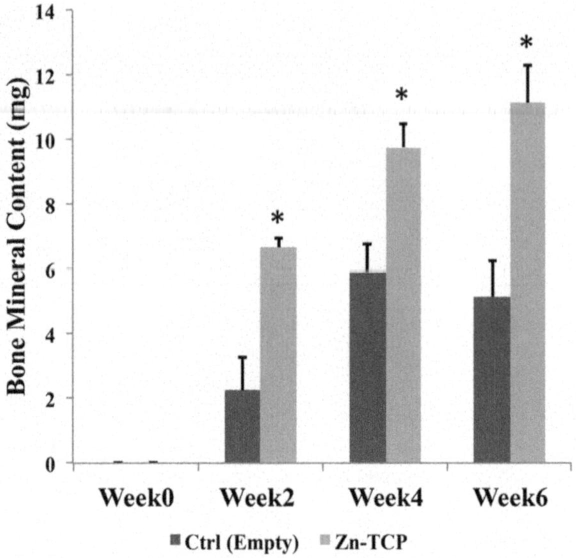

Fig. 14.11 Examination of the bone mineral content of Zn-TCP compared with empty control and β-TCP shows significant bone mineral formation starting at 2 weeks and continuing until 8 weeks where β-TCP had same bone mineral level as Zn-TCP. Asterisk sign represent $p < 0.05$, which was considered statistically significant

was not able to sustain a continual bone growth after 4 weeks, and though the defect may heal after an extended of period of time, the results indicate that the presence of a graft material offers a more improved form of treatment. This study provides a background of what can be achieved using biomimetically modified Zn-TCP. Further studies are required to investigate the material's regenerative abilities with commercially available calcium phosphate bone graft materials before conclusions can be drawn on the clinically applicability of Zn-TCP.

14.4 Conclusion and Future Developments

The development and application of using marine exoskeletons as a precursor material to produce calcium phosphate carriers for drugs has shown to be potentially advantageous. The oceans are still filled with a vast diversity of prospective and innovative structures that are awaiting scientists to explore for tissue engineering applications and learn from their natural synthesis and growth methods. Biomimetics and the hydrothermal conversion method allow us to utilise a wide range of marine-based materials that possess unique structures suitable as carriers for drugs among other biomedical applications. In today's competitive economic climate, the development of drug delivery systems is presented with increased challenges. However, it is not difficult to imagine the use of marine structures as therapeutic materials with synthetic modification in the treatment of current and future bone-related ailments.

References

1. Bose S, Tarafder S (2012) Calcium phosphate ceramic systems in growth factor and drug delivery for bone tissue engineering: a review. Acta Biomater 8(4):1401–1421. doi:10.1016/j.actbio.2011.11.017
2. Fuhrman J, McCallum K, Davis A (1995) Phylogenetic diversity of subsurface marine microbial communities from the Atlantic and Pacific oceans. Appl Environ Microbiol 61(12):4517
3. Rossbach M, Kniewald G (1997) Concepts of marine specimen banking. Chemosphere 34(9–10):1997–2010
4. Leupold J, Barfield W, An Y, Hartsock L (2006) A comparison of ProOsteon, DBX, and collagraft in a rabbit model. J Biomed Mater Res B Appl Biomater 79(2):292–297. doi:10.1002/jbm.b.30541
5. Luesch H, Harrigan G, Goetz G, Horgen F (2002) The cyanobacterial origin of potent anticancer agents originally isolated from sea hares. Curr Med Chem 9(20):1791–1806
6. Pettit G, Xu J, Hogan F, Williams M, Doubek D, Schmidt J et al (1997) Isolation and structure of the human cancer cell growth inhibitory cyclodepsipeptide dolastatin 16. J Nat Prod 60(8):752–754. doi:10.1021/np9700230
7. Simmons T, Coates R, Clark B, Engene N, Gonzalez D, Esquenazi E et al (2008) Biosynthetic origin of natural products isolated from marine microorganism-invertebrate assemblages. Proc Natl Acad Sci U S A 105(12):4587–4594. doi:10.1073/pnas.0709851105
8. Simmons T, Andrianasolo E, McPhail K, Flatt P, Gerwick W (2005) Marine natural products as anticancer drugs. Mol Cancer Ther 4(2):333–342
9. Sithranga Boopathy N, Kathiresan K (2010) Anticancer drugs from marine flora: an overview. J Oncol 2010. doi:10.1155/2010/214186
10. Stanley G (2003) The evolution of modern corals and their early history. Earth Sci Rev 60(3–4):195–225
11. Sethmann I, Worheide G (2008) Structure and composition of calcareous sponge spicules: a review and comparison to structurally related biominerals. Micron 39(3):209–228
12. Wilt F, Kilian C, Livingston B (2003) Development of calcareous skeletal elements in invertebrates. Differentiation 71(4–5):237–250
13. Laine J, Labady M, Albornoz A, Yunes S (2008) Porosities and pore sizes in coralline calcium carbonate. Mater Charact 59(10):1522–1525
14. Chou J, Valenzuela S, Bishop D, Ben-Nissan B, Milthorpe B (2012) Strontium- and magnesium-enriched biomimetic beta-TCP macrospheres with potential for bone tissue morphogenesis. J Tissue Eng Regen Med. doi:10.1002/term.1576/
15. Demers C, Hamdy C, Corsi K, Chellat F, Tabrizian M, Yahia L (2002) Natural coral exoskeleton as a bone graft substitute: a review. Biomed Mater Eng 12:15–35
16. Baudet-Pommel M, Collangettes-Peyrat D, Couvet-Lejczyk V (1988) Autotransplantation: clinical results, radiography, orthodontics, criteria for success. Actual Odontostomatol 163:463–472 (Paris: In French)
17. Patat J, Guillemin G (1989) Natural coral used as a replacement biomaterial in bone grafts. Ann Chir Plast Esthet 34(3):221–225 (French)
18. Bonnelye E, Chabadel A, Saltel F, Jurdic P (2008) Dual effect of strontium ranelate: stimulation of osteoblast differentiation and inhibition of osteoclast formation and resorption in vitro. Bone 42(1):129–138. doi:10.1016/j.bone.2007.08.043
19. LeGeros R (1981) Apatites in biological systems. Prog Cryst Growth Character Mater 41(1–2):1–45
20. Papacharalambous S, Anastasoff K (1993) Natural coral skeleton used as onlay graft for contour augmentation of the face-A preliminary report. Int J Oral Maxillofac Surg 22(5):260–264
21. Ben-Nissan B (2003) Natural bioceramic: from coral to bone and beyond. Curr Opin Solid State Mater Sci 7(4–5):283–288
22. Chou J, Ben-Nissan B, Choi A, Wuhrer R, Green D (2007) Conversion of coral sand to calcium phosphate for biomedical application. J Aust Ceram Soc 43(1):44–48

23. Ben-Nissan B, Milev A, Vago R (2004) Morphology of sol-gel derived nano-coated coralline hydroxyapatite. Biomaterials 25(20):4971–4975
24. Roy D, Linnehan S (1974) Hydroxyapatite formed from coral skeletal carbonate by hydrothermal exchange. Nature 247(438):220–222
25. Damron T, Lisle J, Craig T, Wade M, Silbert W, Cohen H (2013) Ultraporous beta-tricalcium phosphate alone or combined with bone marrow aspirate for benign cavitary lesions: comparison in a prospective randomized clinical trial. J Bone Joint Surg Am 95(2):158–166. doi:10.2106/JBJS.K.00181
26. Guyton G, Miller S (2010) Stem cells in bone grafting: trinity allograft with stem cells and collagen/beta-tricalcium phosphate with concentrated bone marrow aspirate. Foot Ankle Clin 15(4):611–619. doi:10.1016/j.fcl.2010.09.003
27. Barber F, Dockery W (2008) Long-term absorption of beta-tricalcium phosphate poly-L-lactic acid interference screws. Arthroscopy 24(4):441–447. doi:10.1016/j.arthro.2007.10.004
28. Somanathan R, Simunek A (2006) Evaluation of the success of beta-tricalcium phosphate and deproteinized bovine bone in maxillary sinus augmentation using histomorphometry: a review. Acta Medica 49(2):87–89
29. Florczyk S, Leung M, Jana S, Li Z, Bhattarai N, Huang J et al (2012) Enhanced bone tissue formation by alginate gel-assisted cell seeding in porous ceramic scaffolds and sustained release of growth factor. J Biomed Mater Res A 100(12):3408–3415. doi:10.1002/jbm.a.34288
30. Zhou J, Fang T, Wang Y, Dong J (2012) The controlled release of vancomycin in gelatin/beta-TCP composite scaffolds. J Biomed Mater Res A 100(9):2295–2301. doi:10.1002/jbm.a.34170
31. La W, Kwon S, Lee T, Yang H, Park J, Kim B (2012) The effect of the delivery carrier on the quality of bone formed via bone morphogenetic protein-2. Artif Organs 36(7):642–647. doi:10.1111/j.1525-1594.2011.01420.x
32. Suarez-Gonzalez D, Lee J, Lan Levengood S, Vanderby RJ, Murphy W (2012) Mineral coatings modulate beta-TCP stability and enable growth factor binding and release. Acta Biomater 8(3):1117–1124. doi:10.1016/j.actbio.2011.11.028
33. Paschalis E, Wikiel K, Nancollas G (1994) Dual constant composition kinetics characterization of apatitic surfaces. J Biomed Mater Res 28(12):1411–1418. doi:10.1002/jbm.820281205
34. Tang R, Hass M, Wu W, Gulde S, Nancollas G (2003) Constant composition dissolution of mixed phases. II. Selective dissolution of calcium phosphates. J Colloid Interface Sci 260(2):379–384
35. LeGeros R, Lin S, Rohanizadeh R, Mijares D, LeGeros J (2003) Biphasic calcium phosphate bioceramics: preparation, properties and applications. J Mater Sci Mater Med 14(3):201–209
36. Chou J, Ito T, Bishop D, Otsuka M, Ben-Nissan B, Milthorpe B (2013) Controlled release of simvastatin from biomimetic beta-TCP drug delivery system. PLoS One 8(1):e54676. doi:10.1371/journal.pone.0054676
37. Chou J, Ito T, Otsuka M, Ben-Nissan B, Milthorpe B (2013) The effectiveness of the controlled release of simvastatin from β-TCP macrosphere in the treatment of OVX mice. J Tissue Eng Regen Med. doi:10.1002/term.1784
38. Chou J, Ito T, Otsuka M, Ben-Nissan B, Milthorpe B (2012) Simvastatin loaded β-TCP drug delivery system induces bone formation and prevents rhabdomyolysis in OVX mice. Adv Healthc Mater. doi:10.1002/adhm.201200342
39. Chou J, Ben-Nissan B, Green D, Valenzuela S, Kohan L (2010) Targeting and dissolution characteristics of bone forming and antibacterial drugs by harnessing the structure of microspherical shells from coral beach sand. Adv Eng Mater 13(1–2):93–99
40. Kawamura H, Ito A, Miyakawa S, Layrolle P, Ojima K, Ichinose N et al (2000) Stimulatory effect of zinc-releasing calcium phosphate implant on bone formation in rabbit femora. J Biomed Mater Res 50(2):184–190
41. Relea P, Revilla M, Ripoll E, Arribas I, Villa LF, Rico H (1995) Zinc, biochemical markers of nutrition, and type I osteoporosis. Age Ageing 24(4):303–307
42. Yamaguchi M, Oishi H, Suketa Y (1987) Stimulatory effect of zinc on bone formation in tissue culture. Biochem Pharmacol 36(22):4007–4012

43. Moonga B, Dempster D (1995) Zinc is a potent inhibitor of osteoclastic bone resorption in vitro. J Bone Miner Res 10(3):453–457. doi:10.1002/jbmr.5650100317
44. Hernandez-Sierra J, Ruiz F, Pena D, Martinez-Gutierrez F, Martinez A, Guillen Ade J et al (2008) The antimicrobial sensitivity of Streptococcus mutans to nanoparticles of silver, zinc oxide, and gold. Nanomedicine 4(3):237–240. doi:10.1016/j.nano.2008.04.005
45. Chou J, Hao J, Hatoyama H, Ben-Nissan B, Milthorpe B, Otsuka M (2013) The therapeutic effect on bone mineral formation from biomimetic zinc containing tricalcium phosphate (ZnTCP) in zinc-deficient osteoporotic mice. PLoS One. doi:10.1371/journal.pone.0071821
46. Chou J, Hao J, Kuroda S, Ben-Nissan B, Milthorpe B, Otsuka M (2013) Bone regeneration of rat tibial defect by zinc-tricalcium phosphate (Zn-TCP) from porous Foraminifera carbonate macrospheres. Mar Drugs 11(12):5148–5158

Chapter 15
History of Calcium Phosphates in Regenerative Medicine

Sergey Dorozhkin

Abstract The historical development of a scientific knowledge on calcium orthophosphates from the 1770s until 1950 is described. The chosen time scale starts with the earliest available studies of the 1770s (to the best of my findings, calcium orthophosphates had been unknown before), passes through the entire nineteenth century, and finishes in 1950, because since then the amount of publications on calcium orthophosphates rapidly increased and the subject became too broad. In addition, since publications of the second half of the twentieth century are easily accessible, the substantial amount of them has been already reviewed by other scientists. Many forgotten and poorly known historical facts and approaches have been extracted from the old publications. Then they have been analyzed, systematized, and reconsidered from the modern point of view. The reported historical findings clearly demonstrate that many famous scientists of the past contributed to calcium orthophosphate investigations. Furthermore, the significant quantity of the scientific facts and experimental approaches appears to have been known for very many decades, and, in fact, a good deal of the relatively recent investigations on the subject is just either a further development of the earlier studies or a rediscovery of the already forgotten knowledge.

Keywords Apatite • Calcium orthophosphate • Lime phosphate • Calcium phosphate • Calcareous phosphate

S. Dorozhkin (✉)
Kudrinskaja sq. 1-155, Moscow 123242, Russia
e-mail: sedorozhkin@yandex.ru

B. Ben-Nissan (ed.), *Advances in Calcium Phosphate Biomaterials*, Springer Series in Biomaterials Science and Engineering 2, DOI 10.1007/978-3-642-53980-0_15,

15.1 Introduction

By virtue of abundance in the nature and presence in the living organisms, calcium orthophosphates (Table 15.1) appear to be the chemical compounds of a special interest in many fields of science, including geology, chemistry, biology, and medicine [1, 2]. As seen from Table 15.1, calcium orthophosphates with the Ca/P ratio within 1.5–1.67 are called apatites (hydroxyapatite, fluorapatite, and oxyapatite). As a mineral species, apatite was first recognized in 1786 by "the father of German geology" Abraham Gottlob Werner (1750–1817) and named by him from the ancient Greek απατάω (apatao) – "to mislead" or "to deceive" – because it had previously been mistaken for other minerals, such as beryl, tourmaline, chrysolite, amethyst, fluorite, etc. Currently, apatite is the name for a group of minerals with the same crystallographic structure and does not indicate one chemical composition. However, in this review, the term "apatite" is referred to calcium orthophosphates only and means CDHA, HA, FA, and OA (Table 15.1).

As follows from the designation, all calcium orthophosphates contain both calcium (Ca, atomic number 20) and phosphorus (P, atomic number 15) as the major constituencies. The history of both chemical elements is long. Namely, according to Wikipedia, the free encyclopedia, calcium (from Latin *calx*, genitive *calcis*, meaning "lime") compounds were known as early as the first century, when the ancient Romans prepared lime as calcium oxide [3]. However, calcium sulfate (also known as plaster of Paris or lime plaster) had been known much earlier: three statues were discovered in a buried pit at'Ain Ghazal in Jordan; those were sculpted with lime plaster over armatures of reeds and twine. They were made in the pre-pottery Neolithic period, around 7200 BC. However, calcium in a pure state was not isolated until 1808, when the famous British chemist and inventor Sir Humphry Davy (1778–1829) electrolyzed a mixture of lime and mercuric oxide [4, 5].

Phosphorus is a bit younger. The discovery of this element in a pure state (its name given from Greek mythology, Φωσφόρος meaning "light bearer" (Latin: Lucifer), referring to the "Morning Star," the planet Venus) is credited to the German merchant and alchemist Hennig Brand (ca. 1630–ca. 1710) in 1669, although other alchemists might have discovered phosphorus around the same time. Brand experimented with urine, which contained considerable quantities of dissolved phosphates from the normal metabolism [6]. As the matter stands, the earliest research publication containing the word "phosphorus" in the title belongs to M. Krafft from Holland and was printed in 1677 in French *Journal des Sçavans* [7], which was the earliest academic journal published in Europe. In 1680, the famous British natural philosopher, chemist, physicist, and inventor Robert Boyle (1627–1691) also deposited a paper on phosphorus, but it was published only in 1693, shortly after his death [8]. However, it was the famous French chemist Antoine Laurent Lavoisier (1743–1794) who recognized phosphorus as a chemical element in 1777. It turns out that phosphorus was the first element discovered since antiquity [6].

Table 15.1 Existing calcium orthophosphates and their major properties

Ca/P molar ratio	Compounds and their typical abbreviations	Chemical formula	Solubility at 25 °C, −log(K$_s$)	Solubility at 25 °C, g/L	pH stability range in aqueous solutions at
0.5	Monocalcium phosphate monohydrate (MCPM)	$Ca(H_2PO_4)2{\cdot}H_2O$	1.14	~18	0.0–2.0
0.5	Monocalcium phosphate anhydrous (MCPA or MCP)	$Ca(H_2PO_4)_2$	1.14	~17	[c]
1.0	Dicalcium phosphate dihydrate (DCPD), mineral brushite	$CaHPO_4{\cdot}2H_2O$	6.59	~0.088	2.0–6.0
1.0	Dicalcium phosphate anhydrous (DCPA or DCP), mineral monetite	$CaHPO_4$	6.90	~0.048	[c]
1.33	Octacalcium phosphate (OCP)	$Ca_8(HPO_4)_2(PO_4)_4{\cdot}5H_2O$	96.6	~0.0081	5.5–7.0
1.5	α-Tricalcium phosphate (α-TCP)	α-$Ca_3(PO_4)_2$	25.5	~0.0025	[a]
1.5	β-Tricalcium phosphate (β-TCP)	β-$Ca_3(PO_4)_2$	28.9	~0.0005	[a]
1.2–2.2	Amorphous calcium phosphates (ACP)	$Ca_xH_y(PO_4)_z{\cdot}nH_2O$, $n = 3$–4.5; 15–20 %	[b]	[b]	~5–12[d]
1.5–1.67	Calcium-deficient hydroxyapatite (CDHA or Ca-def HA)[e]	$Ca_{10-x}(HPO_4)_x(PO_4)_{6-x}(OH)_{2-x}$ $(0<x<1)$	~85	~0.0094	6.5–9.5
1.67	Hydroxyapatite (HA, Hap or OHAp)	$Ca_{10}(PO_4)_6(OH)_2$	116.8	~0.0003	9.5–12
1.67	Fluorapatite (FA or FAp)	$Ca_{10}(PO_4)_6F_2$	120.0	~0.0002	7–12
1.67	Oxyapatite (OA, OAp or OXA)[f]	$Ca_{10}(PO_4)_6O$	~69	~0.087	[a]
2.0	Tetracalcium phosphate (TTCP or TetCP), mineral hilgenstockite	$Ca_4(PO_4)_2O$	38–44	~0.0007	[a]

Reprinted with permission from Refs. [1, 2]

[a]These compounds cannot be precipitated from aqueous solutions

[b]Cannot be measured precisely. However, the following values were found: 25.7 ± 0.1 (pH = 7.40), 29.9 ± 0.1 (pH = 6.00), and 32.7 ± 0.1 (pH = 5.28). The comparative extent of dissolution in acidic buffer is ACP ≫ α-TCP ≫ β-TCP > CDHA ≫ HA > FA

[c]Stable at temperatures above 100 °C

[d]Always metastable

[e]Occasionally, it is called "precipitated HA (PHA)"

[f]Existence of OA remains questionable

15.2 General Definitions, Major Problems, and Limitations

To begin with, one must define the subject and outline the problems. According to Wikipedia: "History (from Greek ἱστορία – historia, meaning "inquiry, knowledge acquired by investigation") is the discovery, collection, organization, and presentation of information about past events. It is a field of research which uses a narrative to examine and analyse the sequence of events, and it sometimes attempts to investigate objectively the patterns of cause and effect that determine events. The task of historical discourse is to identify the sources which can most usefully contribute to the production of accurate accounts of past" [9].

Unfortunately, the requirement "to identify the sources" meets serious problems, due to the substantial difficulties with accessing to the scientific literature published in the first half of the nineteenth century and before. In addition, that time, both the scientific concepts and the presentation ways were rather different from the modern ones, while the chemical formulae had not been introduced yet. More to the point, scientific journals were rare and just a few of them are currently available in the electronic form. To complicate things further, numerous old journals have been discontinued, merged, and/or renamed, which strongly complicates accessing to the papers published in those journals. Luckily, Google Inc. has scanned a great number of old books as a part of its project to make the world's books discoverable online. This timely project by Google combined with the power of the modern electronic databases of scientific publications allows reconstructing the major historical milestones on calcium orthophosphates, which was often impossible for earlier review writers. For example, a paper of 1994 by Driskell entitled "Early history of calcium phosphate materials and coatings" [10] started with the classical publication of 1920 by Albee assisted by Morrison [11]. In 1999, Shackelford published a paper, "Bioceramics – an historical perspective" [12], in which the same publication by Albee assisted by Morrison [11] was mentioned as the earliest reference. The same is valid for the historical papers by Hulbert et al. [13, 14] and Shepperd [15]. Thus, it might create a false impression that calcium phosphates were unknown before 1920. Certainly, this is not the case; nevertheless, the precise sequence of the scientific events that happened in the first half of the nineteenth century still remains poorly restorable, while the correct historical time scale of even earlier scientific events remains almost irrecoverable. This is mainly due to a lack of the citation practice existing in the scientific literature published at that time. Besides, even nowadays, for the entire eighteenth century and approximately the first quarter of the nineteenth century, only scientific books digitalized by Google are easily accessible. Just a few journal papers devoted to the subject published before ~1820s have been found. Nevertheless, in no case this means that they do not exist; presumably, either they have not been scanned yet (especially, this might be valid for the discontinued journals) or an access to the scanned versions is restricted to a limited amount of subscribers only. Therefore, the historical narrative of the findings and discoveries of the eighteenth century is based dominantly on the available books, and the annals of the nineteenth century are based on both the available books and a limited number of journal papers, while the chronicle of the twentieth century is based on the journal publications only. Here one should also stress that starting from the second half of the nineteenth century, the detailed description of every publication on the subject becomes impossible due to permanently increasing amount of them. Furthermore, since the end of the 1910s, even mentioning all and sundry publications on the subject becomes impossible either (the quantity with moderate novelty breeds ignoring). Therefore, for the twentieth century, the milestone studies have been included only.

15.3 Investigations and Knowledge at the "Pre-calcium Orthophosphate" Time

Prior examination of issues let me briefly report on the earliest scientific publications on bones, teeth, and other types of calcified tissues of mammals, which are the main sources of calcium orthophosphates of the biological origin. Since in those early days the major scientific language was Latin, I am forced to confine myself by the English-language publications only.

According to the second earliest but the world's longest-running scientific journal *Philosophical Transactions* (published in UK), the priority in journal publications on investigations of bones and teeth belongs to the famous Dutch tradesman and scientist Antonie Philips van Leeuwenhoek (1632–1723) from Delft. He is best known for his work on the improvement of a microscope and is often considered as "the father of microbiology." Therefore, within 1674–1695, van Leeuwenhoek published several letters devoted to microscopic investigations of bones and teeth [16–20]. Namely, he wrote (please note the old-fashioned using a long, medial, or descending letter "ſ," which is a form of the minuscule letter "s" formerly used where "s" occurred in the middle or at the beginning of a word) [16]: "I thought likewiſe, I ſaw then alſo, that that Bone conſiſted of united Globuls. Afterwards, I viewed the Shinbone of a *Calf*, in which I found ſeveral little holes, paſſing from without inwards; and I then imagined, that this Bone had divers ſmall pipes going longways" (p. 125). Today these small pipes are known as Haversian canals, named after the British physician Clopton Havers (1657–1702), who did the pioneering research on the microstructure of bones and teeth [21]. Let me continue citing [16]: "But I have ſince obſerved the *Tooth* of a Cow and I found it made up of tranſparent Globuls which I can ſee very perfectly. The ſame I have obſerved in *Ivory* or *Elephants-Teeth*. And having ſeen this ſeveral times, I doubt no longer but that all white Bones do conſiſt of tranſparent Globuls" (p. 125). Obviously, this was the first recognition of the fact that bones and teeth of mammals consist of small units (currently we call them crystals) with a transparent nature. Indeed, single crystals of all known calcium orthophosphates (Table 15.1) are transparent.

Simultaneously, other researchers tried to measure the physical properties and establish the chemical composition of various calcified tissues (both normal and pathological) of humans. For example, let me cite a summary of the experiments performed by the British physician and chemist Frederick Slare (1648–1727) from a publication of 1684 [22]: "Several *Stones* of the *Bladder* and *Kidnies* were diſtill'd, all afforded *volatile urinous Salts*; which *Ferment* upon any *Acids. Bones* were diſtill'd and found to be of agreeable *Principles. Calculi* examined *Hydroſtatically*, were found in proportion to their Bulk of water as 5 to 4. We weigh'd *Bones Hydroſtatically* and found them twice as heavy as their Bulk of water. *Bones* not eaſily wrought on by common *Acids*, only by nitrous ones and that without *Ebullition*." (p. 532). Therefore, scientists dissolved biologically formed calcium orthophosphates in acids as far back as 1684.

Shortly before a discovery of the calcium orthophosphate nature of bones (the next section), Hérissant (presumably, it is referred to either Jean Thomas Hérissant or his son Louis Antoine Prosper Hérissant) and the Swiss anatomist, physiologist, naturalist, and poet Albrecht von Haller (1708–1777) examined a phenomenon that even the weakest acids had the power of softening bones. Namely, according to Fourcroy [23], that study was reported in 1758 and Hérissant "thought he had found in the nitric acid (with which he ſoftened the bones which he ſoaked in it, by diſſolving their earth, which he believed to be cretaceous, without affecting their membraneous cellular part) a means of inſulating the two conſtituent matters of theſe organs. Haller has verified this ſoftening of the bones even by the acetous acid and lemon juice; he ſuſpected that in the ſoftening of the bones by the effect of diſeaſes, there exiſted an acid which thus corroded them. All the chemiſts have afterwards obſerved that a ſolution of bones in an acid precipitated by alkali affords a ſeemingly earthy matter, which does not poſſeſs the property of becoming quick-lime by calcination." (p. 388).

To conclude this part, one can see that the aforementioned few examples clearly demonstrate a scientific importance of the "pre-calcium orthophosphate" epoch, which, ideally, should be investigated in more details. Undoubtedly, one must appreciate the important observations and discoveries made by those early researchers-predecessors.

15.4 Investigations and Knowledge on Calcium Orthophosphates

15.4.1 In the Eighteenth Century

According to the available literature, the history of calcium orthophosphates began in 1769 and was associated with names of the famous Swedish chemist and metallurgist Johan Gottlieb Gahn (1745–1818) and the famous German-Swedish pharmaceutical chemist Carl Wilhelm Scheele (1742–1786). Namely, in 1881, Roscoe and Schorlemmer [24] published the following statement: "Gahn, in 1769, discovered the existence of calcium phosphate in bones, but it was not until this fact was published by Scheele in 1771 that phosphorus was obtained from bone-ash, which has from that time invariably served for its preparation" (p. 458). Furthermore, let me cite a publication of 1777 [25] (again, pay attention to the old-fashioned using a letter "ſ" instead of "s"): "I have only been informed of this diſcovery, by the *Gazette, Salutaire de Bouillon*, October, 1775. It is there ſaid, that Mr. *Henry Gahn*, a phyſician at Stockholm, has communicated a proceſs for extracting from bones the ſaline matter in question; and that Mr. *Scheele* had aſcertained, that the earth of animals was compoſed of a calcareous ſubſtance united with the phoſphoric acid. This diſcovery, continues the author of the article of the Gazette, belongs to Mr. *Gahn*, and has been confirmed by later experiments." (p. 383). Presumably, this citation might be considered as one of the earliest mentioning on calcium phosphates in the history.

The earliest accessible description on how Scheele discovered the chemical composition of bones was given by Fourcroy in 1804 [23]: "After having, like Heriſſant, diſſolved bones in the nitric acid, he filtrated the liquor, and aſcertained that, though always acid, even when ſaturated with all that it could diſſolve of bone, it precipitated ſulphate of lime by the addition of concentrated ſulphuric acid; and that after this precipitation, the ſolution drawn off clear, and evaporated in a retort, afforded volatilized nitric acid, and left phoſphoric acid, which was fuſed into glaſs by the action of a ſufficient heat. He concluded from this experiment that the nitric acid diſſolved the phoſphate of lime, the baſe of the bones; that the ſolution in this acid was a mixture of calcareous nitrate and of phoſphoric acid; that when the firſt was decompoſed by the ſulphuric acid, and the precipitated ſulphate of lime ſeparated from it, there remained only a mixture of the two acids, the phoſphoric and the nitric, and that this latter mixture, when heated, diſengaged volatile nitric acid, whilſt the fixed phoſphoric acid remained at the bottom of the retort." (pp. 388–389). Even more than 200 years afterward, we can add nothing to improve this description. This is an example of how the genius could do!

Simultaneously, the presence of orthophosphates was discovered in blood serum, which follows from a publication of 1770 [26]: "The ſerum conſiſts chemically of a coagulable matter, and water in which common ſal ammoniac and phoſphoric ammoniac, and generally common ſalt, and frequently ſelenites, and, fixed ammoniac, are diſſolved" (p. 309). Obviously, "phoſphoric ammoniac" means ammonium orthophosphate.

Further, according to Shepperd [15], the famous German chemist Martin Heinrich Klaproth (1743–1817) and the famous French chemist Joseph-Louis Proust (1754–1826) also contributed to calcium orthophosphates. Unfortunately, Shepperd has not provided any references to the publications by those great chemists. Nevertheless, a search performed among the Google books has given some results. For example, a short extract from a letter by M. Klaproth was published in 1788 [27], which started with the following words: "Monsieur, Je viens d'analyſer l'apatit de M. Verner (I). J'en ai retiré de la terre calcaire & de l'acide phoſphorique" (p. 313). In addition, in a French book of 1790 [28], one can find a subchapter entitled "Apatite. Phosphate de Chaux" which is started from the following sentence: "C'est Mr. Klaproth, qui à découvert le premier cette combinaison de la terre calcaire avec l'acide phosphorique" (p. 363). Further, "Mr. Proust *dans une Lettre à Mr. d'Arcet* a donné l'Analyse de cette pierre, qui est une combinaison de la terre calcaire avec l'acide phosphorique" (p. 366). Thus, by that time, apatite was already recognized as a calcium phosphate, which is also confirmed by a German book of 1789 [29], in which "Apatit" was called "die Phosphorsaure mit Kalkerde" (p. 2).

More to the point, according to a study, submitted on December 20, 1785 [30], the production process of orthophosphoric acid by decomposition of calcined bones in sulfuric acid was already known. This is how it was described by Lavoisier in 1790 [31]: "The bones of adult animals being calcined to whiteneſs, are pounded, and paſſed through a fine ſilk ſiewe; pour upon the fine powder a quantity of dilute ſulphuric acid, leſs than is ſufficient for diſſolving the whole. This acid unites with the calcareous earth of the bones into a ſulphat of lime, and the phoſphoric acid remains free in the liquor." (p. 205). Further, the production process of white phosphorus has been described [31]: "The liquid is decanted off, and the reſiduum waſhed with boiling water; this water which has been uſed to waſh out the adhering acid is joined with what was before decanted off, and the whole is gradually evaporated; the diſſolved ſulphat of lime criſtallizes in form of ſilky threads, which are removed, and by continuing the evaporation we procure the phoſphoric acid under the appearance of a white pellucid glaſs. When this is powdered, and mixed with one third its weight of charcoal, we procure very pure phoſphorus by ſublimation." (p. 206).

In the last decade of the eighteenth century, very extensive investigations on calcium orthophosphates were performed by two famous French chemists Antoine François, comte de Fourcroy (1755–1809) and Nicolas Louis Vauquelin (1763–1829), who, among other accomplishments, discovered an existence of acidic calcium orthophosphates, currently known as MCPM, MCPA, DCPD, and DCPA (Table 15.1). For example, let me cite a Fourcroy's book of 1789 [32]: "Phoſphoric acid, poured into lime-water, precipitates from it a ſcarce ſoluble ſalt, which does not efferveſce with acids, – is decompoſed by mineral acids, but proof againſt the attacks of cauſtic alkalis. This ſalt is of the ſame nature with the baſe of bones. An exceſs of phoſphoric acid renders calcareous phoſphate ſoluble in water; but magneſia, lime, cauſtic fixed alkalis, and even ammoniac, by carrying off from it the exceſs of acid, precipitate the neutral ſalt. Calcareous phoſphate is not decompoſable by caustic alkalis, but carbonates of potaſh and ſoda decompoſe it. The ſolid matter of bones conſiſts of phoſphate ſuperſaturated with lime." (p. 248). Here we read the correct chemical description of CDHA precipitation from H_3PO_4 and $Ca(OH)_2$, followed by CDHA transformation into soluble MCPM in the presence of an excess of H_3PO_4, which is again transformed into insoluble CDHA by addition of basic compounds MgO, CaO, KOH, NaOH, and NH_4OH. Moreover, the last sentence means that the amount of CaO in bones exceeds the stoichiometry of orthophosphates; therefore, that was the earliest indirect observation of the apatitic ($Ca/P > 1.5$) composition of bones.

Furthermore, in his later book of 1804 [33], Fourcroy wrote: "A FEW years ago this ſalt, which I here denominate the acid phoſphate of lime, was unknown. Scheele very properly remarked that the ſaline earth of bones was diſſolved by an acid in human urine, but he did not obſerve that this union between phoſphoric acid and the bony phofphate, makes a kind of permanent and particular falt different from the latter. It was in the year 1795, the third year of the Republic, that I difcovered it, with Citizen Vauquelin, in a connected feries of experiments upon bony matters; wherein we proved that the calcareous phofphate which conftitutes the folid bafe, is only in part decompofable by acids, and that the portion of phofphoric acid which is feparated, retains in folution phofphate of lime, which it then defends from all fubfequent alteration by other acids." (p. 347). The aforementioned is confirmed by an encyclopedia published in 1816 [34]: "*Super*-Phosphat of Lime was difcovered in 1795, by Fourcroy and Vauquelin. It had indeed been often formed before, but chemifts had neglected to examine it" (p. 458). Thus, the term "superphosphate" has been known since, at least, 1795, and initially it meant calcium phosphates containing an excess (or super quantity) of phosphoric acid. Besides, in the same publication, Fourcroy mentioned other contributors to early studies on calcium orthophosphates [33]: "Citizens Nicholas of Nancy, Pelletrier, Berniard, Bullion, in France; Weftrumb, and feveral chemifts in Germany; Bonviofin, at Turin; Tenant, Pearfon, and fome others in England, multiplied their inquiries and experiments" (p. 337). Thus, one can notice that in the end of the eighteenth century, the subject of calcium orthophosphates was extensively investigated by a number of researchers in several countries of Western Europe.

Finally, it is important to cite a page from an agricultural chemistry book, published in 1795 [35]: "PHOSPHAT OF LIME Is contained in animal matters, such as bones, urine, shells, &c. &c. in some sorts of limestone, and in vegetable substances, particularly in the gluten, or vegeto-animal matter of wheat or other grain. It is a saline compound very insoluble. There is reason to believe, a very considerable proportion of this nearly insoluble salt is contained in most fertile soils, especially those that have been long under cultivation. It is not to be decomposed by pure alkalis; but this may be effected by mild vegetable and mineral alkalis, on the principle of the double electrive attractions; in which case, carbonate of lime (or chalk) will be precipitated, and phosphoric acid will join with the alkali, and form phosphat of potash, or phosphat of soda, according to the alkali applied. These alkaline phosphates will be found to promote vegetation in a very great degree: the substances of which they are composed, viz. alkaline salts and phosphoric acid, are found in the ashes of most vegetables." (p. 75)

To conclude the 1700s, one should recognize that the correct basic knowledge on calcium orthophosphates became available by the end of the eighteenth century.

15.4.2 In the Nineteenth Century

For the nineteenth century, both scientific books and a limited amount of journal publications are available; however, for the first half of the nineteenth century, the quantity of journal publications was very small. Nevertheless, according to the available literature, one can claim on a real explosion of the scientific knowledge on calcium orthophosphates in the nineteenth century. For example, in 1804, Fourcroy stated that the presence of water in acidic calcium orthophosphates was already known (again, pay attention to the old-fashioned using a letter "ſ" instead of "s") [33]: "The acid phoſphate of lime contains a remarkable quantity of water: the cryſtallization immediately ſoftens and becomes liquefied by the fire" (p. 349). The chemical compositions of both neutral and acidic calcium orthophosphates were described as follows [33]: "100 parts of phoſphate of lime contain, according to the analyſis of Citizens Fourcroy and Vauquelin,

Phoſphoric acid	41
Lime	59" (p. 346),

and "An accurate analyſis of this ſalt affords the following proportions of component parts,

Lime	45
Phoſphoric acid	54" (p. 351).

Unfortunately, it is impossible to establish the real meaning of all numerical values. Nevertheless, if we consider the first compound as the stoichiometric HA ($Ca/P = 1.67$), simple calculations using the proportion rules will give $Ca/P = 0.96$ for the acidic phosphate of lime, and if we consider the first compound as TCP ($Ca/P = 1.50$), similar calculations will give $Ca/P = 0.86$ for the acidic phosphate of lime. In both cases, the calculated Ca/P ratios appear to be close to those in DCPD and DCPA. Taking into consideration that the "acid phoſphate of lime contains a remarkable quantity of water," one can conclude that Fourcroy prepared DCPD by 1804. Finally, one more citation from Fourcroy's book is as follows [33]: "The phoſphate of lime is extremely difficult to fuse; neverthelefs, by ſtrong fire, ſuch as that of a glaſs-house, it ſoftens and acquires a ſemi-tranſparence like the grain of porcelain" (p. 341). Thus, calcium phosphate ceramics were prepared by 1804.

Knowledge on acidic calcium orthophosphates was further developed in 1805 [36], "*Acid Phosphate of Lime* is formed either by taking away a part of the base by sulphuric, nitric, or muriatic acid, or by superadding phosphoric acid to the last described phosphate" (p. 195), and in 1806 [37], "In this way were distinguished among the salts two combinations, one neutral, and one with an excess of acid; and these were supposed to be determinate, as in sulphate and super-sulphate of potassa, or the phosphate and super-phosphate of lime" (p. 38). In 1807, a detailed preparation technique of superphosphate of lime was described as follows [38]: "This ſuper-phosphat of lime is prepared with moſt accuracy by digesting phoſphat of lime in phoſphoric acid till it is ſaturated. This ſolution yields the ſalt by evaporation in the form of ſmall ſhining seales or filaments which have almost a gelatinous conſiſtence, and a very ſour taſte" (p. 222). Obviously, this was the earliest description of MCPM preparation; however, an admixture of MCPA was possible due to a partial dehydration at the evaporation stage.

More precise information on acidic calcium orthophosphates became available by 1819 [39]: "XI. *Biphosphate of Lime*. This salt may be formed by digesting phosphate of lime in phosphoric acid, dissolved in hot water" (p. 327). "XII. *Quadriphosphate of Lime. Glassy Phosphoric Acid* of the Apothecaries. This salt may be formed by digesting, for some time, finely powdered phosphate of lime in a quantity of sulphuric acid, sufficient to saturate all the lime of the phosphate, and afterwards diluting the mixture with a sufficient quantity of water, and filtering. Sulphate of lime remains on the filter, and a liquid quadriphosphate passes through." (pp. 327–328). Presumably, aqueous solutions of DCPD and MCPM, respectively, were prepared; therefore, one can claim that MCPM and DCPD were differentiated by 1819. Furthermore, "XIII. *Subphosphate of Lime*. This salt occurs native under the names of apatite or asparagus stone" (p. 328). Since the prefix "sub-" means "incomplete," one can claim that a shortage of orthophosphate ions in apatites (if compared with phosphate of lime) was confirmed.

Various preparation processes of a pure calcium orthophosphate currently known as CDHA were developed by 1807 [38]: "Phosphate of Lime may be obtained quite pure either by ſaturating the pure acid with marble and then evaporating; or by waſhing bone-aſh with hot water to diſſolve out any ſoluble ſalt which it may contain; then adding a little acetous or dilute muriatic acid till the effervefcence ceaſes to engage the carbonat of lime which it contains, and again thoroughly edulcorating. Phoſphat of lime is produced alſo by double decompoſition, on dropping a ſolution of any phoſphated alkali into any ſoluble calcareous ſolution that has not any great exceſs of acid. Vauquelin alſo found that on boiling phoſphat of ſoda with wet and newly precipitated carbonat of lime, the ſame reſult took place, and carbonate of ſoda with phoſphate of lime were produced." (p. 221). One can see that some of these processes are still used to produce chemically pure CDHA. In the fourth edition of *Encyclopædia Britannica* (1810), applications of calcium orthophosphates were described as follows [40]: "The phoſphate of lime is of great importance in chemiſtry, for the purpoſe of extracting phoſphoric acid, to be decompoſed to obtain phoſphorus. It is also employed for making cupels, for poliſhing metals and precious ſtones, and for removing ſpots of greaſy from linen, paper, and ſilk. It is uſed in medicine as a remedy for rickets, to correct the ſuppoſed effects of acids in ſoftening the bones." (p. 585). Although it is slightly beyond the subject, one should mention that calcium orthophosphite ($Ca_3(PO_3)_2$) with trivalent P was also mentioned in that edition of Encyclopædia Britannica, as "phoſphite of lime" (p. 586).

In 1819, the major properties of CDHA were described as follows [39]: "4. Phosphate of lime is a white insoluble powder, destitute of taste, and unaltered by exposure to air. It is soluble in hydrochloric (muriatic) and nitric acids, and may be precipitated from solution in them by means of ammonia. When exposed to a very violent heat, it undergoes a kind of fusion, and is converted into a white semi-transparent porcelain. 5. According to an analysis by Berzelius, calculated in numbers, in which the equivalent number for lime is assumed, phosphate of lime is composed of

Phosphoric acid	34·3
Lime	29·0

one atom; so that it appears that the composition of this salt cannot be reconciled with the atomic theory." (p. 327). Here, one can see the earliest mentioning of the terms "atom" and "atomic theory."

In 1823, W. Henry described the following compounds containing calcium and phosphorus [41]: *phosphuret of lime* obtained by passing phosphorus over red-hot lime (p. 565), which was, obviously, calcium phosphide (Ca_3P_2). It "has the remarkable property of decomposing water and the water afterwards contains phosphite, or hypophosphite, not phosphate of lime.* Drop a small piece of it into a wine-glass of water, and in a short time bubbles of phosphuretted hydrogen gas will be produced; which, rising to the surface, will take fire, and explode" (p. 566), followed by references to two publications written by the famous French chemist and physicist Joseph Louis Gay-Lussac (1778–1850), to whom this discovery was credited. Obviously, the "phosphuretted hydrogen gas" was a mixture of PH_3, P_2H_4, and more complicated PH compounds. Then, W. Henry described *phosphate of lime* [41], which "is constituted, according to Mr. Dalton's experiments, of 49 acid + 51 lime, proportions which authorize us to consider phosphate of lime as consisting of 1 atom of acid = 28, + 1 atom of base = 28, the compound atom being 56" (pp. 566–567). Here, the term "atom" was used again. In addition, this is an evidence that the famous English chemist, meteorologist, and physicist John Dalton (1766–1844), who is best known for his pioneering work in the development of modern atomic theory, as well as his research into color blindness (sometimes referred to as daltonism, in his honor), also contributed to calcium orthophosphates. Afterward, other calcium orthophosphates were mentioned as follows [41]: "*Bi-phosphate of lime* may be formed by digesting phosphate of lime with a quantity of phosphoric acid equivalent to that already engaged in the salt" (p. 567). Obviously, it was DCPD. "*Tri-phosphate of lime.* – This salt, according to Mr. Dalton, perhaps formed by adding pure phosphoric acid to lime water, until a commencement of precipitation appears, when a drop or two of acid must clear the solution. If the solution be evaporated to dryness at a moderate heat, and then dissolved in water again, simple phosphate of lime remains, and a quadri-phosphate exists in the solution." (p. 567). Unfortunately, this description does not allow to identify calcium orthophosphates. They might be DCPD (in solution) and DCPA (evaporated to dryness at a moderate heat) or OCP (in solution) and either ACP or CDHA (evaporated to dryness at a moderate heat): "*Quadri-phosphate of lime.* – If 100 parts of phosphate of lime be digested for 24 hours with 87 parts of sulphuric acid, diluted with a sufficient quantity of water, and be then filtered, the liquid which passes through contains the whole of the phosphoric acid, with only one-fourth of the lime which existed in the original salt ... The dissolved salt is therefore a compound of 1 atom of lime = 28 + 4 atoms of acid = 112. When evaporated it forms, on cooling, pearly scales, which have an acid taste, and dissolve readily in water, giving a solution of the sp. gr. 1,44." (p. 567). Obviously, this was MCPM with a possible admixture of MCPA formed after evaporation. Although the meaning of the statement "1 atom of lime = 28 + 4 atoms of acid = 112" remains unclear, one may guess that the numerical values 28 and 112 should be a kind of molar masses. Indeed, 28 is 50 % of the molar mass of CaO, i.e., this is a gram equivalent (synonym: an equivalent weight). According to Wikipedia, the equivalent weights were established by 1777 [42]; therefore, this suggestion sounds reasonable. Finally, W. Henry [41] mentioned "*Octo-phosphate of lime.* – Mr. Dalton is of opinion that a compound of 8 atoms of acid and 1 atom of lime is the true result of the process described under the last head; and that a compound of as many as 12 atoms of acid with one of lime may exist, forming a dodecaphosphate" (p. 567). Such superacidic calcium orthophosphates are currently unknown; moreover, they were excluded from the books published in 1828 [43] and 1829 [44]. Presumably, chemists quickly found a mistake. In addition, in the latter book, one can read the following [44]: "The *biphosphate of lime* may be prepared by adding one atom of phosphoric acid to one atom of the phosphate of lime" (p. 252). Here, the term "an atom" undoubtedly means either "a molecule" or "a mole," i.e., the correct chemical understanding of the stoichiometry of DCPD preparation from H_3PO_4 and TCP was achieved by 1829.

By 1827, the German mineralogist Gustav Rose (1798–1873) established the correct understanding of the chemical composition of apatites. To demonstrate this, let me cite a publication of 1859, coauthored by the famous French chemist Henri Étienne Sainte-Claire Deville (1818–1881) [45]: "The singular composition of apatite, first determined by M. Gustav Rose in 1827, shows that it is a definite compound of chloride and fluoride of calcium with phosphate of lime" (p. 128). In 1832, a chemical term "tribasic phosphate of lime" (p. 90), which fully corresponds to both α-TCP and β-TCP, was mentioned for the first time [46].

Coincidently, the famous German chemist Eilhard Mitscherlich (1794–1863), who was a learner and a friend of J.J. Berzelius and who today was best remembered for his law of isomorphism (1819), also worked in this area. To prove this, let me cite an introduction from a paper of 1833, written by the Scottish chemist Thomas Graham (1805–1869), clearly demonstrating the established knowledge on phosphates and arsenates by that time [47]: "No classes of salts have more liberally rewarded investigation than the arseniates and the phosphates. Witness the discovery of the extraordinary phosphates of lime by Berzelius; the observation of the identity of form of the corresponding arseniates and phosphates by Mitscherlich, and the doctrine of isomorphism to which that observation led; the discovery by the same chemist of two biphosphates of soda, agreeing in composition but differing in form; and lastly, the discovery of the pyrophosphates by my friend and townsman Mr. Clark. Much, however, still remains to be done to complete the history of these interesting salts." (p. 253). In addition, various modifications of phosphoric acid, currently known as orthophosphoric, pyrophosphoric, and metaphosphoric acids, were already known. On p. 281 of his paper, Graham called them as "a terphosphate, a biphosphate, and phosphate of water," respectively [47].

Concerning chemical formulae of calcium orthophosphates, the earliest ones were discovered in the aforementioned paper by Graham [47] as $\dot{\mathbf{C}}\mathbf{a}^{2}\overset{\cdot\cdot\cdot}{\ddot{\mathbf{P}}}$ and $\dot{\mathbf{C}}\mathbf{a}^{3}\overset{\cdot\cdot\cdot}{\ddot{\mathbf{P}}}$ (p. 265). Another type of the chemical formulae with struck out phosphorus was published in 1844 by Mitscherlich [48] as $2.Ca^2P$ and $5.Ca^2P$ (p. 69^{a}). Furthermore, a combination of both styles with dots above the element's symbols as in Ref. [47]

and striking out phosphorus as in Ref. [48] (additionally, chlorine was written as Cl and fluorine was written as F) was also used [49]. Even such a complicated way of writing with dots, striking out and mathematical fractions as

$$\left(3\dot{Ca}^3\overset{\vdots\vdots}{\not{P}}+\frac{Ca\,F^2}{Ca\,Cl^2}\right)$$

was used on page 399 of Ref. [50] to describe the chemical composition of apatite. One can see that initially neither hydrogen nor oxygen was included into the chemical formulae of calcium orthophosphates. Nevertheless, this topic kept developing. For example, the correct but just strange-looking chemical formula of apatite as $3Ca_3O_3,P_2O_5 + CaCl\ F$ might be found on page 29 of a book published in 1841 [51]. However, in another book of 1841 [52], the numerical subscripts were replaced by superscripts; therefore, the chemical formula for bone phosphate of lime was written as $8CaO + 3P^2O^5$, that for triphosphate of lime as $3CaO + P^2O^5$, that for diphosphate of lime as $2CaO + P^2O^5 + 1$ eq. basic water, and one for phosphate of lime as $CaO + P^2O^5 + 2$ eq. basic water (p. 304). Obviously, the term "basic water" means acidic orthophosphates; therefore, these formulae were the first correct ones for CDHA, TCP, DCPD/DCPA, and MCPM/MCPA, respectively (hydrate water was not mentioned yet). Similar way of writing was used in some later books, such as a publication of 1854 [53], in which the chemical formula of "calcis triphosphas. – triphosphate of lime." was written as $3CaO,PO^5$ (p. 625) and the chemical formulae of other calcium orthophosphates were written as $2CaO,PO^5$ (p. 626) and $8CaO,3PO^5$ (p. 627), as well as a publication of 1859 [45]: "Apatite has the composition $3(PO^5, 3CaO)\{^{Cl}{}_{F}\}Ca$" (p. 128). In the latter formula, anions were placed ahead of cations. In addition, in 1843 and 1845, John Percy published identical papers [54, 55] (the earliest example of redundant publications?), in which he described formation of "a new hydrated phosphate of lime" with a chemical formula $2CaO + PO_5 + 6HO$, with "1 equiv. water being basic and 5 constitutional." Obviously, the "basic water" means existence of HPO_4^-, which is typical for DCPD, OCP, and CDHA, while the "constitutional water" is the hydrate water. Since only OCP contains a combination of HPO_4^- with 5 molecules of hydrate water (Table 15.1), presumably, John Percy prepared OCP.

With a few exceptions [47, 54, 55], the aforementioned information on apatites and other calcium orthophosphates was taken from various books. In addition, a limited amount of journal publications of the first half of the nineteenth century is also available. Namely, research papers on the subject were published by the famous Swedish chemist Jöns Jacob Berzelius (1779–1848) [56, 57], as well as by G.O. Rees [58], M. Baruel [59], the English physician and chemist Henry Bence Jones (1813–1873) [60–62], J.D. Smith [63], and J.L. Lassaigne [64]. Among them, a paper of 1845 by Jones [60] should be noted. Namely, let me cite a figure caption: "Amorphous deposit in alkaline urine. Deposit on boiling phosphate of soda with chloride of calcium, or with sulphate of magnesia" (p. 349). This statement is astonishing because it might be considered as the earliest mentioning on ACP [65], 50 years before discovering X-rays in 1895 by the famous German scientist Wilhelm Conrad Röntgen (1845–1923)! Furthermore, Jones published the earliest-found pictures of precipitated crystals and some of them belonged to calcium orthophosphates (Fig. 15.1). Next early pictures of calcium orthophosphate precipitates from urine might be found in publications of 1859 [66] and 1860 [67].

In the end of the 1840s, the earliest-found solubility experiments of calcium orthophosphates were performed by Lassaigne [64]. Those experiments were carried out in water, saturated with carbon dioxide. The following data were obtained by 1847: "1. *Pure phosphate of lime*, obtained by the double decomposition of a calcareous salt and alkaline phosphate; the solubility was 0·000750. 2. *Fresh* bone, a piece of nearly two inches long, 46/100 dths of an inch wide, and 4/100 dths thick; solubility 0·000166. 3. Bone disinterred after about twenty years' repose in a cemetery, the subsoil of which was sandy; solubility 0·000300." [64]. One can see that the solubility value of pure phosphate of lime (presumably, it was either precipitated ACP or CDHA) was found to be higher than those of bones. In 1849, it was stated that "M.J.L. Lassaigne, at the meeting of the Academy of Sciences of Paris, of the 15th January, presented a memoir upon this subject, showing by experiments that the phosphate and carbonate of lime are introduced into plants in solution in water containing carbonic acid, which had before been shown as to the phosphate by M. Dumas, and has long been known as to the carbonate." [68]. Thus, a higher solubility of both calcium orthophosphates and calcium carbonate in very weak acids was a well-known fact. The solubility data were updated in a publication of 1855 [69]: "Apatite dissolves in 393,000 parts of water saturated with carbonic acid; Artificial neutral phosphate, freshly precipitated, in 1,503 parts; Artificial basic phosphate, freshly precipitated, in 1,102 parts" (p. 27). Furthermore, "apatite requires 356 times as much liquid for its solution, as the same salt artificially prepared" (p. 28). Obviously, the "artificial basic phosphate, freshly precipitated," was ACP, and, indeed, the differences in solubility values between ACP and the stoichiometric well-crystallized HA might be that big. The results of the successive solubility experiments were published in 1866 [70], 1868 [71], 1871 [72, 73], and 1883 [74].

The second half of the nineteenth century started with "Chemistry" by Wilson, published in 1850 [75]. The following parts from that book are worth citing: "797. *Phosphates of Lime*. – There are many compounds of lime and phosphoric acid, owing to the peculiarity of that acid in relation to the number of equivalents of base it combines with at once. The most interesting phosphate of lime is that which occurs in bones, and is distinguished as the bone-earth phosphate, $3CaO,PO_5$." (p. 219). Thus, various types of calcium orthophosphates were known already. However, the preparation technique sounds unusual to the modern readers: "The phosphorus combines in part with the oxygen of the lime, CaO, to form phosphoric acid, and this with undecomposed lime, to form phosphate of lime, CaO,PO_5. At the same time another portion of the phosphorus combines with the calcium of the lime, forming phosphuret of calcium, CaP" (p. 164). Thus, the compositional differences between the chemical formulae of the oxygen-containing calcium

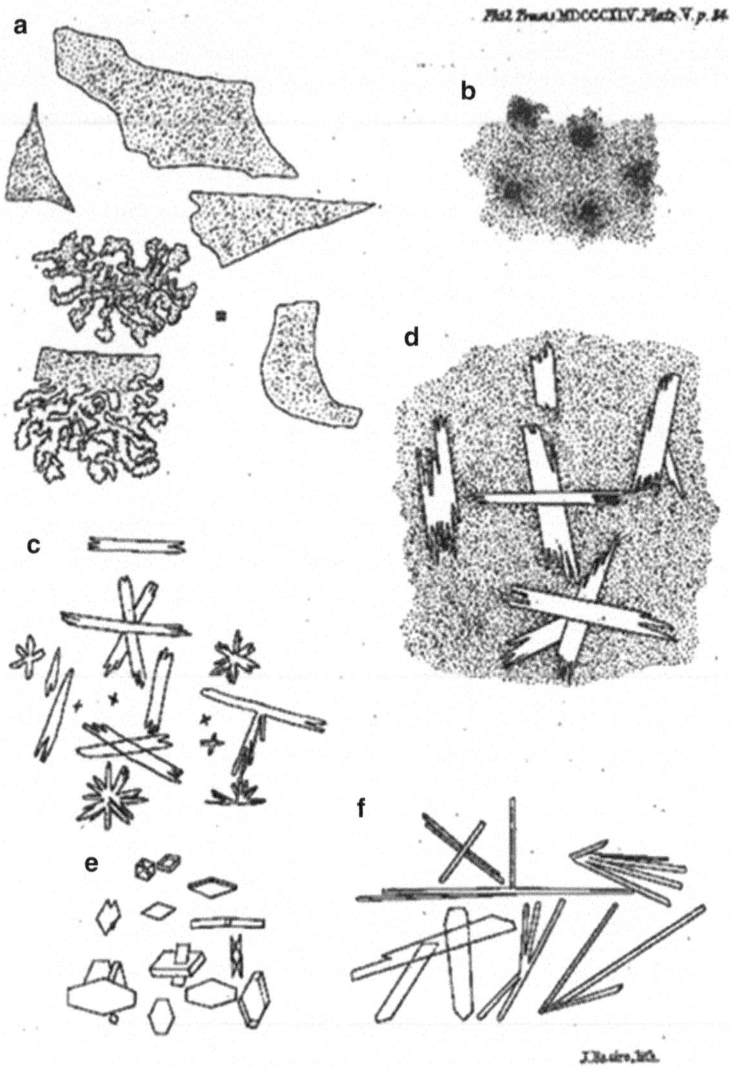

Fig. 15.1 The earliest available pictures of precipitates, some of which contain calcium orthophosphates "(**a**) Iridescent pellicles on some alkaline urine; (**b**) Amorphous deposit in alkaline urine. Deposit on boiling phosphate of soda with chloride of calcium, or with sulphate of magnesia; (**c**) Chloride of calcium with acid phosphate of soda, or with common phosphate of soda, after long standing; (**d**) Phosphate of soda with little chloride of calcium. Bone-earth phosphate; (**e**) On boiling phosphate of soda with sulphate of magnesia and little biphosphate of soda; (**f**) Phosphate of soda with sulphate of magnesia; after long standing" (p. 349). Namely, the precipitates on (**b**) are ACP (in the case, calcium chloride was used) and the crystals on (**c**) and (**d**) are either DCPD or OCP (Reprinted from Ref. [60])

phosphates and the oxygen-free calcium phosphides were clearly established by 1850. The earliest-found thesis on calcium orthophosphates was defended in 1853 [76]. In a publication of 1859, various preparation techniques of apatites were described as follows [45]: "M. Daubrée has prepared apatite by passing chloride of phosphorus over lime; M. Mauross and M. Briegleb, in continuation of the remarkable researchers made in the laboratory of Professor Wöhler, have reproduced apatite in more distinct and more beautiful forms by taking advantage of the double decomposition of alkaline phosphates and chloride of calcium; M. Forchhammer, by acting on phosphate of lime with chloride of sodium, has obtained very beautiful specimens of the same mineral species." (pp. 129–130). Here, the readers' attention was also paid to the names of additional early contributors to calcium orthophosphates.

In "Chemistry" by Brande and Taylor, published in 1863 [77], one can find the following statements: "Common Phosphate of Lime; Tribasic Phosphate of Lime; Bone Phosphate; (3(CaO),PO_5). This salt occurs abundantly in bone-ash, and is found as a mineral product" (p. 331). Furthermore, "*Native phosphate of lime* (bone phosphate) occurs in *apatite*, *moroxite*, *phosphorite*, and *asparagus stone*; its primitive form is a six-sided prism: it also occurs in some volcanic products" (p. 332). Thus, a similarity between the inorganic phase of bones and calcium orthophosphate rocks of natural origin (apatite and phosphorites) was known by 1863. "When a solution of bone-earth in hydrochloric or nitric acid is boiled to expel all carbonic acid, and decomposed by caustic ammonia, the bone-phosphate separates in the form of a bulky precipitate, which, when perfectly dried, is white and amorphous" (p. 331). This seems to be the second earliest mentioning on ACP. Next citation, "The substance known under the name of *coprolites*, and which appear to be the excrements of fossil reptiles, also abound in phosphate of lime" (p. 332), means that by 1863, researchers were aware of this fact.

Further historical description is based on the journal publications only. Namely, C. Morfit [78]; Robert Warington (there were two chemists with this name, presumably, a father (1807–1867) and a son (1838–1907)), who performed the earliest well-documented systematic studies of the outstanding quality [70, 72, 79, 80]; and R. Fresenius [81] also worked with calcium orthophosphates. Interestingly, C. Morfit wrote the chemical symbol of phosphorus as Ph, and, thus, he wrote the chemical formula of tribasic phosphate as 3CaO, PhO_5 [78]. Furthermore, let me cite a paragraph from a Warington's paper of 1866 [70]: "Mitscherlich tells us, that when chloride of calcium is added to ordinary disodic phosphate, the latter being maintained in excess, the precipitate formed is tricalcic phosphate, while the solution becomes acid from the production of monosodic phosphate. Berzelius, on the contrary, states, that the precipitate formed under these conditions is not tricalcic phosphate, but the octocalcic triphosphate, which lie has elsewhere described. All experimenters agree, that when the operation is reversed, and disodic phosphate is poured into an excess of chloride of calcium, the precipitate is neither tricalcic nor octocalcic, but dicalcic phosphate." (pp. 296–297). Thus, TCP, DCP, and OCP have been differentiated from each other by 1866, while, in fact, at least, 20 years earlier because Berzelius died in 1848. Furthermore, the researchers were already aware of the fact that the type of a precipitated calcium orthophosphate depended on a sequence of the mixing reagents.

Among the available publications written by two Robert Waringtons [70, 72, 79, 80], Ref. [70] by Robert Warington Jr. deserves both a special attention and extensive citations. For example, to prove that OCP indeed was already known by 1866, let me make another citation from Ref. [70]: "Octocalcic phosphate can only be produced by the simultaneous formation of monosodic phosphate:

$$8CaCl_2 + 5Na_4H_2P_2O_8 = Ca_8H_2P_6O_{24} + 16NaCl + 2Na_2H_4P_2O_8.\text{" (p. 300)}.$$

One can see a balanced chemical equation, identical to the modern ones. It is hard to believe that it was published in 1866! It is interesting to note that only 22 years appeared to be enough to perform a transition from the primitive chemical formulae without oxygen, such as $2.Ca^2P$ and $5.Ca^2P$ [48], to the modern chemical equations. More to the point, the chemical formulae of hydrated forms of calcium orthophosphates were known by 1866: "8·73 grs. of the vacuum-dried salt, lost on ignition 12·30 grains, or 26·35 per cent.; the formula $Ca_2H_2P_2O_8{\cdot}4H_2O$, demands 26·16 per cent. of water" (p. 299). Needless to explain, "$Ca_2H_2P_2O_8{\cdot}4H_2O$" represents two molecules of DCPD (see Table 15.1). Furthermore, "It is interesting to observe that while disodic phosphate is of an alkaline nature, dicalcic phosphate possesses faint acid properties" (p. 300). More to the point, the form and shape of DCPD crystals were described as well: "The crystalline form of the dicalcic tetrahydrated phosphate has been examined by Professor Church. He describes the crystals as thin rhomboïdal plates, of which the diagonally opposite acute angles are sometimes truncated, hexagonal forms being thus produced. This truncation seems to be occasionally hemihedral, and then may proceed up to the diagonal between obtuse angles; from this change triangular forms arise. Other modifications are also met with." (pp. 300–301). Another interesting conclusion might be found here: "We may then safely affirm that whenever dicalcic phosphate, octocalcic triphosphate, or any phosphate of intermediate composition, is precipitated from solution by ammonia, the salt obtained will be the octocalcic triphosphate; a tricalcic phosphate cannot be obtained in this manner. The following is probably a type of the reaction:

$$4Ca_2H_2P_2O_8 + 6NH_3 = Ca_8H_2P_6O_{24} + 6NH_4.P_2O_8.\text{" (pp. } 301 - 302).$$

This seems to be the earliest mentioning on the fact that TCP cannot be precipitated from the aqueous solutions (currently we know that ACP or CDHA are precipitated instead). In addition, the following citation from the same publication "It is quite possible that precipitated tricalcic phosphate may possess somewhat different solubilities, when prepared by different methods; this difference can, however, scarcely be great" (p. 304) has two important consequences: (1) by 1866, this fact was not quite clear yet; (2) it indirectly points to variability in the Ca/P ratio for the precipitated ACP or CDHA, which is the major reason of different solubilities.

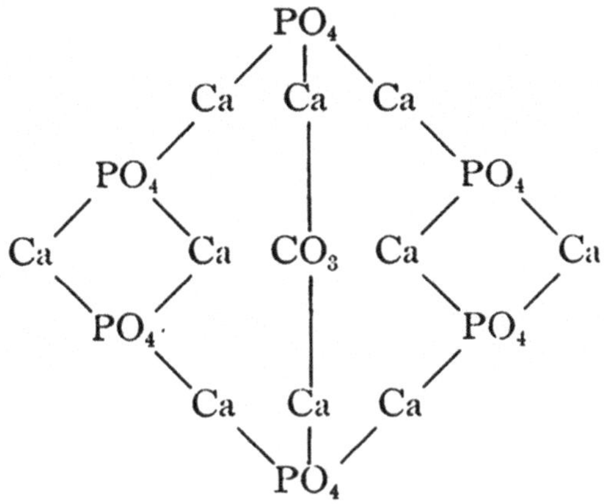

Fig. 15.2 The first available structure of a bone mineral, currently known as carbonate apatite (Reprinted from Ref. [83])

The latest available publication by Warington of 1873 [80] was devoted to the hydrolysis of a freshly precipitated TCP (i.e., either ACP or CDHA) to the stoichiometric HA under continuous (up to 50 h) boiling in distilled water. From the results of numerous chemical analyses, the author concluded that during boiling an aqueous suspension of the TCP was slowly transformed to a suspension of $3Ca_3P_2O_8$. $CaOH_2O$ (i.e., HA – see Table 15.1) and soluble acidic calcium orthophosphates. The following conclusion was made: "Since it appears that all phosphates of calcium less basic than apatite are unstable under the continued action of pure water, it seems probable that a more exact examination of natural phosphates would show that many phosphates now regarded as tricalcic are in fact of a more basic nature" (p. 989). Thus, the apatitic nature of the majority of natural calcium orthophosphates has been predicted in 1873. The next available journal article on the TCP hydrolysis was published in 1929 only [82].

Now it would be logical to cite a publication of 1906 by Wells [83]: "The apparent constancy of the proportion of carbonate and phosphate of calcium in bones made an impression on Hoppe-Seyler in 1862, and we find him speculating on the possibility of the components of the two salts being joined together to form one giant molecule: $3(Ca_3(Po_4)_2)$–$CaCo_3$, which he imagined might be united in some such way" (p. 522) – see Fig. 15.2. Further, Wells mentioned: "This formula is interesting chiefly from the historical standpoint, but it serves to emphasize the tendency of these salts to appear in nearly constant proportions in the animal body, a fact possibly of some importance" (p. 523). Obviously, the atomic arrangement shown in Fig. 15.2 represents the earliest structural drawing of a single molecule of an ion-substituted calcium orthophosphate, currently known as carbonate apatite. An attentive reader will notice two different types of calcium (currently known as Ca(1) and Ca(2)) in that structure. Besides, that time, apatites were considered as combined compounds, which results from this citation of 1879 [84]: "Calcium phosphate, combined with calcium chloride or calcium fluoride, occurs in the well-known minerals, apatite and osteolite" (p. 188). One might guess that, in the nineteenth century, the atomic arrangement of single molecule of carbonate apatite

(Fig. 15.2) could have inspired researchers to compose similar drawings for the single molecules of FA, HA, and/or chlorapatite; unfortunately, I have succeeded to find nothing on this matter.

Chemical equations, describing various interactions between calcium phosphates and other chemicals, have been known since, at least, 1863. For example, the afore-cited production processes of both orthophosphoric acid and white phosphorus from the Lavoisier book [31], in 1863, were written using chemical equations [77]: "When bone-phosphate is digested in dilute sulphuric acid, it is resolved into sulphate of lime and (if a sufficiency of sulphuric acid be used) phosphoric acid:

$$3\,(CaO)\,,PO_5 + 3SO_3 = 3\,[CaO, SO_3] + PO_5.\text{''} \quad (\text{p. } 331)\,.$$

One can see that hydrogen was not included into the chemical formulae yet. Nevertheless, already in 1866, it was included by Robert Warington Jr. [70] (see above). Furthermore, chemical formulae of various types of phosphates (namely, metaphosphate and acid phosphate), as well as differences in their solubility, were known by 1881 [24]: "In order to prepare phosphorus, the bone-ash is first mixed with so much dilute sulphuric acid as to form the acid phosphate:

$$Ca_3(PO_4)_2 + 2H_2SO_4 = CaH_4(PO_4)_2 + 2CaSO_4.$$

The solution of this soluble acid phosphate is next poured off from the precipitated gypsum, and evaporated to dryness, after which, the solid residue heated to redness, water is given off and calcium metaphosphate formed:

$$CaH_4(PO_4)_2 = Ca(PO_3)_2 + 2H_2O.$$

This salt is then carefully mixed with charcoal, and heated to bright redness in earthenware retorts shown in Fig. 15.2, when the following change takes place:–

$$Ca(PO_3)_2 + 10C = P_4 + Ca_3(PO_4)_2 + 10CO.\text{''} \quad (\text{p. } 460)\,.$$

Now, it is time to describe miscellaneous studies on the subject. The first accessible journal paper on detection and preservation techniques of various deposits, including calcium orthophosphates, was published in 1852 [85]. Presence of calcium orthophosphates in teakwood was established in 1862 [86]. Neutral phosphates of lime were further investigated in 1872 [87]. Various analytical topics on calcium orthophosphate chemistry have been studied since, at least, 1863 [88] and remained to be a subject of active research approximately until the 1910s [89–102]. The quantitative analysis of a calcium orthophosphate was performed in 1884 [103], followed by remarks by C. Glaser in 1885 [104]. In the 1880s, occurrence of apatite [105] and TTCP [106–108] in metallurgical slags was discovered. The latter discovery belongs to the German metallurgist Gustav Hilgenstock (1844–1913), after whom TTCP is called hilgenstockite. An attempt of a direct estimation of phosphoric acid as the tribasic phosphate of lime was performed in 1888 [109]. A chemical interaction of TCP with carbon dioxide and iron hydroxide was investigated in 1891 [110].

Besides, in the second half of the nineteenth century, calcium orthophosphates were extensively investigated as fertilizers. As written above, the term "superphosphate" has been known since 1795 [34] and was further developed in 1803 [111]: "The phoſphoric acid ſeparated from that portion of lime, immediately combines with the reſt of the phoſsphate of lime, and forms ſuper phoſphate of lime, which is not farther decompoſable by ſulphuric acid" (pp. 394–395). Obviously, initially it represented just acidic calcium orthophosphates. However, by the second half of the nineteenth century, a fertilizer with the same name became popular. It consisted of "a mixture of the last-mentioned compound and sulphate of lime" [84]. According to Pusey [112], this finding belongs to the famous German chemist Justus Freiherr von Liebig (1803–1873), who is considered as "the father of the fertilizer industry" for his discoveries. Let me cite Pusey [112]: "Dr. Liebig's great discovery of dissolving bones in sulphuric acid for the purpose of manure, has been so clearly established by the experiments as well of the Duke of Richmond as of other farmers, and so fully investigated by Mr. Hannam, that nothing seems now to be wanted but some plan for bringing it within the ordinary routine of farming." (p. 324). In a publication of 1864 [113], one can read the following: "Now, superphosphate of lime is composed, necessarily, of soluble phosphate of lime and plaster, or sulphate of lime formed from a combination of the sulphuric acid employed in the manufacture of superphosphate with the lime of the bones" (p. lv). More than 20 research papers on superphosphate were published by the beginning of the twentieth century, which indicated to the importance of this chemical for the human being [114–136]. One can see that almost all of these studies were performed and published by single researchers (see individual comments to Refs. [115, 121]), while the majority of the investigations were devoted to analytical chemistry.

Although vitrification properties of some forms of calcium orthophosphates upon heating have been known since, at least, 1804 [33], the first accessible journal paper on this topic was published in 1877 [137]. The modern chemical formula of perfectly transparent crystals of natural FA as $Ca_5(PO_4)_3$ F has been known since, at least, 1873 [138], while chemical formulae of DCP (as "mono-hydrogen calcium orthophosphate, $HCaPO_4$") and MCP (as "tetra-hydrogen calcium phosphate, $H_4Ca(PO_4)_2$") [84] have been known since, at least, 1879 (pp. 205–206). Interestingly, in a publication of 1871, the chemical formulae of calcium orthophosphates were written in different ways: as 3CaO PO_5 for apatite and CaO 2HO PO_5 for "some acid phosphate of lime" [73]. Thus, by the 1880s, the rules on how to write chemical formulae of inorganic compounds have not been standardized yet.

Additionally, one should briefly mention the earliest biochemical applications of calcium orthophosphates. Let me cite a couple of self-explanatory sentences from a publication of 1935 [139]: "Calcium phosphate was used for enzyme separation as early as 1860 by Brücke (cited by Effront, 1917). Its use for precipitation of active immunological material was advocated for the purification of diphtheria toxin first by Roux and Yersin in 1889, ..." (p. 150). Thus, the famous French physician, bacteriologist, and immunologist Pierre Paul Émile Roux (1853–1933) and the famous Swiss and French physician and bacteriologist Alexandre Emile Jean Yersin (1863–1943) also contributed to calcium orthophosphates by performing absorption and purification of diphtherial toxin.

Finally, one should report the investigations performed by the British clinician and pharmacologist Sydney Ringer (1836–1910), whose name is remembered in a Ringer's solution. It is an aqueous isotonic solution of several inorganic salts mimicking the body fluids of animals [140]. Within 1882–1885, Ringer determined that a solution perfusing a frog's heart must contain several inorganic salts in a definite proportion if the heart was to be kept beating for long [141–145]. The following citation from his works is worth mentioning [143]: "*(g)* So that we find we possess an excellent circulating fluid capable of maintaining the heart for several hours, which consists of phosphate of calcium saline, with potassium chloride" (p. 19).

To conclude the 1800s, one should recognize that the majority of the fundamental discoveries in chemistry of calcium orthophosphates were made in the nineteenth century.

15.4.3 From 1900 till 1950

As the modern scientific databases comprise of scientific papers published after 1900, the history of calcium orthophosphates in the twentieth century is based on the journal publications only. This approach allows establishing the real chronological order. However, the detailed description of every publication on the subject becomes impossible due to permanently increasing amount of them.

The twentieth century started with the systematic studies performed by F.K. Cameron with co-workers [136, 146–153] and H. Bassett [154–157]. Namely, in 1908, Bassett composed the first version of the solubility diagram $CaO–P_2O_5–H_2O$ (Fig. 15.3) [156]. According to the literature [24, 84, 158], by that time, researchers already worked with the individual calcium orthophosphates; however, not all the chemical formulae appeared in close resemblance to the ones we use today. For example, H. Bassett wrote formulae of MCPM and MCPA as $CaH_4P_2O_8.H_2O$ and $CaH_4P_2O_8$, respectively. In addition, he mentioned hydrated forms for TCP and TTCP as $Ca_3P_2O_8.H_2O$ and $Ca_4P_2O_9.H_2O$, respectively [156], which are currently unknown. A study on dissolution kinetics of several calcium orthophosphates was published in 1910 [159]. Binary salts of calcium orthophosphates with orthophosphates of other chemical elements have been known since, at least, 1911 [160]. The osmotic properties of calcium orthophosphates were investigated in 1915 [161]. Currently well-known chemical route of CDHA preparation by mixing of aqueous solutions of calcium nitrate and K_2HPO_4 (now $(NH_4)_2HPO_4$ is used instead) was investigated conductometrically in 1915 [162], while a neutralization reaction of H_3PO_4 by $Ca(OH)_2$ was investigated in 1923 [163]. Preparation of

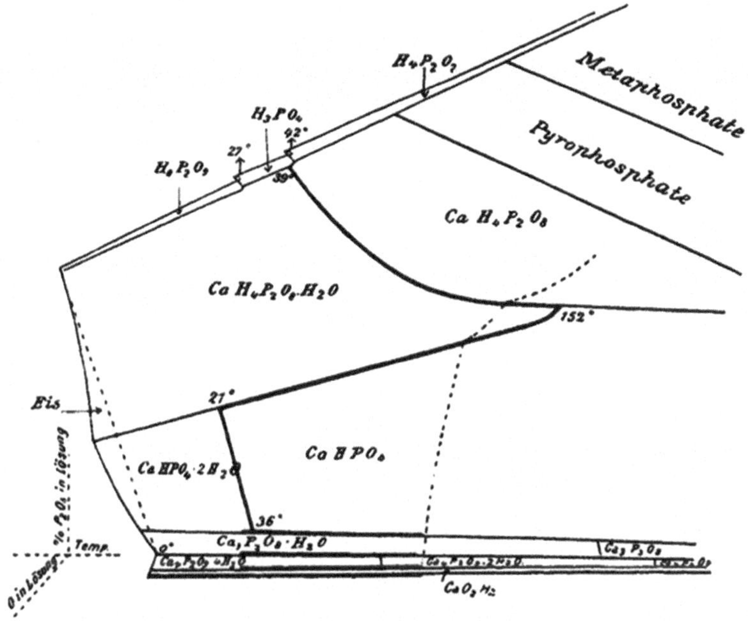

Fig. 15.3 The system CaO–P_2O_5–H_2O in 1908 (Reprinted from Ref. [156]). In 1917, Ramsay published important information on calcium orthophosphates [169]: "1. The substances sold as "Phosphate of lime" and "Calcium Phosphas B.P." are not pure tricalcic phosphate but are mixtures of di- and tricalcic phosphates. 2. Sodium phosphate (Na_2HPO_4) added to ammoniacal calcium chloride and the resulting precipitate washed with water yields a mixture of di- and tricalcic phosphate and calcium hydrate. 3. Bone ash dissolved in hydrochloric acid and precipitated with ammonia, the precipitate being well washed, yields also a mixture of di- and tricalcium phosphate and calcium hydrate. 4. When three equivalents of lime (3CaO) are made to act on one equivalent of phosphoric acid (P_2O_5) and the resulting precipitate removed with little delay pure tricalcium phosphate is obtained." Obviously, the obtained "mixture of di- and tricalcium phosphate and calcium hydrate" was a CDHA; therefore, a nonstoichiometric nature of the precipitates was established by 1917. Furthermore, one can see that chemically pure calcium orthophosphates (B.P. means British Pharmacopoeia) were commercially produced by 1917

calcium orthophosphate (presumably, it was ACP) in a colloid state was reported in 1921 [164]. An interesting note on "liquid crystals of calcium phosphate" was published in 1922 [165]; in fact, the author prepared MCPM. The first paper on in vitro mineralization using aqueous solutions containing ions of calcium and orthophosphate was published in 1926 [166], followed by publications of 1932 [167] and 1933 [168]. These studies might be considered as predecessors of current mineralization investigations using simulating body fluid (SBF) and other artificial simulating solutions.

Furthermore, by 1928, it was clearly known that TCP could not be prepared by wet precipitation [170]: "*We have been unable to find any evidence of the existence of a molecular species with the formula $Ca_3(PO_4)_2$*. Precipitates of this "substance" rarely have the correct empirical composition and they cannot be purified by recrystallization. The evidence is such as to lead us to suspect that there may be no such chemical entity as $Ca_3(PO_4)_2$. No one has succeeded in preparing it by precipitation [12, 35–48], bearing out the theoretical objections to such a reaction on the grounds that fifth order reactions do not occur [49]. We do not take the position that there can be no compound with this formula. It may be found possible to synthesize it by other methods, but so far no one has succeeded in preparing it by precipitation." (p. 128). Other researchers [171] made similar conclusions. Nevertheless, that time this knowledge was not common yet, since, in 1935, a report was published that "Tricalcium phosphate monohydrate was prepared by the slow addition of calcium chloride solution to a constantly agitated alkaline solution of disodium phosphate, maintained at 65° to 70°C" [172]. This controversy was explained in 1940 by a matter of definitions [173]: "The terms "tricalcium phosphate" and "hydroxyapatite" are very widely and very loosely used. For example, some authors use the former for any precipitate more basic than dicalcium phosphate, although such precipitates have been frequently shown to have an apatite lattice or to be mixtures of dicalcium phosphate and an apatite. Others confine the use of the term to those precipitates with P_2O_5:CaO ratios approaching that of $Ca_3(PO_4)_2$." (p. 265). Nevertheless, papers on precipitated TCP [174, 175] and even on precipitated TCP hydrate [176] kept publishing even in the 1940s. An interesting distinction between HA and precipitated TCP hydrate (obviously, it was CDHA with $x = 1$; see Table 15.1) was made in a latter paper [176]: "It seems safe to conclude that a precipitated tricalcium phosphate can be designated as a hydroxyapatite when a 1-gram charge of 900 °C. calcine registers a dissolubility of less than 20 % by a continuously agitated 1-hour digestion in the ammonium citrate reagent at 65 °C. In contradistinction, a tertiary precipitate is identified as a tricalcium phosphate hydrate when a like charge of its calcine shows dissolubility of as much as 50 % by the stipulated citrate digestion." (p. 169). Currently, we are able to explain the solubility differences between these two calcined samples by formation of more soluble β-TCP (Table 15.1).

The crystal structure of apatites was established in 1930 [177, 178], followed by a great study on the structural characteristics of apatite-like calcium orthophosphates of various origins in 1931 [179]. Such terms as hydroxyfluorapatite, $Ca_{10}(F,OH)_2(PO_4)_6$, OA, and carbonate apatite were already known. Besides, the aforementioned "hydrate of tricalcium phosphate, $Ca_9(H_2O)_2(PO_4)_6$," with the molecular weight of 966.4 g and apatite-like diffraction pattern was mentioned as well [179]. The "apatite-like diffraction pattern" clearly indicates that the authors prepared CDHA. The structures of carbonate apatite [180, 181] and DCPD [182] were reported in 1937 and 1938. Furthermore, in 1938, several calcium orthophosphates were X-ray studied to determine their variability and phase purity [183]. The following citation from the abstract is rather interesting: "The commercial tertiary calcium phosphates are probably hydroxylapatite with more or less adsorbed phosphate ions resulting in empirical formulas approaching the theoretical value for $Ca_3P_2O_8$. Secondary calcium phosphate may be admixed" (p. 156). Interestingly, in 1938, the structure of TCP was sometimes considered as that of HA with adsorbed PO_4 ions (presumably, with the counterions) on the surface; still, the chemical formulae were expressed differently to the ones we know today. The detailed investigations on isomorphic substitutions in apatites have been performed since 1938 [184].

In the second quarter of the twentieth century, solubility of apatites and other calcium orthophosphates was investigated extensively. Namely, papers on this topic were published in 1925 [185–187], 1926 [188], 1927 [189–191], 1929 [152], 1931 [192, 193], 1937–1939 [194–197], 1942 [198, 199], 1945 [200, 201], 1948 [202–204], and 1950 [205]. In addition, in 1949, a paperback monograph (or thesis?) on enamel-apatite solubility was published [206]. Buffering abilities of the dissolved calcium orthophosphates have been known since, at least, 1933 [207]. Additionally, in 1931–1933, Bredig et al. [208], Trömel [209], and Schneiderhöhn (a reference was not found) differentiated α- and β-modifications of TCP (see Table 15.1) and created the initial versions of the high-temperature diagram for the binary system $CaO–P_2O_5$. In 1933, reduction experiments of TCP by carbon, carbon monoxide, and hydrogen were performed at temperatures of 900–1,300 °C [210]. In addition, a new set of extensive studies on superphosphate was initiated in the 1930s [211–219] and continued ever since (more recent references are not cited due to their abundance). Besides, in 1934, an important (for fertilizers) reaction between urea and several calcium orthophosphates was investigated [220]. In 1935, the heat capacity values of calcium orthophosphates were measured [221]. Very popular at the turn of this millennium silicon- (or silica-) contained calcium orthophosphates, in fact, appear to have been known since, at least, 1937 [222–224], simultaneously with defluorination studies of natural phosphate rocks [224–226]. Applications of calcium orthophosphates for removal of fluorides from water have been known since, at least, 1938 [227–229], while the earliest research paper on using calcium orthophosphates in chromatography was published in 1942 [230].

In 1940, a fundamental study on the equilibrium in the system $CaO–P_2O_5–H_2O$ was published [231]. Besides, in 1940, the available level of knowledge on basic calcium orthophosphates (TCP, TTCP, and apatites) was summarized into a big review [173], which might be considered as the first comprehensive review on the subject. That time, the existence of OA was uncertain. In addition, the authors of that review wrote about HA that "Existence as a unique stoichiometric compound doubtful" (p. 259, Table 15.1), which was a clear indication to the great difficulties to synthesize HA but not CDHA. Furthermore, the following important assumption was made: "First, between dicalcium phosphate and lime, there exists, in the ternary system, a continuous series of solid solutions having an apatite lattice. It follows from this that tricalcium phosphate and hydroxyapatite do not exist in aqueous systems as unique, stoichiometric compounds" (p. 265). Thus, in 1940, existence of CDHA with variable Ca/P ratio was predicted. The idea on a continuous series of solid solutions was further developed by 1950 [232]: "On structural grounds it appears possible that a continuous series of apatite-like solid solutions can exist between octocalcium phosphate and hydroxy- (or fluor-) apatite. In practice, no two preparations with composition lying between octocalcium phosphate and hydroxyapatite are likely to be identical" (Abstract). Thus, in 1950, the distinct Ca/P borders for CDHA were established between those in OCP (Ca/P = 1.33) and HA (Ca/P = 1.67). In addition, it was noted that calcium orthophosphate precipitates with Ca/P ratios within 1.0–1.33 "consist of at least two phases; dicalcium phosphate and a solid at least as basic as octocalcium phosphate" (Abstract) [232].

The term "whitlockite" (named after an American mineralogist Herbert Percy Whitlock (1868–1948), who was the curator of the American Museum of Natural History, New York, USA) for ion-substituted TCP first appeared in 1941 [233]. Also, in the same year, a study on virus purification by adsorption on calcium orthophosphate was published [234], followed by two other studies in 1945 [235, 236]. An important study on the thermal decomposition of MCPM was published in 1947 [237], while that on high-temperature heat content of HA appeared in 1950 [238].

To finalize the first half of the twentieth century, one should mention on an interesting conclusion, made in 1944. Namely, attempting to explain anomalous pH drop during titration of H_3PO_4 by $Ca(OH)_2$ discovered by earlier researchers [163], Greenwald published a paper on a possibility to precipitate calcium orthophosphates having Ca/P ratio ≥2 [239]: "We may now picture the course of events as follows: after the first equivalent of calcium hydroxide has been added, the solution contains Ca^{++}, $H_2PO_4^-$ and $HPO_4^=$ ions. It also contains some undissociated $CaHPO_4$. This may act as an acid and upon addition of $Ca(OH)_2$ give a precipitate of $Ca(OH){\cdot}CaPO_4$, possibly occluding or adsorbing a little $Ca(OH)_2$ as well." (p. 1306). In fact, precipitation of $Ca(OH){\cdot}CaPO_4$ remained unproven because there is no explanation as to why undissociated $CaHPO_4$ should behave as a stronger acid if compared with $H_2PO_4^-$ ions. Currently, we can explain that anomalous pH drop by formation of ACP, the chemical composition of which may vary in wide ranges (Table 15.1). A similar unproven conclusion on a possibility to precipitate calcium orthophosphates having Ca/P ratio exceeding that in HA due to adsorption of hydroxyl or other anions was published in 1950 [232].

More recent (after 1950) publications on calcium orthophosphates are not considered, since they are well known.

15.5 Calcium Orthophosphates as Bone Grafts

15.5.1 Artificial Grafts in the Nineteenth Century and Before

The artificial generation of tissues, organs, or even entire living organisms has been a matter of myths and dreams throughout the history of humankind. Unfortunately, due to the practice of cremation in many societies, little is known about the prehistoric materials used to replace bones lost to accident or disease. Nevertheless, according to the available literature, introduction of nonbiological materials into the human body was noted far back in prehistory. Namely, according to Ratner [240]: "The remains of a human found near Kennewick, Washington, USA (often referred

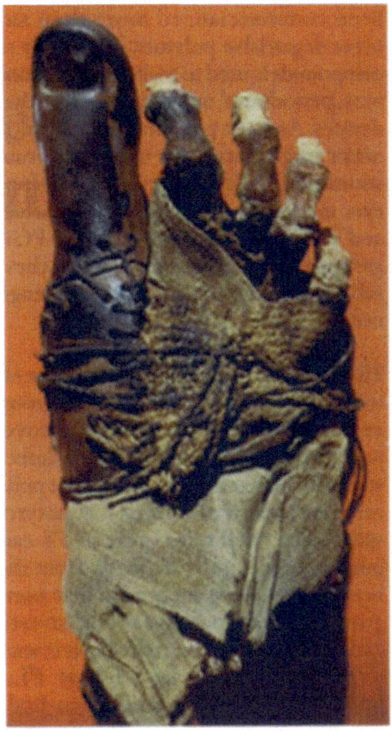

Fig. 15.4 A wooden prosthesis of a hallux of a mummy (Reprinted with permission from Ref. [241]. Copyright 2001, American Chemical Society)

to as the "Kennewick Man") was dated to be up to 9000 years old. That individual, described by archeologists as a tall, healthy, active person, wandered through the region now known as southern Washington with a spear point embedded in his hip. It had apparently healed in and did not significantly impede his activity. This unintended implant illustrates the body's capacity to deal with implanted foreign materials. The spear point has little resemblance to modern biomaterials, but it was a tolerated foreign material implant, just the same. Another example of the introduction of foreign materials into the skin, dated to over 5000 years ago, is the tattoo. The carbon particles and other substances probably elicited a classic foreign-body reaction." (p. xli).

Later, man's attempts to repair the human body with the use of implant materials were recorded in the early medical writings of the Hindu, Egyptian, and Greek civilizations. The earliest successful implants were in the skeletal system. Namely, applying modern pathology methods to an ~3,000-year-old mummy, researchers at Ludwig Maximilians University, Munich, showed that ancient Egyptian physicians designed wooden prostheses to help their ailing patients: in that case, a 50–60-year-old woman whose toe was amputated (Fig. 15.4) [241]. Besides, the famous painting by Fra Angelico (ca. 1395–1455) "The Healing of Justinian by Saint Cosmas and Saint Damian" (Fig. 15.5), a visualization of the legend of twins Sts. Cosmas and Damien (died ca. 287 AD) depicting a transplantation of a homograft limb onto an injured soldier, is one early instance of the vision of a regenerative medicine.

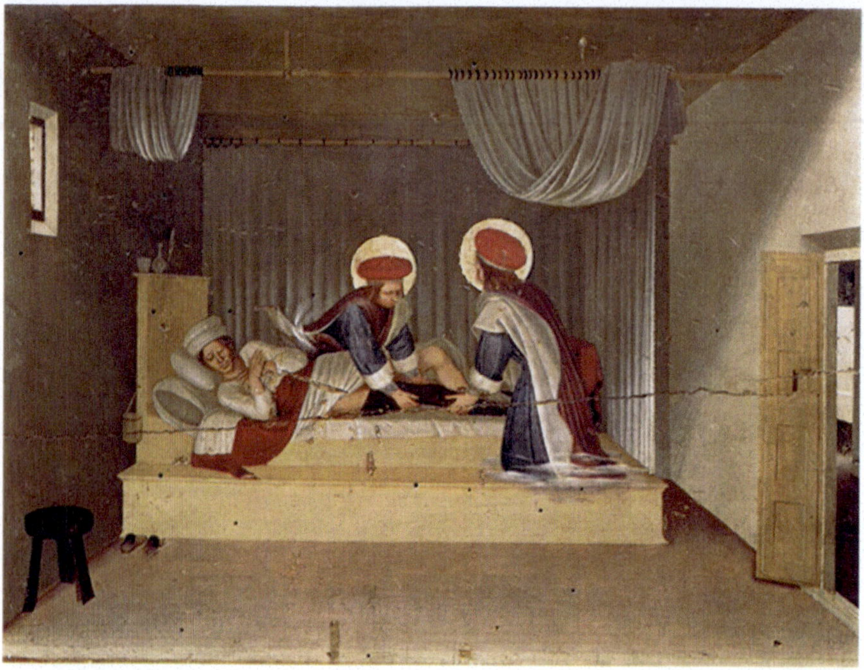

Fig. 15.5 Fra Angelico's (ca. 1395–1455) "The Healing of Justinian by Saint Cosmas and Saint Damian" (approximately 1439) is exhibited at Museo di San Marco, Florence, Italy

Historically, a selection of the materials was based on their availability and an ingenuity of the individual making and applying the prosthetic [242]. Archaeological findings exhibited in museums showed that materials used to replace missing human bones and teeth included animal or human (from corpses) bones and teeth, shells, corals, ivory (elephant tusk), wood (Fig. 15.4), as well as some metals (gold or silver). For instance, "the father of Western medicine" Hippocrates (ca. 460 BC–ca. 370 BC) apparently used gold wire and linen thread for ligatures in the repair of bone fractures. Aulus Cornelius Celsus (ca. 25 BC–ca. 50 AD) recommended the filling of large cavities with lint, lead, and other substances before attempting extraction to prevent the tooth from breaking under the pressure of the instrument. This may have been the beginning of filling materials for carious teeth. The Etruscans learned to substitute missing teeth with bridges made from artificial teeth carved from the bones of oxen, while in ancient Phoenicia, loose teeth were bound together with gold wires for tying artificial ones to neighboring teeth. Popp states that ancient Egyptians also made artificial ears, noses, and eyes [243]. The Chinese recorded the first use of dental amalgam to repair decayed teeth in the year 659 AD, while in the Americas, the pre-Columbian civilizations used gold sheets to heal cranial cavities following trepanation [244]. Besides, while excavating Mayan burial sites in Honduras in 1931, archaeologists found a fragment of mandible of Mayan origin, dating from about 600 AD. This mandible, which is considered to be that of a woman in her twenties, had three tooth-shaped pieces of shell placed into the sockets of three missing lower incisor teeth. In 1970, a Brazilian dental academic Prof. Amadeo Bobbio studied the mandible specimen and took a series of radiographs. He noted compact bone formation around two of the implants, which led him to conclude that the implants were placed during life [245]. This might be the first recorded use of dental implants. More to the point, an iron dental implant in a corpse dated ~200 AD was found in Europe. That implant was also described as properly bone integrated [246].

In the middle ages, one of the first scientific descriptions of congenital and acquired defects of the maxilla and their treatments was given by the famous French barber surgeon Ambroise Paré (ca. 1510–1590), who is considered as one of the "fathers of surgery and modern forensic pathology." In 1564, he published *Dix livres de la chirurgie, avec le magasin des instrumens necessaires à icelle*, where he specifically described defects of the palate with bone destruction caused by harquebus shots, stab wounds, or syphilitic gumma, describing also the accompanying speech deficiency and giving general principles of treatment. He used a flat, vaulted, metallic plate in gold or silver with a sponge attached to it. The sponge was introduced into the defect, where it expanded with readily absorbed nasal and oral secretions, thus holding the obturator base in position. Paré is also credited with having prepared artificial teeth from bones and ivory. In 1668, a book by the Dutch surgeon Job Janszoon van Meekeren (1611–1666) was published [247]. One of the most interesting works, performed by van Meekeren, was a reconstruction of the face of Duke Butterlijn, who received a piece of dog's skull bone to heal his skull defect that was caused by a Tartar sword. The duke recovered well but was banned by Russian priests, who considered that a combination of a Christian head with a dog bone was unacceptable for the church. Therefore, although the graft was completely healed, the duke asked the surgeon to remove it again [247].

In the eighteenth century, the first well-documented studies on autografts and allografts were published. Namely, the first journal paper on clinical use of a bone autograft belongs to the German surgeon and ophthalmologist Philipp Franz von Walther (1782–1849), who replaced surgically removed parts of a skull after trepanation [248], while the first journal paper on clinical use of a bone allograft belongs to the Scottish surgeon Sir William Macewen (1848–1924), who successfully reconstructed an infected humerus of a 4-year-old boy by a graft obtained from the tibia of a child with rickets [249]. Additional historical details on bone grafts are available in literature [250].

Concerning dentistry, at an early stage, a common method to replace teeth was the homologous transplantation of teeth in humans. Namely, the Scottish surgeon John Hunter (1728–1793) not only investigated in his pioneering work the effect of transplantation at a clinical level (he claimed that homologous transplanted teeth lasted for years in the host) but also performed animal experimental work on the fate of transplants, thereby setting the basis for a scientific approach on transplantation medicine [251]. Besides, various restorative materials might be used for feeling defects and capping exposed pulps and dental cavities. Currently they

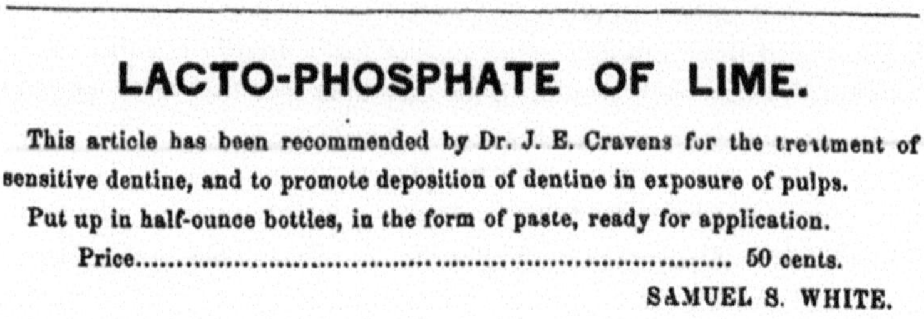

LACTO-PHOSPHATE OF LIME.

This article has been recommended by Dr. J. E. Cravens for the treatment of sensitive dentine, and to promote deposition of dentine in exposure of pulps.

Put up in half-ounce bottles, in the form of paste, ready for application.

Price.. 50 cents.

SAMUEL S. WHITE.

Fig. 15.6 An advertisement of the S.S. White company for "Lacto-Phosphate of Lime" 1873 (Reprinted from Dent. Cosmos 1873, 15, 683)

include zinc orthophosphate, zinc polyacrylate (polycarboxylate), amalgams, glass ionomer cements, calcium hydroxide, etc. [252, 253]; however, within the scope of this review, calcium orthophosphate-based formulations are considered only. According to the available literature, Dr. Junius E. Cravens (1844–1920) from the USA proffered creative concepts in pulp capping in the 1870s. He had the opinion that dentin-like material would be the best to keep the pulp vital. Therefore, Cravens used a calcium orthophosphate powder, which was mixed with lactic acid to low viscosity. The result was a soluble calcium lactic orthophosphate, which was applied onto the exposed pulp tissue [254]. This pulp-capping agent was brought to the market by the S.S. White company with the trade name "Lacto-Phosphate of Lime" (Fig. 15.6). Sugar-containing formulations were known as well [255]. To the best of my findings, that study by Cravens might be considered as the first mentioning on artificial calcium orthophosphate-based biocomposites and hybrid biomaterials (reviewed in Ref. [256]). Thus, one might claim that the grafting history of calcium orthophosphates started in the 1870s.

However, in the past, many implantations failed due to various infections, which tended to be exacerbated in the presence of implants, since they provided a region inaccessible to the body's immunologically competent cells. Therefore, the use of implantable biomaterials did not become practical until the advent of an aseptic surgical technique developed by the British surgeon Sir Joseph Lister (1827–1912) in the 1860s. In addition, there was a lack of knowledge about a toxicity of the selected materials. Since the major inorganic components of the normal calcified tissues of mammals were established by 1808 [257], application of calcium orthophosphates and other calcium-containing compounds as artificial bone grafts became logical.

Historically, plaster of Paris (calcium sulfate) was the first widely tested artificial bioceramics. For example, according to Wikipedia, literature dating back to 975 AD notes that calcium sulfate was useful for setting broken bones. However, those were ex vivo applications. According to the available literature, by the end of the nineteenth century, surgeons already used plaster of Paris as a bone-filling substitute [258]. Nevertheless, it was the famous German surgeon Themistocles Gluck (1853–1942) who, among his range of contributions, on May 20, 1890, performed the first well-documented ivory (virtually pure biological apatite) knee replacement bedded in a calcium sulfate-based cement, which was followed by a total wrist replacement in another patient 3 weeks later [259]. Later in 1890, Gluck presented a further case of a total knee replacement to the Berlin Medical Society: at only 35 days after operation, the patient was pain-free with active knee flexion and extension. All the joint arthroplasties performed by Gluck were remarkably successful in the short term; however, all ultimately failed because of chronic infections [260, 261]. After the abovementioned case of lacto-phosphate of lime (Fig. 15.6), this seems to be the second well-documented grafting application of calcium orthophosphates.

To conclude this part, one should stress that the performance of living tissues is the result of millions of years of evolution, while the performance of acceptable artificial substitutions those humankind has designed to repair damaged tissues is only a few decades old. This explains the greatest differences between them. To get the historical perspective on the development of artificial grafts prepared from other materials, the interested readers are referred to other publications [10, 12–15, 250, 262–265].

15.5.2 The Twentieth Century

According to the previous section, the initial attempts to use calcium orthophosphates for grafting purposes were performed in the end of the nineteenth century. However, in the aforementioned cases, either the biomedical applications of biologically produced calcium orthophosphates (Gluck) or dental applications not requiring any surgery (Cravens) were described. According to both the electronic databases and previous reviews on the subject [10, 12–15, 250, 262–265], the first attempt to implant a laboratory-produced calcium orthophosphate (it was TCP) as an artificial material to repair surgically created defects in rabbit bones was performed in 1920 [11] by the US surgeon Fred Houdlette Albee (1876–1945), who invented bone grafting [266] and some other advances in orthopedic surgery. The researchers injected either 0.5 or 1 c.c. of 5 % slurries of TCP in distilled water (which was then sterilized for three successive days in the Arnold sterilizer, at 60 °C) into surgically created radial bone gaps of rabbits, leaving the periosteum intact [11]. Radiographic analysis revealed that the TCP-injected defect demonstrated more rapid bone growth and union than the control. The average length of time for bony union with TCP was 31 days, compared to 41 days for the controls. No appreciable bone growth was stimulated by injecting TCP beneath the periosteum in non-defective radii or into subcutaneous tissues. Although this seems to be the first scientific study on use of an artificially prepared calcium orthophosphate for in vivo repairing of bone defects, it remains unclear whether that TCP was a precipitated or a ceramic material and whether it was in a powder or a granular form. Unfortunately, the researchers published nothing further on this topic. In 1927, Hey Groves (1872–1944) described pure ivory hip hemi-arthroplasty for fracture [267]. In 1931, Murray also reported an acceleration of healing following implantation of calcium salts composed of 85 % TCP and 15 % $CaCO_3$ in canine long-bone defects [268, 269].

At the beginning of the 1930s, the classic osteoinductive phenomenon was defined well by Huggins [270], who demonstrated that autoimplantation of transitional epithelium of the urinary bladder to abdominal wall muscle in dogs provoked ectopic bone formation. A bit later, Levander demonstrated that crude alcoholic extracts of bones induced a new bone formation when injected into muscle tissue [271, 272].

Simultaneously, in the 1930s, Haldeman and Moore [273], Stewart [274], Key [275], and Shands [276] discovered the fact that only certain types of calcium orthophosphates mentioned in Table 15.1 really influence the bone healing process. Namely, Haldeman and Moore implanted various calcium orthophosphates such as MCP and DCP (it remains unclear whether they were in hydrated or anhydrous forms), TCP, as well as calcium glycerophosphate as dry powdered salts into 0.5–1.0 cm defects in radii of 17 rabbits, while the opposite side served as control. Radiographic analysis demonstrated that in no case did the presence of MCP, DCP, or calcium glycerophosphate had a favorable influence on delayed healing compared to control, while the presence of TCP at the site of the fracture appeared to favor the union [273]. Furthermore, Key [275] suggested that "if a defect in bone could be filled by a non-irritating, slowly soluble mass, which was porous and which contained calcium phosphate and carbonate in a form in which they could be resorbed, it would be reasonable to expect osteoblasts to invade the mass, utilize the calcium, and build new bone which would replace the mass of calcium and cause the bone to be restored to its original form. The ideal material would appear to be rather dense cancellous bone from which a large percentage of the organic material had been removed." (p. 176). However, Key found that "Neither calcium phosphate and carbonate in the proportions in which they occur in bone, nor bone powder, made by removing the organic matter from bone, appear to stimulate osteogenesis of bone when implanted in a bone defect" (p. 184). Stewart [274] concluded that "1. Lime salts and boiled bone when placed into a bone defect with either traumatized muscle or fascia do not serve as a source of available calcium resulting in supersaturation of connective tissue and regeneration of missing bone. 2. Live bone chips placed in bone defects regenerate the missing bone" (p. 871). Shands [276] also reported conflicting effects of several calcium salts (calcium glycerophosphate, a mixture of TCP (3 parts) and $CaCO_3$ (1 part), bone ash, and calcium gluconate) on bone repair. Namely, in defects in the ulna of dogs, the investigated calcium salts appeared to stimulate bone formation, while in operations upon the spine, calcium glycerophosphate did not stimulate bone formation and appeared rather to exert an inhibiting influence. In 1948, Schram and Fosdick confirmed the fact that only certain types of calcium orthophosphates influence the bone healing process [277]. Similar conclusions were obtained in 1951 by Ray and Ward [278].

Due to the reasons mentioned in the abstract, the historical events of the second half of the twentieth century are reported very briefly. Namely, in 1945, the first publication on applications of calcium orthophosphates as dentifrices was published [279]. Two important calcium orthophosphate-containing simulating solutions, namely, Earle's balanced salt solution (EBSS) [280] and Hanks' balanced salt solution (HBSS) [281], became known in 1943 and 1949, respectively. In 1950, the history of self-setting calcium orthophosphate formulations was started [282]. The author of that important publication investigated mixtures of both oxides and hydroxides of various metals with aqueous solutions of orthophosphoric acid and discovered a number of cold-setting formulations. For example, he found that CaO, sintered at 1,100 °C, did not set in H_3PO_4, while that in liquid containing 9.6 % CaO was found to set after ~12 h in the presence of H_3PO_4 [282]. The latter mixture might be considered as the first prototype of the self-setting calcium orthophosphate formulations (reviewed in Refs. [283, 284]). The next publications on this topic appeared in 1975 [285] and 1976 [286]. In the latter study, the authors implanted porous cylinders prepared from mixtures of 80 % TTCP + 20 % MCP, 80 % TCP + 20 % MCP, and 80 % DCP + 20 % MCP (it is unclear whether MCP and DCP were hydrated or not and whether α- or β-TCP was used), which could have possessed some self-setting abilities. Therefore, the study by Köster et al. [286] could probably be considered as the first biomedical application of the self-setting calcium orthophosphate formulations. However, the real history of this subject started in 1982 [287, 288].

The modern history of ACP [65] began in 1955 [289], while, in 1960, the first mentioning on CDHA in the publication's title occurred [290]. In 1963, an important study on HA preparation was published [291], while, in 1964, the crystal structure of HA was refined [292]. In 1965, thorough investigations of carbonated apatites were started [293]. In 1969, an important paper on a forming method of HA prostheses was published [294], in which the authors hot-pressed HA power into dense and useful shapes. That study might be considered as the earliest one on the fabrication of calcium orthophosphate implants. In 1971, the first study on preparation of biodegradable porous β-TCP scaffolds was published [295]. Therefore, it is not surprising that the term "bioceramics" has been introduced simultaneously. Namely, according to the available databases, the first paper with the term "bioceramics" in the abstract was published in 1971 [296], while the first papers with that in the title were published in 1972 [297, 298]. However, application of the ceramic materials as prostheses had been known before [299–302]. Also, in 1972 [303] and 1973 [304], the first publications on lunar apatites were published. In 1973, the work of Graham and van der Eb showed the first application of calcium orthophosphates in condensation of genetic materials [305]. The researchers demonstrated that calcium orthophosphates could condense DNA and increase the transfection efficiency with a relatively simple procedure. In addition, in 1973, the first study on preparation and implantation of resorbable and porous calcium orthophosphate (it was β-TCP) bioceramics was published [306]. Besides, in 1973, an important book by McConnell was published [307]. In 1975, the modern dental application of calcium orthophosphates began. Namely, β-TCP was applied both in surgically created periodontal defects [308] and as an adjunct to apical closure in pulpless permanent teeth [309], followed by a study of 1979, in which dense HA cylinders were used for immediate tooth root replacement [310]. On April 26, 1988, the first international symposium on bioceramics was held in Kyoto, Japan.

The history of calcium orthophosphate coatings, films, and layers (reviewed in Refs. [311, 312]) began in 1976 [313], while that of calcium orthophosphate-based biocomposites and hybrid biomaterials (reviewed in Ref. [256]) initiated in 1981 [314, 315]. An extensive commercialization of the dental and surgical applications of calcium orthophosphate (mainly, HA) bioceramics occurred in the 1980s, largely due to the pioneering efforts by Jarcho [316–319] in the USA, de Groot [320–322] in Europe, and Aoki [323–326] in Japan. Shortly afterward HA has become a bioceramic of reference in the field of calcium orthophosphates for biomedical applications. The early commercial trademarks, composition, producers, and year comprised Synthograft/Synthos (β-TCP), Miter Inc./J&J (1975); CEROS 80 (HA), Mathys (1980); Durapatite (HA), Cook-Waite (<1981); ProOsteon (coralline HA), Interpore (1981); Alveograf (HA), Cook-Waite (1982); Calcitite (HA), Calcitek (1982); CEROS 82 (β-TCP), Mathys (1982); BioBase (α-TCP), Zimmer (1982); and Periograf (HA), Cook-Waite (<1983) [327]. As seen from this list, preparation and biomedical applications of apatites derived from sea corals [328–330] and bovine bone [331] were already known [332]. In 1985, the first publication on drug-loaded calcium orthophosphate bioceramics [333], as well as those on biphasic, triphasic, and multiphasic calcium orthophosphates (reviewed in Ref. [334]), was published [335, 336]. In 1990, the first version of simulated body fluid (SBF) was introduced [337], while the history of nanodimensional and nanocrystalline calcium orthophosphates (reviewed in Refs. [338, 339]) started in 1994 [340–344]. Finally yet importantly, also in 1994, the first paper on use of calcium orthophosphates as scaffolds was published [345], while applications of calcium orthophosphates in tissue engineering began in 1998 [346–348].

To finalize the twentieth century, it is important to mention the early books on the subject. The earliest collected book of 1983 was edited by de Groot [322], followed by a book of 1984 edited by Misra [349], while three most important monographs on apatites and other calcium orthophosphates were published in 1991 by LeGeros [350] and Aoki [351], as well as in 1994 by Elliott [352]. To get further details on the recent history of calcium orthophosphates, bioceramics, and biomaterials in general, the interested readers are referred to other reviews on the subject [10, 12–15, 250, 262–265].

15.6 Conclusions

To finalize this chapter, let me cite Wikipedia once again: “Historians write in the context of their own time, and with due regard to the current dominant ideas of how to interpret the past, and sometimes write to provide lessons for their own society” [9]. Therefore, all the aforementioned historical facts, discoveries, theories, concepts, misconceptions, and approaches are treated according to the current (AD 2013) level of knowledge on calcium orthophosphates. Thus, it is important to bear in mind that the reported treatment of the historical facts and events might be reconsidered in the future due to both new discoveries and updated points of view. Nevertheless, some solid statements can be made.

The subject of apatites and other calcium orthophosphates has been investigated for almost 250 years. This was a long period of great discoveries and impressive mistakes, original concepts and interesting misconceptions, excellent experiments, and various unfortunates initially of the calcified tissues only and afterward of the chemically pure apatites and other calcium orthophosphates. All these years were spent on gaining the initial knowledge on the subject, followed by its further clarification, extension, and development. These eventful years were full of daily and routine hard work performed by many excellent and of moderate abilities scientists and researchers, students and assistants, technicians, and participants, the vast majority of whom have not even been mentioned in this chapter. Nevertheless, by 1950, the combined long-term efforts of all these often-unknown early investigators created the solid background for a real explosion of science, technology, and biomedical applications of apatites and other calcium orthophosphates that started in the 1960s and continuously prospers up to now, which, finally, resulted in the current state of the art.

As seen from the previously mentioned, the substantial amount of currently available scientific facts and experimental approaches has been known for very many decades, and, in fact, the considerable quantity of relatively recent investigations on calcium orthophosphates is just either a further development of the earlier studies or a rediscovery of the already forgotten information. Since the first commercially produced artificial bone grafts and other types of calcium orthophosphate-containing biomaterials appeared just a few decades ago [316–327], a reasonable question arises: why did it take so long (almost 200 years) to translate the initial knowledge into practice? Presumably, this is a matter of the technological development because both the biomedical and mechanical properties of even the most advanced formulations are still unsatisfactory and incomparable with those of natural bones and teeth. Hopefully, the reported historical overview provides the necessary background that will keep encouraging natural scientists, engineers, and clinicians to rethink and reinvestigate the already forgotten and poorly known facts and approaches for further development of calcium orthophosphate-based formulations.

References

1. Dorozhkin SV (2009) Calcium orthophosphates in nature, biology and medicine. Materials 2:399–498
2. Dorozhkin SV (2011) Calcium orthophosphates: occurrence, properties, biomineralization, pathological calcification and biomimetic applications. Biomatter 1:121–164
3. Calcium (2013) http://en.wikipedia.org/wiki/Calcium. Accessed May 2013
4. Davy H (1808) The Bakerian lecture: on some new phenomena of chemical changes produced by electricity, particularly the decomposition of the fixed alkalies, and the exhibition of the new substances which constitute their bases; and on the general nature of alkaline bodies. Philos Trans R Soc Lond 98:1–44

5. Davy H (1808) Electro-chemical researches on the decomposition of the earths; with observations on the metals obtained from the alkaline earths, and on the amalgam procured from ammonia. Philos Trans R Soc Lond 98:333–370
6. Phosphorus (2013) http://en.wikipedia.org/wiki/Phosphorus. Accessed May 2013
7. de Le phosphore M (1677) Krafft ov liqueur & terra ſeiche de ſa compoſition qui iettent continuellement de grands éclats de lumiere. Le Journal des Sçavans:190–191
8. Robert B (1693) A paper of the honourable Robert Boyl's, deposited with the secretaries of the Royal Society, Octob. 14. 1680. and opened since his death; being an account of his making the phosphorus, etc. Philos Trans 17:583–584
9. History (2013) http://en.wikipedia.org/wiki/History. Accessed May 2013
10. Driskell TD (1994) Early history of calcium phosphate materials and coatings. In: Horowitz E, Parr JE (eds) Characterization and performance of calcium phosphate coatings for implants ASTM STP 1196. American Society for Testing and Materials, Philadelphia, pp 1–9
11. Albee FH, Morrison HF (1920) Studies in bone growth triple calcium phosphate as a stimulus to osteogenesis. Ann Surg 71:32–39
12. Shackelford JF (1999) Bioceramics – an historical perspective. Mater Sci Forum 293:1–4
13. Hulbert SF, Hench LL, Forbers D, Bowman LS (1982) History of bioceramics. Ceram Int 8:131–140
14. Hulbert SF, Hench LL, Forbers D, Bowman LS (1983) History of bioceramics. In: Vincenzini P (ed) Ceramics in surgery. Elsevier, Amsterdam, pp 3–29
15. Shepperd J (2004) The early biological history of calcium phosphates. In: Manley MT, Epinete JA (eds) Fifteen years of clinical experience with hydroxyapatite coatings in joint arthroplasty. Springer, Paris, pp 3–8
16. Leeuwenhoeck M (1674) Microscopical observations concerning blood, milk, bones, the brain, spitle, and cuticula, etc. Philos Trans 9:121–128
17. Anthony L (1677) Microscopical observations of the structure of teeth and other bones. Philos Trans 12:133–142
18. Anthony L (1683) Microscopic observations about animals in the scurf of the teeth, the substance called worms in the nose, the cuticura consisting of scale. Philos Trans 14:1568–1574
19. van Anthony L (1693) Animalcules found on the teeth of the scaleyness of the skin. Philos Trans 17:646–649
20. Anthony L (1697) The eggs of snails, roots of vegetables, teeth, and young oysters. Philos Trans 19:790–799
21. Havers C (1729) Osteologia nova: or, some new observations of the bones, and the PARTS belonging to them; with the manner of their accretion and nutrition, 2nd edn. Royal Society Weſt-End of St. Paul's, London, p 293
22. Fre S (1684) An abstract of a treatise of the calculus humanus. Philos Trans 14:523–533
23. Fourcroy AF (1804) A general system of chemical knowledge; and its application to the phenomena of nature and art, vol XI. Cadell and Davies, London, p 561
24. Roscoe HE, Schorlemmer CA (1881) Treatise on chemistry, vol I. The non-metallic elements. Macmillan and Co., London, p 751
25. Cdell T, Elmsly P (1777) A dictionary of chemistry, vol III. Strand, London, p 666
26. Becket T, de Hondt PA (1770) The monthly review, vol XLII. Strand, London, p 584
27. Klaproth M, Ferber M (1788) Conſeiller des Mines de Pruſſe: Sur l'Analyse de l'Apatit. In: Observations sur la physique, sur l'historie naturelle et sur les arts, avec des planches en taille-douce; dédiées a MGR. le comte d'artois; Par M. l'Abbé Rozier, de pluſieurs Académies; par M. J. A. Mongez le jeune, Chanoine Régulier de Sainte Geneviève, des Académies Royales des Sciences de Rouen, de Dijon, de Lyon, etc. etc. et par M. de la Métherie, Doeteur en Médecine, de pluſieurs Académies. Juillet tome XXXIII. A Paris, au bureau du Journal de Phyſique rue & hôtel Serpênte, pp 313–314
28. Catalogue methodique et raisonné de la collection des fossils de MLLE. Éléonore de Raab. Par M^{R}. de Born. Tome premier. A Vienne. Aux Dépens de J.V. Degen, par I. Alberti 1790, p 504

29. Crell L (1789) Chemische Annalen für die Freunde der Naturlehre, Arznengelahrtheit, Haushaltungskunst und Manufakturen. Helmstadt und Leipzig, in ber J O Müllerschen Buchhandlung, p 568
30. Exchaquet HS (1989) Nouvelle méthode d'obtenir l'acide phoſphorique des os, plus pur que par les procédés ordinaries. Histoire et memoires de la société des sciences physiques de Lausanne. Tome second Années 1784, 1785 & 1786, A Lausanne, Chez Mourer, Libraire, pp 219–227
31. Lavoisier AL (1790) Elements of chemistry, in a new systematic order, containing all the modern discoveries (Translated from the French, by Robert Kerr). Printed for William Creech, and sold in London by G.G. and J.J. Robinsons. Edinburgh, 511 pp
32. Fourcroy AF (1790) Elements of natural history and chemistry. Tranſlated from the ſast Paris Edition, 1789, being the third, in 5 vols 8vo. Vol. III. Aaron C. Jewett, London: Printed for C. Elliot and T. Kay, at Dr. Cullen's Head, No 332. Strand; and C. Elliot, Edinburgh, 594 pp
33. Fourcroy AF (1804) A general system of chemical knowledge; and its application to the phenomena of nature and art, vol III. Cadell and Davies, London, p 472
34. Encyclopaedia Perthensis; or Universal dictionary of the arts, Sciences, literature, &c (1816), vol XVII. Edinburgh, p 720
35. Dundonald AC (1795) A treatise, shewing the intimate connection that subsists between agriculture and chemistry. Addressed to the cultivators of the soil, to the proprietors of fens and mosses, in Great Britain and Ireland, and to the proprietors of West India Estates. by the Earl of Dundonald. London: printed for the author, and sold by R. Edwards, No. 142, New Bond street. March 1795, 252 pp
36. Nisbet W (1805) A general dictionary of chemistry, containing the leading principles of the science, in regard to facts, experiments, and nomenclature. For the use of students. Printed for S. Highley (successor to the late Mr. John Murray). London, No. 24, Fleet-street, 415 pp
37. Murray J (1806) A system of chemistry. In four volumes. Vol. I. Printed for Longman, Hurst, Rees & Orme, London; and William Creech, and A. Constable & Co. Edinburgh. Edinburgh, 592 pp
38. A dictionary of chemistry and mineralogy, with an account of the processes employed in many of the most important chemical manufactures. To which are added a description of chemical apparatus, and various useful tables of weights and measures, chemical instruments, &c. &c. Illustrated with fifteen engravings. By A. & C. R. Aikin. Vol. II. London: Printed for John and Arthur Arch, Couninll; and William Phillips, George Yard, Lombard Street. 1807, 176 pp
39. Bache F (1819) A system of chemistry for the use of students of medicine. Printed and published for the author. William Fry, Philadelphia, p 624
40. Encyclopædia Britannica (1810), vol V. Edinburgh/London, p 797
41. Henry W (1823) The elements of experimental chemistry. The ninth edition, comprehending all the recent discoveries; and illustrated with ten plates by lowry, and several engravings on wood. In two volumes. Vol. I. London; Printed for Baldwin, Cradock, and Joy, Paternoster-row, and R. Hunter, St. Paul's church yard, 639 pp
42. Equivalent weight (2013) http://en.wikipedia.org/wiki/Equivalent_weight. Accessed May 2013
43. Webster JW (1828) A manual of chemistry, on the basis of professor Brande's; containing the principle facts of the science, arranged in the order in which they are discussed and illustrated in the lectures at Harvard University, N.E., The United States Military Academy, West Point; Brown University, Amherst, and several other colleges in the United States. Compiled from the works of the most distinguished chemists. Designed as a text book for the use of students, and persons attending lectures on chemistry. The second edition, comprehending the recent discoveries, and illustrated with nine plates and several engravings on wood. Boston: Published by Richardson and Lord, No. 133, Washington Street, 631 pp
44. Green J (1829) A text book of chemical philosophy. RH Smalt, Philadelphia, p 616
45. Sainte-Claire Deville H, Caron H (1859) On apatite, wagnerite, and some artificial species of metallic phosphates. Philos Mag S 17:128–131

46. Muhlenberg WF (1832) Address in hygiene. In: Transactions of the medical society of the state of Pennsylvania, at its thirty-third annual session, held at Titusville, 10–12 May 1832, vol XIV. Times Printing House, Philadelphia, pp 81–102
47. Graham T (1833) Researches on the arseniates, phosphates, and modifications of phosphoric acid. Philos Trans R Soc Lond 123:253–284
48. Mitscherlich E (1844) Lehrbuch der Chemie. Erster Band. Die Metalloïde. Vierte Auflage, Berlin, p 609
49. Joy CA (1853) Miscellaneous chemical researchers. Inaugural dissertation for the degree of doctor of philosophy, addressed to the philosophical faculty of the University of Göttingen. University Press, Göttingen, p 49
50. Daubrée (1841) Extrait d'un mémoir sur le gisement, la constitution et l'origine des amas de minerai d'étain. Bulletin de la Société Géologique de France. Tome 12, 1840 a 1841. Paris, au lieu des séances de la société, aus du Vieux-Colombier 16, p 567
51. von Kobell F (1841) Instructions for the discrimination of minerals by simple chemical experiments. Richard Griffin & Company and Thomas Tegg, London, p 51
52. Gray A (1841) Elements of chemistry. Dayton and Saxton, School Book Publishers, Corner of Fulton and Nassau Streets Saxton and Pierce, Boston, p 396
53. Pereira J (1854) The elements of materia medica and therapeutics, 4th edn, Encyclopaedia of Materia Medica. Longmans, London, p 831
54. Percy J (1843) Notice of a new hydrated phosphate of lime. Mem Proc Chem Soc 2:222–223
55. Percy J (1845) Notice of a new hydrated phosphate of lime. Philos Mag S26:194–195
56. Berzelius J (1816) Untersuchungen über die Zusammensetzung der Phosphorsäure, der phosphorigen Säure und ihrer Salze. Ann Phys 53:393–446
57. Berzelius J (1845) Ueber basische phosphorsaure Kalkerde. Justus Liebigs Ann Chem 53:286–288
58. Rees GO (1883) On separating the phosphates of lime and magnesia. Philos Mag S2:442–443
59. Baruel M (1838) Analysis of a double phosphate of lead and lime. J Franklin Inst 25:343
60. Jones HB (1845) Contributions to the chemistry of the urine. On the variations in the alkaline and earthy phosphates in the healthy state, and on the alkalescence of the urine from fixed alkalies. Philos Trans R Soc Lond 135:335–349
61. Jones HB (1846) Contributions to the chemistry of the urine. Part II. On the variations in the alkaline and earthy phosphates in disease. Philos Trans R Soc Lond 136:449–459
62. Jones HB (1850) Contributions to the chemistry of the urine. Paper III. Part IV. On the variations of the sulphates and phosphates in disease. Philos Trans R Soc Lond 140:661–668
63. Smith JD (1845) Ueber die Zusammensetzung verschiedener Arten von südamerikanischem Guano, nebst der Beschreibung einer neuen Methode, Ammoniak zu bestimmen, so wie Kalk und Magnesia, wenn sie an Phosphorsäure gebunden sind, zu trennen. J Prakt Chem 35:277–291
64. Lassaigne M (1847) Solubility of phosphate of lime in water saturated with carbonic acid. Philos Mag S30:298
65. Dorozhkin SV (2012) Amorphous calcium orthophosphates: nature, chemistry and biomedical applications. Int J Mater Chem 2:19–46
66. Hassall AH (1859) On the frequent occurrence of phosphate of lime, in the crystalline form, in human urine, and on its pathological importance. Proc R Soc Lond 10:281–288
67. Beale L (1860) A course of lectures on urine, urinary deposits, and calculi. BMJ 205:929–932
68. F (1849) On the method by which the phosphate and carbonate of lime is introduced into the organs of plants. J Franklin Inst 48:156
69. Bischof G (1855) Elements of chemical and physical geology. Translated from the manuscript of the author, by Benjamin H. Paul, F.C.S. vol II. Printed for the Cavendish Society by Harrison & Sons, St. Martins' lane, London, p 523
70. Warington R Jr (1866) Researches on the phosphates of calcium, and upon the solubility of tricalcic phosphate. J Chem Soc 19:296–318
71. Voelcker A (1868) On the solubility of phosphatic materials, with special reference to the practical efficacy of the various forms in which bones are used in agriculture. J R Agric Soc Engl Sec Ser 4:176–196

72. Warington R (1871) On the solubility of the phosphates of bone-ash in carbonic water. J Chem Soc 24:80–83
73. Williams CP (1871) On the solubility of some forms of phosphate of lime. J Franklin Inst 92:419–423
74. An inquiry into the degree of solubility requisite in manures, with special reference to precipitated calcic and magnesic phosphates. Nature 27:325–326 (1883)
75. Wilson G (1850) Chemistry. William and Robert Chambers, Edinburgh, p 316
76. Jenkins EE (1853) Phosphate of lime. M.D. thesis, Medical College of the State of South Carolina, p 32
77. Brande WT, Taylor AS (1863) Chemistry. Blanchard and Lea, Philadelphia, p 696
78. Morfit C (1855) On Colombian guano; and certain peculiarities in the chemical behavior of "bone phosphate of lime". J Franklin Inst 30:325–329
79. Warington R (1843) On a curious change in the composition of bones taken from the guano. Mem Proc Chem Soc 2:223–226
80. Warington R (1873) On the decomposition of tricalcic phosphate by water. J Chem Soc 26:983–989
81. Fresenius R (1867) Ueber die Bestimmung der Phosphorsäure im Phosphorit nebst Mittheilung der Analysen des Phosphorits und Staffelits aus dem Lahnthal. Z Anal Chem 6:403–409
82. Lorah JR, Tartar HV, Wood L (1929) A basic phosphate of calcium and of strontium and the adsorption of calcium hydroxide by basic calcium phosphate and by tricalcium phosphate. J Am Chem Soc 51:1097–1106
83. Wells HG (1906) Pathological calcification. J Med Res 14:491–525
84. Roscoe HE, Schorlemmer C (1879) A treatise on chemistry, vol II. Metals. Part 1. Macmillan and Co., London, p 504
85. Hassall A (1852) On the detection and preservation of crystalline deposits of uric acid, urate of ammonia, phosphate of lime, triple phosphate, oxalate of lime, and other salts. Lancet 59:466–467
86. Abel FA (1862) On the occurrence of considerable deposits of crystallized phosphate of lime in teak-wood. J Chem Soc 15:91–93
87. Reichardt E (1872) Ueber neutralen phosphorsauren Kalk, Darstellung und Löslichkeit desselben. Z Anal Chem 11:275–277
88. Stammer C (1863) Bestimmung kohlensauren Kalkes neben phosphorsaurem Kalk. Z Anal Chem 2:96–97
89. Roussin Z (1868) Prüfung des Wismuthsubnitrats auf eine Verfälschung mit Kalkphosphat. Z Anal Chem 7:511
90. Birnbaum K, Chojnacki C (1870) Ueber die Bestimmung der Phosphorsäure in Phosphoriten. Z Anal Chem 9:203–207
91. Graeser P (1870) Maassanalytische Bestimmung der Phosphorsäure in Phosphoriten. Z Anal Chem 9:355–357
92. Janovsky JV (1872) Ueber die verschiedenen Methoden der Phosphorsäure-Bestimmung neben Eisenoxyd, Thonerde, Kalk und Magnesia. Z Anal Chem 11:153–167
93. Zur T (1875) Bestimmung des Jods in Phosphoriten. Z Anal Chem 14:97
94. Maly R (1876) Eine Methode zur alkalimetrischen Bestimmung der Phosphorsäure und der alkalischen Phosphate. Z Anal Chem 15:417–425
95. Pellet H (1882) Die Zusammensetzung des Niederschlags, welcher durch Ammoniak aus sauren Lösungen von Phosphorsäure, Baryt, Kalk und Magnesia gefällt wird. Z Anal Chem 21:261
96. Stokvis BJ, Salkowski E, Smith WG (1888) Ueber die Löslichkeitsverhältnisse des phosphorsauren Kalks im Harn. Z Anal Chem 23:273–274
97. Ott A (1886) Die Löslichkeitsverhältnisse des phosphorsauren Kalks im Harn. Z Anal Chem 25:279–280
98. Kennepohl G (1889) Zur Bestimmung von Eisenoxyd und Thonerde neben Kalk und Phosphorsäure. Z Anal Chem 28:343

99. Immendorff H, Reitmair O (1892) Zur Bestimmung des Kalks in Gegenwart von Phosphorsäure, Eisen, Thonerde und Mangan. Z Anal Chem 31:313–316
100. Fingerling G, Grombach A (1907) Eine neue Modifikation der Bestimmung der zitratlöslichen Phosphorsäure in den Futterkalken nach Petermann. Z Anal Chem 46:756–760
101. Schulze B (1911) Untersuchung des phosphorsauren Futterkalkes. Z Anal Chem 50:126–127
102. Hinden F (1915) Anreicherungsmethode zur Bestimmung der Phosphorsäure in phosphorsäurearmen Kalksteinen. Z Anal Chem 54:214–216
103. Mohr C (1884) Ueber die quantitative Bestimmung der zurückgegangenen Phosphorsäure und der Phosphorsäure im Dicalciumphosphat. Z Anal Chem 23:487–491
104. Glaser C (1885) Bemerkungen zu der Abhandlung des Herrn Carl Mohr über die quantitative Bestimmung der zurückgegangenen Phosphorsäure und der Phosphorsäure im Dicalciumphosphat. Z Anal Chem 24:180
105. Hutchings WM (1887) Occurrence of apatite in slag. Nature 36:460
106. Hilgenstock G (1883) Eine neue Verbindung von P_2O_5 und CaO. Stahl und Eisen 3:498
107. Hilgenstock G (1887) Das vierbasische Kalkphosphat und die Basicitätsstufe des Silicats in der Thomas-Schlacxke. Stahl und Eisen 7:557–560
108. Scheibler C (1886) Ueber die Herstellung reicher Kalkphosphate in Verbindung mit einer Verbesserung des Thomasprocesses. Ber Dtsch Chem Ges 19:1883–1893
109. Tzschucke H (1888) Versuch einer directen Bestimmung der Phosphorsäure als dreibasisch phosphorsauren Kalk. Angew Chem 1:383–385
110. Georgievics GV (1891) Über das Verhalten des Tricalciumphosphats gegen Kohlensäure und Eisenhydroxyd. Monatsh Chem 12:566–581
111. Duncan A Jr (1803) The Edinburgh new dispensatory: containing, I. The Elements of Pharmaceutical Chemistry. II. The Materia Medica; or, the Natural, Pharmaceutical and Medical Hiſtory of the different Subſtances employed in Medicine. III. The Pharmaceutical Preparations and Compositions; including complete and accurate translations of the Octavo Edition of the London Pharmacopoeia, published in 1803. Illuſtrated and Explained in the Language and according to the Principles of Modern Chemistry. Printed for Bell & Bradfute; G. & J. Robinson, London; and Gilbert & Hodges, Dublin. Edinburgh, 710 pp
112. Pusey P (1846) On superphosphate of lime. J R Agric Soc Engl 6:324–328
113. Kennedy JCG (1864) Agriculture of the United States in 1860. GPO, Washington, DC, p 292
114. Fresenius R (1868) Zur Analyse der Superphosphate. Z Anal Chem 1868(7):304–309
115. Chesshire JA, Hughes J, Sutton F, Sibson A (1870) Ueber die Bestimmung des Betrags an "reducirten" Phosphaten in Superphosphaten. Z Anal Chem 9:524–527
116. Rümpler A (1873) Ueber eisen- und thonerdehaltige Superphosphate und deren analytische Untersuchung. Z Anal Chem 12:151–163
117. Albert H, Siegfried L (1877) Beiträge zur Werthbestimmung der Superphosphate. Z Anal Chem 16:182–188
118. Albert H, Siegfried L (1879) Beiträge zur Werthbestimmung der Superphosphate. Z Anal Chem 18:220–224
119. Pavec A (1879) Zur maassanalytischen Bestimmung der Phosphorsäure im Superphosphat und Spodium mittelst Uranlösung. Z Anal Chem 18:360–361
120. Mohr C (1880) Ein maassanalytisches Bestimmungsverfahren der in Rohphosphaten und Superphosphaten enthaltenen Phosphorsäure mit Uran bei Gegenwart von Eisenoxyd. Z Anal Chem 19:150–153
121. Erlenmeyer E, Wattenberg H, Wein E, Rösch L, Lehmann J, Johnson SW, Jenkins EH (1880) Zur Analyse der Superphosphate. Z Anal Chem 19:243–246
122. Meyer CF (1881) Weitere Mittheilungen über das Zurückgehen der eisen- und thonerdehaltigen Superphosphate – Berichtigung. Z Anal Chem 19:309–311
123. Drewsen S (1881) Zur Bestimmung der löslichen Phosphorsäure in Superphosphaten. Z Anal Chem 20:54–57
124. Lloyd FJ (1882) On the estimation of retrograde phosphates. J Chem Soc Trans 41:306–317
125. Mollenda A (1883) Eine neue Methode zur maassanalytischen Bestimmung der Phosphorsäure in den Superphosphaten. Z Anal Chem 22:155–159

126. Phillips WB (1884) Rate of reversion in superphosphates prepared from red Navassa rock. J Am Chem Soc 6:224–228
127. Wagner P (1886) Eine neue Methode zur Feststellung des Handelswerthes der Superphosphate. Z Anal Chem 25:272–278
128. Emmerling A (1887) Eine Methode zur Bestimmung der wasserlöslichen Phosphorsäure in Superphosphaten auf maassanalvtischem Wege. Z Anal Chem 26:244–247
129. Stoklasa J (1890) Bestimmung des Wassers in den Superphosphaten. I Z Anal Chem 29:390–397
130. Crispo D (1891) Belgische Methode zur Bestimmung der in Wasser löslichen Phosphorsäure in den Superphosphaten. Z Anal Chem 30:301–303
131. Güssefeld O (1892) Eine Schüttelmaschine für die Analyse von Superphosphaten. Z Anal Chem 31:556
132. Keller A (1893) Eine Schüttelmaschine für Superphosphaten. Z Anal Chem 32:590–591
133. Kalmann W, Meissels K (1894) Eine Methode zur maassanalytischen Schätzung der wasserlöslichen Phosphorsäure in Superphosphaten. Z Anal Chem 33:764–766
134. Glaser C (1895) Zur maassanalytischen Bestimmung der wasserlöslichen Phosphorsäure in Superphosphaten. Z Anal Chem 34:768–769
135. Seib O (1905) Bestimmung der zitratlöslichen Phosphorsäure in Superphosphaten. Z Anal Chem 44:397–398
136. Cameron FK, Bell JM (1906) The phosphates of calcium, III; Superphosphate. J Am Chem Soc 28:1222–1229
137. C (1877) Vitreous phosphate of lime. J Franklin Inst 104:315
138. Church AH (1873) New analyses of certain mineral arseniates and phosphates. 1. Apatite; 2. Arseniosiderite; 3. Childrenite; 4. Ehlite; 5. Tyrolite; 6. Wavellite. J Chem Soc 26:101–111
139. Felton LD, Kauffmann G, Stahl HJ (1935) The precipitation of bacterial polysaccharides with calcium phosphate. Pneumococcus. J Bacteriol 29:149–161
140. Row R (1903) On some effects of the constituents of Ringer's circulating fluid on skeletal muscular contractions in Rana hexadactyla. J Physiol 29:440–450
141. Ringer S (1882) Concerning the influence exerted by each of the constituents of the blood on the contraction of the ventricle. J Physiol 3:380–393
142. Ringer S (1886) A further contribution regarding the effect of minute quantities of inorganic salts on organised structures. J Physiol 7:118–127
143. Ringer S, Buxton DW (1887) Concerning the action of calcium, potassium, and sodium salts upon the eel's heart and upon the skeletal muscles of the frog. J Physiol 8:15–19
144. Ringer S (1887) Regarding the action of lime potassium and sodium salts on skeletal muscle. J Physiol 8:20–24
145. Ringer S (1893) The influence of carbonic acid dissolved in saline solutions on the ventricle of the frog's heart. J Physiol 14:125–130
146. Cameron FK, Hurst LA (1904) The action of water and saline solutions upon certain slightly soluble phosphates. J Am Chem Soc 26:885–913
147. Cameron FK, Seidell A (1904) The action of water upon the phosphates of calcium. J Am Chem Soc 26:1454–1463
148. Cameron FK, Seidell A (1905) The phosphates of calcium. I. J Am Chem Soc 27:1503–1512
149. Cameron FK, Bell JM (1905) The phosphates of calcium. II. J Am Chem Soc 27:1512–1514
150. Cameron FK, Bell JM (1910) The phosphates of calcium. IV. J Am Chem Soc 32:869–873
151. Cameron FK, McCaughey WJ (1911) Apatite and spodiosite. J Phys Chem 15:463–470
152. Mebane WM, Dobbins JT, Cameron FK (1929) The solubility of the phosphates of calcium in aqueous solutions of sulfur dioxide. J Phys Chem 33:961–969
153. Hughes AE, Cameron FK (1931) Action of sulfur dioxide on phosphates of calcium. Ind Eng Chem 23:1262–1271
154. Bassett H Jr (1907) Beiträge zum Studium der Calciumphosphate. I. Die Hydrate der Calcium-Hydroorthophosphate. Z Anorg Chem 53:34–48
155. Bassett H Jr (1907) Beiträge zum Studium der Calciumphosphate. II. Die Einwirkung von Ammoniakgas auf Calcium-Hydroorthophosphate. Z Anorg Chem 53:49–62

156. Bassett H Jr (1908) Beiträge zum Studium der Calciumphosphate. III. Das System CaO – P2O5–H2O. Z Anorg Chem 59:1–55
157. Bassett H Jr (1917) The phosphates of calcium. Part IV. The basic phosphates. J Chem Soc 111:620–642
158. Norton TH, Newman HE (1897) On a soluble compound of hydrastine with monocalcium phosphate. J Am Chem Soc 19:838–840
159. Bell JM (1910) The rate of extraction of plant food constituents from the phosphates of calcium and from a loam soil. J Am Chem Soc 32:879–884
160. Rolfe BH (1911) Autunite (hydrated uranium-calcium phosphate). Lancet 177:766
161. Meigs EB (1915) The osmotic properties of calcium and magnesium phosphate in relation to those of living cells. Am J Physiol 38:456–489
162. Withers WA, Field AL (1915) A conductivity study of the reaction between calcium nitrate and dipotassium phosphate in dilute solution. J Am Chem Soc 37:1091–1105
163. Wendt GL, Clarke AH (1923) An electrometric study of the neutralization of phosphoric acid by calcium hydroxide. J Am Chem Soc 45:881–887
164. de Toni GM (1921) Ueber kolloides Kalziumphosphat. Kolloid Z 28:145–148
165. Gaubert P (1922) Sur les cristaux liquides de phosphate de calcium. Cr Hebd Acad Sci 174:1115–1117
166. Shipley PG, Kramer B, Howland J (1926) Studies upon calcification *in vitro*. Biochem J 20:379–387
167. von Oettingen WF, Pickett RE (1932) The effect of phosphate and bicarbonate buffers on the ionization of calcium salts in physiologic salt solutions. J Pharmacol Exp Ther 44:435–443
168. Benjamin HR (1933) The forms of the calcium and inorganic phosphorus in human and animal sera II. The nature and significance of the filtrable, adsorbable calcium-phosphorus complex. J Biol Chem 100:57–78
169. Ramsay AA (1917) The solubility of calcium phosphates in citric acid. J Agric Sci 8:277–298
170. Shear MJ, Kramer B (1928) Composition of bone. III Physicochemical mechanism. J Biol Chem 79:125–145
171. Trömel G, Möller H (1932) Die Bildung schwerlöslicher Calciumphosphate aus wäßriger Lösung und die Beziehungen dieser Phosphate zur Apatitgruppe. Z Anorg Allg Chem 206:227–240
172. Larson HWE (1935) Preparation and properties of mono-, di-, and tricalcium phosphates. Ind Eng Chem Anal Ed 7:401–406
173. Elsenberger S, Lehrman A, Turner WD (1940) The basic calcium phosphates and related systems. Some theoretical and practical aspects. Chem Rev 26:257–296
174. MacIntire WH, Wintrerberg SH, Marshall HL, Palmer G, Fetzer WR (1944) Industrial precipitated tricalcium phosphates. Ind Eng Chem 36:547–552
175. Brasseur H, Dallemagne MJ, Melon J (1946) Chemical nature of salts from bones and teeth and of tricalcium phosphate precipitates. Nature 157:453
176. MacIntire WH, Palmer G, Marshall HL (1945) A "reference" precipitated tricalcium phosphate hydrate. Ind Eng Chem 37:164–169
177. Mehmel M (1930) Über die Struktur des Apatits. Z Kristallogr 75:323–331
178. Náray-Szabó S (1930) The structure of apatite $(CaF)Ca_4(PO_4)_3$. Z Kristallogr 75:387–398
179. Hendricks SB, Hill WL, Jacob KD, Jefferson ME (1931) Structural characteristics of apatite-like substances and composition of phosphate rock and bone as determined from microscopical and X-ray diffraction. Ind Eng Chem 23:1413–1418
180. Gruner JW, McConnell D (1937) The problem of the carbonate-apatites. The structure of francolite. Z Kristallogr 97:208–215
181. McConnell D (1938) The problem of the carbonate apatites; a carbonate oxy-apatite (dahllite). Am J Sci 36:296–303
182. Terpstra P (1937) On the crystallography of brushite. Z Kristallogr 97:229–233
183. Hodge HC, Lefevre ML, Bale WF (1938) Chemical and X-ray diffraction studies of calcium phosphates. Ind Eng Chem Anal Ed 10:156–161

184. McConnell D (1938) A structural investigation of the isomorphism of the apatite group. Am Mineral 23:1–19
185. Holt LE, la Mer VK, Chown HB (1925) Studies in calcification I. The solubility product of secondary and tertiary calcium phosphate under various conditions. J Biol Chem 64:509–565
186. Holt LE, la Mer VK, Chown HB (1925) Studies in calcification II. Delayed equilibrium between the calcium phosphates and its biological significance. J Biol Chem 64:567–578
187. Holt LE, Gittleman I (1925) The solubility of tertiary calcium phosphate in cerebrospinal fluid. J Biol Chem 66:23–28
188. Stollenwerk W (1926) Untersuchungen über die Löslichkeit des Monocalciumphosphats in Wasser. Z Anorg Allg Chem 156:37–55
189. Sendroy J, Hastings AB (1927) Studies of the solubility of calcium salts II. The solubility of tertiary calcium phosphate in salt solutions and biological fluids. J Biol Chem 71:783–796
190. Sendroy J, Hastings AB (1927) Studies of the solubility of calcium salts III. The solubility of calcium carbonate and tertiary calcium phosphate under various conditions. J Biol Chem 71:797–846
191. Csapo J (1927) The influence of proteins on the solubility of calcium phosphate. J Biol Chem 75:509–515
192. Clark NA (1931) The system P_2O_5–CaO–H_2O and the recrystallization of monocalcium phosphate. J Phys Chem 35:1232–1238
193. Lugg JWH (1931) A study of aqueous salt solutions in equilibrium with solid secondary calcium phosphate at 40 °C. Trans Faraday Soc 27:297–309
194. Logan MA, Taylor HL (1937) Solubility of bone salt. J Biol Chem 119:293–307
195. Logan MA, Taylor HL (1938) Solubility of bone salt: II Factors affecting its formation. J Biol Chem 125:377–390
196. Logan MA, Taylor HL (1938) Solubility of bone salt: III Partial solution of bone and carbonate-containing calcium phosphate precipitates. J Biol Chem 125:391–397
197. Logan MA, Kane LW (1939) Solubility of bone salt: IV Solubility of bone in biological fluids. J Biol Chem 127:705–710
198. Greenwald I (1942) The solubility of calcium phosphate I The effect of pH and of amount of solid phase. J Biol Chem 143:703–710
199. Greenwald I (1942) The solubility of calcium phosphate II The solubility product. J Biol Chem 143:711–714
200. Kuyper AC (1945) The chemistry of bone formation I. The composition of precipitates formed from salt solutions. J Biol Chem 159:411–416
201. Kuyper AC (1945) The chemistry of bone formation II. Some factors which affect the solubility of calcium phosphate in blood serum. J Biol Chem 159:417–424
202. Jenkins GN, Forster MG (1948) The solubility of calcium phosphate and dental tissues in incubated mixtures of saliva and flours of different extraction rates. Biochem J 42:lvi
203. Rae JJ, Clegg CT (1948) The effect of various inorganic salts on the solubility of calcium phosphate, tooth enamel, and whole teeth in lactic acid. J Dent Res 27:52
204. Rae JJ, Clegg CT (1948) Changes in the calcium and phosphate concentrations of saliva and inorganic salt solutions on shaking with calcium phosphate. J Dent Res 27:54–57
205. Muhler JC, Boyd TM, van Huysen G (1950) Effect of fluorides and other compounds on the solubility of enamel, dentin, and tricalcium phosphate in dilute acids. J Dent Res 29:182–193
206. Ericsson Y (1949) Enamel-apatite solubility: investigations into the calcium phosphate equilibrium between enamel and saliva and its relation to dental caries. Stockholm, p 139
207. Whittier EO (1933) Buffer intensities of milk and milk constituents II. Buffer action of calcium phosphate. J Biol Chem 102:733–747
208. Bredig MA, Franck HH, Fülnder H (1932) Beiträge zur Kenntnis der Kalk-Phosphorsäure-Verbindungen. II. Z Elktrochem Angew 38:158–164
209. Trömel G (1932) Beiträge zur Kenntnis des Systems Kalziumoxyd-Phosphorpentoxyd. Mitt Kaiser-Wilhelm-Inst, Eisenforsch, Düsseldorf 14:25–34
210. Jansen W (1933) Über die Reduktion des Tricalciumphosphates. Z Anorg Allg Chem 210:113–124

211. Keenen FG (1930) Reactions occurring during the ammoniation of superphosphate. Ind Eng Chem 22:1378–1382
212. Keenen FG (1932) Available phosphoric acid content of ammoniated superphosphate. Ind Eng Chem 24:44–49
213. MacIntire WH, Shaw WM (1932) Chemical changes in mixtures of superphosphate with dolomite and with limestone. Ind Eng Chem 24:933–941
214. MacIntire WH, Shaw WM (1932) Reactivity between dolomite and superphosphate components. Ind Eng Chem 24:1401–1409
215. White LM, Hardesty JO, Ross WH (1935) Ammoniation of double superphosphate. Ind Eng Chem 27:563–567
216. Hill WL, Hendricks SB (1936) Composition and properties of superphosphate – calcium phosphate and calcium sulfate constituents as shown by chemical and X-ray diffraction analysis. Ind Eng Chem 28:440–447
217. Copson RL, Newton RH, Lindsay JD (1936) Superphosphate manufacture – mixing phosphate rook with concentrated phosphoric acid. Ind Eng Chem 28:923–927
218. Newton RH, Copson RL (1936) Superphosphate manufacture – composition of superphosphate made from phosphate rock and concentrated phosphoric acid. Ind Eng Chem 28:1182–1186
219. Beeson KC, Jacob KD (1938) Chemical reactions in fertilizer mixtures – reactions of calcined phosphate with ammonium sulfate and superphosphate. Ind Eng Chem 30:304–308
220. Whittaker CW, Lundstrom FO, Shimp JH (1934) Action of urea on calcium orthophosphates. Ind Eng Chem 26:1307–1311
221. Southard JC, Milner RT (1935) Low temperature specific heats. V. The heat capacity of tricalcium phosphate between 15 and 298 degrees K. J Am Chem Soc 57:983–984
222. Nagelschmidt G (1937) A new calcium silicophosphate. J Chem Soc:865–867
223. McConnell D (1937) The substitution of SiO_4- and SO_4-groups for PO_4-groups in the apatite structure; ellestadite, the end-member. Am Mineral 22:977–989
224. Hill WL, Hendricks SB, Jefferson ME, Reynolds DS (1937) Phosphate fertilizers by calcination process. Composition of defluorinated phosphate. Ind Eng Chem 29:1299–1304
225. Marshall HL, Reynolds DS, Jacob KD, Tremearne TH (1937) Phosphate fertilizers by calcination process. Reversion of defluorinated phosphate at temperatures below 1400 °C. Ind Eng Chem 29:1294–1298
226. Curtis HA, Copson RL, Brown EH, Pole GR (1937) Fertilizer from rock phosphate conversion by fusion and treatment with water vapor. Ind Eng Chem 29:766–771
227. MacIntire WH, Hammond JW (1938) Removal of fluorides from natural waters by calcium phosphates. Ind Eng Chem 30:160–162
228. Adler H, Klein G, Lindsay FK (1938) Removal of fluorides from potable water by tricalcium phosphate. Ind Eng Chem 30:163–165
229. Behrman AS, Gustafson H (1938) Removal of fluorine from water – a development in the use of tricalcium phosphate. Ind Eng Chem 30:1011–1013
230. Moore LA (1942) Activation of dicalcium phosphate for the chromatographic determination of carotene. Ind Eng Chem 14:707–708
231. Elmore KL, Farr TD (1940) Equilibrium in the system calcium oxide–phosphorus pentoxide–water. Ind Eng Chem 32:580–586
232. Arnold PW (1950) The nature of precipitated calcium phosphates. Trans Faraday Soc 46:1061–1072
233. Frondel C (1941) Whitlockite: a new calcium phosphate, $Ca_3(PO_4)_2$. Am Mineral 26:145–152
234. Salk JE (1941) Partial purification of the virus of epidemic influenza by adsorption on calcium phosphate. Proc Soc Exp Biol Med 46:709–712
235. Salk JE (1945) The immunizing effect of calcium phosphate adsorbed influenza virus. Science 101:122–124
236. Stanley WM (1945) The precipitation of purified concentrated influenza virus and vaccine on calcium phosphate. Science 101:332–335

237. Hill WL, Hendricks SB, Fox EJ, Cady JG (1947) Acid pyro- and metaphosphates produced by thermal decomposition of monocalcium phosphate. Ind Eng Chem 39:1667–1672
238. Egan EP Jr, Wakefield ZT, Elmore KL (1950) High-temperature heat content of hydroxyapatite. J Am Chem Soc 72:2418–2421
239. Greenwald I (1944) Anomalous effects in the titration of phosphoric acid with calcium hydroxide. J Am Chem Soc 66:1305–1306
240. Ratner BD (2012) A history of biomaterials. In: Ratner BD, Hoffman AS, Schoen FJ, Lemons JE (eds) Biomaterials science: an introduction to materials in medicine, 3rd edn. Academic Press, San Diego, pp xli–liii
241. Jacoby M (2001) Custom-made biomaterials. Chem Eng News 79:30–35
242. Huebsch N, Mooney DJ (2009) Inspiration and application in the evolution of biomaterials. Nature 462:426–432
243. Popp H (1939) Zur Geschichte der Prosthesen. Med Welt 13:961–964
244. Ring ME (1992) Dentistry: an illustrated history. Harry N Abrams, New York, p 320
245. Bobbio A (1972) The first endosseous alloplastic implant in the history of man. Bull Hist Dent 20:1–6
246. Crubezy E, Murail P, Girard L, Bernadou JP (1998) False teeth of the Roman world. Nature 391:29
247. van Meekeren J (1668) Heel'-en geneeskonstige aanmerkingen. Commelijn, Amsterdam
248. von Walter P (1821) Wiedereinheilung der bei der Trapanation ausgebohrten Knochenscheibe. J Chir Augen Heilkunde 2:571
249. Macewen W (1881) Observations concerning transplantation of bone. Illustrated by a case of inter-human osseous transplantation, whereby over two-thirds of the shaft of a humerus was restored. Proc R Soc Lond 32:232–247
250. de Boer HH (1988) The history of bone grafts. Clin Orthop Relat Res 226:292–298
251. Hunter J (1771) The natural history of the human teeth: explaining their structure, use, formation, growth, and diseases. Printed for J. Johnson, No 72. St. Paul's Church-yard, London, 191 pp
252. Hoffman-Axthelm W (1981) History of dentistry. Quintessence, Chicago, p 436
253. Wildgoose DG, Johnson A, Winstanley RB (2004) Glass/ceramic/refractory techniques, their development and introduction into dentistry: a historical literature review. J Prosthet Dent 91:136–143
254. Cravens JE (1876) Lacto-phosphate of lime; pathology and treatment of exposed dental pulps and sensitive dentine. Dent Cosmos 18:463–476
255. Pendleton LW (1873) The lacto-phosphate of lime. Trans Maine Med Assoc 4:313–318
256. Dorozhkin SV (2011) Biocomposites and hybrid biomaterials based on calcium orthophosphates. Biomatter 1:3–56
257. Nicholson W (1808) A dictionary of practical and theoretical chemistry, with its application to the arts and manufactures, and to the explanation of the phænomena of nature: including throughout the latest discoveries, and the present state of knowledge on those subjects. With plates and tables. Printed for Richard Phillips, No. 6, Bridge-street
258. Dreesmann H (1892) Ueber Knochenplombierung. Beitr Klin Chir 9:804–810
259. Gluck T (1891) Referat über die durch das moderne chirurgische. Langenbecks Arch Klin Chir 41:187–239
260. Muster D (1990) Themistocles Gluck, Berlin 1890: a pioneer of multidisciplinary applied research into biomaterials for endoprostheses. Bull Hist Dent 38:3–6
261. Eynon-Lewis NJ, Ferry D, Pearse MF (1992) Themistocles Gluck: an unrecognised genius. BMJ 305:1534–1536
262. Weinberger BW (1948) An introduction to the history of dentistry with medical and dental chronology and bibliographic data. The CV Mosby Company, St. Louis, p 992
263. Baden E (1955) Prosthetic therapy of congenital and acquired clefts on the palate: an historical essay. J Hist Med Alld Sci 10:290–301
264. Ratner BD, Bryant SJ (2004) Biomaterials: where we have been and where we are going. Annu Rev Biomed Eng 6:41–75

265. Dammaschke T (2008) The history of direct pulp capping. J Hist Dent 56:9–23
266. Albee FH (1915) Bone-graft surgery. WB Saunders Company, Philadelphia/London, p 417
267. Hey Groves EW (1927) Some contributions to the reconstructive surgery of the hip. Br J Surg 14:486–517
268. Murray CR (1931) Delayed and non-union in fractures in the adult. Ann Surg 93:961–967
269. Murray CR (1931) The modern conception of bone formation and its relation to surgery. J Dent Res 11:837–845
270. Huggins C (1931) The formation of bone under the influence of epithelium of the urinary tract. Arch Surg 22:377–408
271. Levander G (1934) On the formation of new bone in bone transplantation. Acta Chir Scand 74:425–426
272. Levander G (1938) A study of bone regeneration. Surg Gynecol Obstet 67:705–714
273. Haldeman KO, Moore JM (1934) Influence of a local excess of calcium and phosphorus on the healing of fractures-an experimental study. Arch Surg 29:385–396
274. Stewart WJ (1934) Experimental bone regeneration using lime salts and autogenous grafts as sources of available calcium. Surg Gynecol Obstet 59:867–871
275. Key JA (1934) The effect of a local calcium depot on osteogenesis and healing of fractures. J Bone Joint Surg 16:176–184
276. Shands AR Jr (1937) Studies in bone formation: the effect of the local presence of calcium salts on osteogenesis. J Bone Joint Surg 19:1065–1076
277. Schram WR, Fosdick LS (1948) Stimulation of healing in long bones by use of artificial material. J Oral Surg 6:209–217
278. Ray RD, Ward AA Jr (1951) A preliminary report on studies of basic calcium phosphate in bone replacement. Surg Form 3:429–434
279. McClendon JF, Carpousis A (1945) Prevention of dental caries by brushing the teeth with powdered fluorapatite. J Dent Res 24:199
280. Earle WR, Schilling EL, Stark TH, Straus NP, Brown MF, Shelton E (1943) Production of malignancy *in vitro* IV. The mouse fibroblast cultures and changes seen in the living cells. J Natl Cancer Inst 4:165–212
281. Hanks JH, Wallace RE (1949) Relation of oxygen and temperature in the preservation of tissues by refrigeration. Proc Soc Exp Biol Med 71:196–200
282. Kingery WD II (1950) Cold-setting properties. J Am Ceram Soc 33:242–246
283. Dorozhkin SV (2009) Calcium orthophosphate cements and concretes. Materials 2:221–291
284. Dorozhkin SV (2011) Self-setting calcium orthophosphate formulations: cements, concretes, pastes and putties. Int J Mater Chem 1:1–48
285. Driskell TD, Heller AL, Koenigs JF (1975) Dental treatments. US Patent 3,913,229, 21 Oct 1975
286. Köster K, Karbe E, Kramer H, Heide H, König R (1976) Experimenteller Knochenersatz durch resorbierbare Calciumphosphat-Keramik. Langenbecks Arch Chir 341:77–86
287. LeGeros RZ, Chohayeb A, Shulman A (1982) Apatitic calcium phosphates: possible dental restorative materials. J Dent Res Spec Iss 61:343
288. Brown WE, Chow LC (1983) A new calcium phosphate setting cement. J Dent Res Spec Iss 62:672
289. Robinson RA, Watson ML (1955) Crystal-collagen relationships in bone as observed in the electron microscope III Crystal and collagen morphology as a function of age. Ann NY Acad Sci 60:596–660
290. Posner AS, Stutman JM, Lippincott ER (1960) Hydrogen-bonding in calcium-deficient hydroxyapatites. Nature 188:486–487
291. Hayek E, Newesely H (1963) Pentacalcium monohydroxyorthophosphate (hydroxylapatite). In: Kleinberg J (ed) Inorganic syntheses, vol VII. McGraw-Hill Book Company Inc., New York, pp 63–65
292. Kay MI, Young RA, Posner AS (1964) Crystal structure of hydroxyapatite. Nature 204:1050–1052

293. LeGeros RZ (1965) Effect of carbonate on the lattice parameters of apatite. Nature 206:403–404
294. Levitt SR, Crayton PH, Monroe EA, Condrate RA (1969) Forming methods for apatite prostheses. J Biomed Mater Res 3:683–684
295. Bhaskar SN, Brady JM, Getter L, Grower MF, Driskell T (1971) Biodegradable ceramic implants in bone. Electron and light microscopic analysis. Oral Surg Oral Med Oral Pathol 32:336–346
296. Blakeslee KC, Condrate RA Sr (1971) Vibrational spectra of hydrothermally prepared hydroxyapatites. J Am Ceram Soc 54:559–563
297. Garrington GE, Lightbody PM (1972) Bioceramics and dentistry. J Biomed Mater Res 6:333–343
298. Cini L, Sandrolini S, Paltrinieri M, Pizzoferrato A, Trentani C (1972) Materiali bioceramici in funzione sostitutiva. Nota preventiva. [Bioceramic materials for replacement purposes. Preliminary note]. Chir Organi Mov 60:423–430
299. Rivault MA (1966) Evolution, conception et technologie des travaux de prothèse fixe, réalisés en céramo-métallique. [Evolution, conception and technology of fixed prosthesis made of ceramic and metal]. Rev Fr Odontostomatol 13:1367–1402
300. Dumont A, Appel M, Favard E (1968) Prothèses plurales en céramique sur métal. Soudage et artifices de jonction. [Multiple prostheses made of ceramics on metal. Soldering and artifacts of the junction]. Ann Odontostomatol (Lyon) 25:231–240
301. Hulbert SF, Young FA, Mathews RS, Klawitter JJ, Talbert CD, Stelling FH (1970) Potential of ceramic materials as permanently implantable skeletal prostheses. J Biomed Mater Res 4:433–456
302. Hench LL, Splinter RJ, Allen WC, Greenlee TK (1971) Bonding mechanisms at the interface of ceramic prosthetic materials. J Biomed Mater Res 2:117–141
303. Griffin WL, Åmli R, Heier KS (1972) Whitlockite and apatite from lunar rock 14310 and from Ödegården, Norway. Earth Planet Sci Lett 15:53–58
304. Reed GW Jr, Jovanovic S (1973) Fluorine in lunar samples: implications concerning lunar fluorapatite. Geochim Cosmochim Acta 37:1457–1462
305. Graham FL, van der Eb AJ (1973) A new technique for the assay of infectivity of human adenovirus 5 DNA. Virology 52:456–467
306. Driskell TD, Hassler CR, Tennery VJ, McCoy LR, Clarke WJ (1973) Calcium phosphate resorbable ceramics: a potential alternative to bone grafting. J Dent Res 52:123
307. McConnell D (1973) Apatite its crystal chemistry, mineralogy, utilization, and geologic and biologic occurrences, vol 5, Applied mineralogy. Springer, New York, p 111
308. Nery EB, Lynch KL, Hirthe WM, Mueller KH (1975) Bioceramic implants in surgically produced infrabony defects. J Periodontol 46:328–347
309. Roberts SC Jr, Brilliant JD (1975) Tricalcium phosphate as an adjunct to apical closure in pulpless permanent teeth. J Endod 1:263–269
310. Denissen HW, de Groot K (1979) Immediate dental root implants from synthetic dense calcium hydroxylapatite. J Prosthet Dent 42:551–556
311. León B, Jansen JA (eds) (2009) Thin calcium phosphate coatings for medical implants. Springer, New York, p 326
312. Dorozhkn SV (2012) Calcium orthophosphate coatings, films and layers. Prog Biomater 1:1–40
313. Sudo SZ, Schotzko NK, Folke LEA (1976) Use of hydroxyapatite coated glass beads for preclinical testing of potential antiplaque agents. Appl Environ Microbiol 32:428–437
314. Bonfield W, Grynpas MD, Tully AE, Bowman J, Abram J (1981) Hydroxyapatite reinforced polyethylene – a mechanically compatible implant material for bone replacement. Biomaterials 2:185–189
315. Bonfield W, Bowman J, Grynpas MD (1981) Composite material for use in orthopaedics. UK Patent 8,032,647
316. Jarcho M, Bolen CH, Thomas MB, Bobick J, Kay JF, Doremus RH (1976) Hydroxylapatite synthesis and characterization in dense polycrystalline form. J Mater Sci 11:2027–2035

317. Jarcho M, O'Connor JR, Paris DA (1977) Ceramic hydroxylapatite as a plaque growth and drug screening substrate. J Dent Res 56:151–156
318. Jarcho M, Salsbury RL, Thomas MB, Doremus RH (1979) Synthesis and fabrication of β-tricalcium phosphate ceramics for potential prosthetic applications. J Mater Sci 14:142–150
319. Jarcho M (1981) Calcium phosphate ceramics as hard tissue prosthetics. Clin Orthop Rel Res 157:259–278
320. Rejda BV, Peelen JGJ, de Groot K (1977) Tricalcium phosphate as a bone substitute. J Bioeng 1:93–97
321. de Groot K (1980) Bioceramics consisting of calcium phosphate salts. Biomaterials 1:47–50
322. de Groot K (ed) (1983) Bioceramics of calcium phosphate. CRC Press, Boca Raton, p 146
323. Aoki H, Kato KM, Ogiso M, Tabata T (1977) Studies on the application of apatite to dental materials. J Dent Eng 18:86–89
324. Kato K, Aoki H, Tabata T, Ogiso M (1959) Biocompatibility of apatite ceramics in mandibles. Biomater Med Dev Artif Organs 7:291–297
325. Akao M, Aoki H, Kato K (1981) Mechanical properties of sintered hydroxyapatite for prosthetic applications. J Mater Sci 16:809–812
326. Akao M, Aoki H, Kato K, Sato A (1982) Dense polycrystalline β-tricalcium phosphate for prosthetic applications. J Mater Sci 17:343–346
327. Bohner M (2011) Private communication
328. Roy DM, Linnehan SK (1974) Hydroxyapatite formed from coral skeletal carbonate by hydrothermal exchange. Nature 247:220–222
329. Holmes RE (1979) Bone regeneration within a coralline hydroxyapatite implant. Plast Reconstr Surg 63:626–633
330. Elsinger EC, Leal L (1996) Coralline hydroxyapatite bone graft substitutes. J Foot Ankle Surg 35:396–399
331. Shipman P, Foster G, Schoeninger M (1984) Burnt bones and teeth: an experimental study of color, morphology, crystal structure and shrinkage. J Archaeol Sci 11:307–325
332. LeGeros RZ, LeGeros JP (2003) Calcium phosphate bioceramics: past, present, future. Key Eng Mater 240–242:3–10
333. Randzio J, Thoma K, Alex R, Rhomberg B (1985) Einheilung und Pharmakokinetik einer β-Trikalziumphosphat-Gentamicin-Kombination im Tierversuch (vorläufige Mitteilung). Dtsch Zahnarztl Z40:668–671
334. Dorozhkin SV (2012) Biphasic, triphasic and multiphasic calcium orthophosphates. Acta Biomater 8:963–977
335. Anuta DA, Richardson D (1985) Biphasic hydroxyapatite/beta-tricalcium phosphate granules bound in polymerized methyl methacrylate: bone substitute studies. In: Transactions of the annual meeting of the society for biomaterials in conjunction with the internal, vol 8, p 62
336. Moore DC, Chapman MW, Manske DJ (1985) Evaluation of a new biphasic calcium phosphate ceramic for use in grafting long bone diaphyseal defects. Transactions of the annual meeting of the society for biomaterials in conjunction with the Internal, vol 8, p 160
337. Kokubo T, Kushitani H, Sakka S, Kitsugi T, Yamamuro T (1990) Solutions able to reproduce *in vivo* surface-structure changes in bioactive glass-ceramic A-W3. J Biomed Mater Res 24:721–734
338. Dorozhkin SV (2009) Nanodimensional and nanocrystalline apatites and other calcium orthophosphates in biomedical engineering, biology and medicine. Materials 2:1975–2045
339. Dorozhkin SV (2012) Nanodimensional and nanocrystalline calcium orthophosphates. Am J Biomed Eng 2:48–97
340. Layrolle P, Lebugle A (1994) Characterization and reactivity of nanosized calcium phosphate prepared in anhydrous ethanol. Chem Mater 6:1996–2004
341. Cui FZ, Wen HB, Zhang HB, Ma CL, Li HD (1994) Nanophase hydroxyapatite-like crystallites in natural ivory. J Mater Sci Lett 13:1042–1044
342. Li YB, de Wijn J, Klein CPAT, de Meer SV, de Groot K (1994) Preparation and characterization of nanograde osteoapatite-like rod crystals. J Mater Sci Mater Med 5:252–255

343. Li YB, de Groot K, de Wijn J, Klein CPAT, de Meer SV (1994) Morphology and composition of nanograde calcium phosphate needle-like crystals formed by simple hydrothermal treatment. J Mater Sci Mater Med 5:326–331
344. Shirkhanzadeh M (1994) X-ray diffraction and Fourier transform infrared analysis of nanophase apatite coatings prepared by electrocrystallization. Nanostruct Mater 4:677–684
345. Norman ME, Elgendy HM, Shors EC, El-Amin SF, Laurencin CT (1994) An in-vitro evaluation of coralline porous hydroxyapatite as a scaffold for osteoblast growth. Clin Mater 17:85–91
346. Dekker RJ, de Bruijn JD, van den Brink I, Bovell YP, Layrolle P, van Blitterswijk CA (1998) Bone tissue engineering on calcium phosphate-coated titanium plates utilizing cultured rat bone marrow cells: a preliminary study. J Mater Sci Mater Med 9:859–863
347. Friedman CD, Costantino PD (1998) Hydroxyapatite cement, a smart biomaterial for craniofacial skeletal tissue engineering. Surg Technol Int 7:421–423
348. Friedman CD, Costantino PD, Takagi S, Chow LC (1998) BoneSource™ hydroxyapatite cement: a novel biomaterial for craniofacial skeletal tissue engineering and reconstruction. J Biomed Mater Res 43:428–432
349. Misra DN (ed) (1984) Adsorption on and surface chemistry of hydroxyapatite. Plenum Press, New York, p 192
350. LeGeros RZ (1991) Calcium phosphates in oral biology and medicine, vol 15, Monographs in oral science. Karger, Basel, p 201
351. Aoki H (1991) Science and medical applications of hydroxyapatite. JAAS, Tokyo, pp 214–352
352. Elliott JC (1994) Structure and chemistry of the apatites and other calcium orthophosphates: studies in inorganic chemistry, vol 18. Elsevier, Amsterdam, p 389

Chapter 16
Advances in Calcium Phosphate Nanocoatings and Nanocomposites

Andy H. Choi, Besim Ben-Nissan, Richard C. Conway, and Innocent J. Macha

Abstract It is possible by using nanocomposite approach to control the strength and Young's modulus of the composite to become close to those of human cortical or cancellous bone. This is made possible with the help of secondary substitution phases. Various materials have been applied as biomaterials and tissue regeneration materials, and the in vivo cytotoxicity and biocompatibility have been the main consideration in their use and their long-term success. This chapter aims to give a brief introduction and current applications of calcium phosphate nanocomposites as tissue engineering and as a delivery vehicle for drugs, genes, and proteins. Furthermore, the chapter will also examine the potential use of calcium phosphate nanocomposite coatings for tissue engineering scaffolds.

Keywords Nanocomposites • Hydroxyapatite • Tissue engineering • Scaffolds • Drug delivery

16.1 Introduction

Nanocomposites and nanocomposite coatings can be described as combination of two or more materials, which includes a matrix material and nanoscale secondary particles. The matrix can be a biocompatible polymeric, metallic, or ceramic material. By using the composite approach, it is possible to manipulate the mechanical properties such as strength and Young's modulus of the composites closer to those of natural bone, with incorporation of secondary nanoparticles. Nanomaterials and their modified forms such as nanocoatings and nanocomposites offer a number

A.H. Choi (✉) • B. Ben-Nissan • R.C. Conway • I.J. Macha
School of Chemistry and Forensic Science, Faculty of Science, University of Technology, Broadway, Ultimo, PO BOX 123, Sydney, NSW 2007, Australia
e-mail: ahchoi@hotmail.com

B. Ben-Nissan (ed.), *Advances in Calcium Phosphate Biomaterials*, Springer Series in Biomaterials Science and Engineering 2, DOI 10.1007/978-3-642-53980-0_16,

of attractive possibilities in the field of tissue and implant engineering for oral, maxillofacial, and orthopaedic applications [1, 2].

The current emphasis at the moment is on the production of new nanomaterials and nanocomposites that are relevant to a wide range of applications including to increase bioactivity, drug, and gene delivery; implantable surface-modified medical devices for better tissue attachment; treatment of bacterial and viral infections; tissue regeneration and engineering; cancer treatment; and materials for minimally invasive surgery.

A number of research groups have reported the use of a self-assembly mechanism to produce novel bone nanocomposites of hydroxyapatite (HAp) and collagen, gelatin, or chondroitin sulphate. These self-assembled experimental bone nanocomposites have been reported to exhibit similarities to natural bone in both structures and physiological properties [3, 4]. Nanocomposites can be produced by either physically mixing or the introduction of a new component into an existing material inducing changes in properties and may even offer new material functions. For example, some man-made and naturally found biopolymers and biomolecules, such as *poly*(lactic acid) (PLA), *poly*(lactic-*co*-glycolic acid) (PLGA), *poly*amide, collagen, silk fibrin, chitosan, and alginate, have been reported widely to mix into nano-HAp systems.

In the past, the development of bone tissue engineering has been directly related to changes in the materials used. A number of clinical reasons arise from the development of bone tissue engineering replacements, for example, the necessity in dental and biomedical implants that are mechanically more well suited to their biological environment and a need for better filler materials when reconstructing large orthopaedic defects. Stem cells have been incorporated into a range of bioceramics and together with mineralised 3-D scaffolds can form highly vascularised bone tissues when implanted.

Nanocomposites and nanocomposite coatings offer a number of attractive possibilities in the fields of tissue and implant engineering for oral and maxillofacial applications, taking advantage of the use of 3-D scaffolds to deliver cells to support tissue regeneration or to supply metal ions such as calcium and phosphate and at the same time the release of antibacterial materials to promote osseointegration and stimulate the growth of bone tissue towards the implant surface.

This chapter aims to provide a review on the recent advancements in calcium phosphate-based nanocomposites and coatings, for tissue engineering and regeneration.

16.2 Calcium Phosphates for Drug, Gene, and Protein Delivery

The primary aim for drug delivery is to target drugs to specific sites within the human body and to release the pharmaceuticals in a controllable fashion. However, for many current delivery systems, release is sudden rather than steady state. This type of release is particularly undesirable and problematic when the guest molecule such as an anti-tumour drug that is cytotoxic and might potentially harm healthy cells and tissues before being delivered to the affected sites [5].

In the case of ceramics such as calcium phosphate, the phase composition and the critical pore and grain size may be varied from a few nanometers up to microns in order to control the ease of delivery and dispersion of a material to the targeted area. A variety of calcium phosphate nanoceramic-based drug delivery systems are currently undergoing clinical evaluation. In addition to reducing toxicity to non-diseased or healthy cells, these systems have the potential to increase drug efficiency, which translates to significant cost savings for the expensive drug treatment that currently are being engineered.

The main concern for nanoparticle drug carriers is the appropriate circulation time within the body. The surface modification of nanoparticles with a range of biocompatible non-ionic surfactant or polymeric macromolecules has proved to be the most successful for maintaining nanoparticle presence in the blood for prolonged periods [6].

Calcium phosphates are characterised by particular solubilities and their ability to degrade and be replaced by advancing bone growth; they also widen the effective means of administration for successful treatment of bone diseases [7].

16.2.1 Drug Delivery

Due to their favourable properties in cancer chemotherapy, a variety of nanoceramic drug delivery systems such as those that are based on calcium phosphate are currently undergoing clinical evaluation. It has been theorised that besides factors such as particle size and roughness, the morphology of the particles also plays an important consideration when it comes to drug loading and release capacity as well as obtaining the highest cell viability and reducing negative cell responses [8]. The effects of four morphologically different calcium phosphate particles (flaky, elongated orthogonal, brick-shaped, and spherical) on sustained drug release profiles were carried out by Uskoković et al. [8]. The spherical nanosized particles were observed to be the most effective in both drug loading and release. Moreover, the spherical nanoparticles also possess the highest cell viability, the largest gene expression upregulation of three different osteogenic markers, and the least disrupted cell cytoskeleton and cell morphologies. Kester et al. [9] hypothesised the possibility of using a 20–30 nm diameter, pH-responsive, non-agglomerating, and non-toxic calcium phosphate nanoparticle matrix to encapsulate hydrophobic antineoplastic chemotherapeutics. The nanoparticles were found to be capable of encapsulating both fluorophores and chemotherapeutics and are colloidally stable in physiological solution for an extended time at 37 °C.

Bastakoti and co-workers [10] suggested that sub-100 nm colloidal nanoparticles loaded with fluorescent dyes and anticancer drugs, along with a controlled mineralisation technology, could lead to the successful development of robust, biocompatible hybrid nanocarriers for the simultaneous delivery of drugs and imaging agents.

Various factors relating to the materials of the drug delivery vehicle such as immune reaction of the host against the system and poor control over the release of drugs influence the success of the delivery system in cancer treatment [11]. A range of anticancer drugs have been examined including docetaxel, doxorubicin hydrochloride, methotrexate, and 5-fluorouracil [11–16]. Zhao et al. [12] investigated the drug loading and release behaviour of lipid-coated calcium phosphate hybrid nanoparticles synthesised through self-assembly loaded with the anticancer drug docetaxel. The average diameter of the hybrid nanoparticles was approximately 72 nm. They reported that the nanoparticles showed excellent biocompatibility and high drug loading capacity; Liang et al. [13] also attempted to examine the in vitro drug release and cell inhibition effect of calcium phosphate hybrid nanoparticles. Heparin/$CaCO_3$/calcium phosphate nanoparticles with a size of less than 50 nm were prepared through co-precipitation technique and loaded with the anticancer drug doxorubicin hydrochloride. From their in vitro cellular cytotoxicity study, the unloaded hybrid nanoparticles possessed good biocompatibility, whereas the drug-loaded nanoparticles exhibited a strong cell inhibition effect. An efficient drug delivery system consisted of an amphiphilic gelatin-iron oxide core, and calcium phosphate shells were also attempted [14].

Highly water-soluble magnetic mesoporous amorphous calcium phosphate nanoparticles with a diameter of 41 nm were prepared by Rout et al. [15]. Platinum pharmacophore *cis*-diaquadiamine platinum (II), folic acid, and rhodamine isothiocyanate were conjugated on these nanoparticles and its antitumour potential investigated against human cervical carcinoma cells by MTT assay. They discovered the nanoparticles can effectively target cancer cells and optimally deliver cisplatin and resulting in cell death following the induction of apoptosis.

The therapeutic efficacy of a porous silica-calcium phosphate nanocomposites was also investigated as a new delivery system for the anticancer drug 5-fluorouracil [11]. Based on the results of their in vitro studies, they noticed that the nanocomposites were very cytotoxic for 4T1 mammary tumour cells. Release kinetics studies showed the nanocomposites containing 5-fluorouracil provided a burst release of the anticancer drug in the first 24 h followed by a sustained release of a therapeutic dose of the drug for up to 32 days. The in vivo subcutaneous implantation in an immunocompetent murine model of breast cancer also suggested that the nanocomposites containing 5-fluorouracil can cease the growth of 4T1 tumour. Calcium phosphate nanoparticle containing an anticancer drug methotrexate was synthesised and characterised by Mukesh et al. [16]. The average size of the nanoparticles was approximately 262 nm, and they have an entrapment efficiency of 58 %. In vitro release study revealed slow release of methotrexate at physiological pH, while greater than 90 % release was observed within 3–4 h at endosomal pH.

Using a biomimetic approach, Chen et al. [17] attempted to engineer mesoporous silica nanoparticles with calcium phosphate-hyaluronic acid hybrid shell to be used as a pH-responsive targeted drug delivery vehicle. They noticed that the addition of another layer of hyaluronic acid on the calcium phosphate surfaces not only stabilises the nanocomposites but also confers target ability towards CD44 overexpressed cancer cells. Furthermore, the nanomaterials were found to possess the ability to control the release of loaded anticancer drugs in acidic subcellular environments after receptor-mediated endocytosis. Chiu et al. [18] hypothesised that small calcium phosphate core-protein shell nanoparticles might be effective vehicles for the delivery of adjuvanted antigen to dendritic cells. They utilised cell surface display to identify disulfide-constrained calcium phosphate binding peptides that, when inserted within the active site loop of *E. coli* thioredoxin 1 (TrxA), readily and reproducibly drive the production of nanoparticles which were 50–70 nm in hydrodynamic diameter and consisted of an approximately 25 nm amorphous calcium phosphate core stabilised by the protein shell. When compared to a commercial aluminium phosphate adjuvant, they observed the small core-shell assemblies led to a threefold increase in mice anti-TrxA titres 3 weeks post-injection.

In addition to delivering anticancer chemotherapeutics, calcium phosphate nanoparticle-based systems were also investigated for the potential delivery of common drugs such as aspirin, insulin, and vitamins [19–22]. To address the problem of stomach irrigation caused by aspirin, the use of a composite microsphere delivery vehicle composed of porous nano-HAp particles and *poly*(styrene-divinylbenzene) (P(St-DVB)) was explored [19]. The aspirin-loaded microspheres were observed to exhibited excellent buoyancy with relatively short instantaneous floating time and a long sustained floating time in simulated gastric juice. The microspheres also offered good sustained release of aspirin of up to 8 h. Ignjatović et al. [20] examined the effects of the local delivery of cholecalciferol (vitamin D_3) using nanoparticulate carriers composed of HAp and PLGA. Two types of multifunctional nanoparticulate HAp-based powders were prepared and tested: HAp nanoparticles as direct cholecalciferol delivery agents and HAp nanoparticles coated with cholecalciferol-loaded PLGA for sustained delivery. They observed the fast delivery was achieved by desorption of the drug from the HAp particle surface, while the slow delivery was conditioned by the rather slow degradation of PLGA in physiological conditions.

The methazolamide-loaded calcium phosphate nanoparticles with a mean diameter of approximately 256 nm were prepared by Chen et al. [21]. From the in vitro release studies, they observed diffusion-controlled release of methazolamide from the nanoparticles over a period of 4 h, while in vivo studies showed the intraocular pressure-lowering effect of the nanoparticle eye drops lasted for 18 h. Ramachandran et al. [22] examined the possibility of PEGylated calcium phosphate nanoparticles with an average particle size of 48 nm as oral carriers for insulin. The non-cytotoxic nature of the PEGylated calcium phosphate nanoparticles has been established through the MTT assay. The release profiles revealed negligible release in gastric pH after the nanoparticles were coated with a pH-sensitive polymer, while a sustained release of insulin at intestinal pH for over 8 h was recorded. They also discovered the insulin loading process in the PEG-conjugated calcium phosphate nanoparticles did not affect the conformation and stability of insulin.

16.2.2 Gene Delivery

In the field of tissue engineering, the role of gene therapy in aiding wound healing and treating various diseases or defects has become increasingly important. The use of calcium phosphate nanoparticles in gene delivery has emerged as a popular and necessary delivery vehicle for obtaining controlled gene delivery [23, 24]. The main challenge for any successful small interfering ribonucleic acid (siRNA)-based therapies is the research and development of an efficient in vivo delivery vehicle. Pittella et al. [23] examined the possibility of utilising smart polymer/calcium phosphate/siRNA hybrid nanoparticles approximately 100 nm in size for siRNA-based cancer treatment. According to the authors, the nanoparticle showed high gene silencing efficiency in cultured pancreatic cancer cells without associated cytotoxicity. Intravenously injected nanoparticles incorporating vascular endothelium growth factor siRNA led to significant reduction in tumour growth. Li et al. [24] suggested the efficient delivery via intravenous administration of siRNA to a xenograft tumour model using a calcium phosphate nanoparticle with an average diameter of about 60–80 nm coated with liposome. They observed untargeted nanoparticles had a very low silencing effect, while a three- to four-fold in vitro silencing effect was observed with the lipid-coated calcium phosphate nanoparticle. They hypothesised that after entering the cells, the lipid-coated calcium phosphate nanoparticle would dissemble at low pH in the endosome, which would cause endosome swelling and bursting to release the entrapped siRNA.

Currently, calcium phosphate is one of the most attractive nonviral vectors being investigated for the in vitro delivery of plasmid DNA (pDNA) into cultured cells due to factors such as ease of handling, biodegradability, biocompatibility, and known adsorption capacity for pDNA. On the other hand, when compared to viral approaches, traditional calcium phosphate synthesis methods often lead to lower and less consistent transfection efficiency [25–27]. Olton et al. [25] claimed more consistent levels of gene expression could be achieved by optimising both the stoichiometry (Ca/P ratio) of the calcium phosphate particles in addition to the mode in which the precursor solutions are mixed. The optimised forms of these calcium phosphate particles were approximately 25–50 nm in size (when complexed with pDNA) and maximum transfection efficiencies in both HeLa and MC3T3-E1 cell lines were obtained when a Ca/P ratio between 100 and 300 was used.

In an attempt to improve the transfection efficiency and to stabilise the particle size and inhibit further growth of the particle, Liu et al. [26] coated calcium phosphate nanoparticles with protamine sulphate, and based on atomic force microscopy, the protamine sulphate-coated calcium phosphate nanoparticles were observed to be much smaller than classical calcium phosphate particles, and in vitro studies showed the smaller nanoparticles enhanced the transfection efficiency by promoting the endocytic delivery of DNA into cells.

Furthermore, growth factors such as transforming growth factor beta-1 (TGF-β1), in general, have been used to enhance the tissue-forming efficiency and to accomplish the goal of tissue regeneration. TGF-β1, which possesses multifunctional capacities that regulate many aspects of cellular activity, including cell proliferation, differentiation, and extracellular matrix metabolism, in a time- and concentration-dependent manner, was selected by Cao et al. [28] to stimulate cartilage tissue formation. A three-dimensional nanocomposite gene delivery system based on collagen/chitosan scaffolds, in which plasmid TGF-β1/calcium phosphate nanoparticles mixed with fibronectin were used to transfect mesenchymal stem cells (MSCs). They noticed the MSCs transfected with nanocomposite system showed remarkably high levels of the growth factor over long periods. Observations made based on an immunohistochemistry analysis revealed greater amounts of collagen II was produced by the nanocomposite-transfected MSCs than MSCs transfected by the Lipofectamine 2000 method. The authors hypothesised that transfection with the nanocomposite gene delivery system could successfully induce MSC chondrogenic differentiation in vitro without dexamethasone.

For any practical application of a nanoscale medical delivery system, it is essential that no dissolved biomolecules are accompanying the delivery system as well as knowing precisely the dose of the applied biomolecules. An efficient delivery system based on biodegradable multi-shell calcium phosphate-oligonucleotide nanoparticles as carriers for the immunoactive toll-like receptor ligands CpG and polyinosinic-polycytidylic acid for the activation of dendritic cells (DC) combined with the viral antigen haemagglutinin was attempted by Sokolova et al. [29]. They discovered that the purified calcium phosphate nanoparticles (without dissolved biomolecules) are capable of inducing adaptive immunity by activation of DC. Immunostimulatory effects of purified calcium phosphate nanoparticles on DC were demonstrated by increased expression of co-stimulatory molecules and MHC II and by cytokine secretion. Furthermore, DC treated with purified functionalised calcium phosphate nanoparticles induced an antigen-specific T-cell response in vitro.

16.2.3 Protein Delivery

Nanocarriers such as those based on calcium phosphate provide improvement in effectiveness during the delivery of therapeutic proteins for cancer therapy compared to naked protein drugs [30, 31]. The loading of proteins (bovine serum albumin and lysozyme) into calcium phosphate nanoparticles approximately 50 nm in size was attempted by Han et al. [30] through an inverse micelle technique and the protein loading efficiency and release profiles at different pH conditions investigated. X-ray photoelectron spectroscopy revealed the proteins were not adsorbed onto the surface of the nanoparticles suggesting the proteins were entrapped within the particle matrix. Release studies showed that protein release was more rapid at lower pH conditions than at physiological pH. Paul and Sharma [31] also examined the option of using calcium phosphate-based nanoparticles as oral delivery carriers for their model protein drug insulin. The majority of the nanoparticles were less than 100 nm in size and were shown to be non-cytotoxic. They discovered lauric acid-conjugated calcium phosphate nanoparticles were highly compatible with insulin and it is possible to use the nanoparticle system to deliver insulin in a sustained manner in the physiological pH of the intestine with no degradation or conformational changes of entrapped insulin.

16.3 Calcium Phosphate-Based Nanocomposite Coatings

By combining HAp with other micro- and nanoscale-based materials as a secondary phase, the mechanical properties of the HAp coating can be further increased through the formation of HAp nanocomposite coatings. This approach is currently being explored in the development of a new generation of nanocomposite coatings containing nanomaterials such as carbon nanotube (CNT), titanium oxide, and collagen to promote osseointegration.

16.3.1 Carbon Nanotubes

Due to their exceptional mechanical properties, both single- and multi-walled carbon nanotubes (MWCNT) have been extensively investigated, and from the time the concept that can be used in conjunction with HAp, their use in the biomedical industry has been anticipated [32–35] (Fig. 16.1). On the other hand, the chemical inertness and hydrophobicity of CNT severely restrict their applications [36]. Furthermore, by taking advantage of their excellent mechanical and biological characteristics, a new area of research into CNT-reinforced HAp composite coating has been initiated in an attempt to reduce premature fracture of the HAp coating layer as a result of the low fracture toughness and brittle nature of thick layer plasma-coated HAp [37–40]. The addition of reinforcement materials such as CNT to HAp has been reported by Kealley et al. [32–34, 37] to have significant effects in the improvement of mechanical properties. Using nanoindentation technique, they observed an increase in hardness as the percentages of CNT mixed with HAp increases.

The introduction of MWCNTs into the HAp matrix and dip coating of nanocomposite on titanium alloy (Ti-6Al-4V) plate was applied by Abrishamchian et al. [38] in an attempt to improve the performance of the HAp-plasma-coated implants. They noticed that the addition of low concentrations of MWCNTs to HAp improved the mechanical properties and reduced the surface roughness of the coating. Furthermore, biological evaluation revealed normal cell adhesion and growth process on the HAp/MWCNT composite coating, comparable with that of pure HAp coating.

The in vivo behaviour of plasma-sprayed CNT-reinforced HAp coating on titanium alloy implants embedded in rodents' bone was examined by Facca et al. [39], who observed no adverse effects or cytotoxicity attributed to the addition of CNT to bone tissues. Balani et al. [40] also investigated the non-toxicity of

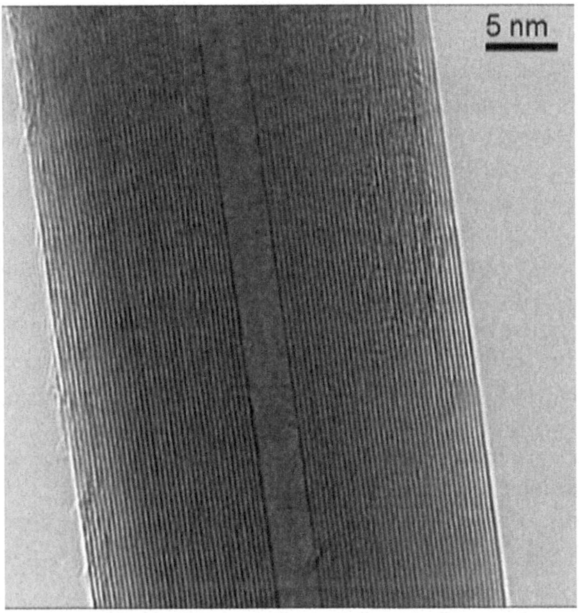

Fig. 16.1 TEM image of a multi-walled CNT

HAp-CNT coating on Ti-6Al-4V implants, and the results of those cell culture studies showed unrestricted growth of human osteoblast hFOB 1.19 cells near CNT regions.

The in vitro bioactivity of a HAp-TiO_2-CNT nanocomposite coating was investigated by Zhang and Kwok [41], who observed that, after immersion in Hanks's solution for 4 weeks, thick layers of apatite were formed on the surfaces of the monolithic HAp and HAp-CNT and HAp-TiO_2-CNT nanocomposite coatings. They noted that the addition of TiO_2 and CNT in HAp did not affect the apatite-forming ability on their surfaces.

16.3.2 Collagen

Considered to be one of the most useful biomaterials for applications such as tissue scaffolding, collagen is readily available and biocompatible and exhibits properties such as negligible cytotoxicity and hydrophilicity and has good haemostatic properties [42]. The seminal experiment that demonstrated bonding of bone collagen to bioactive glass composition 45S5 was published by Hench et al. in 1971 [43]. Bone is a composite of an organic collagen matrix and inorganic calcium phosphate crystal reinforcements which have inspired researchers to theorise that a collagen-calcium phosphate composite coating mimicking the unique nanocomposite structure of native bone tissue could present an added value over the individual components. Fan et al. [44] and later Wahl et al. [45] hypothesised that the poor fracture toughness of calcium phosphate can be compensated by the ductile properties of collagen and the use of collagen-calcium phosphate composite coatings also offers an added advantage in that the coating resembles the unique nanocomposite structure of native bone tissue.

Uezono et al. [46] investigated bone formation around Ti samples with a machined surface, HAp coating, and HAp-collagen nanocomposite coating. Their histomorphometric analyses revealed that the HAp-collagen group had the greatest bone contact ratio among all candidates. Furthermore, the results from bonding strength tests indicated that the HAp-collagen group exhibited the greatest bonding strength to bone.

In an attempt to improve the anchoring and long-term behaviour of Ti implant materials, nanoscale calcium phosphate and collagen-calcium phosphate composite coatings were examined by de Jonge et al. [47]. The biological property of the coatings was characterised by in vitro cell culture. According to their findings, improvements in both osteoblast differentiation and mineral deposition were most prominent when collagen was co-deposited with calcium phosphate. Osteogenic effects were also displayed for coatings with thicknesses well below 100 nm.

16.3.3 Titanium Dioxide (TiO_2)

The use of titanium dioxide or titania (TiO_2) as a bioactive coating has attracted much interest, and it was believed that using TiO_2 within the coating as reinforcement was one method for improving the mechanical reliability of HAp. Furthermore, it was also believed that TiO_2 is capable of inducing cell growth and enhancing osteoblast adhesion [48, 49]. In 1999, Webster et al. [48] observed an increase in osteoblast adhesion with decreasing titania grain size, correlating to the greater surface area displayed by the nanomaterial. They hypothesised that an increase in the surface area would lead to an increase in osteoblast adhesion. To improve the strength and adhesion of the coating, to reduce loosening of implants due to failure at the metal-coating interface, and to increase biological responses, researchers have used various approaches to fabricate a TiO_2-HAp nanocomposite coating. Such a coating is capable of supporting osteogenic differentiation of osteoblast-like and mesenchymal stem cells (MSCs) [50–52].

Kuwabara et al. [51] attempted to investigate the biological response associated with bone formation on HAp-TiO_2 composite coatings with a thickness of approximately 100 nm. Rat bone marrow-derived osteoblast-like cells were cultured on the coated surfaces with different electric charges. They discovered surfaces coated with both HAp and TiO_2 have greater effects on cell attachment and spreading, as well as bone-titanium integration, as compared with either HAp- or TiO_2-coated surfaces. Dimitrievska et al. [52] also investigated the mechanical and biological properties of TiO_2-HAp nanocomposite coatings. They also observed an increase in proliferation and osteoblastic differentiation of human mesenchymal stem cells (hMSCs) on the nanocomposite coatings.

16.4 Advances in Calcium Phosphate Scaffolds for Tissue Engineering

The development of bone tissue engineering in the past has been directly related to changes in materials and nanotechnology. While the inclusion of materials requirements is standard in the design process of engineered bone substitutes, it is also vital to incorporate clinical requirements such that clinically relevant devices can be engineered.

Traditionally, biological methods for the management of bone defects consist of autografting and allografting. In addition to design and material factors, four biologically important components are needed for bone regeneration: (1) a morphogenetic signal, (2) responsive host cells that will respond to the signal, (3) an appropriate carrier of this signal and delivering it to specific sites, (4) scaffolding for the growth of the responsive host cells, and a well-vascularised host bed [53–55]. The purpose of scaffolding material is to act as a carrier or template for implanted bone cells or other agents. They can also be used to induce the formation of bone from the surrounding tissues.

The process of bone regeneration is common to the repair of fractures. The incorporation of bone grafts, the skeletal homeostasis, and the cascading sequence of biological events are often described as the remodelling cycle. Stem cells have been incorporated into a range of bioceramics and, when implanted, can combine with mineralised 3-D scaffolds to form highly vascularised bone tissue. These nanoscale cultured cell-bioceramic composites can be used to treat full-thickness gaps in long bone shafts, providing an excellent integration of the ceramic scaffold with bone and a good functional recovery. In a HAp-tricalcium phosphate composite, it was observed that the nano-sheet architecture promoted primary human osteoblast adhesion as reflected by the activation of focal adhesion kinase and expression of actin in human osteoblasts [56].

Bioactive composite grafts consisting of bioactive ceramic filler in a polymeric matrix have attracted a significant amount of attention during the past three decades. These bioactive composite grafts are designed essentially to achieve interfacial bonding between the graft and the host tissues. HAp-collagen, HAp/*poly*ethylene (PE), and HAp/Ti-6Al-4V are notable examples of bioactive composite grafts [57, 58]. Of particular interest is the combination of HAp with collagen as a bioactive composite, as this appears to be a natural choice for bone grafting [59].

Skeletal bones are composed mainly of collagen and carbonate-substituted HAp, both of which are osteoconductive components. A composite matrix, when embedded with human-like osteoblast cells, showed better osteoconductive properties compared to monolithic HAp and produced calcification of an identical bone matrix [60].

The reconstruction of bone tissue using nanocomposite bone grafts with composition, biomechanical, structure, physiochemical, and biological features that mimic those of natural bone is an objective to be achieved. It has been well established that natural bone is made up of platelike nanosized crystals of HAp grown in intimate contact with an organic matrix which is rich in collagen fibres. Utilising strategies found in nature to produce nanocomposite bone grafts has received much attention recently and is perceived to be beneficial over conventional methods. Several methods have been used for the production of collagen-HAp composite gels, films, collagen-coated ceramics, ceramic-coated collagen matrices, and composite scaffolds for spine and hard tissue repair [45].

Based on the works of Daculsi et al. [61] and LeGeros et al. [62, 63], Ebrahimi et al. [64] proposed the utilisation of nano-HAp-TCP biphasic composites and that simple incorporation of collagen may improve physical properties of biphasic calcium phosphate (BCP) scaffolds and increase their bioactivity. The dimensional shrinkage after sintering of large scaffolds was found to be lower than small ones and scaffolds with high nano-HAp ratios experienced higher dimensional changes than those with higher β-tricalcium phosphate ratios.

Various biodegradable synthetic and natural polymeric materials have been proposed by Reis et al. [57, 65] and investigated in conjunction with HAp as scaffolding materials for tissue engineering applications. Man-made or synthetic polymers possess a number of advantages such as the physical-chemical properties can be modified and, by changing the chemical composition, the degradation and mechanical properties can be tailored to specific needs. Another advantage of synthetic polymers is its ability to be bioactivated with specific molecules by combining side chains and functional groups.

16.4.1 Calcium Phosphate Nanocoated Coralline Apatite

A number of natural and synthetic bone-graft materials currently in use are produced from coralline HAp. As a result of the conversion process, commercial coralline HAp has retained coral or $CaCO_3$ and the structure possesses nanopores within the inter-pore trabeculae, resulting in high dissolution rates.

Under certain conditions, these features reduce durability and strength, respectively, and are not utilised where high structural strength is required. To overcome these limitations, a double-stage conversion technique was developed by Ben-Nissan and co-workers [1, 2]. The method involves a two-stage application route whereby, in the first stage, a complete conversion of coral to 100 % HAp is achieved. In the second stage, a sol-gel-derived HAp nanocoating is applied directly to cover the meso- and nanopores within the intra-pore material, while maintaining the large pores for appropriate bone growth (Fig. 16.2).

Mechanical properties such as fracture toughness, Young's modulus, and compression and biaxial strengths were each improved as a result of this unique double treatment. Application of the treatment method is expected to result in an enhanced bioactivity due to the nanograin size – and hence large surface area – that increases the reactivity of the nanocoating. It is anticipated that this material could be applied to load-bearing bone-graft applications where high-strength requirements are pertinent.

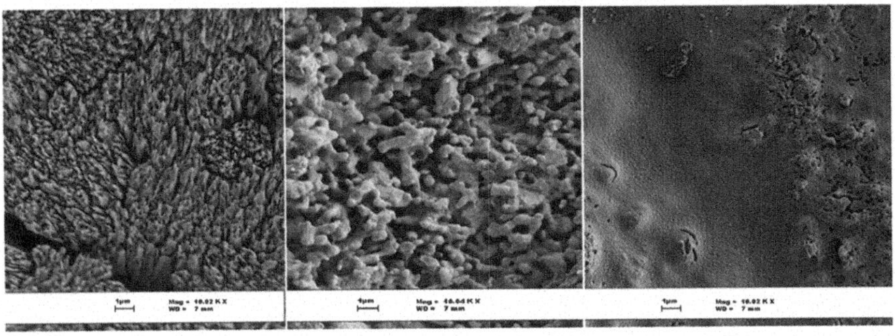

Fig. 16.2 Stages of nanocystalline HAp-coated coralline apatite formation. The *first* figure shows an enlarged micrograph of a coral skeleton spine area that has very sharp meso- and nanopore platelet regions. The *middle* micrograph shows surface morphological changes of the coral after conversion to hydroxyapatite, while the *last* one is the converted coral coated with HAp nanocoating, modifying the surface features to more bioactive nanoscale grains

For these studies, the coral was obtained from the Australian Great Barrier Reef and contained micropores of 100–300 μm size. The coral was shaped and treated with boiling water and 5 % NaClO solution. A hydrothermal conversion was carried out in a Parr reactor with a Teflon liner at 220 °C and 3.8 MPa pressure with excess $(NH_4)_2HPO_4$. A total conversion to HAp was achieved in this way. Nanocrystalline ceramic coatings were produced using the sol-gel process. For this, the precursor solution was formed using the previously reported method [1, 2]. Coatings were formed using these solutions, followed by subsequent heat treatments. Mechanical testing involved a standard, four-point bend test according to ASTM C1161, to measure the flexural strength and flexural modulus of the natural coral. Comparative compression and biaxial strength tests were also carried out.

Characterisation studies of the natural and converted corals using XRD, SEM, DTA/TGA, nuclear magnetic resonance (NMR), and Raman spectroscopy have been previously reported. These results showed a large increase in all mechanical properties, specifically the compression strength, due to hydrothermal conversion and nanocoatings methods. The bioactivity was enhanced through the nanocrystalline formation, due to the HAp nanocoating [66].

In addition to enhancing the bioactivity and the mechanical properties, HAp coatings can also be used in controlling the rate of drug release from coralline apatite delivery system. A bone-stimulator drug, simvastatin, was successfully loaded with the coral-derived β-tricalcium phosphate, and in an attempt to control the release of simvastatin and reduce its release rate, a lipid coating was utilised [67].

16.4.2 Liposomes and Calcium Phosphates

Liposomes are one of the most clinically established nanometer-scale systems currently employed to deliver non-toxic and antifungal drugs, genes, and vaccines.

Liposomes consist of a single layer, or multiple concentric lipid bilayers, that encapsulate an aqueous compartment. When compared to other delivery systems, the outstanding clinical profile of liposomes is based on their biocompatibility, biodegradability, reduced toxicity, and capacity for size and surface manipulations [68].

The encapsulation of nanoparticles such as calcium phosphate within liposomes may lead to an increase in nanoparticle hydrophilicity, stability in plasma, and an overall improvement in their biocompatibility [68–70]. Moreover, by utilising the ability of liposomes to carry hydrophilic and hydrophobic moieties, combinatory therapy/imaging modalities can be achieved by incorporating therapeutic and diagnostic agents into a single liposome delivery system [68].

Based on their excellent biocompatibility, calcium phosphate-based hybrid nanoparticles have shown great promise as candidates for drug delivery and bone regeneration systems [71–73]. Recently, composite scaffolds composed of collagen and HAp with liposomes were proposed by Wang et al. [72] to provide a sustained drug release platform in bone regeneration and repair. The liposomes were composed of distearoylphosphodioline, cholesterol, distearoylphosphoethanolamine-*poly*(ethylene glycol), and a bone-binding bisphosphonate attached to the liposome. By taking advantage of the specific interaction between the liposomal bisphosphonate and the HAp incorporated into the scaffold, the bisphosphonate-decorated liposomes were shown to display a strong affinity to collagen-HAp scaffolds. They reported there were no differences in drug release from the liposomes whether the liposomes were bisphosphonate decorated or not. Whereas unencapsulated drugs and drugs encapsulated in PEG-liposomes displayed rapid release from the scaffolds, the drugs entrapped in bisphosphonate liposomes showed a slower release from the collagen-HAp scaffolds.

HAp-coated liposomes were successfully manufactured by Xu et al. [71] and filled with a model hydrophobic (lipophilic) drug, namely, indomethacin (IMC). In this process, the HAp layer was precipitated onto the liposomes, the aim being to provide the HAp-coated liposomes with two functions: (1) that the inner core liposome provides a sustained drug release and (2) that the outer HAp layer provides the osteoconductivity for bone cells. The liposomes were formed from 1,2-dimyristoyl-sn-glycero-3-phosphate (DMPA) and 1,2-dimyristoyl-sn-glycero-3-phosphocholine (DMPC). The results reported by the authors indicated that precipitating HAp onto the liposome reduced the release rate of IMC compared to uncoated liposomes. In fact, under the conditions used, the 5 h period required to release 70 % of the IMC from the liposomes was extended to 20 h when the liposomes were coated with HAp. Perhaps, more importantly, IMC release from the uncoated liposomes occurred more rapidly at pH 7.4 than at pH 4, whereas the HAp coating reduced the release rate at pH 7.4 compared to that at pH 4. Based on these findings, they suggested that this effect might open up the possibility of creating "smart" (pH-controlled) targeted drug delivery devices.

Osteoporosis, a degenerative bone disorder, is one of the leading causes of morbidity in the elderly. Lewis [73] examined the possibility of using liposomes to encapsulate various micro- and nanosized calcium-based mineral compounds

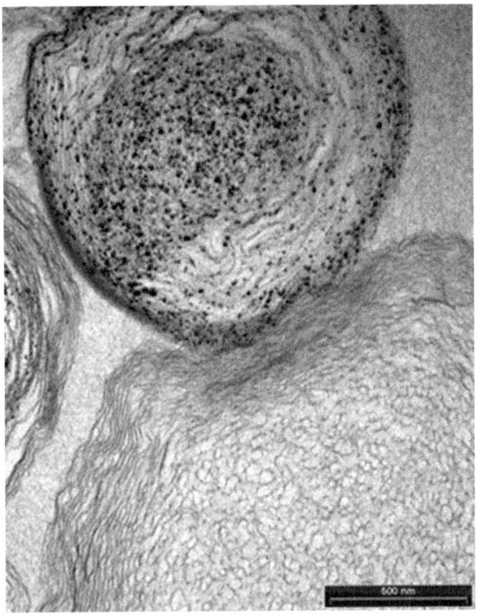

Fig. 16.3 Multilayer liposome with nano-HAp particles (Courtesy of Dr. K. Lewis)

for direct delivery to the bone which may be beneficial to bone health. Calcium phosphate mineral including HAp, dicalcium phosphate dihydrate, as well as multiphase and substituted calcium phosphates was produced using biomimetic process. Preliminary cell culture studies showed no direct effect on osteoblast-like Mg63 or Saos-2 cells or osteoclast resorption, measured by bone collagen release. Macrophage response was explored using U937 cell line. Expression of TNF-α and IL-1, markers of inflammation, increased with liposome treatments compared to the negative control but decreased compared the positive control. The Mg63 cells given U937 supernatants showed liposomes increased OPG production, but this was regardless of mineralisation (Fig. 16.3).

The clinical significance of hydroxyapatite (HAp) as a bone substitute has become apparent in recent years, and bone morphogenetic protein (BMP) has attracted much attention. In a study conducted by Ono et al. [74], 1.2 cm-diameter bone defects created on rabbit cranium were treated with the BMP-2 gene (cDNA plasmid) introduced with porous HAp after completion of haemostasis, and the effect of using cationic liposomes as a vector to the amounts of new bone formation was examined. Four groups of rabbits were compared. In the HAp group, the cranial bone defect was treated with HAp containing 40 μg of liposomes and a dummy gene. The BMP gene HAp group was treated with HAp soaked in liposomes and 10 μg of the BMP-2 gene. Although new bone formation was evident surrounding the scaffold 3 weeks post-operation, the induced bone tissue did not fill all the pores of the scaffold even at 9 weeks post-operation. They hypothesised the clinical usefulness of gene therapy for bone formation, using the BMP-2 gene combined with cationic liposomes as a vector.

When Huang et al. [75] used liposome-coated HAp and tricalcium phosphate as bone implants in the mandibular bony defect of miniature swine; they found the liposome-coated materials to be biocompatible. Moreover, the clinical endpoint was enhanced compared to that in the absence of liposomes. It was hypothesised that HAP coating and tricalcium phosphate with negatively charged liposomes might improve the nucleation process for new bone formation. In experiments conducted in miniature swine, artificial bony defects on one side were implanted with either HAp-coated or tricalcium phosphate-coated liposomes, while defects on the other side served as controls. Histology and radiography performed at 3 and 6 weeks after surgery showed the coated liposome materials to be biocompatible. At 3 weeks, the implant material was surrounded by dense connective tissues, while by 6 weeks new bone formation was visible near the implanted material. Liposomes immobilised in agarose gel and implanted in the defects also showed new bony bridge formation.

16.4.3 Chitosan and Calcium Phosphate Composites

Despite being one of the most extensively investigated biomaterial in tissue engineering, the bioactivity of chitosan needs to be enhanced for specific tissues and making them not as ideal when used as a stand-alone material [76]. As a result, new composites are created by combining chitosan with other bioactive materials such as HAp [76–79]. Nano-HAp and its composites with variety of chitosan content were investigated by Tavakol et al. [76], and they observed that the degree of bone regeneration potential was greater in nano-HAp powder than in nano-HAp-chitosan composites. Cell culture studies were attempted by Tomoaia et al. [77] on fibrous biocomposite scaffolds made of nano-HAp particles, chitosan, and type I collagen. They noticed that the incorporation of small amounts of silicon, magnesium, and zinc within the nano-HAP lattice could improve the in vitro biological activity of human osteoblasts on these scaffolds. Im et al. [78] hypothesised that chitosan nanocomposite with both nano-HAp and single-walled carbon nanotubes (SWCNT) could significantly enhance the mechanical properties of the scaffold and synergistically improve scaffold cytocompatibility for osteoblast adhesion and proliferation. Nanocomposites containing magnetically synthesised single-walled CNT (SWCNT) had superior cytocompatibility when compared with nonmagnetically synthesised SWCNT. Their study also revealed that osteoblasts favoured magnetically synthesised SWCNT which has smaller diameters and were twice as long as their nonmagnetically prepared counterparts indicating that the dimensions of SWCNTs can have a substantial effect on osteoblast attachment.

Electrospun composite nanofibrous substrates of chitosan and HAp nanoparticles were fabricated by Venugopal et al. [79] with an aim towards the lowest level of hierarchical organisation similar to bone, for the mineralisation of osteoblasts in vitro in bone tissue regeneration. The interaction of human fetal osteoblasts and nanofibrous substrates was analysed for cell morphology and mineralisation, and the results showed mineralisation was increased significantly in chitosan/nano-HAp compared with chitosan nanofibres.

A major component of bone scaffolds containing HAp and collagen has also been used as scaffold for bone regeneration, and it has been reported that the use of HAp-collagen composite could induce bony growth into the porous structure [80]. Rodrigues et al. [81] investigated the possible application of collagen and nano-HAp as scaffolds for bone regeneration. They noticed an improvement in the mechanical properties as the nano-HAp content increases. In vitro studies with osteoblasts cells showed collagen-nano-HAp composites resulted in higher overall cellular proliferation compared to pure collagen scaffold. Ou et al. [80] examined the cell-material interaction of bone regenerative nanocomposites consisting of nano-HAp, nano-amorphous calcium phosphate, and reconstituted collagen. Bone marrow-derived MSCs were selected to evaluate the nanoporous HAp-collagen effect on osteogenic differentiation. They observed the incorporation of reconstituted collagen with the composite significantly facilitated the osteogenic differentiation of MSCs. Reconstituted collagen was covered with nano-HAp and nano-amorphous calcium phosphate profoundly impacted the improvement of biocompatibility on application of implant and tissue engineering.

16.4.4 Synthetic Polymer and Calcium Phosphate Composites

Due to its high toughness, researchers have examined the possibility of enhancing the brittleness of HAp with the addition of *poly*amide for applications such as bone defect reconstruction. Ideally, a composite biomaterial consisting of HAp and *poly*amide would combine the advantages of the two materials where *poly*amide would improve the toughness of the composite and HAp would increase the bioactivity of the resulting composite [82, 83]. Guo et al. [82] assessed the in vitro and in vivo biological activity of nano HAp/*poly*amide composite using bone marrow stromal cells (BMSCs). The composite showed great bioactivity with significant BMSC proliferation, active alkaline phosphatase secretion, and stimulating the expression of osteogenic proteins. The in vivo rabbit model revealed the amount of new bone formation around the composite was significant at marrow-rich implantation sites, but BMSC was necessary at marrow-poor sites. Huang et al. [83] attempted to improve the mechanical and biological properties of the highly porous scaffold of nano-HAp/*poly*amide66 by coating it with chitosan. They noticed a five-fold increase in the compressive strength when the scaffold was coated with chitosan. The biological evaluation demonstrated chitosan coating on the scaffolds had no negative effect on osteoblast-like MG63 cells and showed good cytocompatibility.

PLGA can be considered as one of the commonly used biodegradable polymer that can be easily processed. Unfortunately, the application of PLGA has been greatly limited for its weak mechanical strength, hydrophobic surface, and poor bioactivity. In view of the physiochemical and structural benefits of nano-HAp in the formation of new bone and the biodegradable and biocompatible nature of polymers such as PLGA, nanocomposites composed of HAp and PLGA have been hypothesised and considered as a solution by researchers in controlling the adhesion and the osteogenic differentiation of hMSCs [84, 85]. An in vitro study was carried out by Lock et al. [84], and they discovered nano-HAp/PLGA nanocomposites promoted hMSC adhesion better than PLGA alone. The effect of PLGA/HAp composite nanofibres on the osteogenic differentiation of hMSCs was investigated by Lee et al. [85]. The presence of HAp increased alkaline phosphatase activity and enhanced the expression of genes related to osteogenic differentiation including ALP, bone sialoprotein, and osteocalcin. Buschmann et al. [86] reported the in vitro and in vivo behaviour of an electrospun nanocomposite based on PLGA and amorphous calcium phosphate nanoparticles seeded with human adipose-derived stem cells (ASC) compared to PLGA. They discovered the cells retained their morphology when ASC were seeded on the nanocomposite. The in vivo behaviour was confirmed by avian vessels from the chick chorioallantoic membrane which has completely penetrated the nanocomposite within 1 week.

Composites of *poly*vinyl alcohol (PVA) and HAp have been suggested to lack the complex hierarchical nanostructures and high mechanical property to meet the demand of bone substitute [87, 88]. Ba Linh et al. [87] investigated the biological and mechanical properties of a biodegradable nanofibre mat composed of functional PVA/gelatin fibres and biphasic calcium phosphate (BCP) nanoparticles for bone regeneration. The addition of BCP nanoparticles was found to be responsible for an increase in fibre diameter, tensile strength, osteoblast cell adhesion, proliferation, and protein expression. Porous BCP nanoparticle/PVA scaffolds were also characterised by Nie et al. [88]. The in vitro degradation analysis revealed the scaffolds have a low variation of pH values in simulated body fluid (SBF) solution and the biodegradation rate decreases with increasing concentration of PVA. MTT assay indicated that the scaffold has no negative effects on cell growth and proliferation.

To enhance the biocompatibility and mechanical properties, gelatine [89, 90] and hydrogels [8] were investigated to be used in conjunction with HAP and *poly*caprolactone (PCL) for the production of nanocomposite scaffolds. Jaiswal et al. [89] hypothesised that nano-HAp-coated PCL-gelatin nanofibrous scaffolds resemble more closely to bone environment and enhance the cellular activity towards bone formation as compared to HAp-blended PCL-gelatin scaffolds. Nano-HAp-coated PCL-gelatin nanofibrous scaffolds exhibited better mechanical strength, proliferation and cellular adhesion of MG-63 cells, and osteostimulation than PCL-gelatin and HAp-blended PCL-gelatin scaffolds. Yang et al. [90] also utilised scaffolds composed of electrospun PCL, gelatin, and nano-HAp to examine their in vitro and in vivo behaviour when seeded with dental pulp stem cells (DPSCs). They discovered the addition of nano-HAp significantly increased the odontogenic differentiation of the seeded rat DPSCs. Juhasz et al. [91] attempted to combine a synthetic hydrogel *poly*-2-hydroxyethylmethacrylate (PHEMA) with PCL and to investigate the potential of nano-HAp and carbonate-substituted nano-HAp in providing the PHEMA/PCL composite with greater biologically suitable properties. The addition of both HAp and carbonate-substituted HAp in nano-form was reported to increase the bioactivity and biocompatibility of the PHEMA/PCL composite.

The potential use of high-density *poly*ethylene in conjunction with calcium phosphate nanoparticles as scaffolds was investigated by Hild et al. [92]. Viability assays revealed the absence of cytotoxic effects of the scaffolds. Microscopic images after haematoxylin and eosin staining also confirmed typical growth and morphology.

Electrospun mats of *poly*(vinylpyrrolidone) and amorphous calcium phosphate were prepared by Fletcher et al. [93] in an effort to guide and promote in vitro remineralisation of dental enamel in the presence of fluoride. Crystallisation of amorphous calcium phosphate is promoted specifically in the presence of the enamel surface to produce a firmly adhered contiguous overlayer of HAP crystallites that is approximately 500 nm thick after 1 h of treatment. They suggested the mats can be used as high-concentration reservoirs of amorphous calcium phosphate for the remineralisation of acid-etched dental enamel and occlusion of exposed dentinal tubules in vitro.

16.5 Concluding Remarks

A major increase in interest has been witnessed in nanostructured materials in medicine and dentistry during the last 10 years. It is strongly envisaged that the biomedical applications of materials and devices containing nanocoatings and composites will increase throughout the next decade to be used in tissue engineering, slow drug delivery systems, biologically active membranes, implantable materials, and robotics.

Materials utilising encapsulation or coating of therapeutic and nutritional products will increase. Targeted cancer treatment and slow drug delivery will make use of nanopowders, nanocoatings, and nanocomposites. In drug delivery systems, there are numerous possibilities that contribute to suitable approaches to a range of major medical applications. The nanoparticle approach and hence the increased surface area usually improve solubility, targeting tissues, cells, and cellular receptors.

Nanocomposite coatings and surface modifications of nanocomposite scaffolds are currently being employed to create body-interactive materials that promote the regeneration of tissues and help the body to heal, therefore restoring physiological function. The same coatings are searched, developed, and applied against bacteria, viruses, and infection after operation. This approach is currently being explored in the development of a new generation of nanocoatings that mimic the nature, with a widened range of applications in dentistry and maxillofacial surgery.

Stem cells have been incorporated into a range of calcium phosphate-based scaffolds. Cultured bone marrow cells derived from adult stem cells can be thought of as mesenchymal precursor cell population and are similar to stem cells in that they can also differentiate into different lineages, which are osteoblasts, chondrocytes, adipocytes, and myocytes. When implanted into the body, these cells can combine with mineralised three-dimensional scaffolds to create highly vascularised bone tissue. These nanoscale cultured cell-bioceramic composites can be used for the treatment of large gap in long bone shafts, providing excellent integration of the ceramic scaffold with bone and good functional recovery.

The scope of the application of nanomedical coatings in diagnostics, drug delivery, and implant applications may cover a number of important factors, such as design, engineering, and surgical aspects. At the moment, synthetic dental and orthopaedic implants suffer from a major disadvantage of failing to adapt to the local tissue environment. The purpose of utilising nanocoatings and nanocomposite coatings is to reduce corrosion and ion release and at the same time modifying the surfaces of implant materials to help the body to heal and to promote regeneration of tissues, thus restoring physiological function.

Even though the effect of nanotechnology is widely considered to be extremely beneficial, consideration has to be given to the potential risk associated with such structures. At the moment, there seems to be an absence in the standards of using nanomaterials in dentistry, with no effective techniques to determine and assess exposure risks to nanoparticles in patients or the clinician. Problems may also arise from incomplete nanomaterial safety and toxicity profiles, which sequentially may influence a large range of long-term medical problems. The main point in these discussions is the size of these nanomaterials which is close to a DNA molecular in diameter, and concerns have been raised that these dimensions might permit the nanomaterials to penetrate the skin and enter into the bloodstream and the possibility of escaping the immune system to reach vital organs including the brain.

For now, the relationship between biological responses and surface properties of nanomaterials is one of the main issues in biomedical materials research. The modification of surfaces has become a vital tool for research aimed at understanding how the properties of chemical and structural surface influence material-biosystem interactions. One can expect that surface modifications for the purpose of controlling tissue response will open up avenues for the development of new and superior dental and maxillofacial implants and devices in a more systematic manner and at a faster rate than at present as better understanding is achieved.

References

1. Ben-Nissan B, Choi AH (2006) Sol-gel production of bioactive nanocoatings for medical applications: Part I: An introduction. Nanomedicine 1:311–319
2. Choi AH, Ben-Nissan B (2007) Sol-gel production of bioactive nanocoatings for medical applications: Part II: Current research and development. Nanomedicine 2:51–61
3. Chang MC, Ko CC, Douglas WH (2003) Conformational change of hydroxyapatite/gelatin nanocomposite by glutaraldehyde. Biomaterials 24:3087–3094
4. Zhang W, Liao SS, Cui FZ (2003) Hierarchical self-assembly of nano-fibrils in mineralized collagen. Chem Mater 15:3221–3226
5. Giri S, Trewyn BG, Lin VS (2007) Mesoporous silica nanomaterial-based biotechnological and biomedical delivery systems. Nanomedicine 2:99–111

6. Wu C, Chang J, Zhai W et al (2007) A novel bioactive porous bredigite ($Ca_7MgSi_4O_{16}$) scaffold with biomimetic apatite layer for bone tissue engineering. J Mater Sci Mater Med 18:857–864
7. Victor SP, Sharma CP (2012) Calcium phosphates as drug delivery systems. J Biomater Tissue Eng 2:269–279
8. Uskoković V, Batarni SS, Schweicher J et al (2013) Effect of calcium phosphate particle shape and size on their antibacterial and osteogenic activity in the delivery of antibiotics in vitro. ACS Appl Mater Interfaces 5:2422–2431
9. Kester M, Heakal Y, Fox T et al (2008) Calcium phosphate nanocomposite particles for in vitro imaging and encapsulated chemotherapeutic drug delivery to cancer cells. Nano Lett 8:4116–4121
10. Bastakoti BP, Hsu YC, Liao SH et al (2013) Inorganic-organic hybrid nanoparticles with biocompatible calcium phosphate thin shells for fluorescence enhancement. Chem Asian J 8:1301–1305
11. El-Ghannam A, Ricci K, Malkawi A et al (2010) A ceramic-based anticancer drug delivery system to treat breast cancer. J Mater Sci Mater Med 21:2701–2710
12. Zhao XY, Zhu YJ, Chen F et al (2013) Calcium phosphate hybrid nanoparticles: self-assembly formation, characterization, and application as an anticancer drug nanocarrier. Chem Asian J 8:1306–1312
13. Liang P, Zhao D, Wang CQ et al (2013) Facile preparation of heparin/$CaCO_3$/CaP hybrid nano-carriers with controllable size for anticancer drug delivery. Colloids Surf B Biointerfaces 102:783–788
14. Li WM, Chen SY, Liu DM (2013) In situ doxorubicin-CaP shell formation on amphiphilic gelatin-iron oxide core as a multifunctional drug delivery system with improved cytocompatibility, pH-responsive drug release and MR imaging. Acta Biomater 9:5360–5368
15. Rout SR, Behera B, Maiti TK et al (2012) Multifunctional magnetic calcium phosphate nanoparticles for targeted platin delivery. Dalton Trans 41:10777–10783
16. Mukesh U, Kulkarni V, Tushar R et al (2009) Methotrexate loaded self stabilized calcium phosphate nanoparticles: a novel inorganic carrier for intracellular drug delivery. J Biomed Nanotechnol 5:99–105
17. Chen Z, Li Z, Lin Y et al (2013) Biomineralization inspired surface engineering of nanocarriers for pH-responsive, targeted drug delivery. Biomaterials 34:1364–1371
18. Chiu D, Zhou W, Kitayaporn S et al (2012) Biomineralization and size control of stable calcium phosphate core-protein shell nanoparticles: potential for vaccine applications. Bioconjug Chem 23:610–617
19. Li S, Wang K, Chang K-C et al (2012) Preparation and evaluation of nano-hydroxyapatite/poly(styrene-divinylbenzene) porous microsphere for aspirin carrier. Sci China Chem 55:1134–1139
20. Ignjatović N, Uskoković V, Ajduković Z et al (2013) Multifunctional hydroxyapatite and poly(D, L-lactide-co-glycolide) nanoparticles for the local delivery of cholecalciferol. Mater Sci Eng C 33:943–950
21. Chen R, Qian Y, Li R et al (2010) Methazolamide calcium phosphate nanoparticles in an ocular delivery system. Yakugaku Zasshi 130:419–424
22. Ramachandran R, Paul W, Sharma CP (2009) Synthesis and characterization of PEGylated calcium phosphate nanoparticles for oral insulin delivery. J Biomed Mater Res B Appl Biomater 88:41–48
23. Pittella F, Miyata K, Maeda Y et al (2012) Pancreatic cancer therapy by systemic administration of VEGF siRNA contained in calcium phosphate/charge-conversional polymer hybrid nanoparticles. J Control Release 161:868–874
24. Li J, Chen YC, Tseng YC et al (2010) Biodegradable calcium phosphate nanoparticle with lipid coating for systemic siRNA delivery. J Control Release 142:416–421
25. Olton D, Li J, Wilson ME et al (2007) Nanostructured calcium phosphates (NanoCaPs) for non-viral gene delivery: influence of the synthesis parameters on transfection efficiency. Biomaterials 28:1267–1279

26. Liu Y, Wang T, He F et al (2011) An efficient calcium phosphate nanoparticle-based nonviral vector for gene delivery. Int J Nanomedicine 6:721–727
27. Zhou C, Yu B, Yang X et al (2010) Lipid-coated nano-calcium-phosphate (LNCP) for gene delivery. Int J Pharm 392:201–208
28. Cao X, Deng W, Wei Y et al (2012) Incorporating pTGF-β1/calcium phosphate nanoparticles with fibronectin into 3-dimensional collagen/chitosan scaffolds: efficient, sustained gene delivery to stem cells for chondrogenic differentiation. Eur Cell Mater 23:81–93
29. Sokolova V, Knuschke T, Buer J et al (2011) Quantitative determination of the composition of multi-shell calcium phosphate-oligonucleotide nanoparticles and their application for the activation of dendritic cells. Acta Biomater 7:4029–4036
30. Han JY, Tan TTY, Loo JSC (2011) Utilizing inverse micelles to synthesize calcium phosphate nanoparticles as nano-carriers. J Nanopart Res 13:3441–3454
31. Paul W, Sharma CP (2010) Fatty acid conjugated calcium phosphate nanoparticles for protein delivery. Int J Appl Ceram Technol 7:129–138
32. Kealley CS, Ben-Nissan B, van Riessen A et al (2006) Development of carbon nanotube reinforced hydroxyapatite bioceramics. Key Eng Mater 309–311:597–600
33. Kealley CS, Elcombe MM, van Riessen A et al (2006) Development of carbon nanotube reinforced hydroxyapatite bioceramics. Phys Condens Mater 385–386:897–899
34. Kealley CS, Latella BA, van Riessen A et al (2008) Micro- and nano-indentation of a hydroxyapatite-carbon nanotube composite. J Nanosci Nanotechnol 8:3936–3941
35. Hahn BD, Lee JM, Park DS et al (2009) Mechanical and in vitro biological performances of hydroxyapatite-carbon nanotube composite coatings deposited on Ti by aerosol deposition. Acta Biomater 5:3205–3214
36. Wepasnick KA, Smith BA, Bitter JL et al (2010) Chemical and structural characterization of carbon nanotube surfaces. Anal Bioanal Chem 396:1003–1014
37. Kealley CS, Elcombe MM, van Riessen A et al (2007) Development of carbon nanotube reinforced hydroxyapatite bioceramics. Phys Condens Matter 385–386:897–899
38. Abrishamchian A, Hooshmand T, Mohammadi M et al (2013) Preparation and characterization of multi-walled carbon nanotube/hydroxyapatite nanocomposite film dip coated on Ti-6Al-4V by sol-gel method for biomedical applications: an in vitro study. Mater Sci Eng C Mater Biol Appl 33:2002–2010
39. Facca S, Lahiri D, Fioretti F et al (2011) In vivo osseointegration of nano-designed composite coatings on titanium implants. ACS Nano 5:4790–4799
40. Balani K, Anderson R, Laha T et al (2007) Plasma-sprayed carbon nanotube reinforced hydroxyapatite coatings and their interaction with human osteoblasts in vitro. Biomaterials 28:618–624
41. Zhang B, Kwok CT (2011) Hydroxyapatite-anatase-carbon nanotube nanocomposite coatings fabricated by electrophoretic codeposition for biomedical applications. J Mater Sci Mater Med 22:2249–2259
42. Stylianou A, Yova D, Politopoulos K (2012) Atomic force microscopy surface nanocharacterization of UV-irradiated collagen thin films. In: Kyriacou E, Promponas V, Loizou C et al (eds) Proceedings of the IEEE 12th international conference on bioinformatics and bioengineering. IEEE, New York, pp 603–608
43. Hench LL, Splinter RJ, Greenlee TK et al (1971) Bonding mechanisms at the interface of ceramic prosthetic materials. J Biomed Mater Res 2:117–141
44. Fan Y, Duan K, Wang R (2005) A composite coating by electrolysis-induced collagen self-assembly and calcium phosphate mineralization. Biomaterials 26:1623–1632
45. Wahl DA, Czernuszka JT (2006) Collagen-hydroxyapatite composites for hard tissue repair. Eur Cell Mater 11:43–56
46. Uezono M, Takakuda K, Kikuchi M et al (2013) Hydroxyapatite/collagen nanocomposite-coated titanium rod for achieving rapid osseointegration onto bone surface. J Biomed Mater Res B Appl Biomater. doi:10.1002/jbm.b.32913

47. de Jonge LT, Leeuwenburgh SC, van den Beucken JJ et al (2010) The osteogenic effect of electrosprayed nanoscale collagen/calcium phosphate coatings on titanium. Biomaterials 31:2461–2469
48. Webster TJ, Siegel RW, Bizios R (1999) Osteoblast adhesion on nanophase ceramics. Biomaterials 20:1221–1227
49. Li H, Khor KA, Cheang P (2003) Impact formation and microstructure characterization of thermal sprayed hydroxyapatite/titania composite coatings. Biomaterials 24:949–957
50. Siddharthan A, Sampath Kumar TS, Seshadri SK (2010) In situ composite coating of titania-hydroxyapatite on commercially pure titanium by microwave processing. Surf Coat Technol 204:1755–1763
51. Kuwabara A, Hori N, Sawada T et al (2012) Enhanced biological responses of a hydroxyapatite/TiO_2 hybrid structure when surface electric charge is controlled using radiofrequency sputtering. Dent Mater J 31:368–376
52. Dimitrievska S, Bureau MN, Antoniou J et al (2011) Titania-hydroxyapatite nanocomposite coatings support human mesenchymal stem cells osteogenic differentiation. J Biomed Mater Res A 98:576–588
53. Croteau S, Rauch F, Silvestri A et al (1999) Bone morphogenetic proteins in orthopedics: from basic science to clinical practice. Orthopedics 22:686–695
54. Harakas NK (1984) Demineralized bone-matrix-induced osteogenesis. Clin Orthop Relat Res 188:239–251
55. Zhang N, Nichols HL, Taylor S et al (2007) Fabrication of nanocrystalline hydroxyapatite doped degradable composite hollow fiber for guided and biomimetic bone tissue engineering. Mater Sci Eng 27:599–606
56. Wang GC, Lu ZF, Zhao XB et al (2013) Ordered HAp nanoarchitecture formed on HAp-TCP bioceramics by "nanocarving" and mineralization deposition and its potential use for guiding cell behaviours. J Mater Chem B 1:2455–2462
57. Oliveira JM, Rodrigues MT, Silva SS et al (2006) Novel hydroxyapatite/chitosan bilayered scaffold for osteochondral tissue-engineering applications: Scaffold design and its performance when seeded with goat bone marrow stromal cells. Biomaterials 27:6123–6137
58. Murugan R, Ramakrishna S (2005) Development of nanocomposites for bone grafting. Compos Sci Technol 65:2385–2406
59. TenHuisen KS, Martin RI, Klimkiewicz M et al (1995) Formation and properties of a synthetic bone composite: hydroxyapatite-collagen. J Biomed Mater Res 29:803–810
60. Scabbia A, Trombelli L (2004) A comparative study on the use of a HA/collagen/chondroitin sulphate biomaterial (Biostite) and a bovine-derived HA xenograft (Bio-Oss) in the treatment of deep intra-osseous defects. J Clin Periodontol 31:348–355
61. Daculsi G, Passuti N, Martin S, LeGeros RZ (1990) Macroporous biphasic calcium phosphate ceramic for long bone surgery in human and dogs: clinical and histological study. J Biomed Mater Res 4:379–396
62. LeGeros RZ, Lin S, Rohanizadeh R, Mijares D, LeGeros JP (2003) Biphasic calcium phosphate bioceramics: preparation, properties and applications. J Mater Sci Mater Med 14:201–210
63. Nery E, LeGeros RZ, Lynch KL, Lee K (1992) Tissue response to biphasic calcium phosphate ceramic with different ratios of HA/β-TCP in periodontal osseous defects. J Periodontol 63:729–735
64. Ebrahimi M, Pripatnanont P, Monmaturapoj N et al (2012) Fabrication and characterization of novel nano hydroxyapatite/β-tricalcium phosphate scaffolds in three different composition ratios. J Biomed Mater Res A 100:2260–2268
65. Azevedo MC, Reis RL, Claase MB, Grijpma DW, Feijen J (2003) Development and properties of polycaprolactone/hydroxyapatite composite biomaterials. J Mater Sci Mater Med 14:103–107
66. Ben-Nissan B (2003) Natural bioceramics: from coral to bone and beyond. Curr Opin Solid State Mater Sci 7:283–288
67. Chou J, Ito T, Bishop D, Otsuka M et al (2013) Controlled release of simvastatin from biomimetic beta-TCP drug delivery system. PLoS One 8:e54676. doi:10.1371/journal.pone.0054676

68. Al-Jamal WT, Kostarelos K (2007) Liposome-nanoparticle hybrids for multimodal diagnostic and therapeutic applications. Nanomedicine 2:85–98
69. Schmidt HT, Ostafin AE (2002) Liposome directed growth of calcium phosphate nanoshells. Adv Mater 14:532–535
70. Moura SP, Carmona-Ribeiro AM (2006) Biomimetic particles for isolation and reconstitution of receptor function. Cell Biochem Biophys 44:446–452
71. Xu Q, Tanaka Y, Czernuszka JT (2007) Encapsulation and release of a hydrophobic drug from hydroxyapatite coated liposomes. Biomaterials 28:2687–2694
72. Wang G, Babadağli ME, Uludağ H (2011) Bisphosphonate-derivatized liposomes to control drug release from collagen/hydroxyapatite scaffolds. Mol Pharm 8:1025–1034
73. Lewis K (2010) The development of liposome encapsulated calcium phosphates for bone regeneration. Ph.D. thesis, University of Technology, Sydney, Australia
74. Ono I, Yamashita T, Jin HY et al (2004) Combination of porous hydroxyapatite and cationic liposomes as a vector for BMP-2 gene therapy. Biomaterials 25:4709–4718
75. Huang JS, Liu KM, Chen CC et al (1997) Liposomes-coated hydroxyapatite and tricalcium phosphate implanted in the mandibular bony defect of miniature swine. Kaohsiung J Med Sci 13:213–228
76. Tavakol S, Nikpour MR, Amani A et al (2013) Bone regeneration based on nano-hydroxyapatite and hydroxyapatite/chitosan nanocomposites: an in vitro and in vivo comparative study. J Nanopart Res 15:1373
77. Tomoaia G, Soritau O, Tomoaia-Cotisel M et al (2013) Scaffolds made of nanostructured phosphates, collagen and chitosan for cell culture. Powder Technol 238:99–107
78. Im O, Li J, Wang M et al (2012) Biomimetic three-dimensional nanocrystalline hydroxyapatite and magnetically synthesized single-walled carbon nanotube chitosan nanocomposite for bone regeneration. Int J Nanomedicine 7:2087–2099
79. Venugopal JR, Dev VRG, Senthilram T et al (2011) Osteoblast mineralization with composite nanofibrous substrate for bone tissue regeneration. Cell Biol Int 35:73–80
80. Ou KL, Wu J, Lai WF et al (2010) Effects of the nanostructure and nanoporosity on bioactive nanohydroxyapatite/reconstituted collagen by electrodeposition. J Biomed Mater Res A 92:906–912
81. Rodrigues SC, Salgado CL, Sahu A et al (2013) Preparation and characterization of collagen-nanohydroxyapatite biocomposite scaffolds by cryogelation method for bone tissue engineering applications. J Biomed Mater Res A 101A:1080–1094
82. Guo J, Meng Z, Chen G et al (2012) Restoration of critical-size defects in the rabbit mandible using porous nanohydroxyapatite-polyamide scaffolds. Tissue Eng Part A 18:1239–1252
83. Huang D, Zuo Y, Zou Q et al (2012) Reinforced nanohydroxyapatite/polyamide66 scaffolds by chitosan coating for bone tissue engineering. J Biomed Mater Res B 100B:51–57
84. Lock J, Nguyen TY, Liu H (2012) Nanophase hydroxyapatite and poly(lactide-co-glycolide) composites promote human mesenchymal stem cell adhesion and osteogenic differentiation in vitro. J Mater Sci Mater Med 23:2543–2552
85. Lee JH, Rim NG, Jung HS et al (2010) Control of osteogenic differentiation and mineralization of human mesenchymal stem cells on composite nanofibers containing poly[lactic-co-(glycolic acid)] and hydroxyapatite. Macromol Biosci 10:173–182
86. Buschmann J, Härter L, Gao S et al (2012) Tissue engineered bone grafts based on biomimetic nanocomposite PLGA/amorphous calcium phosphate scaffold and human adipose-derived stem cells. Injury 43:1689–1697
87. Ba Linh NT, Lee KH, Lee BT (2013) Functional nanofiber mat of polyvinyl alcohol/gelatin containing nanoparticles of biphasic calcium phosphate for bone regeneration in rat calvaria defects. J Biomed Mater Res A 101:2412–2423
88. Nie L, Chen D, Suo J et al (2012) Physicochemical characterization and biocompatibility in vitro of biphasic calcium phosphate/polyvinyl alcohol scaffolds prepared by freeze-drying method for bone tissue engineering applications. Colloids Surf B Biointerfaces 100:169–176

89. Jaiswal AK, Chhabra H, Soni VP et al (2013) Enhanced mechanical strength and biocompatibility of electrospun polycaprolactone-gelatin scaffold with surface deposited nanohydroxyapatite. Mater Sci Eng C 33:2376–2385
90. Yang X, Yang F, Walboomers XF et al (2010) The performance of dental pulp stem cells on nanofibrous PCL/gelatin/nHA scaffolds. J Biomed Mater Res A 93:247–257
91. Juhasz JA, Best SM, Bonfield W (2010) Preparation of novel bioactive nano-calcium phosphate-hydrogel composites. Sci Technol Adv Mater 11:014103
92. Hild N, Fuhrer R, Mohn D et al (2012) Nanocomposites of high-density polyethylene with amorphous calcium phosphate: in vitro biomineralization and cytocompatibility of human mesenchymal stem cells. Biomed Mater 7:054103
93. Fletcher J, Walsh D, Fowler CM et al (2011) Electrospun mats of PVP/ACP nanofibres for remineralization of enamel tooth surfaces. Cryst Eng Commun 13:3692–3697

Chapter 17
Fundamental Structure and Properties of Enamel, Dentin and Cementum

Mahdi Shahmoradi, Luiz E. Bertassoni, Hunida M. Elfallah, and Michael Swain

Abstract In this chapter, the fundamental structure of dental tissue at different scale levels and its concurrent role in determining the mechanical properties of the tooth are discussed. The main emphasis is on the role of the organic phase in determining the mechanical properties of enamel and dentin. In this regard, the results of nanoindentation experiments following different treatments of enamel and dentin are presented. These treatments include selective removal of matrix proteins and water of enamel and dentin tissue. The findings indicate that peptides and organic remnants not only play a significant role in the formation and structure of enamel and dentin, but also they regulate the mechanical response and functional integrity of the tooth tissue. In addition, these findings provide a basis for further investigation of the adverse effect of some current clinical treatments, such as bleaching, on the health and properties of dental tissue.

Keywords Nanoindentation • Enamel • Dentin • Bleaching • Matrix proteins

17.1 Introduction

Calcium phosphate research is one of the major fields of research in oral and dental sciences. Naturally, calcium phosphates comprise the main building block of dental hard tissues and alveolar bone and exist in saliva and gingival crevicular fluid precipitations for the whole of life. Pathological calcifications and disturbances in the dynamics of calcium phosphates are the main causes of a variety of oral and dental pathological states. Salivary stone formation (sialolithiasis) and dental calculus formation, which leads to periodontal diseases and dental tissue

---

M. Shahmoradi • L.E. Bertassoni • H.M. Elfallah • M. Swain (✉)
Biomaterials Science Research Unit, Department of Dental Biomaterials, Faculty of Dentistry, University of Sydney, 2 Chalmers Street, Surry Hills, NSW 2010, Australia
e-mail: mswain@mail.usyd.edu.au

B. Ben-Nissan (ed.), *Advances in Calcium Phosphate Biomaterials*, Springer Series in Biomaterials Science and Engineering 2, DOI 10.1007/978-3-642-53980-0_17,

Table 17.1 Calcium phosphates in oral and dental system [1]

Calcium phosphate	Chemical formula	Occurrences
Apatite	$(Ca,Z)_{10}(PO_4,Y)_6(OH,X)_2$	Enamel, dentin cementum, bone, and dental calculi
Octacalcium phosphate, OCP	$Ca_8H_2(PO_4)_6.5H_2O$	Dental calculi
Brushit, dicalcium phosphate dehydrate, DCPD	$CaHPO_4.2H_2O$	Dental calculi
Whitlockite, tricalcium phosphate, β-TCP	$(Ca,Mg)_9(PO_4)_6$	Dentinal caries, salivary stones, and dental calculi

Z = Na, Mg, K, Sr, etc.; Y = CO_3, HPO_4; X = Cl, F

demineralisation resulting in tooth caries, are common presentations of calcium phosphate pathologies in the mouth. These various forms of calcium phosphates in biological structure and pathological states of oral and dental tissues are summarised in Table 17.1. Therapeutic applications of calcium phosphates are another extensive scientific domain, which has gained considerable popularity in recent decades. Calcium phosphate-based restorative dental materials, dental implant coatings, enamel remineralisation systems and periodontal regeneration biomaterials are among the most common oral and dental therapeutics [1].

Our main focus in this chapter is on dental hard tissue-based calcium phosphates, which are mainly in the form of biological apatite. Dental hard tissue comprises enamel, dentin and cementum. The bulk of the dental hard tissue is dentin, which covers the dental soft tissue (dental pulp) lying at the core of the tooth. Enamel is the outer layer that covers the dentin in the crown area, and cementum is the outer layer, covering the dentin in the root area [2]. Enamel, as the masterpiece of biological mineralised tissues and bioceramics, has been of a great interest for material scientists and biologists. Specific features of enamel, including aesthetic, strength and durability, have inspired scientists to develop materials based on these nature-optimised designs. Natural beauty of enamel has inspired the development of direct and indirect tooth-coloured restorative materials. Resin composites and dental porcelain are the materials that have been developed to fulfil the growing demand for beauty and aesthetics in dentistry. Dentin has been a focus of research due to its well-designed hybrid structure, which represents an excellent biocomposite material. However, the most significant aspects of dental tissue structure, which are its exclusive mechanical properties and lifelong durability, have many features that remain to be clarified.

The need for functionally strong and durable dental materials capable of withstanding chronic mechanical, thermal and chemical stresses has created a long-term challenge for researchers in this discipline. The key to potentially unlocking this challenge is to gain an understanding of the magnificent structure and design of the naturally crafted (evolved) structure of dental tissues. The mechanical properties of dental tissues can be studied from two aspects: first, the effect of different compositional elements of this tissue on mechanical response of the tooth and, second, the role of structure and design of the building blocks of this tissue.

Among various methods that have been proposed for the study of mechanical features, nanoindentation has proven to be a reliable nondestructive mechanical testing method that enables the study of spatial variation of materials properties at submicron levels. A great benefit of this technique in studying dental hard tissues is its ability to investigate the materials with heterogeneous structures such as dentin and to some degree enamel. This ability of nanoindentation when coupled with recent structural analysis and microscopy techniques that reveal submicron structure of dental tissue has created unique opportunities to study the mechanical properties in relation to compositional and structural elements.

The aim of this chapter is to review the fundamental structure and properties of enamel, dentin and cementum, with an emphasis on their mechanical features. Most of the presented data are the results of nanoindentation studies on human dental tissue samples. Moreover, data from recent studies by the authors will provide new insights on the role of enamel matrix protein remnants and dentin matrix proteins on the excellent mechanical performance and durability of dental hard tissues. Furthermore, the effect of bleaching treatments, which has become a highly popular treatment of demand by patients, on the features and structure of the tooth will be discussed.

17.2 Structure of Dental Hard Tissues

Histologically, dental hard tissues include enamel, dentin and cementum. Enamel is a rigid, inert and acellular tissue that covers the tooth crown. Dentin forms the bulk of the tooth and as a tougher foundation provides enough support for the more rigid and brittle enamel [3]. In the root area, dentin is covered by cementum, which anchors periodontal ligament fibres that provide the support for a range of dental movements during mastication and function [2]. These tissues form a highly organised and complex structure with ideal functional and structural capabilities, which assist in sustaining mastication-induced mechanical loading and preventing their mechanical failures during function. For achieving a better understanding of these highly organised tissues, the structure and composition of enamel, dentin and cementum are reviewed in this section.

17.2.1 Structure of Enamel

Dental enamel, as the most highly mineralised tissue in the human body, consists of 96 wt% inorganic materials, which are mainly organised in the form of carbonated hydroxyapatite crystals. Other components of enamel include remnants of the organic matrix and loosely bound water molecules [2]. Enamel has an acellular and avascular structure without the ability to regenerate or repair itself. These features reflect the exclusive processes, which occur during the formation of enamel.

Enamel formation (amelogenesis) happens during three primary stages, namely, cytodifferentiation, matrix secretion and maturation.

Amelogenesis is initiated by secretion of the organic matrix from the ameloblasts (enamel-forming cells) into the extracellular space adjacent to the dentinoenamel junction (DEJ). This protein-rich matrix controls enamel biomineralisation by self-assembling into supramolecular assemblies that initiate, regulate and organise the precipitation and growth of the hydroxyapatite crystals. Enamel matrix proteins are noncollagenous proteins composed of hydrophobic amelogenins and non-amelogenin proteins including ameloblastin, enamelin and tuftelin [4]. At the time of mineral deposition, enamel proteinases, enamelysin (MMP 20) and Kallikrein 4 actively participate in the selective degradation and removal process of the protein-rich matrix [5]. Throughout the long maturation stage, the initially protein-rich matrix of enamel is broken down by proteases and replaced by mineral deposition onto the pre-existing apatite crystals, allowing them to grow in width and thickness. After the maturation stage, enamel-forming cells (ameloblasts) disappear thereby preventing any further enamel deposition or repair [5]. This makes the preservation and care of dental enamel of paramount importance.

The result of the maturation stage of amelogenesis is a very hard, highly mineralised tissue, which consists of extremely long high-aspect-ratio hydroxyapatite crystals, and small amount of organic components and water. Enamel crystallites are principally composed of calcium and phosphorus as hydroxyapatite (HAp), $Ca_{10}(PO_4)_6(OH)_2$, with traces of sodium, magnesium, chlorine, carbonate, potassium and fluoride. The organic matrix of mature enamel constitutes 1–2 % of total enamel and functions as the glue for the apatite crystallites [2].

Structurally, the HAp crystals are tightly packed in three levels of hierarchical organisation, which explains some aspects of enamel's mechanical strength [6, 7]. At the largest structural level, bundles combining dozens of enamel rods form the Hunter–Schreger bands. These bands are approximately 50 μm wide and are visible because of the different directions that adjacent bands of prisms reflect or transmit the light [8]. At the next level, enamel rods (prisms) and interrods (interprismatic substance) are visible which represent the primary and fundamental structural units of tooth enamel. Enamel rods are 5–8 μm in diameter cylindrical-like structures [9] that run continuously through the enamel from the dentinoenamel junction (DEJ) to the outer surface of enamel. Close to the DEJ, they are initially in a tortuous course, which follows the movement of the ameloblasts during initial cell growth and enamel deposition [2]. The diameter of the rods almost doubles from dentinoenamel junction to the surface of enamel [10]. In longitudinal section, each rod is near cylindrical in shape and made up of tightly packed apatite crystals with their long axis approximately parallel to the longitudinal axis of the rod (Fig. 17.1). A thin rod sheath surrounds each rod and separates it from adjacent rods by an interrod substance [11]. The line of demarcation between rod and interrod enamel can be identified by the change in crystallite orientation [2].

In cross section, enamel rods have a fish-scale- or keyhole-like pattern. The keyhole shape is made of a head and tail portions (Fig. 17.1). The head is rounded and defined by a thin proteinaceous rod sheath about 0.5 μm thick [2]. However, the rod

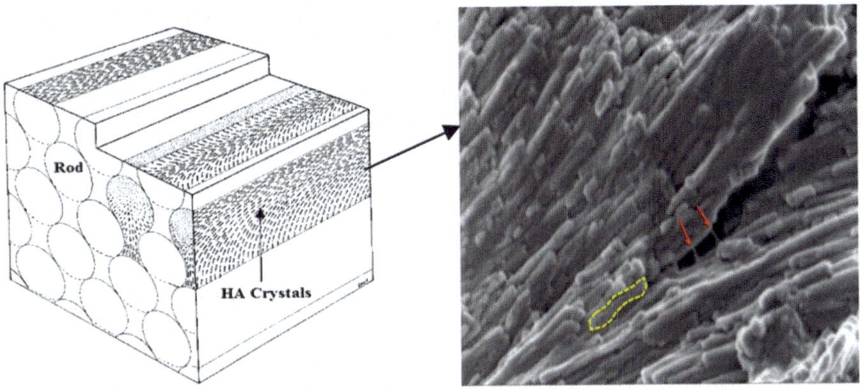

Fig. 17.1 Schematic of enamel rod and interrod structure (Modified and incorporated from Nanci [2]), composed of enamel proteins (*red arrows*) and HAp crystallites (*yellow dotted line*)

tail is less defined and becomes continuous with the interrod enamel [9]. At the last structural level, the nanoscale level, each rod consists of extremely long carbonated HAp crystals which are thin ribbon-like structures with around 60–70 nm wide and ~20 nm thick [12]. In the central part of the rod, the apatite crystallites are arranged with their long axis (*c*-axis) parallel to the longitudinal axis of the rod, whereas in the tail portion they diverge from the longitudinal axis of the rod by up to 65° [8]. Each calcium phosphate unit cell in the maturing enamel appears hexagonal. However, in fully mature enamel, the crystal outline looks more irregular due to the interaction with other growing crystals during the last stages of crystal growth.

Upon tooth eruption, although most of the enamel organic matrix is removed during mineralisation and maturation by the activity of enamel proteinases [5], some proteins are retained between the HAp crystallites and in the rod sheath [13]. In fact, some of the matrix proteins are resistant to protein degradation due to their strong binding to the HAp crystals and are retained in the mature enamel. These matrix proteins remain trapped between the crystallites and around the rods in mature enamel. This remnant matrix of mature enamel is a multicomponent protein/peptide mix formed by the association of different monomeric proteins [14]. Those proteins lying between crystallites have the function of 'gluing' HAp crystallites together, maintaining the hierarchical structure and enabling enamel to sustain the mechanical loading during function. The presence of remnant matrix proteins in mature enamel has been shown to influence its optical and mechanical properties. The minor components of enamel, protein remnants and water, have a profound plasticising effect [9]. Enamel is now known to be much more flexible and softer than its major component, crystalline HAp [15]. Structural changes in these protein components can reduce the ability of enamel to dissipate stresses [16]. In the later parts of this chapter, the effect of protein matrix modification of enamel on its mechanical response will be discussed. The presence of this organic matrix along with the mentioned hierarchical organisation of enamel has been shown to regulate the mechanical properties of enamel by forming a structure whereby flexural strength and elastic modulus decrease with increasing hierarchical dimension along with a change from linear–elastic to elastic–inelastic mechanical behaviour. This complex structural arrangement also makes enamel the hardest tissue in the human body [16]. Mechanical properties vary at different regions of enamel. The surface layer of enamel is stiffer, denser and less permeable than the rest of the enamel [8]. In spite of its hardness, enamel is extremely brittle especially when the underlying resilient dentin is lost.

Enamel is translucent and varies in shade from light yellow to grey white. At the incisal edge of a recently erupted tooth, enamel appears bluish white [11]. In cervical areas, enamel reflects the yellow colour of the underlying dentin, which determines the tooth colour along with the enamel thickness and translucency. The enamel translucency increases with age and therefore transmits the yellow colour of the underlying dentin and appears darker. Despite the fact that enamel is composed of tightly packed hydroxyapatite crystals, enamel is selectively permeable by way of the protein 'glue' structure to certain substances such as calcium and fluoride for remineralisation of demineralised enamel. Fluoride ions can penetrate the enamel from saliva and form fluorapatite crystal-rich layers at the surface, which are larger and more chemically resistant to bacterial acid dissolution [11]. Ions can penetrate enamel either from saliva, food and beverages, and then become incorporated into the interprismatic region or internally from the pulp through the DEJ and change its chemical composition [10]. In addition to small inorganic molecules, enamel is also permeable to larger molecules associated with stains and pigments. These large molecules diffuse through pores found at the prism boundaries and interprismatic enamel [8].

17.2.2 Structure of Dentin

Dentin and pulp tissue are generally regarded as a single functional and histological unit, termed the dentin–pulp complex [2]. However, we will only consider dentin in this chapter, as the subject of this book is about calcium phosphates. Dentin is a highly organised biological structure composed of complex protein assemblies and organised mineral components, which collectively form a rigid and durable mineral-rich biocomposite [17]. Dentin is formed through the process of dentinogenesis, by odontoblasts that differentiate from ectomesenchymal cells of the dental papilla. The dental papilla primarily induces the formation of dentin until it is finally surrounded by secreted dentin, thus forming the dental pulp [2]. A complex group of synchronised biological events regulates the formation and maturation of dentin. The main stages of dentinogenesis include the cytodifferentiation of the odontoblasts, the formation of mantle dentin, the control of mineralisation of the primary dentin organic matrix and, finally, the secretion of secondary and tertiary dentin. Primary dentin is the outermost layer of the dentin, which includes the mantle and the circumpulpal components. Secondary dentin is a layer that is secreted after the root formation. Tertiary dentin is the type of dentin that is secreted after full formation of the tooth, as a response to a stimulus, such as carious attack or wear.

Compositionally, dentin is a hydrated tissue comprised of approximately 50 vol% of carbonated hydroxyapatite minerals, 30 vol% of collagen and noncollagenous molecules and the remainder fluids. 90 wt% of the organic phase in dentin is almost exclusively composed of collagen type I, although other types of collagen have also been identified [18]. The remainder of the dentin organic matrix includes noncollagenous structures, of which proteoglycans (PG) are of a greater structural and mechanical importance [17]; other dentin matrix proteins, such as phosphoproteins and γ-carboxyglutamate-containing proteins, are believed to be more involved in mineral–matrix binding events [19]. Decorin and biglycan, two members of the small leucine-rich repeat (SLRP) family, are the PGs predominantly expressed in dentin. The most frequently found GAGs, in turn, are chondroitin 4-sulphate and a relatively lower content of chondroitin 6-sulphate.

Structurally, dentin is composed of packed dentinal tubules, measuring about 1–2 μm diameter surrounded by a hypermineralised layer called peritubular dentin, and a softer intertubular matrix, where the organic material is concentrated [20]. Dentinal tubules contain cytoplasmic extensions of odontoblasts, which lie in the pulp and originally were involved in the secretion of dentin matrix. In addition to this odontoblastic process, dentinal tubules contain dentinal fluid, which contains proteins and proteoglycans. The peritubular dentin is a highly mineralised composite material constituted of phosphorylated proteins [21, 22], proteoglycans and glycosaminoglycans [22], which lacks collagen fibrils [22, 23]. The intertubular dentin, on the other hand, is composed of supramolecular aggregates of collagen molecules, which are assembled into type I fibrils interconnected by noncollagenous components and water [24]. This array of organic molecules forms a hydrated organic network serving as a scaffold for the nucleation and growth of carbonated apatite mineral crystals [25]. The result of this organic–inorganic interplay is an intricate biocomposite that exhibits outstanding longevity and serves as a tough and resilient foundation for the brittle enamel, as well as a protective layer for the living pulpal soft tissue. This foundation prevents the propagation of catastrophic cracks from the brittle enamel further into the dentin [3, 26].

Dentin and enamel are bound strongly at their common interface, which is called the dentinoenamel junction (DEJ). Dentinoenamel junction is a hypermineralised area that appears like a well-defined scalloped area under the microscope. The presence and the form of this area have an important role in the structural and functional integrity of enamel and dentin. Due to the presence of dentinal tubules, dentin is far more permeable than enamel (Fig. 17.2).

17.2.3 Structure of Cementum

Cementum is a mineralised avascular connective tissue, which is primarily composed of HAp minerals (65 wt%), with the addition of organic matrix (23 wt%)

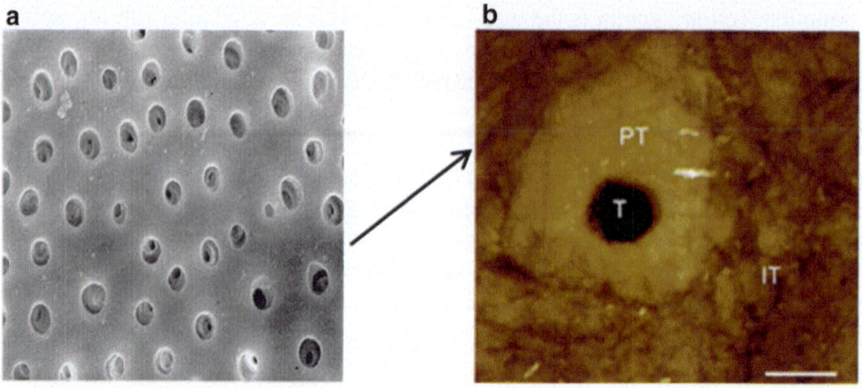

Fig. 17.2 (**a**) SEM of a transverse section of dentin. (**b**) Atomic force microscopy (*AFM*) image showing the cross-sectional view of the general structure of dentin tubule and peritubular and intertubular dentin (1 μm scale bar)

and water (12 wt%). The composition of cementum is very similar to bone. HAp minerals in cementum have a uniform small plate shape. The organic matrix is composed of collagen and noncollagenous proteins. Type I collagen fibrils comprise about 90 % of the organic cementum matrix. During cementogenesis, cementum is secreted by cementoblasts and after the completion of tooth development; it covers the roots of the tooth tightly in an interlocking manner. There are two types of cementum, which includes cellular and acellular cementum. Cellular cementum, which covers the apical third of the root, has an organised lacunar structure similar to bone and includes cementocytes. Acellular cementum covers the cervical portion of the root and has no organised structure and cells. It is assumed that cellular cementum anchors the periodontal ligament (PDL) fibre bundles and the acellular cementum has a more adaptive role [2]. Cementum, along with alveolar bone and periodontal ligament, forms the dental periodontium, which is the attachment apparatus of the tooth. Collagen fibrils within the cementum matrix play a crucial role in the attachment of periodontal ligament fibres to the tooth. The mastication forces exerted on the teeth are directed and distributed into the alveolar bone through these fibres.

17.3 Mechanical Properties of Enamel

Among various methods for studying the mechanical properties of dental tissues, nanoindentation has emerged as a nondestructive, precise method which is very useful in examining materials with small specimen size. Due to the differences which exist in the structure, mineral density, age and type among different teeth and also among different regions of each tooth, nanoindentation can provide a nondestructive method for studying a very small area of the specimen, therefore preserving other parts of the specimen for comparative studies.

Based on the load–displacement response of nanoindentation tests and its related calculations, several mechanical features of the test material can be measured. These parameters include hardness and elastic modulus, energy expenditure and creep behaviour.

In this chapter, we do not present the detailed calculation and theoretical basis for all of the nanoindentation experiments. Rather, we mostly emphasise on the presentation of the data and interpretation of the results which are of more interest for the readers of this chapter and are related to the scope of this book. Interested readers are encouraged to refer to available literature [27, 28] on nanoindentation and its application in studying biological tissues and other materials.

17.3.1 Mechanical Properties of Sound Enamel

In this section, we first discuss the basic mechanical properties of sound enamel, and later we will present the data on the contributing role of each structural element of enamel, including HAp, water and protein remnants in determining the mechanical behaviour of dental enamel.

17.3.1.1 Hardness and Elastic Modulus

Hardness is defined as the resistance of the material to permanent deformation under the indentation [29]. The nanoindentation hardness (H) is the contact pressure of the indenter divided by the projected contact area (A) of the sample at maximum load (P_{max}) which can be estimated from [30]

$$H = \frac{P_{\mathrm{max}}}{A} \tag{17.1}$$

Elastic modulus or Young's modulus is the rigidity of a material within the elastic range. In nanoindentation experiments, the elastic modulus of the specimen E_{s} can be calculated from [30]

$$E = \left(\frac{1-\nu_{\mathrm{s}}^{2}}{E_{\mathrm{s}}} + \frac{1-\nu_{\mathrm{i}}^{2}}{E_{\mathrm{i}}}\right)^{-1} \tag{17.2}$$

where E is the indentation elastic modulus (reduced modulus) and E_{i} and ν_{i} are the elastic modulus and Poisson's ratio of the indenter, respectively. ν_{s} is the Poisson's ratio of the sample which is 0.3 for enamel [31].

Unlike the great variability in the results of hardness and elastic modulus tests of macroscale experiments, the results of nanoindentation tests show better consistency. However, these results depend on several factors related to sample properties and testing conditions. For example, the hardness for the top surface of enamel has been reported in a range of 3.39 ± 0.18 to 4.9 ± 0.5 GPa and the elastic modulus in the range of 83.4 ± 7.1 to 105.2 ± 1.3 GPa [27]. Lower values are reported for the cross-sectional surface [27]. Observed trends in the results of different measurements of hardness and elastic modulus can be summarised as follows:

1. The hardness and elastic modulus of enamel are dependent on the direction of the load relative to its rod and interrod orientation [32]. The values are significantly higher at top (occlusal) surface of enamel compared with the cross-sectional lateral surface. These results are reflective of the anisotropic microstructure of the enamel. In fact, higher hardness and elastic modulus values are observed when the direction of the load is parallel with the direction of enamel rods and is resisted by thousands of aligned HAp crystals. Lower values are obtained when the force is applied perpendicular to the rods, allowing more displacement and movement due to the presence of less stiff organic sheathe.
2. The hardness and elastic modulus are dependent on the site of the indentation within each tooth. Enamel is more mineralised in the surface and becomes less mineralised towards the DEJ [33]. The size of enamel rods is larger at the surface, while in the inner portion of enamel, softer interrods which contain more protein become larger and comprise a higher volume fraction of enamel. This difference in the amount of mineralisation and rod–interrod size is reflected in the mechanical features of enamel, as surface enamel has higher hardness and elastic modulus values compared with inner enamel.
3. The elastic modulus is dependent on the type and size of the indenter tip and the applied load [34]. It has been suggested that with increased load of the indenter tip, more interrod area is involved in the indenter contact area which leads to inclusion of more organic sheath area with less elastic modulus value [27].

17.3.1.2 Stress–Strain Relationship of Enamel

The stress–strain curves of enamel and several dental materials were plotted from nanoindentation experiments [35]. There were several findings when comparing stress–strain curve of enamel with other materials. Firstly, the resultant curve for enamel is fairly smooth, and unlike pure HAp, no prominent elastic–plastic transition point is observed. This shows that enamel response to mechanical stress is different from that of HAp which is enamel's main building block. This different mechanical response is attributed to the presence of organic component which makes the enamel a viscoelastic material.

Secondly, the surface perpendicular to the rod orientation shows a higher stress–strain response than lateral cross-sectional surfaces. This finding confirms the anisotropic nature of dental enamel and is explained by the response of protein-rich interrod area to mechanical stress.

Thirdly, the stress–strain curve of enamel is more similar to metallic materials than HAp and ceramics (Fig. 17.3). This behaviour of enamel is also caused by the

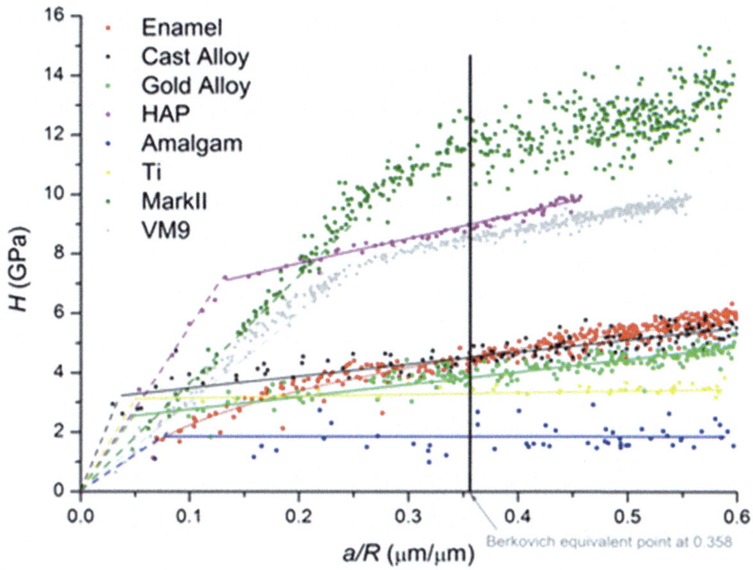

Fig. 17.3 Stress–strain relationship of different materials (*solid lines* show plastic part and *short dots lines* show elastic part of materials calculated from Hertz equation) [34]

presence of organic components and the hierarchical structure of enamel in different scale levels which imparts enamel with the ability to dissipate stress without losing its structural integrity by cracking.

17.3.1.3 Indentation Creep Behaviour

Inelastic strain of a material is caused by slow flow of its structure when it is held at a fixed load below its conventional yield strength for a period of time. This viscoelastic response may also be reversible, as is the case for enamel, which enables it to tolerate and redistribute the loading stresses during function [27].

The constant load indentation creep analysis is considered the most commonly used method for testing the creep behaviour of different materials including mineralised biological materials such as teeth [6]. With this method, the viscoelastic properties are recorded as the change in penetration depth with time under constant applied load. The difference between the displacement during creep at maximum load and recovery at minimum load represents the amount of unrecovered deformation during a hold period at constant force. In addition, the relative recovery of the material in relation to the deformation is calculated as a percentage by the relationship

$$\% \text{ Recovery} = h_2/h_1 \times 100 \tag{17.3}$$

where h_1 is the indentation depth displacement during hold at maximum load and h_2 is the displacement recovery during the holding time at a specific portion (typically 1 %) of the maximum load upon unloading.

This relative recovery indicates the amount of the deformation that occurs during loading and is recovered towards its normal state during a specific time interval upon unloading.

Comparison of the creep response of enamel, compared with HAp and dental materials, showed it exhibited a relatively stable creep response. In contrast, HAp did not show a viscous behaviour, and its creep deformation was very limited (Fig. 17.4).

Similarly the response of enamel upon unloading was significant, while HAp exhibited limited creep recovery. The reversible creep behaviour of enamel is considered as a mechanism to withstand functional stresses during mastication which helps the teeth to distribute the localised high masticatory forces and sliding contact forces between teeth.

The mechanisms responsible for this behaviour are mostly related to the presence of the minor organic phase and water components of enamel. These organic protein/peptide biopolymers possess viscoelastic deformation and recovery features gained through sacrificial bond mechanism [35]. Similar explanations were proposed by Schneider et al. who suggested that the creep behaviour of enamel is due to flow of the protein in the interrod sheath layer under stress application [36].

17.3.1.4 Energy Absorption of Enamel

As mentioned above, enamel is not an ideal elastic material, and it shows inelastic behaviour due to the presence of organic phase and water content. For studying inelastic behaviour of dental enamel using nanoindentation, energy absorption and creep response of enamel are considered reliable test parameters which can properly measure the plastic response of the material.

One of the defined parameters which relates to the energy absorption of enamel is energy expenditure index, ψ, which is the ratio of the dissipated energy, U_d, to the total energy, U_t. This parameter describes the relative elastic–inelastic behaviour of a material when it undergoes stresses and inelastic strains. This parameter can be calculated based on the following equation for normalising different test results:

$$\psi = \left(\frac{U_d}{U_t}\right) 100\,\% \tag{17.4}$$

The resultant value of ψ ranges from 0 for an ideal elastic material to 100 for an ideal plastic material.

Energy expenditure ratios of enamel and hydroxyapatite were calculated from nanoindentation experiments and were plotted against the contact strain values [37]. The results indicated that enamel exhibits an energy expenditure ratio beginning at 30 % which has a monotonic increase with the contact strain without any obvious

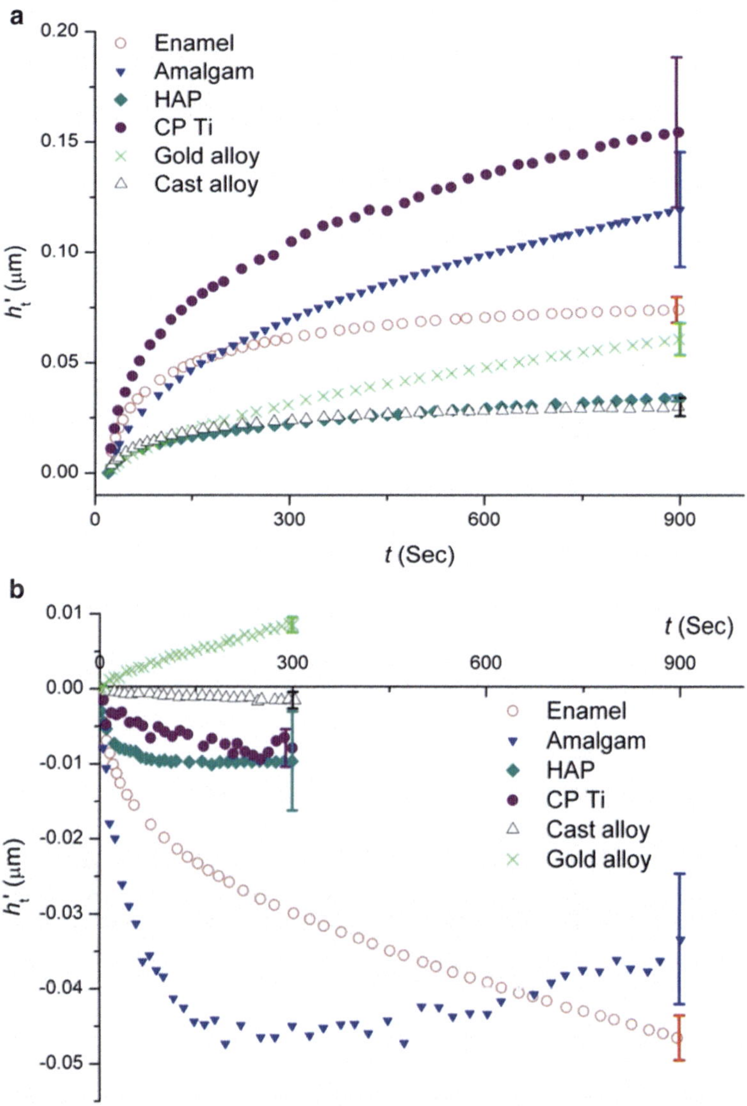

Fig. 17.4 Curves of (**a**) creep and (**b**) creep recovery of different materials. (h_t' values of amalgam in (**a**) were divided by 10 to fit onto the diagram.) (Reprinted from He and Swain [35]. Copyright 2007, with permission from Elsevier)

elastic part. In comparison, in the case of HAp, the curve started from 0 %, and it possessed a linear portion for strain values less than 0.5. When comparing the amount of energy dissipation between enamel and HAp, it was observed that enamel had a somewhat higher (10 %) capability to dissipate energy than HAp at the same strain level (Fig. 17.5).

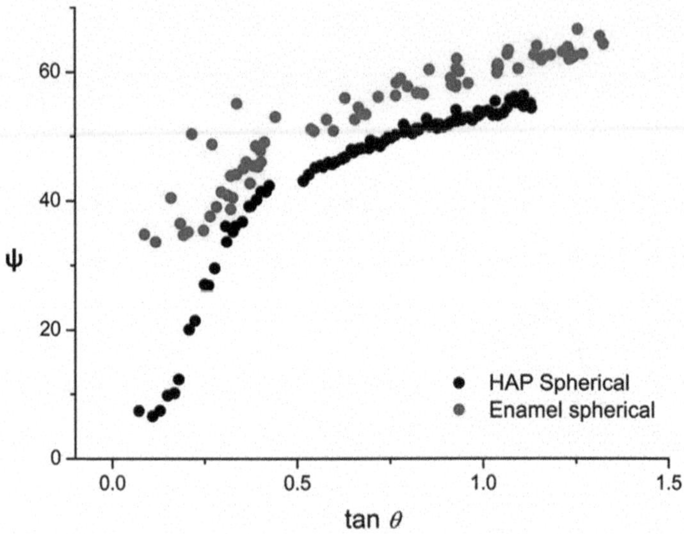

Fig. 17.5 Comparison of energy absorption ability between enamel and HAp disc [34]

This difference between the energy expenditure of enamel and HAp has been attributed to the presence of organic phase and water component in the structure of enamel. It has been suggested [37] that these two components contribute to this energy dissipation role through the following possible mechanisms:

1. Fluid flow within the sheath structure based on Fox's stiff sponge model [38]: based on this mechanism, enamel acts like a stiff sponge from which liquid is expelled in compression and drawn in again once the load is removed.
2. Temporary sacrifice of inter- and intramolecular bonds of enamel protein fragments based on Smith's model [39]: with this mechanism, the remaining protein fragments consume the energy to enable configuration rearrangements. As these new configurations are thermodynamically unstable, these molecules regain their original configuration after removal of the external strain.
3. Nanoscale friction and slippage within sheath which is related to the presence of cleavage planes and degustation of enamel rods [40].

Higher energy expenditure of enamel is one of the keys to its long-lasting function and resistance against considerable mechanical stresses which are exerted on dental enamel during the whole life of an individual.

17.3.2 Mechanical Properties of Heated and Ethanol-Treated Enamel

Dental tissue is subjected to a variety of external materials and environmental conditions which affect its structural and mechanical properties. Some of these conditions like acid treatment influence the mechanical properties of enamel through their effect on mineral content of this tissue. Other factors, like heating and ethanol treatment, exclusively affect the water content and organic content of enamel, therefore providing a suitable method for studying the contributing role of water molecules and organic phase in mechanical properties of dental enamel.

In a series of experiments, nanoindentation tests were performed on samples which were placed in a dental ceramic furnace and were heated to a temperature of 300 °C for 5 min. Other samples were treated by immersion into ethanol [41]. Mechanical properties including nanoindentation elastic modulus, hardness and creep behaviour of sound and burnt enamel specimens were tested in water and dry environment. The sound enamel samples were then immersed in pure ethanol for 24 h for achieving dehydration, and the same indentation tests were performed. Then, for rehydrating the samples, they were returned into distilled water for another 24 h period before the same tests were repeated. In the last stage, the samples were dried in ambient environment for another 24 h (dry), and indentation tests were repeated again. The data from nanoindentation tests were used to determine hardness, elastic modulus and creep behaviour of enamel specimens.

17.3.2.1 Hardness and Elastic Modulus

The results of the experiments demonstrated that sound and burnt enamel had the highest hardness values followed by the ethanol-dehydrated samples (Fig. 17.6). Rehydrated samples were the softest, while drying of the rehydrated samples raised their hardness values [41].

The results for E modulus calculations indicated that the values of the alcohol-dehydrated and dry enamel are significantly higher than sound enamel. In contrast, rehydrated samples have a much lower value than sound enamel. Because matrix proteins and other organic components have been denatured during the heating procedure, the modulus for burnt sample was not calculated. Heat treatment destroys matrix proteins inside enamel, while pure ethanol partially blocks functions of matrix proteins by dehydrating the system. As a result, without deformable matrix proteins, the mechanical behaviour of different enamel samples noticeably changed.

Different responses of ethanol-dehydrated group are result of the change in the structure and function of enamel matrix proteins. This change may be assigned to the biochemical function of ethanol. The small radius of ethanol molecule ($\sim$0.17 nm) allows this small molecule to penetrate into most pores of the molecular-sieve-like enamel [42]. Moreover, ethanol has a strong dehydrating function and can change the conformation of a peptide chain within proteins [43, 44]. Ethanol's amphiphilic properties enable it to be attracted simultaneously to both hydrophobic and hydrophilic targets, displace water and bind to specific targets favourably and lead to conformational changes of peptide chains of proteins [43]. Comparison of the mechanical behaviour of sound and treated enamel samples demonstrates that matrix proteins improve the performance of enamel as a load-bearing calcified tissue.

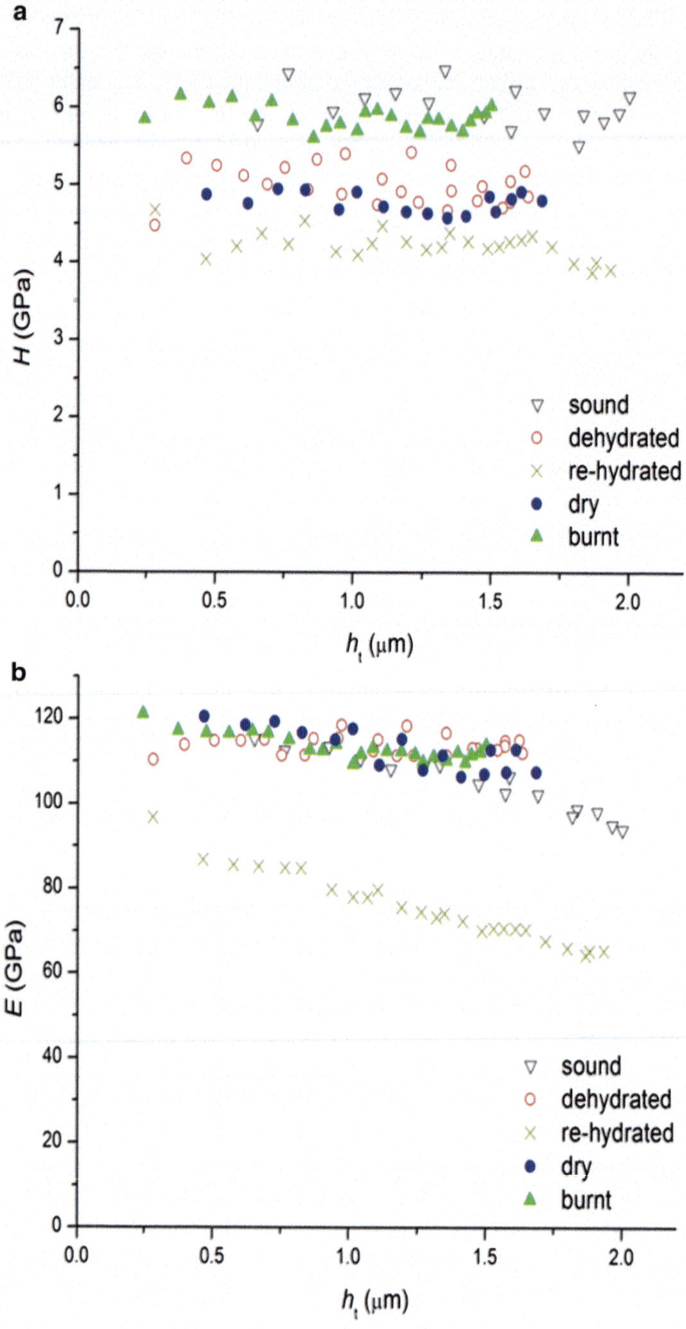

Fig. 17.6 (**a**) Hardness and (**b**) elastic modulus of enamel under different treatments [34]

17.3.2.2 Indentation Creep Behaviour

Creep test results of sound and treated specimens indicated that at maximum-load holding (creep period), rehydrated enamel had the highest creep displacement followed by sound enamel [41]. Alcohol-dehydrated and burnt samples had similar creep curves, which were much lower than the other two samples. Dried enamel had a value between burnt and sound samples. At the minimum-load-holding period (creep recovery period), the recovery was again highest for the rehydrated sample, which was more than sound enamel. Dehydrated sample had very limited creep recovery, while that for burnt enamel was negligible after the first 100 s (Fig. 17.7).

These results show that at both the maximum and minimum loads, different environment mediums affect the creep behaviour of enamel. As HAp has minimal viscous behaviour, it can be assumed that creep and creep recovery are consequences of the protein matrix deformation. A possible explanation for high creep and creep recovery value of rehydrated sample may be the oversaturation of water within the enamel microstructure following rehydration. Additional water may have contributed to more extensive creep and creep recovery responses of the sample by softening or plasticising the entire biocomposite system.

It can be suggested that the rehydration procedure may have resulted in hyper-hydration of the peptide chains and swelling of the enamel matrix. However, following 24 h drying of the rehydrated sample in an ambient environment, creep and creep recovery behaviour decreased and were slightly lower than sound enamel.

Similar studies on bone and enamel [45, 46] have shown that heat treatment denatured matrix protein and collagen fibres, therefore affecting the mechanical properties of heated samples significantly. Similarly, it is reasonable to assume that the protein matrix and water within burnt enamel specimens have been destroyed and eliminated. This supports the notion that creep recovery arises mainly from the presence of the protein matrix. By comparing burnt with dehydrated samples, the limited creep recovery of dehydrated samples may be explained as follows: although the biological functions of protein matrix have been disrupted by ethanol, these protein remnants may still act as biopolymers with some degree of viscoelastic behaviour. In addition, although free water and loosely bound water were released from burnt enamel, ethanol liquid inside dehydrated samples may have some lubricating function which contributes to viscoelastic behaviour.

The protein components of ethanol-dehydrated and dry samples became stiffer than sound enamel due to the loss of water and/or changing of conformation. With higher E values, indicating that the biopolymer proteins are less plasticised, it is reasonable to anticipate less creep and creep recovery for these two groups. On the other hand, additional plasticising agents such as water in rehydrated group may not only recover the protein responses but also lubricate the biocomposite system, therefore, resulting in increased creep and creep recovery. In addition, as heating results in the loss of the biological functions of organic matrix, therefore crystallite-boundary sliding and densification may remain as the main creep and deformation mechanisms of heated enamel with its fine microstructure and considerable porosity existing between the crystallites [47].

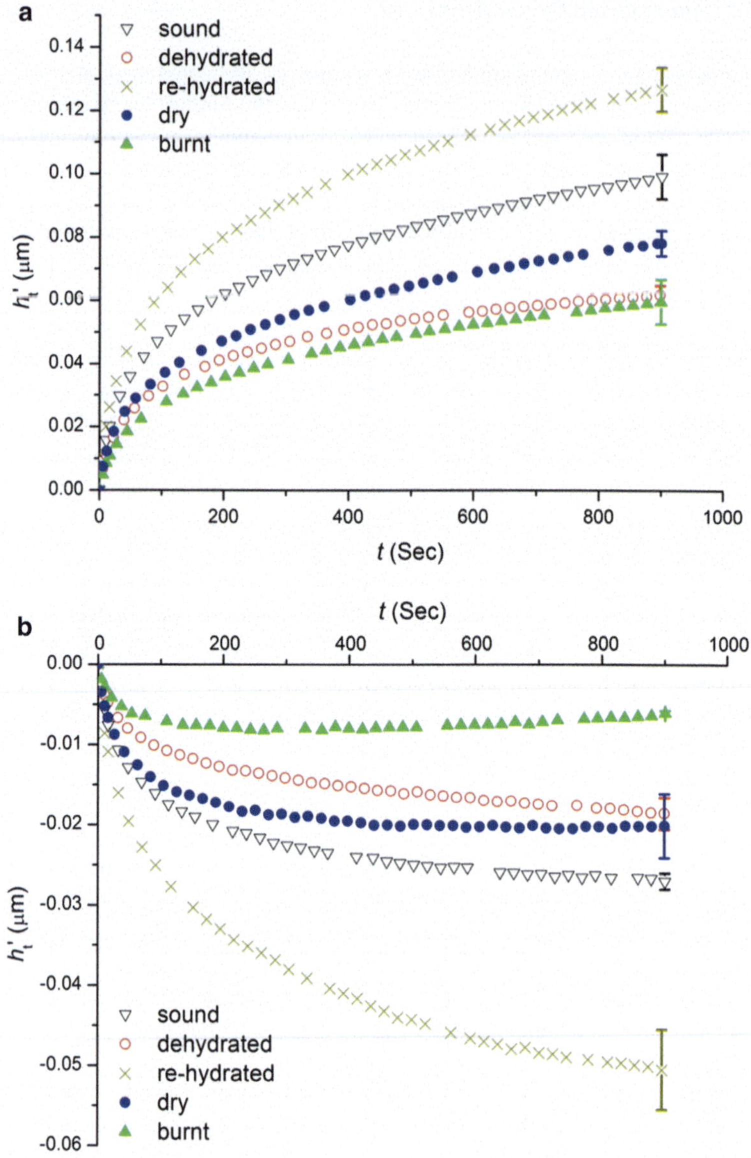

Fig. 17.7 Indentation depth against time, h_t'–t, curves of (**a**) creep and (**b**) creep recovery of enamel under different treatments (Reprinted from He and Swain [41]. Copyright 2007, with permission from Elsevier)

In order to ensure that heating does not change the chemical and compositional features of dental enamel, elemental analysis (EDX) was performed on sound and burnt specimens (Fig. 17.8). The results showed that sound and burnt enamel had exactly the same elemental composition, including the Ca to P ratio, which indicates

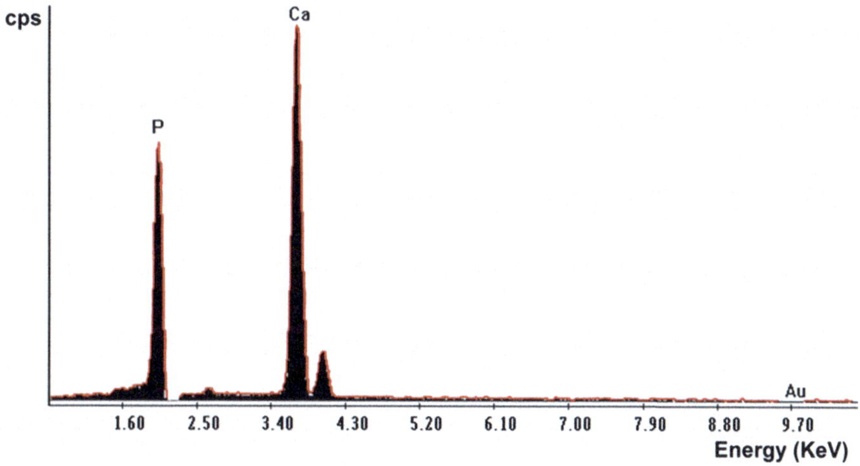

Fig. 17.8 Comparison of EDX spectrum on sound (*black area*) and burnt enamel (*red line*). (Two spectra completely overlapped.) (Reprinted from He and Swain [41]. Copyright 2007, with permission from Elsevier)

no chemical changes of the inorganic component of enamel occurred during the heating procedure [47].

As HAp crystals are considered chemically and thermally stable under the above-mentioned test conditions, these findings indicate the changes that occurred in the mechanical properties of enamel are not related to mineral composition, and therefore, it is only the changed small amount of protein and water inside enamel which has affected the mechanical properties of the specimen.

17.3.3 Mechanical Properties of Bleached Enamel

Bleaching of dental surfaces is a process in which oxidising agents are applied on the external surfaces of vital teeth or internal surfaces of endodontically treated teeth in order to remove the external and/or internal discoloration caused by various pigment molecules. The main component of the bleaching agents is hydrogen peroxide which acts as a strong oxidising agent through the formation of oxygen free radicals such as superoxide, peroxyl and alkoxyl [48]. These free radicals have the ability to oxidise chromophores to produce shorter-chain and less-pigmented molecules [49]. Tooth bleaching occurs by diffusion of these peroxide agents into and through the discoloured enamel.

Associated with the fact that these agents contact and interact with the protein remnants of the enamel, it is expected that the application of these oxidising agents may influence the mechanical properties of enamel through their effect on its organic components. As a result, studying the effect of bleaching agents on mechanical properties of enamel may shed further light on the role of protein content to mechanical behaviour of this tissue exclusively.

However, there is considerable controversy in the literature regarding the effect of bleaching agents especially on the hardness of dental enamel. Some of these studies have found no adverse effect of bleaching products on the enamel [50–52]. Almost all those studies have used microhardness techniques such as Vickers and Knoop tests that rely upon visual measurement of the contact dimensions [53, 54]. Only relatively few studies have used the nanoindentation system to investigate the changes in enamel hardness after treatment with tooth bleaching products [55–57].

In our experiments [58], we applied a range of loads to normal and bleached enamel samples to measure the hardness and elastic modulus of bleached enamel. In addition, the ability of sound and bleached enamel to recover the viscoelastic strains was evaluated. For a better understanding of the effect of bleaching agent concentration on mechanical features of enamel, two bleaching regimes, home and office bleaching, were applied.

17.3.3.1 Hardness and Elastic Modulus

The results of hardness and elastic modulus under different indentation loads indicated that a significant reduction of enamel hardness and elastic modulus occurs after application of H_2O_2 (Fig. 17.9). These changes in mechanical properties are attributed to the compositional and structural changes in enamel proteins caused by the oxidation reaction of the hydrogen peroxide free radicals. These results are supported by other studies which have shown a reduction of mechanical properties of enamel and dentin following bleaching treatment [57].

The results also indicate that the effect of tooth bleaching is more obvious in the surface and adjacent subsurface layer of enamel. The greatest reduction was observed at the surface layer of enamel (less than 2 μm) and the values returned to normal with increasing depth below the surface. The reduction of the mechanical properties with increasing contact depth (load) of the indentation, which was seen in the sound and bleached enamel, supports the concept that bleaching effect is more significant in the surface enamel. The difference in mechanical properties between the control and the bleached enamel is greater at lower loads. As the load and subsequent contact depths increase, the differences between the control and bleached groups decrease. This observation also helps explain why negative results were seen in most previous studies that used high indentation loads.

17.3.3.2 Indentation Creep Behaviour

Following different bleaching treatments, sound enamel exhibited higher creep deformation than untreated teeth (Fig. 17.10). The creep deformation behaviour of dental enamel has been found, as mentioned above, to originate principally from its protein components [16]. Under constant loading, the indenter produces tension on

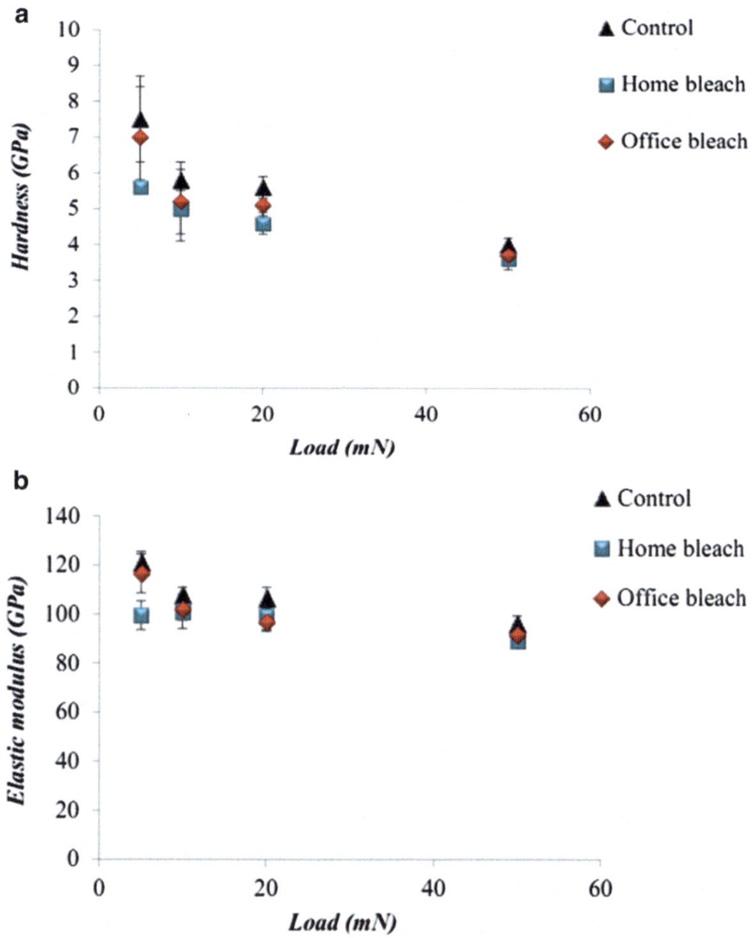

Fig. 17.9 (**a**) Hardness and (**b**) elastic modulus elastic for sound and bleached enamel at different indentation loads

the hydroxyapatite crystallites that is transferred as shear to the proteins between the crystals and in the rod sheath.

The protein shearing results in unfolding of its domain structure and permits limited sliding of the hydroxyapatite crystals. The higher creep deformation seen in bleached enamel is due to conformational changes in its protein structure and loss or denaturing of its domain bonds caused by the oxidation reaction of the peroxides. These structural changes of the protein can lead to increased slippage at the protein–mineral interface which was seen as increased deformation.

Regarding the creep recovery response of sound and bleached enamel, it was observed that treated enamel with home and in-office bleaching agents show limited recovery of the creep deformation in comparison with the sound enamel. This is

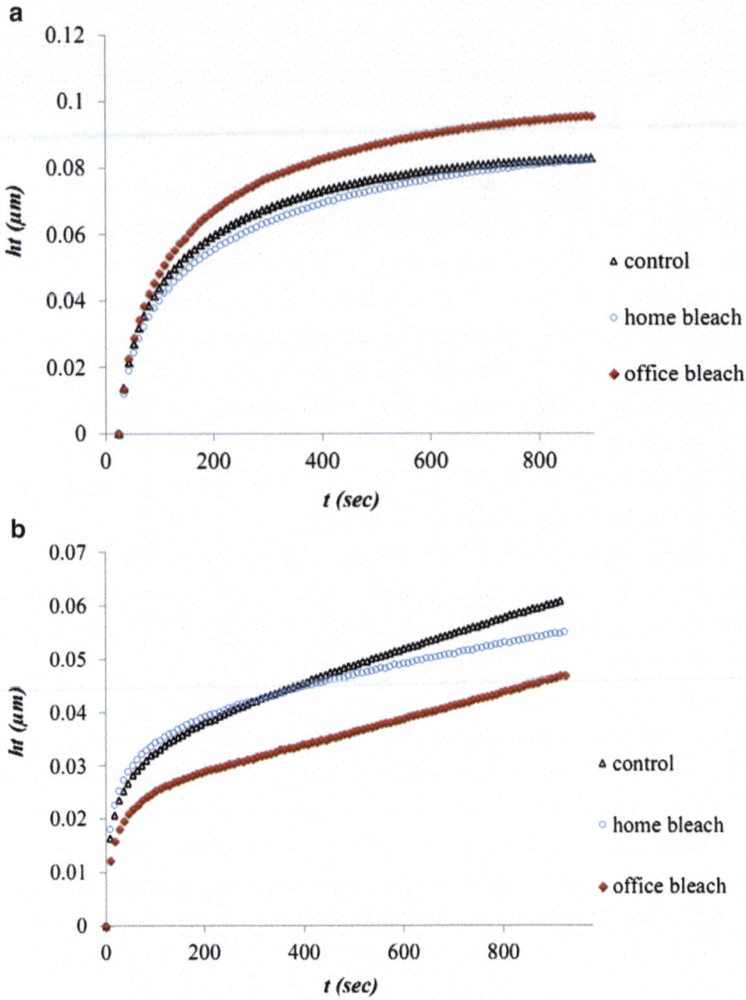

Fig. 17.10 (**a**) The creep behaviour of dental enamel for different treatment groups and (**b**) the recovery behaviour of control, home-bleached and in-office-bleached enamel

because refolding of the protein domain bond does not take place in the bleached enamel due to conformational changes and damage to the protein content caused by peroxide free radicals. This limited ability of refolding results in reduced creep recovery of bleached enamel.

For the purpose of demonstrating the relation between sound and bleached enamel protein content with its mechanical properties, a detailed biochemical investigation of the bleached and sound enamel proteins was conducted. A considerable reduction of the protein contents of the home-bleached (CP) and in-office (HP)-bleached enamel was observed by the SDS-PAGE electrophoresis and Western

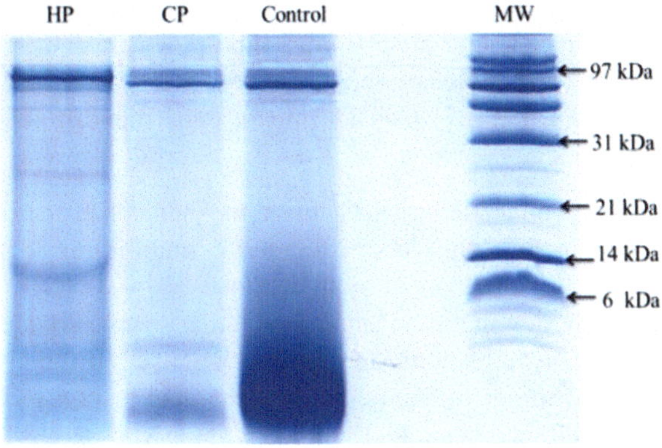

Fig. 17.11 SDS-PAGE profile of protein extracted from human enamel from control, home-bleached (*CP*) and in-office (*HP*)-bleached teeth with standard molecular weight marker (*MW*)

immunoblotting study (Fig. 17.11). Significant reduction of immunogold-labelled enamel proteins in the home-bleached and in-office-bleached enamel sections was also observed under FEG-SEM.

From a clinical perspective, these results indicate that bleaching treatment considerably affects the mechanical behaviour of dental enamel and its ability to tolerate applied loadings through obvious damage to its deformable matrix proteins by the peroxide free radicals. Therefore, it is necessary that the aesthetic benefits of such treatment be weighed against its harmful effects on enamel mechanical properties prior to its routine application.

17.4 Mechanical Properties of Dentin

Dentin is a natural biocomposite with a high level of structural complexity and hierarchical organisation. This complexity makes the understanding of the exact governing mechanisms of its mechanical performance rather challenging. Due to its heterogeneous structure at the micro and nano level, conventional macro tests are not suitable for studying the mechanical features of dentin with regard to its structural components; therefore, nanoindentation testing is the method of interest in our studies on dentin specimens. In the first part of this section, we present the data on nanoindentation-based mechanical properties of dentin, and later we will provide recent findings on the role of supramolecular components that constitute its organic matrix, namely, proteoglycans and glycosaminoglycans, in the mechanical behaviour of dentin.

17.4.1 Mechanical Properties of Sound Dentin

Similar to enamel, the results of various nanoindentation hardness and elastic modulus tests exhibit variation based on the test condition and features of the dentin specimen. The hardness value of dentin has been reported from 0.15 ± 0.03 GPa for the intertubular area of inner dentin to 2.45 ± 0.14 GPa for peritubular dentin. The elastic modulus of dentin has been reported to be in a range of 11.59 ± 3.95 to 29.8 ± 8.9 GPa [27]. Considering the data from different experiments, the following points can be concluded:

Firstly, primary dentin has lower mechanical properties compared to permanent dentin [59, 60]. This difference is mainly due to the higher level of mineral content in permanent tooth dentin.

Secondly, dentin has an anisotropic microstructure which is reflected in its different mechanical response to applied loads from different directions to the specimen [61]. Similar to enamel, the mechanical response of dentin is higher when the applied load is parallel with dentinal tubules and is lower when the applied load is perpendicular to these tubules [62]. In addition, the difference in mechanical response of peritubular and intertubular dentin is significant [63]. The peritubular dentin shows higher hardness and elastic modulus than intertubular dentin which is attributed to its higher degree of mineralisation.

Thirdly, the outer dentin close to the dentinoenamel junction has higher hardness and elastic modulus compared to inner dentin [64]. This difference is due to the lower density and dimension of dentinal tubules and higher thickness of peritubular dentin in outer dentin. In addition, the results of hardness and elastic modulus tests are influenced by the age of the dentin sample and its degree of mineralisation [65]. Aged dentin specimens are usually more mineralised with less water and organic content resulting in higher hardness and elastic modulus.

17.4.2 Mechanical Properties of Dehydrated Dentin

17.4.2.1 Hardness and Elastic Modulus

Water comprises about 20 % of dentin; therefore, hydration and dehydration of this tissue are expected to affect its mechanical properties significantly. In this regard, we did a series of nanoindentation experiments on dry and wet dentin to evaluate the effect of environmental changes on dentin mechanical behaviour [24]. For this purpose, the top surface of dry dentin samples was indented with a Berkovich indenter at the maximum load of 50 mN with no hold period at maximum or minimum loads. Twelve indentations were performed on each specimen. Subsequently, de-ionised water was added to a fluid cell containing the samples, fully covering specimen surfaces and the indenter. Twelve indentations were performed with the specimens fully immersed in water and represented the wet state. For studying the creep and creep recovery, indentations were performed using a two-step loading and unloading method. A maximum load of 50 mN was selected, and a holding time of 120 s at maximum load was used for all tests to measure creep. After an unloading segment, another holding period of 120 s at 1 mN was used to measure viscoelastic recovery.

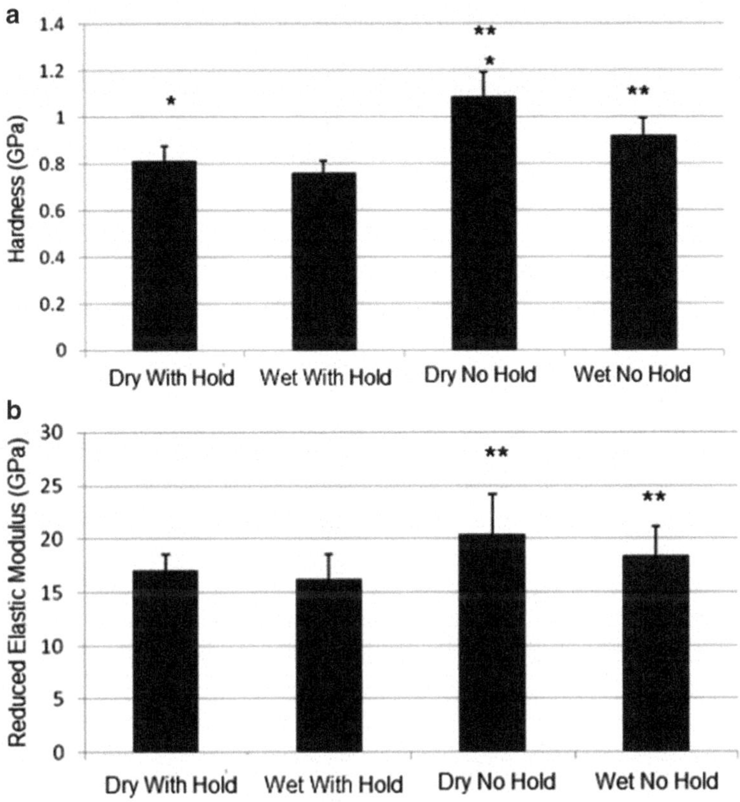

Fig. 17.12 (**a**) Hardness and (**b**) elastic modulus for the dry and wet specimens both with and without creep

The results indicated that in tests without a holding time, dry dentin had an average hardness of 1.1 ± 0.1 GPa, whereas wet dentin had an average hardness value of 0.91 ± 0.07 GPa ($p < 0.05$). With the incorporation of holding time, dry dentin showed an average hardness of 0.80 ± 0.06 GPa, which was significantly higher than wet dentin, with a hardness value of 0.75 ± 0.05 GPa ($p < 0.05$). Comparing the indentation results between tests with creep and test without creep, it was observed that holding at maximum load resulted in a significant decrease in hardness for both wet and dry dentin ($p < 0.05$) (Fig. 17.12).

The results of this experiment are consistent with the results obtained in previous investigations. Guidoni et al. [66] reported an approximately 35 % decrease in elastic modulus and nearly 30 % decrease in the hardness of dry dentin when specimens were measured in Hank's solution. Kinney et al. [67] also reported a decrease in elastic modulus from ~24 to ~20 GPa with hydration.

Our results also indicate that adding a holding time at maximum load causes a decrease in modulus and a more significant decrease in hardness for both dry and wet dentin. Since no chemical desiccation method was used and drying was achieved by placing the specimens in a desiccating chamber for relatively short periods of time, the dry samples may still have some water trapped within their interfibrillar spaces. Therefore, the plasticising effect of water on the collagen that contributes to the increased compliance of the organic matrix could have resulted in a less significant change which was observed in the dry specimens.

17.4.2.2 Indentation Creep Behaviour

Regarding the creep behaviour of dentin, both dry and wet specimens exhibited an increasing penetration depth with time, which is typical for viscoelastic materials (Fig. 17.13). Comparison between wet and dry dentin [24] showed that the dry tissue behaves similarly to the wet tissue, with an averaged normalised displacement of nearly 0.15 μm at maximum load. The normalised recovery at minimum load was not as extensive as the deformation at maximum load, therefore indicating a viscoelastic–plastic type of response. In addition, the normalised recovery of wet dentin (0.09 μm) was greater than that observed for dry dentin (0.06 μm).

Hydration, as a known plasticiser of the collagen in the dentin matrix, resulted in higher creep rate sensitivity for wet dentin compared with dry dentin. This result is also expected, as the plasticised organic matrix accounts for an increase in localised shear flow beneath the contact area of the indenter.

We suggest that the increased localised shear flow beneath the indenter associated with the wet tissue might be a potential explanation for a more significant viscoelastic recovery of wet dentin in comparison to the dry and more collapsed matrix of the dry tissue.

In addition, the creep rate sensitivity, m, of wet and dry dentin specimens was calculated using contact pressure (hardness) versus the strain rate (Fig. 17.14). It has been proposed [68] that the creep rate sensitivity is a value that reflects the flowability of a material. For a given material, if $m = 1$, the material is considered viscous, with a Newtonian flow response; m values less than 1 indicate inhomogeneous non-Newtonian flow. Similar to the reports by He and Swain [69] for enamel, the very small creep rate sensitivity obtained for dentin suggests that strong localised shear flow occurs inside the material under loading.

17.4.2.3 Indentation Energy Absorption

In terms of energy absorption, hydration caused the unloading curve to exhibit a characteristic 'bowing out' [70] followed by a lower residual depth of penetration, which was translated into a significantly higher value of recovered energy, U_e, during the indentation process. As a result, hydration caused a significant increase of ~15 % in U_e values ($p < 0.0001$). There was not a significant difference in the values of dissipated energy, U_d, between dry and wet dentin (Figs. 17.15 and 17.16).

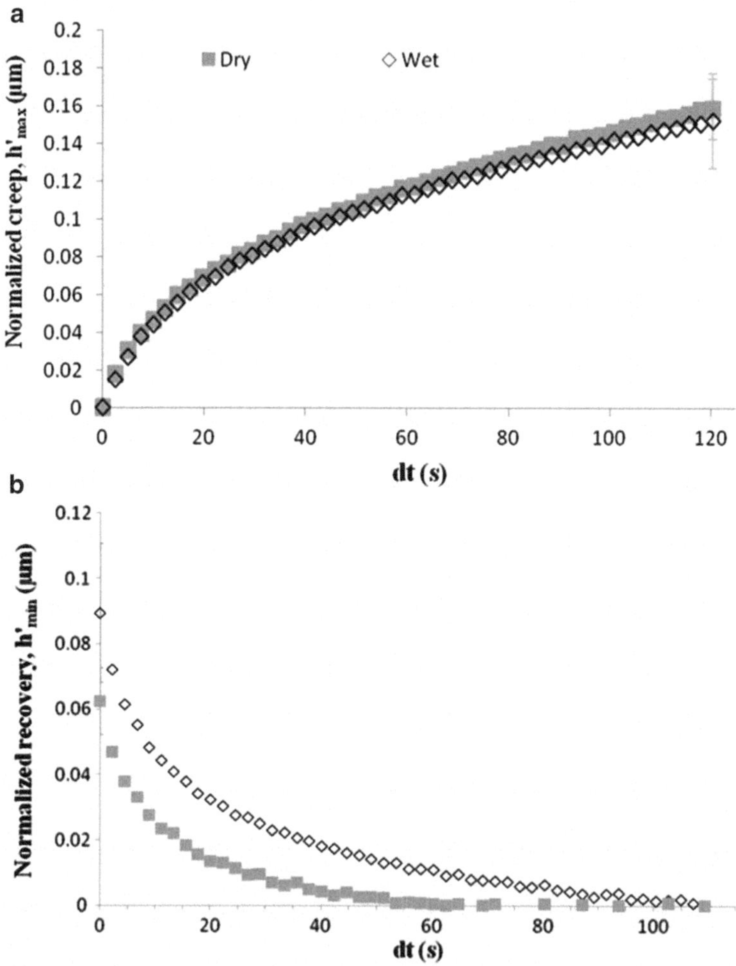

Fig. 17.13 Averaged creep (**a**) and recovery (**b**) for dry and wet dentin

Comparing the results obtained for energy expenditure index, ψ, and penetration depth, h_p, of dry and wet dentin, it is suggested that drying leads to an increase in energy expenditure index of dentin. Dry dentin exhibited a dissipation index of 69.3 % (1.2), whereas wet dentin yielded 66.5 % (1.6). Dry dentin also offered a significantly lower depth of penetration than wet dentin. This was reflected on the significantly lower hardness, H, of the hydrated tissue. It is suggested that this increase associated with drying was primarily associated with the lower recovered energy values, U_e, of dry dentin, which appeared to be related to the more restricted ability of the dry tissue to recover stored elastic energy surrounding the area of contact during nanoindentation.

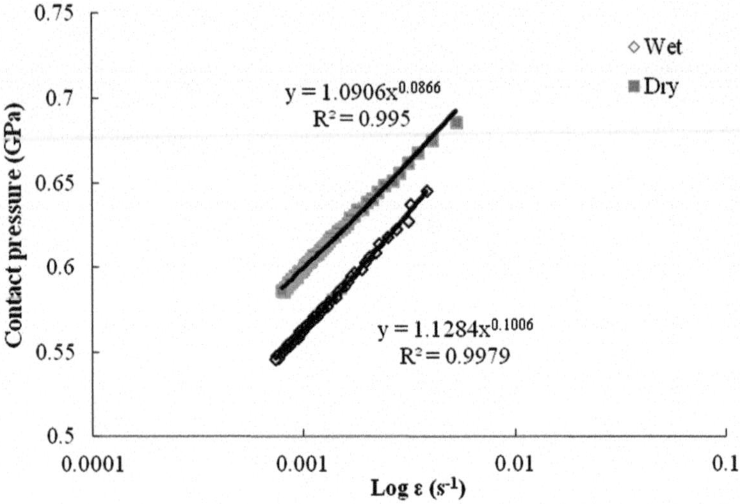

Fig. 17.14 Curve of contact pressure (hardness) versus log of indentation strain rate for dry and wet dentin

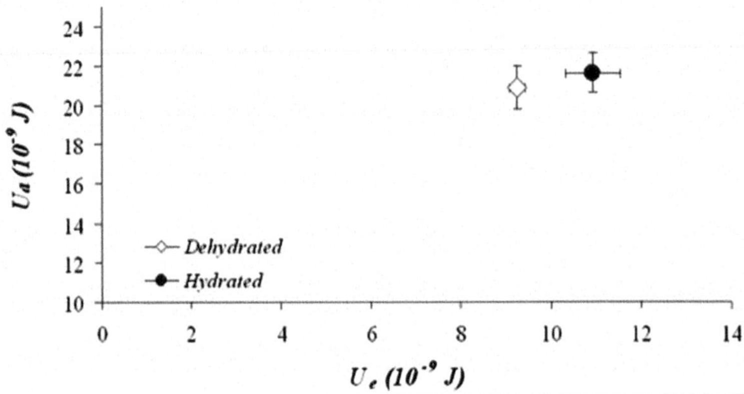

Fig. 17.15 The energy spent during indentation, which is the deconvolution of dissipated energy, U_d, and recovered energy, U_e. Dry dentin showed a significantly lower U_e than wet dentin (Reprinted from Bertassoni and Swain [71]. Copyright 2012, with permission from Elsevier)

Higher values of recovered energy of the hydrated group demonstrate an important difference between dry and wet dentin, which may be associated with an increase in the viscoelastic response of the hydrated tissue. However, the specific contribution of viscoelastic effects to the energy expenditure behaviour of the indented tissue is rather difficult to assess using our analysis methods.

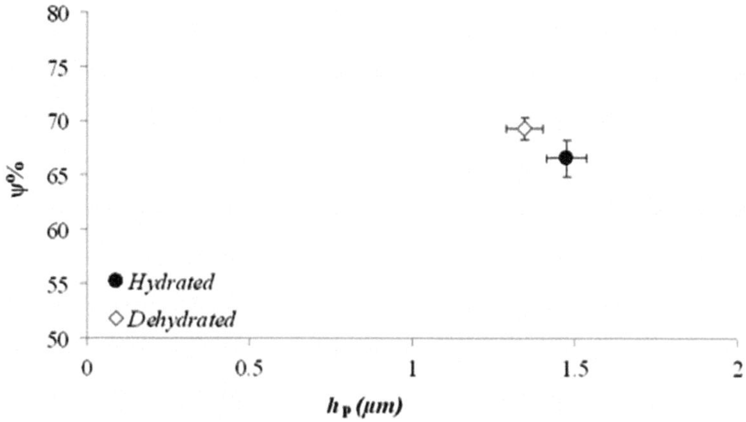

Fig. 17.16 Normalised energy dissipation index, ψ %, was significantly lower for wet dentin in comparison to dry dentin ($p < 0.0001$). Dry dentin also presented a significantly lower effective contact depth, hp ($p < 0.0001$) (Reprinted from Bertassoni and Swain [71]. Copyright 2012, with permission from Elsevier)

17.4.3 Mechanical Properties of Proteoglycan-Digested Dentin

As mentioned earlier, dentin is composed of apatite mineral crystallites (50 vol%), collagen and noncollagenous components (25–30 vol%) and water (~20 vol%). In the previous section, we demonstrated the role of water content on mechanical response of dentin. Several studies had investigated the role of the main building blocks of the dentin, including collagen and HAp mineral [72]; however, the role of the supramolecular assemblies formed by proteoglycans, which contribute to securing the dentin collagenous network as a stable unit, was rather elusive thus far. Although proteoglycans represent less than 3 vol% of the dentin matrix, they have been shown to play an important role in the mutual interaction between collagen fibrils of nearly all connective human.

In a series of experiments, we tried to demonstrate the role of these supramolecular aggregates on dentin mechanical behaviour by selectively digesting different portions of these interfibrillar structures. Consequently, nanoindentation tests were performed on enzymatically treated specimens to provide data on mechanical properties of dentin tissue.

The results of the hardness testing of sound versus proteoglycan-digested dentin specimens showed a significant decrease in the apparent hardness of dentin after the removal of PGs with trypsin (Fig. 17.17). The sound dentin had an average value of 0.74 ± 0.15 GPa, and the enzymatic digestion caused a significant decrease to 0.53 ± 0.09 GPa ($p < 0.001$). These results are in agreement with observations from another study using enzymatic digestions (chondroitinase ABC) to break down the glycosaminoglycan (GAG) side chain of PGs in the cementum–dentin junction [73].

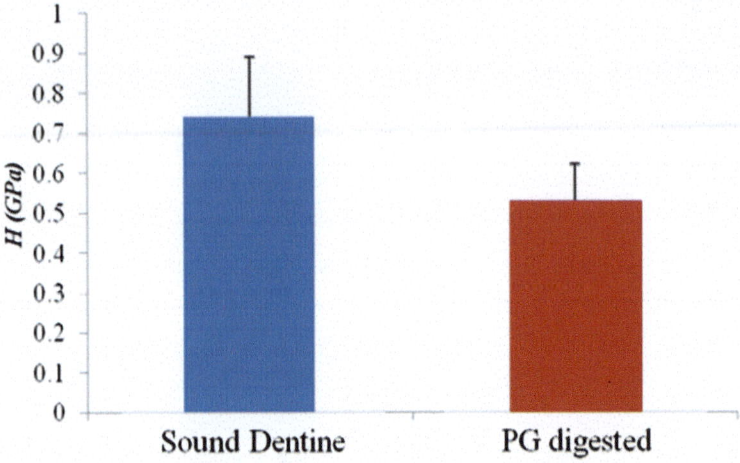

Fig. 17.17 Apparent hardness of dentin before and after trypsin treatment to remove PGs. Normal dentin yielded 0.74 ± 0.15 GPa and the removal of PGs decreased hardness to 0.53 ± 0.09 GPa ($p < 0.001$)

Our interpretation for the decrease in apparent hardness of sound dentin after the trypsin treatment is that once PGs and GAGs are digested by the trypsin, the network that contributed to the 'securing' of mineral crystals is disrupted, and hence the granular crystallites may achieve greater mobility to be displaced within the collagenous matrix by the moving probe tip during indentation. In addition, Ho et al. [73] suggested that the decrease in hardness of the cementum–dentin junction associated with the digestion of GAGs was due to a decrease in the osmotic pressure and hydrophilic nature of the organic matrix in that region.

Regarding the creep behaviour of dentin specimens, it was observed that the removal of PGs led to a significantly higher depth of penetration of the indenter when the loads were held constant during the holding period (Fig. 17.18). In addition, while the creep curve of sound dentin appeared to saturate within about 25 s, the trypsin-treated specimens exhibited significant viscoelastic deformation until the end of the holding period. These observations suggest that PGs, possibly via the interconnection of their GAG side chains, may function as sites of interfibrillar anchorage, therefore limiting further creep deformation of dentin at a constant load.

One limitation of mentioned experiment is that in fully mineralised dentin, the noncollagenous structures, such as PGs, are surrounded by mineral crystals and are therefore difficult to be accessed by digestive activity of the enzymes. Therefore in the next experiments, dentin specimens were partially demineralised before trypsin treatment in order to provide better access for the acting enzymes.

The results in all cases indicated that the demineralised specimens had higher deformation and recovery displacement, which is consistent with the increased viscoelastic behaviour of mineral-free organic scaffolds. PG digestion caused an even

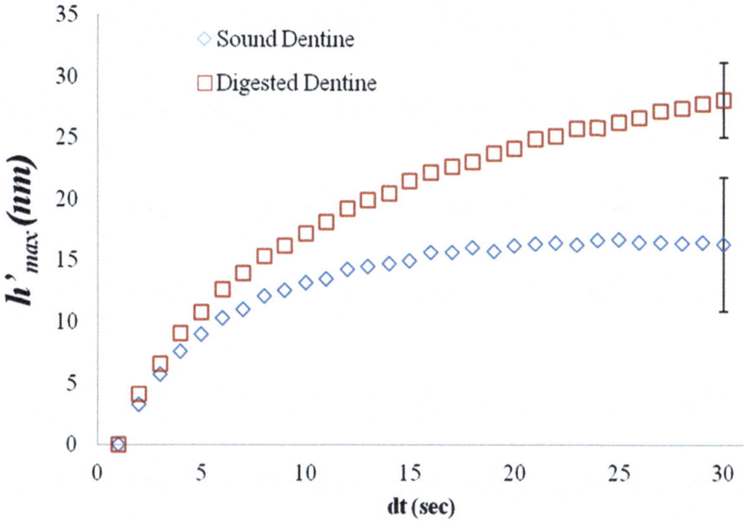

Fig. 17.18 The normalised creep displacement, h'_{max}, of sound and digested dentin before and after the digestion with trypsin

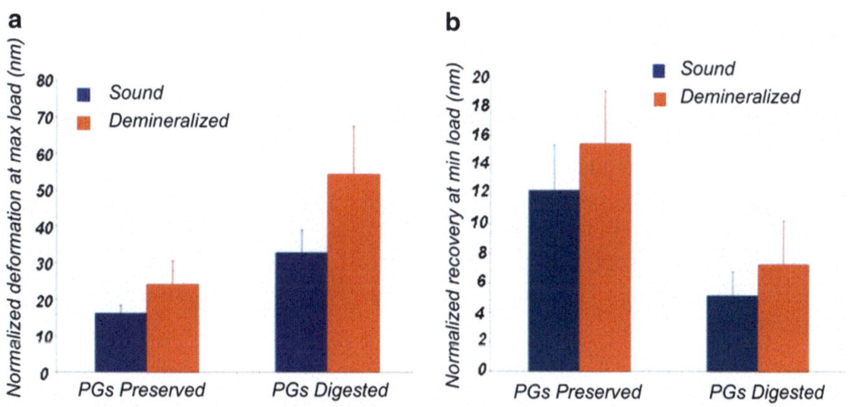

Fig. 17.19 (**a**) Normalised creep deformation and (**b**) recovery of sound and demineralised dentin under different treatments

higher increase in normalised creep deformation of the demineralised specimens (Fig. 17.19). These results suggest that proteoglycans contribute significantly to the ability of dentin to resist time-dependent deformation. Similarly, both sound and demineralised dentin suffered nearly a twofold reduction in normalised recovery after trypsin treatment in comparison to the sound and demineralised control groups.

Collectively, these observations suggest that GAGs and PGs participate via a nanoscale mechanism that limits the deformation of dentin under load, and most importantly, it implies that these structures are key elements responsible for the ability of dentin to recover following time-dependent deformation. As a possible explanation, it has been suggested that GAGs and PGs form interfibrillar supramolecular assemblies that function as damped 'nano-springs' within the dentin matrix. Accordingly, these biological 'nano-springs' would be key elements responsible for preventing the accumulation of sub-micrometre permanent deformation within dentin beneath the enamel.

17.5 Mechanical Properties of Cementum

The cementum is different from enamel and dentin as it is a live tissue that has various types in different areas of the root. It is vascular and cellular and may have the ability to undergo remodelling under mechanical stress. The remodelling activity of cementum is similar to bone tissue and is a distinctive feature of cementum among dental hard tissues. The nature of the exerted forces on the cementum is also different from dentin and enamel. While the majority of exerted mechanical forces on enamel and dentin are compressive, a significant amount of exerted forces on cementum are tensile. As a result of these differences, cementum uses different response mechanisms against external loading compared with dentin and enamel. These mechanisms in cementum are mostly remodelling activities which are performed through controlled resorption and secretion processes. The remodelling activity of cementum along with stress-breaking role of periodontal ligament and adaptive response of supporting bone tissue plays a critical role in managing exerted masticatory forces during function [74].

Considering the fact that cementum is a relatively thin layer, it is hard to study its mechanical features using macroscale tests. As a result, the nanoindentation method has been used as the main method for quantifying its mechanical features. However, preparing proper cementum specimens for nanoindentation still remained a challenging practice. The findings from several nanoindentation tests can be summarised as follows:

1. Firstly, the results of hardness and elastic modulus testing of cementum are variable. This variability can be attributed to the presence of different cementum types in different root sections. For example, the hardness value of cementum has been reported from 0.25 ± 0.09 GPa to 0.63 ± 0.06 GPa [27]. Its elastic modulus has been reported from 2.4 ± 1.8 GPa for the outer surface of the apical third portion of the root to 20.8 GPa for the polished transversal section [27].
2. Secondly, the outer layer of cementum exhibited various values of hardness and elastic modulus in different areas of the root which can be the result of different amounts of protein and collagen fibres in each area [75]. Similarly the cementum–dentin junction has a lower hardness and elastic modulus compared with dentin and the rest of the cementum [76] which is again due to its higher content of collagenous proteins.

3. Lastly, similar to enamel and dentin, the mechanical features of cementum are affected by the storage media and environment [77]. Storing the sample in ethanol or keeping it in dry environment affects the results of mechanical tests. The effect of dehydration seems to be more significant in the case of cementum compared with enamel and dentin as cementum has a higher level of water and organic components.

From a clinical point of view, mechanical behaviour of cementum in pathological states, like periodontal disease and following treatments like orthodontic therapy, undergoes considerable alteration. Although there are some reports on the nanoindentation testing of pathologically or iatrogenic cementum [78], however, further research seems necessary to create more reliable results regarding the effect of these conditions on its mechanical features.

17.6 Conclusion

Application of nondestructive mechanical testing methods such as nanoindentation along with new peptide and protein analysis methods has enabled us to expand our knowledge about the mechanisms and regulating factors of the mechanical behaviour of biological mineralised tissues.

Water and organic molecules comprise a minor fraction of dental enamel structure. However, their critical role in improving the mechanical properties of enamel has been suggested following various studies. Remaining peptide fragments from developmental and formational stages of dental enamel exert a softening effect on mature enamel structure and form a very thin layer around HAp crystals which acts like a glue. These proteins are located with a greater amount in the interrod area. The water molecules are mostly located within the protein matrix and have an influence on enamel's compressibility, permeability and ionic conductivity.

Our current perception of the role of organic components in determining the mechanical behaviour of natural materials like enamel and dentin will provide excellent clues for designing biomaterials with superior structure and improved function. In addition, the hierarchical organisation of enamel and dentin is an important structural feature which is of great importance in determining unique mechanical and physical strength for enamel and dentin. Any attempt to develop biomimetic substitutes for calcium phosphate-based tissues such as enamel and dentin needs to consider these compositional and structural features in order to create materials with rational structure and efficient performance.

Acknowledgement The authors would like to acknowledge and remember the late Dr Lihong He, whose data and scientific work in this area helped us to write this chapter.

References

1. LeGeros RZ (1990) Calcium phosphates in oral biology and medicine. Monogr Oral Sci 15:2
2. Nanci A (2007) Ten Cate's oral histology: development, structure and function. Mosby, St. Louis
3. Kahler B, Swain MV, Moule A (2003) Fracture-toughening mechanisms responsible for differences in work to fracture of hydrated and dehydrated dentine. J Biomech 36(2):229–237
4. Zeichner-David M (2001) Is there more to enamel matrix proteins than biomineralization? Matrix Biol 20(5):307–316
5. Smith C, Pompura J, Borenstein S, Fazel A, Nanci A (1989) Degradation and loss of matrix proteins from developing enamel. Anat Rec 224(2).292–316
6. Bechtle S, Habelitz S, Klocke A, Fett T, Schneider GA (2010) The fracture behaviour of dental enamel. Biomaterials 31(2):375–384
7. Bechtle S, Özcoban H, Lilleodden ET, Huber N, Schreyer A, Swain MV, Schneider GA (2012) Hierarchical flexural strength of enamel: transition from brittle to damage-tolerant behaviour. J R Soc Interface 9(71):1265–1274
8. Berkovitz BK, Holland GR, Moxham B (2002) Oral anatomy, embryology and histology. Mosby, Edinburgh
9. White S, Luo W, Paine M, Fong H, Sarikaya M, Snead M (2001) Biological organization of hydroxyapatite crystallites into a fibrous continuum toughens and controls anisotropy in human enamel. J Dent Res 80(1):321–326
10. Schroeder HN (1991) Oral structural biology: embryology, structure and function of normal hard and soft tissues of the oral cavity and temporomandibular joints. Thieme Medical Publisher, New York
11. Bath-Balogh M, Fehrenbach MJ, Thomas P (1997) Illustrated dental embryology, histology, and anatomy. Saunders, St. Louis, Philadelphia
12. Avery JK, Steele PF, Avery N (2002) Oral development and histology. Thieme, New York
13. Hu CC, Fukae M, Uchida T, Qian Q, Zhang CH, Ryu OH, Simmer JP (1997) Sheathlin: cloning, cDNA/polypeptide sequences, and immunolocalization of porcine enamel sheath proteins. J Dent Res 76(2):648–657
14. Klein JP, Schöller M, Frank RM (1982) Soluble and insoluble proteins of normal human mature enamel. Arch Oral Biol 27(2):133–139
15. Xu HHK, Smith DT, Jahanmir S, Romberg E, Kelly JR, Thompson VP, Rekow ED (1998) Indentation damage and mechanical properties of human enamel and dentin. J Dent Res 77(3):472–480
16. He LH, Swain MV (2008) Understanding the mechanical behaviour of human enamel from its structural and compositional characteristics. J Mech Behav Biomed Mater 1(1):18–29
17. Bertassoni LE, Orgel JP, Antipova O, Swain MV (2012) The dentin organic matrix–limitations of restorative dentistry hidden on the nanometer scale. Acta Biomater 8(7):2419
18. Goldberg M, Takagi M (1993) Dentine proteoglycans: composition, ultrastructure and functions. Histochem J 25(11):781–806
19. Boskey AL (1991) The role of extracellular matrix components in dentin mineralization. Crit Rev Oral Biol Med 2(3):369–387
20. Bertassoni LE, Stankoska K, Swain MV (2012) Insights into the structure and composition of the peritubular dentin organic matrix and the lamina limitans. Micron 43(2):229–236
21. Gotliv B-A, Veis A (2007) Peritubular dentin, a vertebrate apatitic mineralized tissue without collagen: role of a phospholipid-proteolipid complex. Calcif Tissue Int 81(3):191–205
22. Gotliv B-A, Robach JS, Veis A (2006) The composition and structure of bovine peritubular dentin: mapping by time of flight secondary ion mass spectroscopy. J Struct Biol 156(2):320–333
23. Habelitz S, Rodriguez B, Marshall S, Marshall G, Kalinin S, Gruverman A (2007) Peritubular dentin lacks piezoelectricity. J Dent Res 86(9):908–1011

24. Bertassoni LE (2012) Nanomechanical and nanostructural properties of human dentine: an improved understanding of the role of proteoglycans. University of Sydney, Sydney
25. Marshall GW Jr, Marshall SJ, Kinney JH, Balooch M (1997) The dentin substrate: structure and properties related to bonding. J Dent 25(6):441–458
26. Imbeni V, Kruzic J, Marshall G, Marshall S, Ritchie R (2005) The dentin–enamel junction and the fracture of human teeth. Nat Mater 4(3):229–232
27. Oyen ML (2010) Handbook of nanoindentation: with biological applications. Pan Stanford Publishing, Singapore
28. Haque F (2003) Application of nanoindentation development of biomedical to materials. Surf Eng 19(4):255–268
29. Lucas PW (2004) Dental functional morphology: how teeth work. Cambridge University Press, Cambridge
30. Oliver WC, Pharr GM (1992) Improved technique for determining hardness and elastic modulus using load and displacement sensing indentation experiments. J Mater Res 7(6):1564–1583
31. Haines D (1968) Physical properties of human tooth enamel and enamel sheath material under load. J Biomech 1(2):117–125
32. Habelitz S, Marshall SJ, Marshall GW Jr, Balooch M (2001) Mechanical properties of human dental enamel on the nanometre scale. Arch Oral Biol 46:173–183
33. Cuy JL, Mann AB, Livi KJ, Teaford MF, Weihs TP (2002) Nanoindentation mapping of the mechanical properties of human molar tooth enamel. Arch Oral Biol 47:281–291
34. He LH (2008) Mechanical behaviour of human enamel and the relationship to its structural and compositional characteristics. University of Sydney, Sydney
35. He LH, Swain MV (2007) Enamel—a "metallic-like" deformable biocomposite. J Dent 35(5):431–437
36. Schneider G, He LH, Swain M (2008) Viscous flow model of creep in enamel. J Appl Phys 103(1):014701–014705
37. He LH, Swain MV (2007) Energy absorption characterization of human enamel using nanoindentation. J Biomed Mater Res A 81(2):484–492
38. Fox P (1980) The toughness of tooth enamel, a natural fibrous composite. J Mater Sci 15(12):3113–3121
39. Smith BL, Schäffer TE, Viani M, Thompson JB, Frederick NA, Kindt J et al (1999) Molecular mechanistic origin of the toughness of natural adhesives, fibres and composites. Nature 399(6738):761–763
40. Macho GA, Jiang Y, Spears IR (2003) Enamel microstructure—a truly three-dimensional structure. J Hum Evol 45(1):81–90
41. He LH, Swain MV (2007) Influence of environment on the mechanical behaviour of mature human enamel. Biomaterials 28(30):4512–4520
42. Darling A, Mortimer K, Poole D, Ollis W (1961) Molecular sieve behaviour of normal and carious human dental enamel. Arch Oral Biol 5(3):251–273
43. Klemm W (1990) Dehydration: a new alcohol theory. Alcohol 17(1):49–59
44. Klemm W (1998) Biological water and its role in the effects of alcohol. Alcohol 15(3):249–267
45. Catanese J, Featherstone J, Keaveny TM (1999) Characterization of the mechanical and ultrastructural properties of heat-treated cortical bone for use as a bone substitute. J Biomed Mater Res 45(4):327–336
46. Holcomb D, Young R (1980) Thermal decomposition of human tooth enamel. Calcif Tissue Int 31(1):189–201
47. He LH, Fujisawa N, Swain MV (2006) Elastic modulus and stress-strain response of human enamel by nanoindentation. Biomaterials 27:4388–4398
48. Dahl J, Pallesen U (2003) Tooth bleaching—a critical review of the biological aspects. Crit Rev Oral Biol Med 14(4):292–304
49. Minoux M, Serfaty R (2008) Vital tooth bleaching: biologic adverse effects-a review. Quintessence Int 39(8):645–659

50. White DJ, Kozak KM, Zoladz JR, Duschner HJ, Götz H (2004) Effects of Crest Whitestrips bleaching on subsurface microhardness and ultrastructure of tooth enamel and coronal dentin. Am J Dent 17(1):5
51. Sasaki RT, Arcanjo AJ, Flório FM, Basting RT (2009) Micromorphology and microhardness of enamel after treatment with home-use bleaching agents containing 10 % carbamide peroxide and 7.5 % hydrogen peroxide. J Appl Oral Sci 17(6):611–666
52. Götz H, Duschner H, White DJ, Klukowska MA (2007) Effects of elevated hydrogen peroxide 'strip' bleaching on surface and subsurface enamel including subsurface histomorphology, micro-chemical composition and fluorescence changes. J Dent 35(6):457–466
53. Faraoni-Romano JJ, Turssi CP, Serra MC (2009) Effect of a 10 % carbamide peroxide on wear resistance of enamel and dentine: in situ study. J Dent 37(4):273–278
54. Götz H, Klukowska MA, Duschner H, White DJ (2006) Physical, morphological, and micro-Raman chemical studies on bleaching strip effects on enamel, coronal dentin, and root dentin. J Clin Dent 18(4):112–119
55. Azer SS, Machado C, Sanchez E, Rashid R (2009) Effect of home bleaching systems on enamel nanohardness and elastic modulus. J Dent 37(3):185–190
56. Hairul Nizam B, Lim C, Chng H, Yap A (2005) Nanoindentation study of human premolars subjected to bleaching agent. J Biomech 38(11):2204–2211
57. Zimmerman B, Datko L, Cupelli M, Alapati S, Dean D, Kennedy M (2010) Alteration of dentin–enamel mechanical properties due to dental whitening treatments. J Mech Behav Biomed Mater 3(4):339–346
58. Elfallah H (2013) The effect of tooth bleaching agents on mechanical properties and protein contents of dental enamel. University of Sydney, Sydney
59. Poolthong S (1998) Determination of the mechanical properties of enamel, dentine and cementum by an ultra micro-indentation system. University of Sydney, Sydney
60. Mahoney E, Holt A, Swain M, Kilpatrick N (2000) The hardness and modulus of elasticity of primary molar teeth: an ultra-micro-indentation study. J Dent 28:589–594
61. Poolthong S, Swain M, Sumii T, Mori T (eds) (1998) Effect of tubule orientation on some mechanical properties of dentine. J Dent Res. American Association for Dental Research, Alexandria
62. Poolthong S, Low D, Swain M, Sumii T, Mori T (eds) (1998) Prediction of positional dependence of mechanical properties of dentine. J Dent Res. American Association for Dental Research, Alexandria
63. Kinney J, Balooch M, Marshall S, Marshall G Jr, Weihs T (1996) Atomic force microscope measurements of the hardness and elasticity of peritubular and intertubular human dentin. J Biomech Eng 118(1):133–135
64. Angker L, Swain MV, Kilpatrick N (2003) Micro-mechanical characterisation of the properties of primary tooth dentine. J Dent 31(4):261–267
65. Arola D, Reprogel R (2005) Effects of aging on the mechanical behavior of human dentin. Biomaterials 26(18):4051–4061
66. Guidoni G, Denkmayr J, Schöberl T, Jäger I (2006) Nanoindentation in teeth: influence of experimental conditions on local mechanical properties. Philos Mag 86(33–35):5705–5714
67. Kinney J, Marshall S, Marshall G (2003) The mechanical properties of human dentin: a critical review and re-evaluation of the dental literature. Crit Rev Oral Biol Med 14(1):13–29
68. Wei B, Zhang T, Li W, Xing D, Zhang L, Wang Y (2005) Indentation creep behavior in Ce-based bulk metallic glasses at room temperature. Mater Trans 46(12):2959–2962
69. He LH, Swain MV (2009) Nanoindentation creep behavior of human enamel. J Biomed Mater Res A 91(2):352–359
70. Bushby A, Ferguson V, Boyde A (2004) Nanoindentation of bone: Comparison of specimens tested in liquid and embedded in polymethylmethacrylate. J Mater Res 19(01):249–259
71. Bertassoni LE, Swain MV (2012) Influence of hydration on nanoindentation induced energy expenditure of dentin. J Biomech 45(9):1679–1683

72. Kinney J, Habelitz S, Marshall S, Marshall G (2003) The importance of intrafibrillar mineralization of collagen on the mechanical properties of dentin. J Dent Res 82(12):957–9561
73. Ho SP, Sulyanto RM, Marshall SJ, Marshall GW (2005) The cementum–dentin junction also contains glycosaminoglycans and collagen fibrils. J Struct Biol 151(1):69–78
74. Herring SW (2012) Biomechanics of teeth in bone: function, movement, and prosthetic rehabilitation. In: McCauley LK, Somerman MJ (eds) Mineralized tissue in oral and craniofacial science: biological principles and clinical correlates, 1st edn. Wiley, Ames, pp 255–268
75. Malek S, Darendeliler MA, Swain MV (2001) Physical properties of root cementum: Part I. A new method for 3-dimensional evaluation. Am J Orthod Dentofacial Orthop 120(2):198–208
76. Ho S, Balooch M, Goodis H, Marshall G, Marshall S (2004) Ultrastructure and nanomechanical properties of cementum dentin junction. J Biomed Mater Res A 68(2):343–351
77. Malek S, Darendeliler MA, Rex T, Kharbanda OP, Srivicharnkul P, Swain MV (2003) Physical properties of root cementum: Part 2. Effect of different storage methods. Am J Orthod Dentofacial Orthop 124(5):561–570
78. Chutimanutskul W, Darendeliler MA, Shen G, Petocz P, Swain M (2006) Changes in the physical properties of human premolar cementum after application of 4 weeks of controlled orthodontic forces. Eur J Orthod 28(4):313–318

The manufacturer's authorised representative in the EU is Springer Nature Customer Service Centre GmbH, Europaplatz 3, 69115 Heidelberg, Germany. If you have any concerns regarding our products, please contact ProductSafety@springernature.com

Printed and bound by CPI Group (UK) Ltd, Croydon, CR0 4YY
25/09/2026
02222847-0007